AF449224

ADVANCES IN

Pediatric Infectious Diseases®

VOLUME 11

ADVANCES IN

Pediatric Infectious Diseases®

VOLUMES 1 THROUGH 8 (OUT OF PRINT)

VOLUME 9

ADVANCES IN

Pediatric Infectious Diseases®

VOLUME 11

Editor-in-Chief
Stephen C. Aronoff, M.D.
Professor, Department of Pediatrics and Microbiology/Immunology, West Virginia University School of Medicine; Chief, Pediatric Infectious Diseases, West Virginia University Children's Hospital, Morgantown, West Virginia

Editorial Board
Walter T. Hughes, M.D.
Professor of Pediatrics, Department of Pediatrics, University of Tennessee, College of Medicine; Chairman, Department of Infectious Diseases, St. Jude Children's Research Hospital, Memphis, Tennessee

Steve Kohl, M.D.
Professor of Pediatrics, Department of Pediatrics; Chief, Division of Pediatric Infectious Diseases, University of California, San Francisco General Hospital, San Francisco, California

William T. Speck, M.D.
Clinical Professor of Pediatrics, College of Physicians and Surgeons, Columbia University; President and CEO, The Presbyterian Hospital at Columbia Presbyterian Medical Center, New York, New York

Ellen R. Wald, M.D.
Professor of Pediatrics, Department of Pediatrics, University of Pittsburgh School of Medicine; Chief, Divisions of Ambulatory Care and Infectious Diseases, Children's Hospital of Pittsburgh, Pittsburgh, Pennsylvania

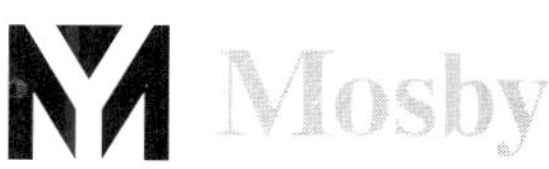

St. Louis   Baltimore   Boston   Carlsbad   Chicago   Naples   New York   Philadelphia   Portland
London   Madrid   Mexico City   Singapore   Sydney   Tokyo   Toronto   Wiesbaden

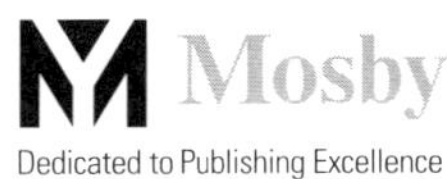

Dedicated to Publishing Excellence

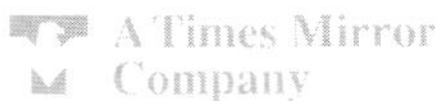

Vice President and Publisher, Continuity Publishing: Kenneth H. Killion
Director, Editorial Development: Gretchen C. Murphy
Developmental Editor: Kelly Poirier
Acquisitions Editor: Linda Steiner
Manager, Continuity–EDP: Maria Nevinger
Associate Production Editor: Gary Howard
Assistant Project Supervisor: Sandra Rogers
Proofreading Supervisor: Barbara M. Kelly
Vice President, Professional Sales and Marketing: George M. Parker
Senior Marketing Manager: Eileen M. Lynch
Marketing Specialist: Lynn D. Stevenson

Printed in the United States of America
Composition by The Clarinda Company
Printing/binding by The Maple-Vail Book Manufacturing Group

Mosby–Year Book, Inc.
11830 Westline Industrial Drive
St. Louis, Missouri 63146

Editorial Office:
Mosby–Year Book, Inc.
200 North La Salle Street
Chicago, Illinois 60601

International Standard Serial Number: 0884-9404
International Standard Book Number: 0-8151-0314-X

Contributors

Michael J. Bangs, M.S.P.H.
Division of Tropical Public Health, Department of Preventive Medicine and Biometrics, Uniformed Services University of the Health Sciences, Bethesda, Maryland

Kenneth M. Boyer, M.D.
Director, Section of Pediatric Infectious Diseases, Rush-Presbyterian-St. Luke's Medical Center, Professor and Associate Chairman, Department of Pediatrics, Rush Medical College of Rush University, Chicago, Illinois

Stephen J. Chanock, M.D.
Infectious Diseases Section, Pediatric Branch, National Cancer Institute, Bethesda, Maryland

Thomas G. Cleary, M.D.
Professor of Pediatrics, Director, Pediatric Infectious Diseases, University of Texas–Houston Health Science Center, Department of Pediatrics, Infectious Diseases Division, Houston, Texas

John H. Cross, Ph.D.
Professor, Department of Preventive Medicine and Biometrics, Uniformed Services University of the Health Sciences, Bethesda, Maryland

Steven J. Czinn, M.D.
Department of Pediatrics, School of Medicine, Case Western Reserve University, Rainbow Babies and Children's Hospital, Cleveland, Ohio

Gail J. Demmler, M.D.
Associate Professor of Pediatrics (Section of Infectious Diseases) and Pathology, Baylor College of Medicine; Director, Diagnostic Virology Laboratory, Texas Children's Hospital, Houston, Texas

Mark S. Glassman, M.D.
Professor, Department of Pediatrics, New York Medical College, Valhalla, New York

Corina Gonzalez, M.D.
Infectious Diseases Section, Pediatric Branch, National Cancer Institute, Bethesda, Maryland

Barry M. Gray, M.D.
Professor of Pediatrics and Microbiology, University of Alabama at Birmingham, Birmingham, Alabama

David P. Greenberg, M.D.
Assistant Professor of Pediatrics, UCLA School of Medicine, Harbor-UCLA Medical Center, Associate Director, UCLA Center for Vaccine Research, Torrance, California

Willem A. Hanekom, M.B., Ch.B, D.C.H.(S.A.), F.C.P.(S.A.)
Instructor of Pediatrics, Northwestern University Medical School, Fellow, Division of Infectious Diseases, The Children's Memorial Hospital, Chicago, Illinois

Walter T. Hughes, M.D.
Chairman, Department of Infectious Disease, St. Jude Children's Research Hospital, Memphis, Tennessee

Niranjan Kanesa-thasan, M.D., M.T.M.H.
Division of Communicable Diseases & Immunology, Walter Reed Army Institute of Research, Washington, D.C.

Jane E. Koehler, M.D.
Assistant Professor of Medicine, Division of Infectious Diseases, University of California at San Francisco, San Francisco, California

Jay M. Lieberman, M.D.
Assistant Professor of Pediatrics, UCLA School of Medicine; Harbor-UCLA Medical Center, UCLA Center for Vaccine Research, Torrance, California

Caron A. Lyman, M.D.
Infectious Diseases Section, Pediatric Branch, National Cancer Institute, Bethesda, Maryland

Martin A. Nash, M.D.
Associate Professor of Clinical Pediatrics, Columbia University College of Physicians and Surgeons, Director of Pediatric Nephrology, Babies and Children's Hospital of New York, Columbia-Presbyterian Medical Center, New York, New York

Philip A. Pizzo, M.D.
Head, Infectious Diseases Section, Chief, Pediatric Branch, National Cancer Institute, Bethesda, Maryland

Idalia R. Rivera-Matos, M.D.
Fellow, Pediatric Infectious Diseases, University of Texas–Houston Health Science Center, Department of Pediatrics, Infectious Diseases Division, Houston, Texas

William Rodriguez, M.D., Ph.D.

Professor of Pediatrics, George Washington University School of Medicine and Health Sciences, Children's National Medical Center, Washington, D.C.

Robert L. Seigle, M.D.

Assistant Professor of Clinical Pediatrics, Columbia University College of Physicians and Surgeons, Division of Pediatric Nephrology, Babies and Children's Hospital of New York, Columbia-Presbyterian Medical Center, New York, New York

Nalini Singh-Naz, M.D., M.P.H.

Associate Professor of Pediatrics, George Washington University School of Medicine and Health Sciences, Children's National Medical Center, Washington, D.C.

Thomas J. Walsh, M.D.

Head, Mycology Unit, Infectious Diseases Section, Pediatric Branch, National Cancer Institute, Bethesda, Maryland

Ram Yogev, M.D.

Professor of Pediatrics, Northwestern University Medical School, Director, Section of Pediatric and Maternal HIV Infection, The Children's Memorial Hospital, Chicago, Illinois

Contents

Nematode Infections in Children.
*By Niranjan Kanesa-thasan, Michael J. Bangs, and
John H. Cross*

Diagnosis and Treatment of Congenital Toxoplasmosis.

Mosby Document Express

Copies of the full text of journal articles referenced in this book are available by calling Mosby Document Express, toll-free, at 1-800-55-MOSBY.

With Mosby Document Express, you have convenient 24-hour-a-day access to literally every journal reference within this book. In fact, through Mosby Document Express, virtually any medical or scientific article can be located and delivered by FAX, overnight delivery service, international airmail, electronic transmission of bit-mapped images (via Internet), or regular mail. The average cost of a complete delivered copy of an article, including copyright clearance charges and first-class mail delivery, is $12.

For inquiries and pricing information, please call the toll-free number shown above.

Bartonella Infections*

Jane E. Koehler, M.D.
Assistant Professor of Medicine, Division of Infectious Diseases,
University of California at San Francisco, San Francisco, California

HISTORICAL OVERVIEW OF *BARTONELLA* SPECIES

The spectrum of syndromes resulting from human infection with *Bartonella* species (formerly *Rochalimaea* species[1]) has expanded rapidly since the first *Bartonella* infection was identified in the United States in the 1980s. Bacillary angiomatosis (BA) lesions occurring in a human immunodeficiency virus (HIV)–infected patient were first described by Stoler et al.[2] in 1983, although the name BA was not proposed until 1989 by LeBoit et al.[3] and the etiologic agents were not identified until several years later. In 1990, three simultaneous publications in the *New England Journal of Medicine* described isolation of a fastidious gram-negative rod from five patients with bacteremia,[4] association of bacillary forms with an unusual histopathologic entity known as peliosis hepatis,[5] and the identification of DNA closely related to *Bartonella* (formerly *Rochalimaea*) *quintana* in the lesions of BA.[6] In 1992, this new species was further characterized and named *Rochalimaea henselae*.[7, 8]

In 1993, the four species belonging to the genus *Rochalimaea* were moved to the genus *Bartonella* based on the close genetic relatedness of *Rochalimaea* species to *B. bacilliformis*. In addition, the family Bartonellaceae was removed from the order Rickettsiales because of the more distant relationship of bartonellae to rickettsiae.[1] The genus *Bartonella* takes precedence over the genus *Rochalimaea* because it was named first. There are now five species of *Bartonella* identified, including the four former members of the genus *Rochalimaea* (*Bartonella henselae*, *Bartonella quintana*, *Bartonella elizabethae*, and *Bartonella vinsonii*) and the original member of the genus, *Bartonella bacilliformis*. The relationship between *Bartonella* species and other closely related gen-

---

*The author is a Pew Scholar and was supported by the NIH R29 AI36075 and the University of California AIDS Research Program.

era of the alpha subdivision of *Proteobacteria* is shown in Figure 1.[9]

BARTONELLA HENSELAE

As an indirect result of the study of *Bartonella* infections in immunocompromised patients, it became evident that all or the majority of cat-scratch disease (CSD) infections are caused by this newly described organism, *B. henselae*. In the late 1980s, BA in HIV-infected patients was associated anecdotally with cat scratches in many case reports and series.[10] In 1987, LeBoit et al.[11] noted that the bacilli in BA lesions had an identical appearance to those

Alpha-Proteobacteria

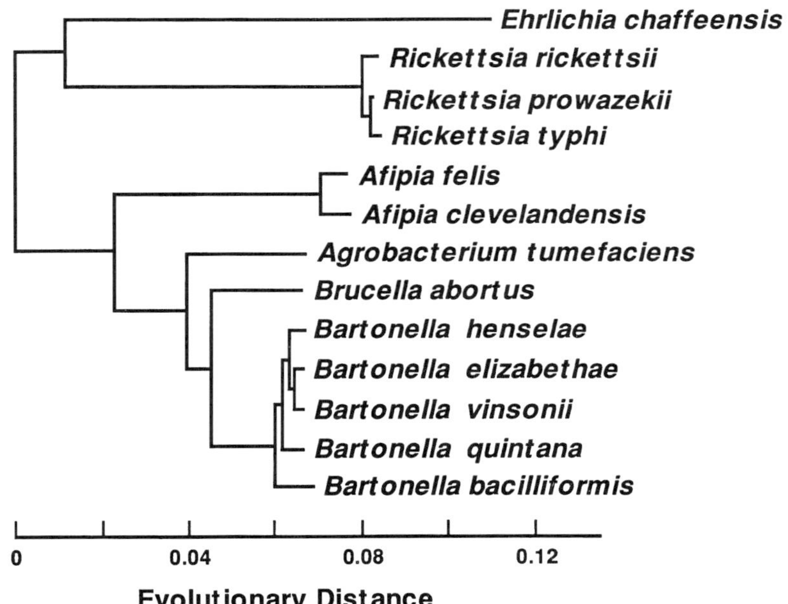

FIGURE 1.

Members of the *Bartonella* genus and their relationship to other members of the alpha subdivision of *Proteobacteria*, based on 16S ribosomal RNA gene sequences. Evolutionary distance between bacteria is proportional to the summed lengths of the horizontal segments from a branch point. (From Slater LN, Welch DF: *Rochalimaea* species [recently renamed *Bartonella*]. In *Principles and Practice of Infectious Diseases*, ed 4. New York, Churchill Livingstone, 1994. Used by permission.)

described in CSD by Wear et al.[12] in 1983. These bacilli were clearly demonstrated in both the lymph nodes of CSD patients and in BA lesions by the Warthin-Starry stain. In 1988, an organism called the CSD bacillus was isolated at the Armed Forces Institute of Pathology[13] and subsequently named *Afipia felis*.[14] However, in the past several years, no subsequent isolations of this organism from CSD-related tissues have been reported. In 1992, after the agent of BA was identified as what was then known as a *Rochalimaea* species, an indirect fluorescence antibody (IFA) test developed to detect *Bartonella* antibodies in BA patients revealed the presence of these antibodies in 88% of banked sera from CSD patients but in only 3% of controls.[15] In 1993, two studies systematically studied the epidemiology of BA[16] and CSD.[17] Both found a statistical association between traumatic cat contact and development of either BA (predominantly immunocompromised patients[16]) or CSD (immunocompetent patients[17]). Subsequently, *B. henselae* DNA was shown to be present in CSD skin test material.[18] *Bartonella henselae* also was isolated from the lymph nodes of two patients with apparent CSD lymphadenopathy.[19] Finally, a major reservoir for *B. henselae* was identified as the domestic cat when *B. henselae* bacteremia was documented in 41% of a random sampling of pet and pound cats in the San Francisco Bay area.[20] The now well-established relationship between *B. henselae* and CSD will be discussed in greater detail later.

BARTONELLA QUINTANA

When direct isolation of *Bartonella* species from cutaneous BA lesions was accomplished for the first time, *B. quintana* was identified as an additional species, which can cause these vascular proliferative lesions in HIV-infected patients.[21] Although HIV-associated infections constituted the first documentation of *B. quintana* infection in the United States in the early 1990s, hundreds of thousands of troops in Europe were infected with *B. quintana* during the epidemic outbreaks of World War I.[22] The syndrome was known as trench fever and before the onset of the influenza epidemic, was described as the leading cause of morbidity (without mortality) during this conflict. Manifestations of trench fever included relapsing high fever, generalized myalgias with focal shin pain, headache, and splenomegaly, which resulted in debilitation of the affected soldier for 10 to 12 weeks.[23] Scientists studied trench fever intensively during the early part of this century and discovered that *B. quintana* was carried by the body louse

Pediculus humanus. Researchers determined that transmission of *B. quintana* occurred as the result of louse infestation among troops confined to battle trenches. After biting the human, the infected louse defecated material containing viable *B. quintana* bacilli. The organisms were subsequently inoculated into the bite wound by the human during scratching of the wound. Because *B. quintana* could not be propagated on solid agar or in laboratory animals, it was maintained in infected lice, which were then used to experimentally infect humans. Swift[23] commented that "in the investigation of no other disease have so many men submitted themselves to artificial inoculation." After World Wars I and II, sporadic outbreaks and isolated cases of trench fever continued to occur in Mexico and Europe. *Bartonella quintana* (at the time known as *Rickettsia quintana*) was first isolated from the blood of a human with trench fever in 1961.[24]

BARTONELLA BACILLIFORMIS, BARTONELLA ELIZABETHAE, AND *BARTONELLA VINSONII*

Bartonella bacilliformis infection, also known as bartonellosis, has never been reported to occur outside of a very restricted geographic region in the Andes of western South America. Infection occurs in humans residing at specific altitudes between 2,500 and 8,000 ft, the geographic region coinciding with the distribution of the *Phlebotomus* sandfly, which transmits *B. bacilliformis*.[25] Two different manifestations of bartonellosis have been identified: an acute form known as Oroya fever and a chronic form called verruga peruana. The acute infection can produce a severe febrile illness with hemolysis, anemia, and lymphadenopathy, which, when left untreated, can result in mortality in 40% of patients.[25] People who survive the acute phase without treatment often develop intercurrent infections with intracellular pathogens such as *Salmonella* or *Mycobacterium tuberculosis*, apparently as the result of depressed cellular immune function.[26] Verruga peruana, the chronic phase of infection, is characterized by warty, vascular cutaneous lesions. Of note, these verrugas are clinically indistinguishable from the cutaneous lesions of BA due to *B. quintana* and *B. henselae.*

Bartonella vinsonii was isolated in 1946 from Canadian voles (*Microtus pennsylvanicus*) on Grosse Isle off Newfoundland but has never been associated with human disease.[27] Recently a novel *B. vinsonii* subspecies (*B. vinsonii* subsp. *berkhoffi*) was isolated from a dog with severe aortic and mitral valvular endocarditis.[28] *Bartonella elizabethae* was isolated only once from an immunocompetent patient with endocarditis in 1993.[29]

MANIFESTATIONS OF *BARTONELLA* INFECTION IN THE IMMUNOCOMPROMISED PATIENT

Two *Bartonella* species are known to cause disease in the immunocompromised host: *B. henselae* and *B. quintana.* Individuals with impaired immune function due to HIV infection are at highest risk for developing severe sequelae from *Bartonella* infection. Prolonged and even fatal infections can occur, usually as a late manifestation of HIV infection.[30] In one review, the median $CD_4{}^+$ cell count for 15 BA patients was 57/mm^3.[10] Patients with immunocompromise due to cancer chemotherapy or pharmacologic immunosuppression after organ transplantation have also experienced severe sequelae from *Bartonella* infection. The manifestations of *B. quintana* and *B. henselae* infections in the immunocompromised host can be quite diverse[10] and include BA, bacillary peliosis hepatis, endocarditis, isolated bacteremia, and central nervous system (CNS) parenchymal mass lesions. Delayed diagnosis is common because of the diverse presentations and the difficulty in recognizing and confirming *Bartonella* infection. In one study of four HIV-infected patients, cutaneous BA lesions were present in two of the patients for a minimum of 8 months before diagnosis.[21]

CUTANEOUS AND OSSEOUS BACILLARY ANGIOMATOSIS LESIONS

Cutaneous BA lesions are the most easily identified and therefore most frequently recognized form of *Bartonella* infection in the immunocompromised host. The clinical appearance can be extremely diverse,[31] and in HIV-infected patients, the vascular cutaneous lesions of BA can be clinically indistinguishable from Kaposi's sarcoma (KS).[32] The vascular proliferative lesions of BA may be cutaneous (Fig 2) or subcutaneous (Fig 3) and enlarge to form large pedunculated structures. The most characteristic BA lesion is papular and red, with an erythematous base and a collarette of scale (Fig 4). Ulceration occurs with older lesions, and trauma to these painful lesions often results in profuse bleeding. In addition to KS, the vascular cutaneous lesions of BA can be clinically indistinguishable from verruga peruana and pyogenic granuloma. Histopathologic examination of biopsy specimens can distinguish between BA and KS or pyogenic granuloma, and verruga peruana can be eliminated from the differential diagnosis by obtaining a travel history. Deep soft tissue masses due to BA also have been described (Fig 5); these lesions are remarkable for the high degree of vascularity, which often resembles a malignant process.

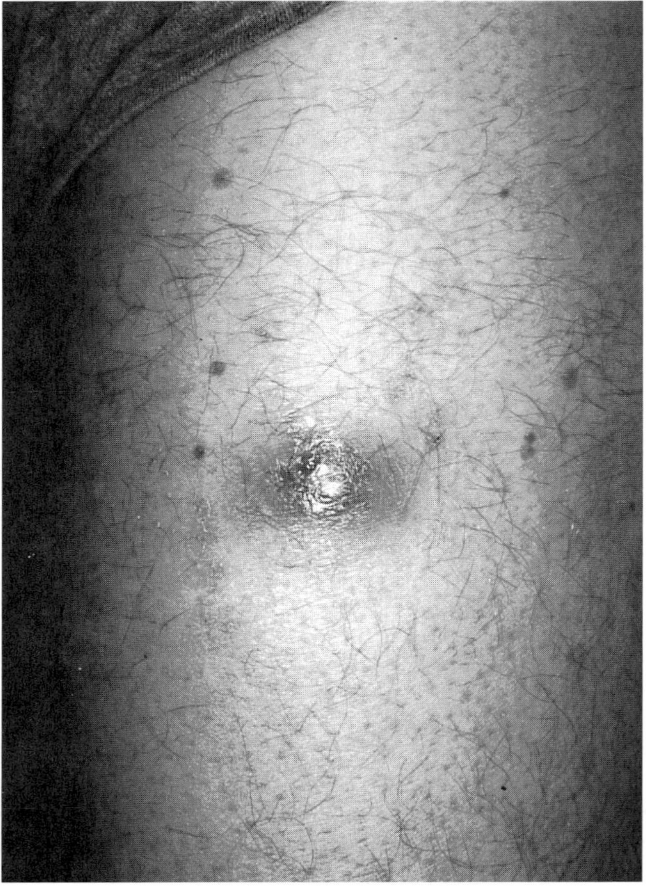

FIGURE 2.

Unusual-appearing erythematous, dry, scaling plaque of cutaneous bacillary angiomatosis mimicking staphylococcal pyoderma. *Bartonella quintana* was isolated from this lesion. (From Koehler JE, Tappero JW: *Clin Infect Dis* 17:612–624, 1993. Used by permission.)

Bartonella osteomyelitis most commonly involves the long bones such as the tibia, fibula, and radius (Fig 6, A). The largest series was reported by Baron et al.,[33] but a number of additional cases, including BA of the rib and vertebrae, have been reported.[10] These lytic lesions are extremely painful and highly vascular; because of the vascularity they are often misdiagnosed as malignancy. The technetium 99m methylene diphosphonate bone scan is invariably positive at the affected site, and occasionally there is an erythematous cellulitic cutaneous plaque overlying the osteolytic lesion, as shown in Figure 6, B.

BACILLARY PELIOSIS HEPATIS

Bacillary peliosis hepatis was described for the first time in 1990 by Perkocha et al.[5] Although peliosis hepatis had been described

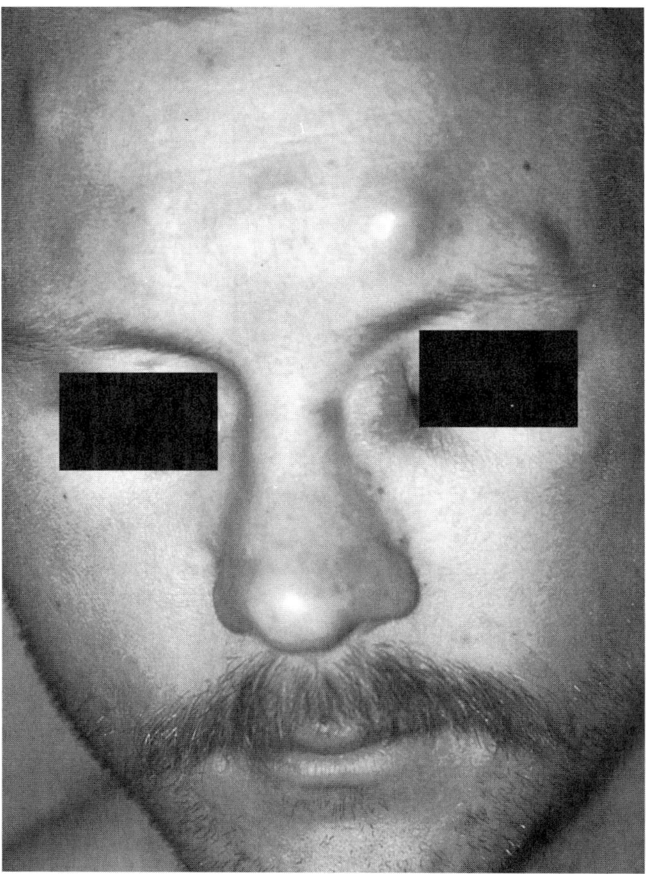

FIGURE 3.

Numerous subcutaneous bacillary angiomatosis (BA) nodules in a patient with concomitant Kaposi's sarcoma (KS) of the medial left eye canthus. Biopsy and histopathologic examination were necessary to distinguish between the BA and KS lesions. (From Koehler JE, Tappero JW: *Clin Infect Dis* 17:612–624, 1993. Used by permission.)

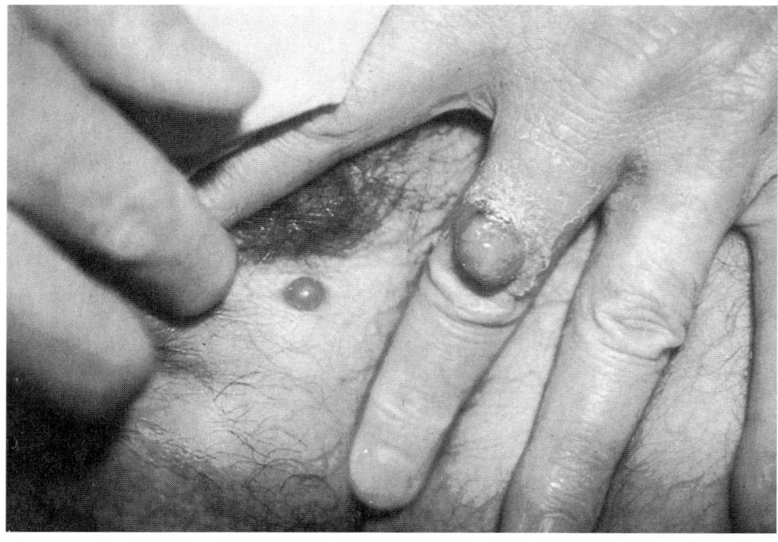

FIGURE 4.

A friable, exophytic angiomatous bacillary angiomatosis nodule of the finger. A collarette of scale is evident at the base of the lesion. A newer dome-shaped vascular papule, without erosion, is present in the same patient. (From Koehler JE, LeBoit PE, Egbert BM, et al: *Ann Intern Med* 109:449–455, 1988. Used by permission.)

previously in patients with terminal malignancy or during treatment with anabolic steroids, Perkocha et al.[5] noted that the peliosis hepatis observed in HIV-infected patients was associated with numerous bacillary organisms located adjacent to the peliotic or blood-filled cysts. The clinical symptoms of the eight patients they described included fever and abdominal pain, and the laboratory findings were notable for increased liver function tests, with the alkaline phosphatase level elevated out of proportion to the level of the transaminases. Two of these patients had cutaneous BA lesions, and two had concomitant splenomegaly. Thrombocytopenia or pancytopenia developed in several patients with splenomegaly and resolved after treatment of the *Bartonella* infection. The vascular proliferative lesions in liver and spleen appear as hypodense lesions scattered throughout the parenchyma on abdominal computed tomography (Fig 7), but this pattern also can be seen with many other conditions such as hepatic KS, lymphoma, extrapulmonary pneumocystosis, and infection with *Mycobacterium avium-intracellulare.*

BACILLARY ANGIOMATOSIS LESIONS AFFECTING OTHER ORGANS

Bacillary angiomatosis lesions have been identified in almost every organ,[10] including the respiratory tract, gastrointestinal tract, lymph nodes, bone marrow, and brain. The vascular proliferative lesions of BA can be visualized in the respiratory tract during bronchoscopy[34] and the gastrointestinal tract during endoscopy as raised, nodular, ulcerated mucosal abnormalities of the stomach and large and small intestines.[35] In one untreated patient, an angioma reached sufficient size to occlude the respiratory tract and result in asphyxiative death.[36] Bacillary angiomatosis may occur in lymph nodes draining a cutaneous BA lesion or present as a single, enlarged lymph node, which on biopsy shows characteristic angiomatous changes. Spach et al.[37] described an HIV-infected man with a left temporal lobe mass and focal neurologic symptoms caused by BA; the mass did not resolve with treatment for toxoplasmosis. A cutaneous BA lesion developed subsequently, and

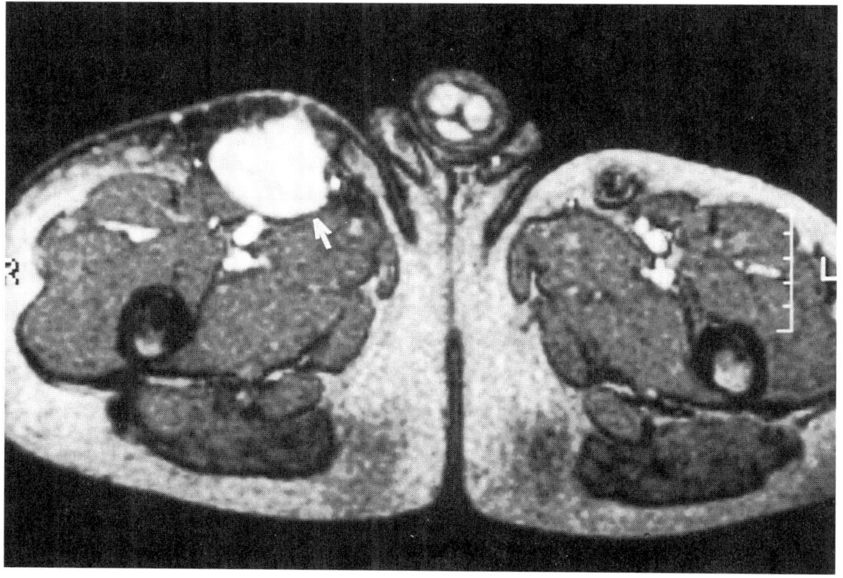

FIGURE 5.

Magnetic resonance imaging showing a deep, highly vascular soft tissue mass of bacillary angiomatosis in the anterior right thigh *(arrow)*. *Bartonella quintana* was the causative species. (From Koehler JE, Tappero JW: *Clin Infect Dis* 17:612–624, 1993. Used by permission.)

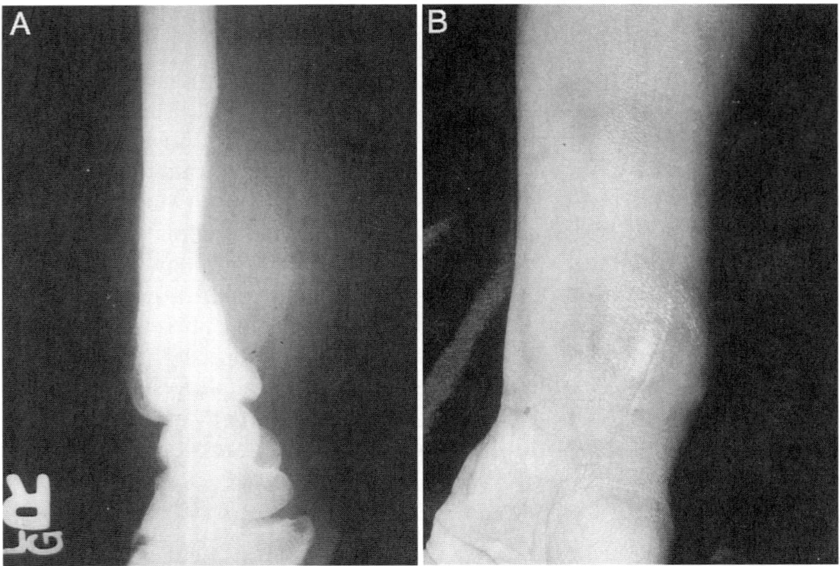

FIGURE 6.
A, roentgenogram demonstrating cortical bone erosion of the radius, with active periostitis, adjacent to the vascular soft tissue mass. **B,** tense, firm, erythematous, and cellulitic-appearing wrist mass of same patient due to BA. (From Koehler JE, LeBoit PE, Egbert BM, et al: *Ann Intern Med* 109:449–455, 1988. Used by permission.)

both the cutaneous lesion and brain parenchymal mass resolved during erythromycin therapy. Antibodies have also been detected in the cerebrospinal fluid and serum of some HIV-infected patients with neurologic disease,[38] and the contribution of *Bartonella* infection to neuropsychiatric deterioration in these patients warrants further investigation.

BARTONELLA BACTEREMIA AND ENDOCARDITIS

Bacteremia in the absence of cutaneous or other focal BA lesions may be the most common *Bartonella* infection in the immunocompromised host but is only rarely diagnosed. In the initial report of isolation of *B. henselae*, Slater et al.[4] described five patients with *B. henselae* bacteremia. Three of these patients were immunocompromised (two with HIV infection and one with a history of bone marrow transplant for chronic myelogenous leukemia), but none had cutaneous BA lesions. One of the HIV-infected patients reported fevers for greater than 40 days and a weight loss of 12 kg before diagnosis. For this latter patient, permanent remission from fevers occurred after 8 weeks of appropriate antibiotic therapy; for the other patient with HIV infection, resolution of fevers occurred after 4 weeks of erythromycin therapy.

Endocarditis may complicate bacteremia with *Bartonella* species in the immunocompromised host. One HIV-infected patient had fatigue, weight loss, night sweats, a holosystolic murmur, splenomegaly, anemia, and mild renal insufficiency.[39] Cardiac echocardiography revealed mitral and aortic valvular vegetations with both aortic and mitral regurgitation. Blood cultures grew *B. quintana*, and after prolonged antibiotic treatment, constitutional symptoms, anemia, and renal insufficiency resolved.

BARTONELLA INFECTIONS IN PEDIATRIC PRACTICE

Although BA is diagnosed most frequently in men with HIV infection, two case reports are of special interest from the perspective of the pediatrician: one describing BA in an immunocompromised child and one in an HIV-infected pregnant woman. The 12-year-

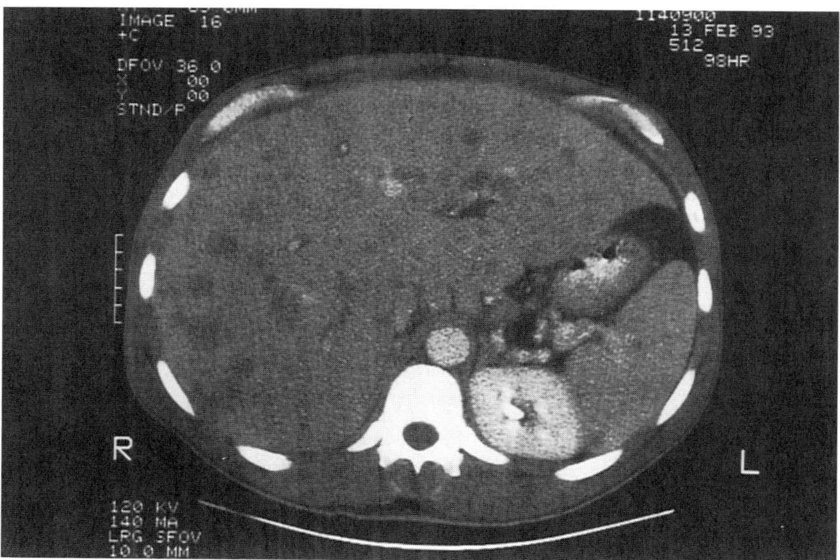

FIGURE 7.

Computed tomography of the abdomen showing hepatosplenomegaly with numerous low-density hepatic parenchymal lesions, in addition to pelvic ascites and pulmonary effusions. Histopathologic examination of a biopsy specimen of percutaneous liver tissue from this patient demonstrated peliosis hepatis. (From Koehler JE, Tappero JW: *Clin Infect Dis* 17:612–624, 1993. Used by permission.)

old pediatric patient was diagnosed with lymphocytic leukemia and received induction chemotherapy.[40] He developed a cutaneous BA lesion above the left eye during maintenance therapy 11 months after the diagnosis of leukemia. He was afebrile at the time of BA diagnosis and received appropriate antibiotic therapy, with complete resolution of the lesions over the subsequent 6 weeks. An HIV-infected Haitian woman who was 26 weeks pregnant had anemia, weight loss, diarrhea, and several violaceous, nontender cutaneous nodules on the thumb, elbow, and thigh. She received intravenous antibiotics for 2 weeks with complete resolution of the cutaneous lesions and had an uneventful spontaneous vaginal delivery at term.[41]

MANIFESTATIONS OF *BARTONELLA* INFECTION IN THE IMMUNOCOMPETENT PATIENT

BACILLARY ANGIOMATOSIS

Virtually all cases of BA have occurred in immunocompromised patients, most frequently in HIV-infected patients. However, five apparently immunocompetent patients with BA (four patients) or bacillary splenitis (one patient) were identified by Tappero et al.[42] Extensive evaluation of immune system function, including testing for HIV infection (Western blotting, culture, and polymerase chain reaction [PCR]), complement, immunoglobulin levels, lymphocyte subset percentages, and T- and B-lymphocyte activation studies, were negative, or normal. Bacilli were detected by Warthin-Starry staining and by electron microscopy in biopsy specimens from each of these patients. Probes known to specifically amplify *Bartonella* DNA[6] were used to demonstrate presence of *B. henselae* DNA in the tissue of the three patients for whom sufficient tissue was available.[42] One patient had hereditary spherocytosis and diabetes mellitus, another was diagnosed with idiopathic hemochromatosis at the time of BA diagnosis, and a third patient was elderly (age 74). These three patients may have had subtle defects in immune function, but the remaining two patients had no evidence of any chronic disease. It is thus evident that BA may develop in the absence of profound immune dysfunction.

BACTEREMIA

In the past 5 years, infections with *B. henselae*, *B. elizabethae*, and *B. quintana* have been reported in immunocompetent individuals in the United States. Isolation of *B. henselae* from two patients with fever was reported in 1990[4] and 1992.[43] The two immunocompe-

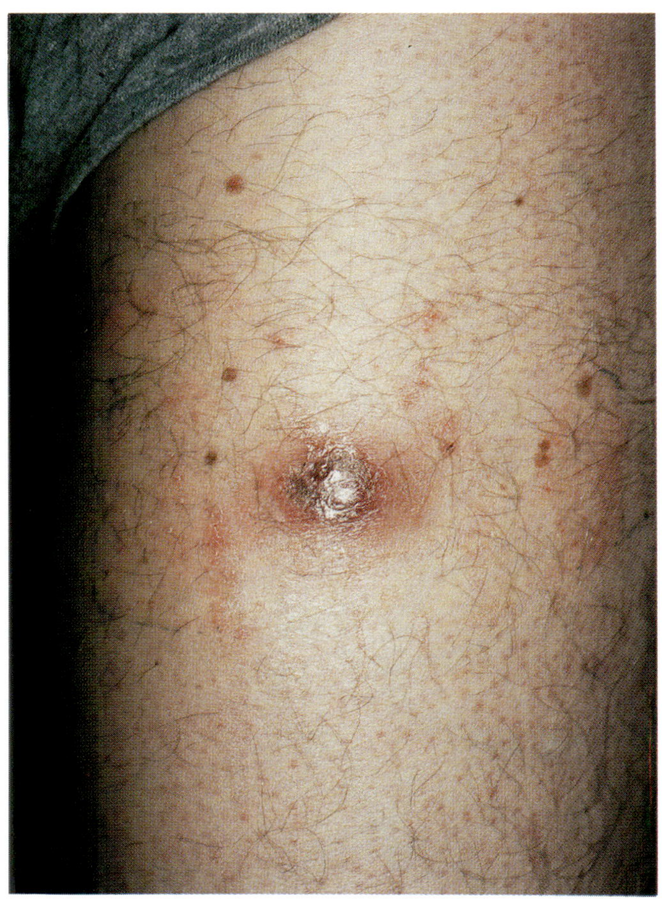

Color Plate I (See page 6.)
Unusual-appearing erythematous, dry, scaling plaque of cutaneous bacillary angiomatosis mimicking staphylococcal pyoderma. *Bartonella quintana* was isolated from this lesion. (From Koehler JE, Tappero JW: *Clin Infect Dis* 17:612-624, 1993. Used by permission.)

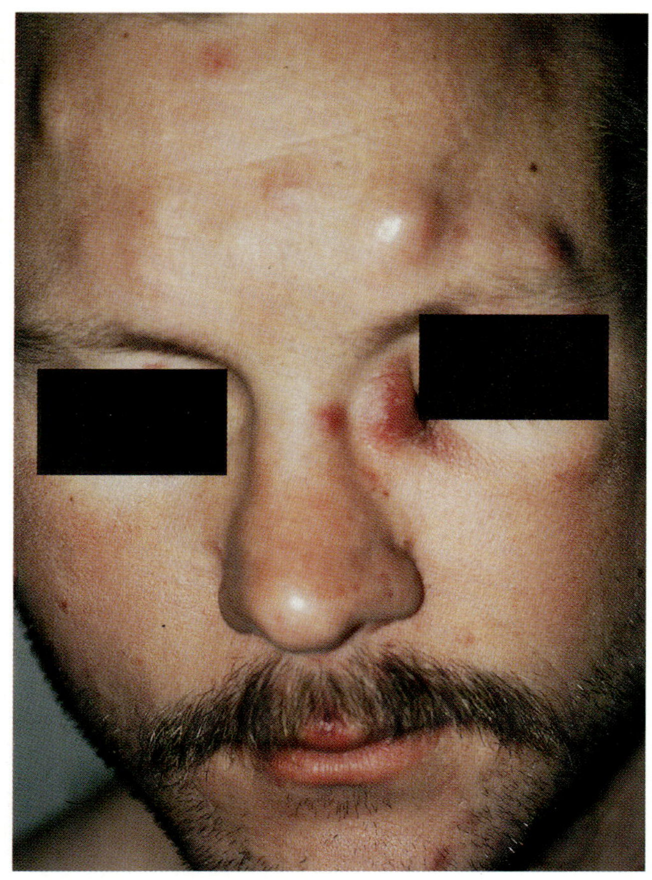

Color Plate II (See page 7.)
Numerous subcutaneous bacillary angiomatosis (BA) nodules in a patient with concomitant Kaposi's sarcoma (KS) of the medial left eye canthus. Biopsy and histopathologic examination were necessary to distinguish between the BA and KS lesions. (From Koehler JE, Tappero JW: *Clin Infect Dis* 17:612-624, 1993. Used by permission.)

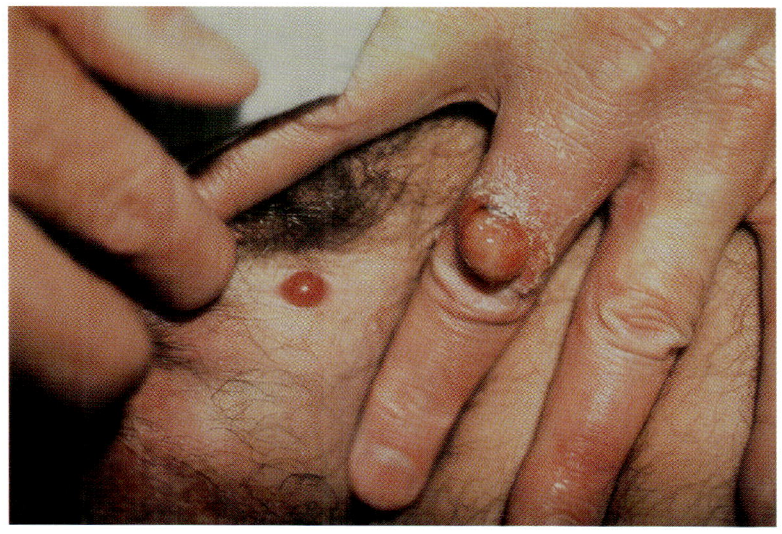

Color Plate III (See page 8.)
A friable, exophytic angiomatous bacillary angiomatosis nodule of the finger. A collarette of scale is evident at the base of the lesion. A newer dome-shaped vascular papule, without erosion, is present in the same patient. (From Koehler JE, LeBoit PE, Egbert BM, et al: *Ann Intern Med* 109:449-455, 1988. Used by permission.)

Color Plate IV (See page 10.)
A, roentgenogram demonstrating cortical bone erosion of the radius, with active periostitis, adjacent to the vascular soft tissue mass. B, tense, firm, erythematous, and cellulitic-appearing wrist mass of same patient due to BA. (From Koehler JE, LeBoit PE, Egbert BM, et al: *Ann Intern Med* 109:449-455, 1988. Used by permission.)

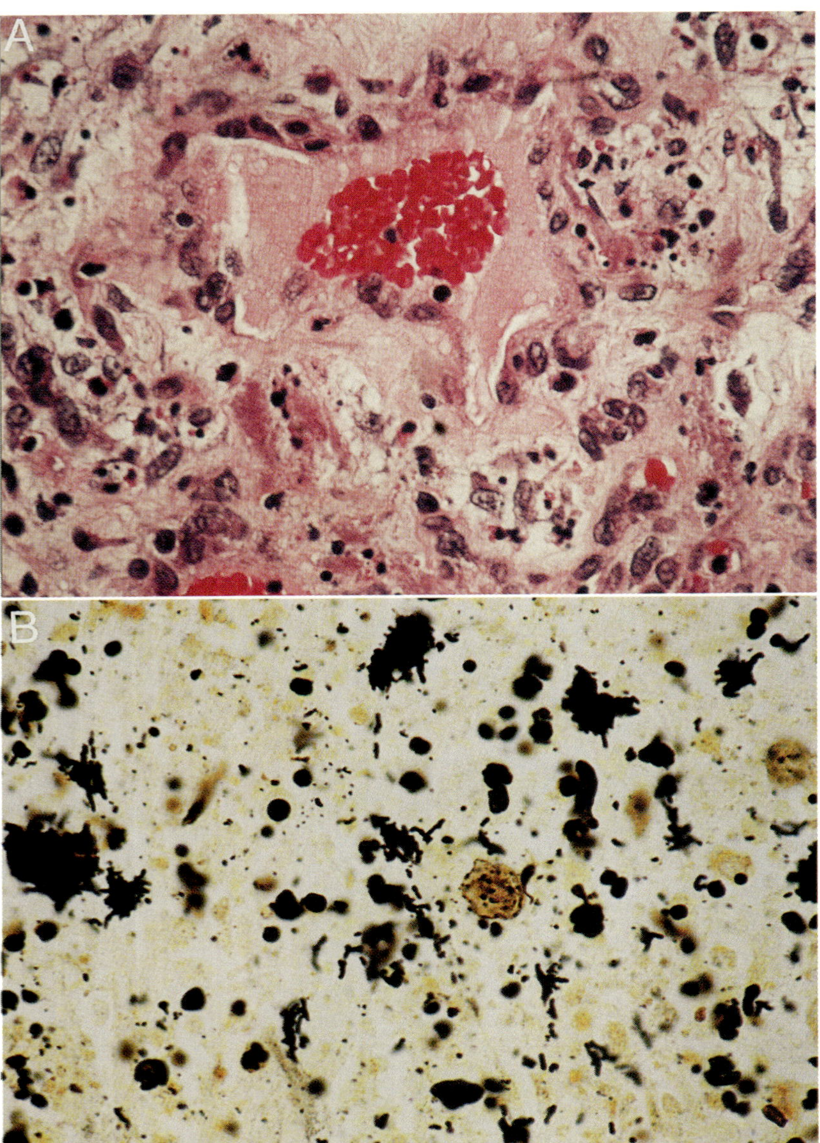

Color Plate V (See page 18.)
A, hematoxylin-eosin staining of a biopsy specimen from a cutaneous bacillary angiomatosis lesion demonstrates a dermal vessel. The vessel is lined with protuberant endothelial cells surrounded by myxoid connective tissue containing neutrophils and amphophilic granular material in close proximity to the vascular lumen (original magnification x 240). The granular material represents clumps of *Bartonella* bacilli, visualized more clearly with Warthin-Starry staining. (From Koehler JE, LeBoit PE, Egbert BM, et al: *Ann Intern Med* 109:449-455, 1988. Used by permission.) **B,** Warthin-Starry silver staining of a cutaneous bacillary angiomatosis biopsy specimen reveals multiple clumps of tangled, dark silver-staining bacillary organisms (bar = 10 µm). (From Koehler JE, Tappero JW: *Clin Infect Dis* 17:612-624, 1993. Used by permission.)

tent patients described by Lucey et al.[43] had a prolonged illness complicated by neurologic symptoms. These two previously healthy patients developed relapsing fever and a clinical syndrome consistent with aseptic meningitis. Blood cultures were positive for *B. henselae* over a prolonged period (4 weeks in one case, 6 weeks in the other) despite treatment with tetracycline, doxycycline, or erythromycin for variable periods. For one patient, the blood cultures remained positive 5 weeks after resolution of fever in the absence of any symptoms. The patient had two transthoracic echocardiograms, both of which failed to demonstrate valvular lesions or other abnormalities. Prolonged *B. quintana* bacteremia in the absence of symptoms was also reported by Swift[23] in 1920. In several of these trench fever patients, bacteremia was reported to have persisted as long as 1 year after initial infection.

In 1993, a cluster of cases with culture-proven *B. quintana* bacteremia was identified in Seattle over a 6-month period by Spach et al.[44] Almost all of these 10 patients were homeless people with chronic alcoholism, and most had a temperature greater than 39.0° C or hypothermia. Six of the patients were tested for HIV antibodies; none was positive. This series of patients appears to represent an outbreak of "urban trench fever." Unlike the World War I trench fever epidemics, however, there was no definite association with body louse infestation in these contemporary patients. *Bartonella quintana* bacteremia also was reported recently in a French patient with chronic lymphadenopathy; *B. quintana* DNA was not detected in the lymph node tissue.[45] Neither the patient's immune status nor the patient's treatment was documented, but this case report documents the continuing presence of *B. quintana* infection in Europe.

ENDOCARDITIS

A 31-year-old man without significant medical problems had symptoms of subacute bacterial endocarditis.[29] Severe aortic regurgitation and valvular vegetations were present, necessitating replacement of the aortic valve. A diagnosis of *B. elizabethae* endocarditis was made on the basis of a positive blood culture and amplification of *Bartonella*-specific DNA from the patient's resected heart valve tissue. This is the only reported infection with *B. elizabethae* to date. In addition to this patient, one other immunocompetent patient with endocarditis has been reported. This patient, one of the cluster of *B. quintana* patients reported by Spach et al.,[44] had subacute bacterial endocarditis and also required aortic valve replacement. Positive blood cultures in both of these cases were detected only when unusual microbiologic methods were used: blind subculturing of a routine Bactec blood culture after 1 week *(B. elizabethae)*[29] or acridine orange staining of a routine Bactec blood culture after 8 days *(B. quintana)*.[44] Because of the difficulty in detection and isolation of *Bartonella* species under routine culture conditions, it is probable that some cases of culture negative subacute bacterial endocarditis actually represent *Bartonella* endocarditis.

CAT-SCRATCH DISEASE

Cat-scratch disease is probably the most common *Bartonella* infection in the United States, as well as the *Bartonella* infection seen most frequently by pediatricians. Historically the diagnosis of CSD is confirmed by three of the four following criteria[46]: (1) a history of cat contact and the presence of a primary lesion (e.g., scratch); (2) development of lymphadenopathy approximately 2 weeks after the primary inoculation, with the exclusion of other causes of lymphadenopathy; (3) a positive CSD skin test result; and (4) histopathologic findings on lymph node biopsy specimens showing a granulomatous process with stellate necrosis and pleomorphic bacilli visualized by Warthin-Starry silver staining.

The true incidence of CSD in the United States is unknown, but a recent data base analysis study by the Centers for Disease Control and Prevention (CDC) indicates that it is much more common than previously thought.[47] It is estimated that 22,000 patients visit ambulatory care clinics and 2,000 patients are hospitalized each year because of CSD. The annual total health care cost related to CSD is more than $12 million in 1992 dollars. This study also estimated a higher incidence in adults than previous studies: Carithers[48] found 87% of his 1,200 CSD patients were 18 years old or younger; Margileth[49] found 83% of 1,400 were less than 21 years old, but the 1993 CDC study found that only an estimated 56% of CSD patients were 18 years old or younger.[47] Both of the studies showing a higher percentage of CSD in children were from pediatricians, and this may have biased these earlier reports toward a younger age of CSD patient. Nevertheless, CSD remains one of the most common causes of chronic lymphadenopathy in children.

Although CSD was first recognized by Debré et al.[50] in 1950, the causative organism was identified only recently as *B. henselae*. The pathway to the true microbiologic identity of this microorganism has been circuitous and included descriptions of the causative organism as a subviral particle,[51] then as a Warthin-Starry-staining bacillus[12] followed by reports of isolation of *Rothia dentocariosa*,[52] then *Afipia felis*[13] and, ultimately, *B. henselae.*[15, 19] The final identification of *B. henselae* represents the convergence of fascinating data from eclectic fields of study, including acquired immunodeficiency syndrome (AIDS)–related opportunistic infections, epidemiology, pathology, molecular biology, microbiology, and veterinary medicine.

After *B. henselae* was identified as an agent of BA, the IFA test was developed at the CDC to test sera of BA patients for antibodies to *B. henselae*. A set of blinded serum samples from HIV-infected patients with biopsy-documented BA or CSD were submitted for testing; surprisingly, the two CSD patients were found to have high titer *B. henselae* antibodies. Subsequent testing of banked CSD patient sera demonstrated that a high percentage had antibodies to *B. henselae,*[15] and the relationship between *B. henselae* and CSD was confirmed thereafter by microbiologic and molecular biologic investigations. In 1993, *B. henselae* was isolated from the lymph nodes of two immunocompetent patients with lymphadenopathy.[19] One was a 68-year-old man with fever and an enlarged, tender epitrochlear lymph node; the other was a 27-year-old man who developed fever and tender left axillary lymphadenopathy. Although there was no mention of a specific cat scratch, the patients had contact with cats, and each was noted to have an eschar on the ipsilateral hand at the time lymphadenopathy developed. The nodes were excised and showed necrotizing granulomas and no organisms on Warthin-Starry staining, but in each case, culture of the lymph node biopsy specimen grew *B. henselae*. Although the patient histories and histopathologic findings are not pathognomonic for CSD, it is likely that both of these cases represented *B. henselae* culture-positive CSD lymphadenitis.

Several months later, another group demonstrated the presence of *B. henselae* DNA in CSD skin test material.[18] Skin testing has been used for years to aid in the diagnosis of CSD in thousands of patients since it was originally developed by Hangar and Rose in 1946.[53] The skin test material consists of pus aspirated from the suppurated lymph node of a patient with CSD, cultured on media for bacteria, fungi, and acid-fast organisms, diluted with sterile saline solution, incubated at 60°C for 72 hours, and recultured.[54] The material is then tested by intradermal injection of 0.1 mL in patients with a known previous response. The skin test result is positive in 92% to 99% of patients with the diagnostic criteria of CSD and 89% of patients with bacilli seen on biopsy.[54] Anderson et al.[18] tested two lots of CSD skin test antigen used by clinicians for the diagnosis of CSD. DNA was extracted from the skin test material and evaluated using techniques that amplify the DNA of any bacterium that might be present. The DNA detected in the skin test antigen was then sequenced and found to be *B. henselae,* and no other bacterial DNA was detected, including *A. felis.*

The same group evaluated lymph node tissue from CSD patients by PCR.[55] The 25 patients had regional lymphadenopathy and cat contact, without any other obvious diagnosis. The DNA was extracted and amplified, and the PCR product was probed to detect the presence of *B. henselae* DNA in the lymph node biopsy or aspirate specimens. *Bartonella henselae* DNA was detected in 21 of the 25 samples, including 100% (9/9) of the aspirates and 75% (12/16) of the lymph node biopsy specimens.

ATYPICAL CAT-SCRATCH DISEASE

Rarely, systemic or severe disease can complicate CSD. An estimated 5% to 14% of patients have atypical manifestations of CSD and without lymphadenopathy.[48, 53] Of the atypical manifestations of CSD, CNS and hepatosplenic manifestations now have been linked convincingly to *Bartonella* infection by microbiologic culture, serologic titer, or both.

Although neurologic manifestations are rare (approximately 2% of all cases) they are a well-described complication of CSD. These syndromes include encephalopathy, seizures, neuroretinitis, myelitis, radiculitis, polyneuritis, paraplegia, and cerebral arteritis.[53] Neuroretinitis, one of the most frequently reported neurologic syndromes, has been serologically and microbiologically linked to *B. henselae* infection recently.[56] The syndrome of Leber's idiopathic stellate neuroretinitis is characterized by visual loss, stellate macular exudates, and optic disc edema. It has been associated with CSD in both children and adults. A report describes two adult patients with cat contact who developed high fevers, visual loss, and stellate neuroretinitis whose blood cultures grew *B. henselae.*[56] High titers of antibodies against *B. henselae* were also present in the serum of both patients. A culture of blood from the couple's pet cat also grew *B. henselae.* Additional evidence supporting the association of *B. henselae* and this syndrome was reported by Golnik et al.[57] Three unrelated adults and one child, each of whom was exposed to a pet cat, developed neuroretinitis and had high titer antibodies against *B. henselae.* Thus, the neuroretinitis syndrome previously identified as one of the more severe manifestations of CSD has been associated directly with *B. henselae* infection.

A cluster of five CSD encephalitis cases was reported in December 1994.[58] Three children were admitted to the same hospital within a 26-hour period after sudden onset of generalized seizures, coma, and respiratory depression necessitating intubation. In the following month, two additional children were admitted to hospitals in the same area with similar symptoms. None of these children had documented cat scratches or bites before becoming ill, but all had direct contact with stray cats or kittens. Each child developed regional lymphadenopathy and markedly elevated antibody titers to *B. henselae*. As has been described previously with most CSD encephalitis cases, all five of these children recovered completely. The reason for this clustering of CSD encephalitis cases remains unknown, but clustering of CSD cases was also reported in Connecticut.[17]

Another atypical manifestation of CSD is hepatosplenic granulomatous disease.[53] In many reports of this syndrome, a presumptive diagnosis of CSD granulomatous hepatitis was made after visualization of bacilli in the hepatic granulomas of patients with cat exposure and positive CSD skin test results. A recent report described two pediatric patients with high fevers for approximately 3 weeks, anorexia, fatigue, and hypoechoic lesions of the liver, spleen, or both.[59] Each child had markedly elevated antibody titers to *Bartonella* species. As diagnostic tests for culture and serology are improved and become more widely available, the association between *B. henselae* and the different manifestations of typical and atypical CSD will be further elucidated.

DIAGNOSIS

HISTOPATHOLOGY

In many reported cases of suspected *Bartonella* infection, including those in the immunocompromised patient (e.g., BA), as well as in the immunocompetent patient (e.g., CSD), there is no molecular or microbiologic documentation of *Bartonella* infection. At the minimum, characteristic histopathology (especially positive Warthin-Starry staining) must be present to confirm *Bartonella* infection.

With histopathologic examination, BA lesions are characterized by proliferation of small blood vessels lined with protuberant endothelial cells (Fig 8, A). There is usually a mixed inflammatory cell response consisting of lymphocytes and neutrophils.[3] Clumps of amphophilic or basophilic material adjacent to the newly formed vessels represent the *Bartonella* bacilli, which are better visualized by Warthin-Starry silver staining (Fig 8, B). The histopathologic ap-

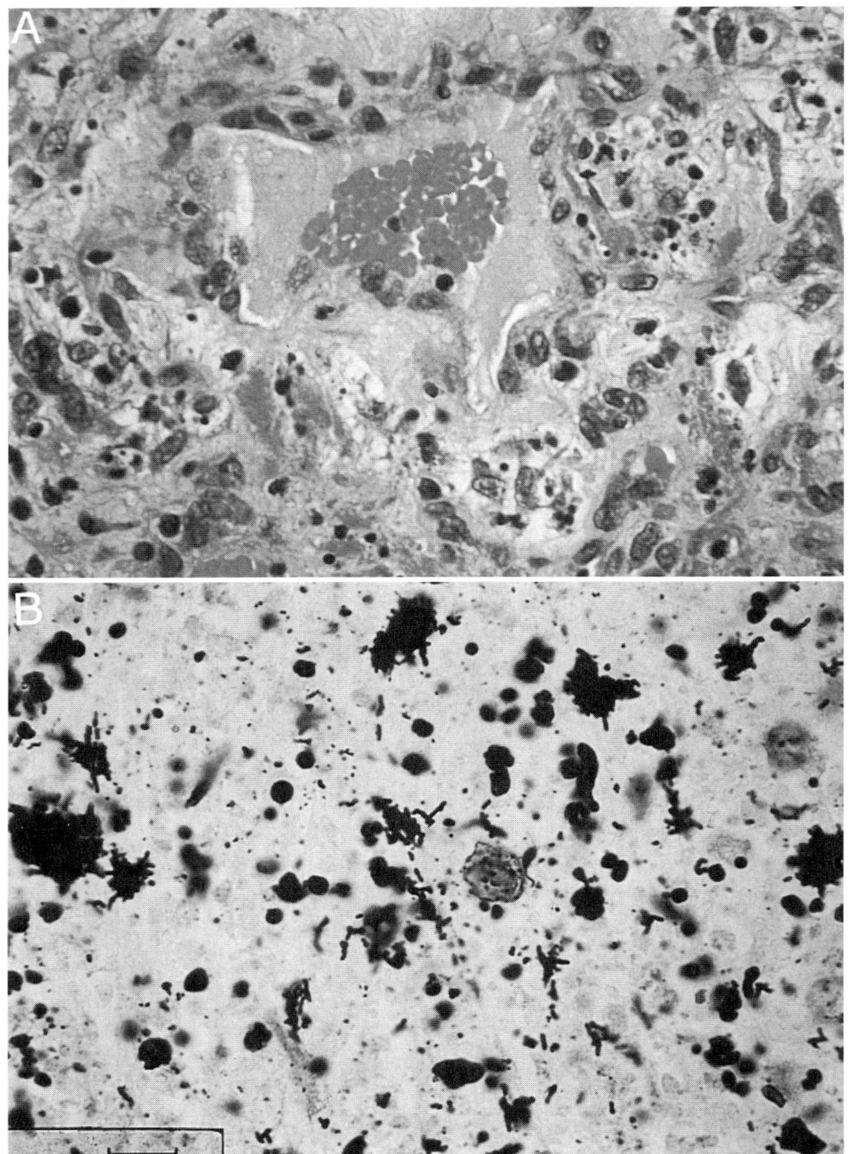

FIGURE 8.

A, hematoxylin-eosin staining of a biopsy specimen from a cutaneous bacillary angiomatosis lesion demonstrates a dermal vessel. The vessel is lined with protuberant endothelial cells surrounded by myxoid connec-
(Continued.)

pearance of CSD differs markedly from that of BA. Biopsy specimens of CSD lymph node tissue often exhibits scattered microabscesses, larger abscesses, and granulomas.[53] Although the host tissue inflammatory response differs markedly between BA and CSD, Warthin-Starry staining reveals similar-appearing bacilli for both infections, although there is usually a much larger number of bacilli in BA lesions.

CULTURE

Isolation of *Bartonella* species remains difficult because of the fastidious nature of these organisms. Recovery of *Bartonella* bacilli on solid agar is best achieved by inoculating tissue homogenate onto very fresh agar plates. Isolation from blood can be achieved using the lysis-centrifugation tubes.[4] Chocolate agar or heart infusion agar with 5% rabbit blood have been used successfully for recovery of *B. henselae* from blood,[4] *B. quintana* and *B. henselae* from cutaneous BA lesions,[21] *B. elizabethae* from blood,[29] and *B. henselae* from CSD lymph nodes.[19] Cocultivation of tissue homogenate from biopsy and eukaryotic endothelial cells has also been used for the isolation of *Bartonella* species.[21] Inoculated agar plates should be incubated in 5% CO_2 at 35°C for a prolonged period (14−28 days).

SEROLOGY

The serologic test for *Bartonella* antibodies, which was developed at the CDC,[15] has been assessed most extensively. Although this serologic test does not distinguish between antibody response to *B. quintana* and *B. henselae,* it has been useful in the detection of *Bartonella* antibodies in both CSD[17] and BA.[60] In the study of CSD patients in Connecticut, 84% (34/38) had positive antibody titers for *B. henselae* compared with only 3.6% (4/112) of controls.[17] Testing of serum from seven patients with biopsy-proven cutane-

---

FIGURE 8 (cont.).

tive tissue containing neutrophils and amphophilic granular material in close proximity to the vascular lumen (original magnification × 240). The granular material represents clumps of *Bartonella* bacilli, visualized more clearly with Warthin-Starry staining. (From Koehler JE, LeBoit PE, Egbert BM, et al: *Ann Intern Med* 109:449−455, 1988. Used by permission.) **B,** Warthin-Starry silver staining of a cutaneous bacillary angiomatosis biopsy specimen reveals multiple clumps of tangled, dark silver-staining bacillary organisms (bar = 10 μm). (From Koehler JE, Tappero JW: *Clin Infect Dis* 17:612−624, 1993. Used by permission.)

ous BA revealed that all had antibodies to *B. henselae*, but seven HIV-positive patients without evidence of *Bartonella* infection did not have antibodies.[60]

TREATMENT

The clinical response of CSD and BA to antibiotic treatment differs markedly, even though both syndromes can be caused by the same organism, *B. henselae*. Bacillary angiomatosis responds rapidly to antibiotic treatment and is potentially fatal if untreated, but CSD is almost uniformly a self-limiting illness, regardless of antibiotic treatment. Several differences in the characteristics of the host response to *B. henselae* in these two syndromes may be relevant to this difference in response to antibiotics. First, the number of bacteria seen in BA lesions in the immunocompromised host is much greater than that seen in CSD. Second, the nature of the host response differs markedly, with an angiogenic response in BA and a granulomatous response in CSD. The histopathologic manifestations of CSD may result from a more predominant cell-mediated immunologic response of the host[61]; this host response apparently continues even after bacilli can no longer be visualized.

For *Bartonella* infection in the immunocompromised host, antibiotic therapy is guided by clinical experience because treatment has never been studied systematically. The drug of first choice is erythromycin, with doxycycline prescribed for patients intolerant of erythromycin (Table 1).[10] Tetracycline and minocycline also have been used to successfully treat patients with BA. Patients who are immunocompromised and severely ill (e.g., peliosis hepatis, en-

TABLE 1.
Clinical Efficacy of Antibiotics in the Treatment of Bacillary Angiomatosis and Bacillary Peliosis*

Definite	Possible	Inconclusive	None
Erythromycin	Gentamicin	Ciprofloxacin	Penicillin
Doxycycline	Rifampin	Ceftriaxone	Ceph[1]
Tetracycline		Ceftizoxime	PCN-D
Minocycline		TMP-SMX	

*TMP-SMX = trimethoprim-sulfamethoxazole; Ceph[1] = first-generation cephalosporins; PCN-D = penicillin derivatives (PCNase-resistant penicillins and aminopenicillins).

docarditis, osteomyelitis) should be treated initially with intravenous antibiotics, including a primary drug (erythromycin or doxycycline) plus a secondary drug (rifampin or gentamicin). Initiation of treatment may be followed by a Jarisch-Herxheimer reaction.[21] It is evident that the penicillins and first-generation cephalosporins have no clinical efficacy in the treatment of *Bartonella* in the immunocompromised host. Progression of BA disease during ciprofloxacin therapy has been reported.[62] Immunocompromised patients may develop relapsing infection; therefore, prolonged treatment (at least 4 months for severe disease) is necessary, with closely monitored follow-up after discontinuation of antibiotic therapy.

Treatment of CSD is not clearly beneficial and also has not been evaluated prospectively. For the majority of patients with CSD, management should include conservative symptomatic care and observation.[63] Complete resolution of lymphadenopathy usually occurs after 2 to 6 months. Patients with severe CSD (e.g., encephalopathy, neuroretinitis) may have a shortened course and thus benefit from antibiotic therapy, but choice of antibiotics is unclear. Margileth[63] studied 268 cases of CSD retrospectively and found that rifampin, ciprofloxacin, gentamicin, and trimethoprim-sulfamethoxazole (TMP-SMX) appeared to have clinical efficacy in patients with CSD (listed in order of clinical efficacy from greatest to least), but failures also have been reported after treatment of CSD patients with gentamicin and TMP-SMX.[63] The retrospective studies are difficult to interpret because atypical and typical CSD resolve without antibiotic therapy, and patients often receive multiple courses of different antibiotics. In addition, in vitro and in vivo antibiotic susceptibilities of *Bartonella* species often do not correlate and cannot be used to guide antibiotic recommendations.[10]

PREVENTION

Recommendations for the prevention of *Bartonella* infections depend on identification of the vertebrate reservoirs, vectors, and route of transmission for each of the species. The only known vertebrate host for *B. quintana* and *B. bacilliformis* is the human. Prolonged periods (months) of asymptomatic human bacteremia have been reported for both of these species, providing a reservoir from which the body louse and sandfly, respectively, can transmit the bacilli to another human host. The arthropod vector involved in transmission of *B. quintana* in contemporary times is unknown, but it is suspected to be the body louse, as occurred in World War I. At present, recommendations for prevention of *B. quintana* infection are limited to avoiding contact with lice and promptly eradicating any lice infestation. The primary vertebrate reservoir and vector or vectors for *B. elizabethae* remain undiscovered. The Canadian vole is chronically infected with *B. vinsonii*, but transmission to humans has not been documented.

The domestic cat is a major reservoir for *B. henselae*, from which transmission to humans apparently occurs. A prevalence of *B. henselae* bacteremia in 41% (25/61) of pet and impounded cats in the San Francisco area was reported in 1994.[20] The cats were all asymptomatic, and prolonged bacteremia was documented to be 2.5 months in one cat and was suspected to be 17 months in another. Prevalence of *Bartonella*-specific antibodies in cats living in other regions of the United States ranges from 14% to 50%[17, 64] and indicates that *Bartonella* infection is also common in other areas of the United States. In addition to serving as the reservoir for *B. henselae*, the domestic cat also appears to be a major vector involved in the transmission of *B. henselae* to humans. Most patients develop CSD after sustaining a cat scratch and developing a primary lesion at the site of the scratch. It is presumed that the cat's claws become contaminated with *B. henselae*, with subsequent introduction to the human by a cat scratch. It is estimated that there are 57 million pet cats in the United States residing in nearly one third of all households,[65] and thus the potential for exposure of humans to *B. henselae* is great. It is noteworthy that although there are probably many more than 24,000 cases of CSD in the United States annually, it is still a very rare disease considering the magnitude of the reservoir and the number of exposures (e.g., scratches and bites) suffered by cat owners.

The cat flea, *Ctenocephalides felis*, may be an additional vector that transmits *B. henselae* to humans, cats, or both. In one epidemiologic study, development of CSD was associated with kittens infested with fleas.[17] Subsequently, viable *B. henselae* bacilli were isolated from fleas combed from a cat bacteremic with *B. henselae*, suggesting that transmission might occur via this arthropod.[20] Several reports also mention tick bites preceding documented *B. henselae* bacteremia in two immunocompetent individuals, raising the possibility of yet another arthropod vector for *B. henselae*.[8, 43]

The potential transmission of *B. henselae* from pet cats to humans is of particular concern for immunocompromised patients. An epidemiologic study of numerous environmental exposures experienced by patients in the 6 months before developing BA revealed that the only risk factor statistically associated with developing BA was traumatic cat contact (e.g., cat scratches and bites).[16] In a later study, all seven cats belonging to four patients with BA were found to be bacteremic with *B. henselae*.[20] The BA lesions of these patients (elderly or HIV infected) were caused by *B. henselae*, not *B. quintana*. Although pet cats pose some risk to immunocompromised patients, it is evident that these pets provide invaluable, even life-sustaining companionship, and that the potential risk is outweighed by the benefit.[66] With our current knowledge about *B. henselae*, some measures can be suggested to decrease exposure of pet cat owners to *B. henselae*.[67] Rough play likely to result in scratches should be avoided. Scratches should be immediately washed with soap and water, and flea infestation should be controlled. More definitive recommendations for prevention of infection from all *Bartonella* species will be forthcoming as research elucidates more information about the reservoirs, vectors, and transmission of these important and emerging pathogens.

REFERENCES

1. Brenner DJ, O'Connor SP, Winkler HH, et al: Proposals to unify the genera *Bartonella* and *Rochalimaea*, with descriptions of *Bartonella quintana* comb. nov., *Bartonella vinsonii* comb. nov., *Bartonella henselae* comb. nov., and *Bartonella elizabethae* comb. nov., and to remove the family Bartonellaceae from the order Rickettsiales. *Int J System Bact* 43:777–786, 1993.
2. Stoler MH, Bonfiglio TA, Steigbigel RT, et al: An atypical subcutaneous infection associated with acquired immune deficiency syndrome. *Am J Clin Pathol* 80:714–718, 1983.
3. LeBoit PE, Berger TG, Egbert BM, et al: Bacillary angiomatosis: The histopathology and differential diagnosis of a pseudoneoplastic infection in patients with human immunodeficiency virus disease. *Am J Surg Pathol* 13:909–920, 1989.
4. Slater LN, Welch DF, Hensel D, et al: A newly recognized fastidious gram-negative pathogen as a cause of fever and bacteremia. *N Engl J Med* 323:1587–1593, 1990.
5. Perkocha LA, Geaghan SM, Yen TSB, et al: Clinical and pathological features of bacillary peliosis hepatis in association with human immunodeficiency virus infection. *N Engl J Med* 323:1581–1586, 1990.
6. Relman DA, Loutit JS, Schmidt TM, et al: The agent of bacillary angiomatosis: An approach to the identification of uncultured pathogens. *N Engl J Med* 323:1573–1580, 1990.
7. Regnery RL, Anderson BE, Clarridge JE III, et al: Characterization of a novel *Rochalimaea* species, *R. henselae*, sp. nov., isolated from blood of a febrile, HIV-positive patient. *J Clin Microbiol* 30:265–274, 1992.

8. Welch DF, Pickett DA, Slater LN, et al: *Rochalimaea henselae* sp. nov., a cause of septicemia, bacillary angiomatosis, and parenchymal bacillary peliosis. *J Clin Microbiol* 30:275–280, 1992.

9. Slater LN, Welch DF: *Rochalimaea* species (recently renamed *Bartonella*). In Mandell GL, Bennett JE, Dolin R (eds): *Principles and Practice of Infectious Diseases*, ed 4. New York, Churchill Livingstone, 1994, pp 1741–1747.

10. Koehler JE, Tappero JW: AIDS commentary: Bacillary angiomatosis and bacillary peliosis in patients infected with human immunodeficiency virus. *Clin Infect Dis* 17:612–624, 1993.

11. LeBoit PE, Berger TG, Egbert BM, et al: Epithelioid haemangioma-like vascular proliferation in AIDS: Manifestation of cat-scratch disease bacillus infection? *Lancet* 1:960–963, 1988.

12. Wear DJ, Margileth AM, Hadfield TL, et al: Cat scratch disease: A bacterial infection. *Science* 221:1403–1405, 1983.

13. English CK, Wear DJ, Margileth AM, et al: Cat-scratch disease: Isolation and culture of the bacterial agent. *JAMA* 259:1347–1352, 1988.

14. Brenner DJ, Hollis DG, Moss CW, et al: Proposal of *Afipia* gen. nov., with *Afipia felis* sp. nov. (formerly the cat scratch disease bacillus), *Afipia clevelandensis* sp. nov. (formerly the Cleveland Clinic Foundation Strain), *Afipia broomeae* sp. nov., and three unnamed genospecies. *J Clin Microbiol* 29:2450–2460, 1991.

15. Regnery RL, Olson JG, Perkins BA, et al: Serological response to "*Rochalimaea henselae*" antigen in suspected cat-scratch disease. *Lancet* 339:1443–1445, 1992.

16. Tappero JW, Mohle-Boetani J, Koehler JE, et al: The epidemiology of bacillary angiomatosis and bacillary peliosis. *JAMA* 269:770–775, 1993.

17. Zangwill KM, Hamilton DH, Perkins BA, et al: Cat scratch disease in Connecticut: Epidemiology, risk factors, and evaluation of a new diagnostic test. *N Engl J Med* 329:8–13, 1993.

18. Anderson B, Kelly C, Threlkel R, et al: Detection of *Rochalimaea henselae* in cat-scratch disease skin test antigens. *J Infect Dis* 168:1034–1036, 1993.

19. Dolan MJ, Wong MT, Regnery RL, et al: Syndrome of *Rochalimaea henselae* adenitis suggesting cat scratch disease. *Ann Intern Med* 118:331–336, 1993.

20. Koehler JE, Glaser CA, Tappero JW: *Rochalimaea henselae* infection: A new zoonosis with the domestic cat as reservoir. *JAMA* 271:531–535, 1994.

21. Koehler JE, Quinn FD, Berger TG, et al: Isolation of *Rochalimaea* species from cutaneous and osseous lesions of bacillary angiomatosis. *N Engl J Med* 327:1625–1631, 1992.

22. Strong RP (ed): *Trench Fever: Report of Commission, Medical Research Committee, American Red Cross*. New York, Oxford University Press, 1918, pp 40–60.

23. Swift HF: Trench fever. *Arch Intern Med* 26:76–98, 1920.
24. Vinson JW, Fuller HS: Studies on trench fever: I. Propagation of *Rickettsia*-like microorganisms from a patient's blood. *Pathol Microbiol (Suppl)* 152–166, 1961.
25. Weinman D: Bartonellosis. In Weinman D, Ristoc M (eds): *Infectious Blood Diseases of Man and Animals*. New York, Academic Press, 1968, pp 3–24.
26. Garcia-Caceres U, Garcia FU: Bartonellosis: An immunodepressive disease and the life of Daniel Alcides Carrion. *Am J Clin Pathol* 959(suppl):S58–S66, 1991.
27. Baker JA: A rickettsial infection in Canadian voles. *J Exp Med* 84:37–51, 1946.
28. Breitschwerdt EB, Kordick DL, Malarkey DE, et al: Endocarditis in a dog due to infection with a novel *Bartonella* subspecies. *J Clin Microbiol* 33:154–160, 1995.
29. Daly JS, Worthington MG, Brenner DJ, et al: *Rochalimaea elizabethae* sp. nov. isolated from a patient with endocarditis. *J Clin Microbiol* 31:872–881, 1993.
30. Mohle-Boetani J, Reingold A, LeBoit P, et al: Bacillary angiomatosis: Spectrum of disease and clinical characteristics in HIV+ patients [abstract no 372]. In *Program and Abstracts of the 32nd Interscience Conference on Antimicrobial Agents and Chemotherapy*. Washington, DC, American Society for Microbiology, 1992, p 173.
31. Koehler JE, LeBoit PE, Egbert BM, et al: Cutaneous vascular lesions and disseminated cat-scratch disease in patients with the acquired immunodeficiency syndrome (AIDS) and AIDS-related complex. *Ann Intern Med* 109:449–455, 1988.
32. Berger TG, Tappero JW, Kaymen A, et al: Bacillary (epithelioid) angiomatosis and concurrent Kaposi's sarcoma in acquired immunodeficiency syndrome. *Arch Dermatol* 125:1543–1547, 1989.
33. Baron AL, Steinbach LS, LeBoit PE, et al: Osteolytic lesions and bacillary angiomatosis in HIV infection: Radiologic differentiation from AIDS-related Kaposi sarcoma. *Radiology* 177:77–81, 1990.
34. Slater LN, Min K-W: Polypoid endobronchial lesions: A manifestation of bacillary angiomatosis. *Chest* 102:972–974, 1992.
35. Tuur SM, Macher AM, Angritt P, et al: AIDS case for diagnosis series, 1988. *Milit Med* 153:M57–M64, 1988.
36. Cockerell CJ, Whitlow MA, Webster GF, et al: Epithelioid angiomatosis: A distinct vascular disorder in patients with the acquired immunodeficiency syndrome or AIDS-related complex. *Lancet* 2:654–656, 1987.
37. Spach DH, Panther LA, Thorning DR, et al: Intracerebral bacillary angiomatosis in a patient infected with human immunodeficiency virus. *Ann Intern Med* 116:740–742, 1992.
38. Schwartzman WA, Patnaik M, Barka NE, et al: *Rochalimaea* antibodies in HIV-associated neurologic disease. *Neurology* 44:1312–1316, 1994.

39. Spach DH, Callis KP, Paauw DS, et al: Endocarditis caused by *Rochalimaea quintana* in a patient infected with human immunodeficiency virus. *J Clin Microbiol* 31:692–694, 1993.

40. Myers SA, Prose NS, Garcia JA, et al: Bacillary angiomatosis in a child undergoing chemotherapy. *J Pediatr* 121:574–578, 1992.

41. Riley LE, Tuomala RE: Bacillary angiomatosis in a pregnant patient with acquired immunodeficiency syndrome. *Obstet Gynecol* 79:818–819, 1992.

42. Tappero JW, Koehler JE, Berger TG, et al: Bacillary angiomatosis and bacillary splenitis in immunocompetent adults. *Ann Intern Med* 118:363–365, 1993.

43. Lucey D, Dolan MJ, Moss CW, et al: Relapsing illness due to *Rochalimaea henselae* in immunocompetent hosts: Implication for therapy and new epidemiological associations. *Clin Infect Dis* 14:683–688, 1992.

44. Spach DH, Larson AM, Coyle MB, et al: Unanticipated *Rochalimaea quintana* bacteremia in patients with chronic alcoholism [Late Breaker Abstracts]. In *Program and Abstracts of the 33rd Interscience Conference on Antimicrobial Agents and Chemotherapy*. Washington, DC, American Society for Microbiology, 1993.

45. Raoult D, Drancourt M, Carta A, et al: Bartonella (*Rochalimaea*) quintana isolation in patient with chronic adenopathy, lymphopenia, and a cat [letter]. *Lancet* 343:997, 1994.

46. Margileth AM: Cat scratch disease: A therapeutic dilemma. *Vet Clin North Am* 17:91–103, 1987.

47. Jackson LA, Perkins BA, Wenger JD: Cat scratch disease in the United States: An analysis of three national databases. *Am J Public Health* 83:1707–1711, 1993.

48. Carithers HA: Cat-scratch disease: An overview based on a study of 1,200 patients. *Am J Dis Child* 139:1124–1133, 1985.

49. Margileth AM: Dermatologic manifestations and update of cat scratch disease. *Pediatr Dermatol* 5:1–9, 1988.

50. Debré R, Lamy M, Jammet M-L, et al: La maladie des griffes de chat. *Bull Soc Med Hop Paris* 66:76–79, 1950.

51. Kalter SS, Kim CS, Heberling RL: Herpes-like virus particles associated with cat scratch disease. *Nature* 224:190, 1969.

52. Gerber MA, MacAlister TJ, Ballow M, et al: The aetiological agent of cat scratch disease. *Lancet* 1:236–239, 1985.

53. Margileth AM: Cat scratch disease. *Adv Pediatr Infect Dis* 8:1–21, 1993.

54. Moriarity RA, Margileth AM: Cat scratch disease. *Infect Dis Clin North Am* 1:575–590, 1987.

55. Anderson B, Sims K, Regnery R, et al: Detection of *Rochalimaea henselae* DNA in specimens from cat scratch disease patients by PCR. *J Clin Microbiol* 32:942–948, 1994.

56. Lattuada C Jr, Garcia M, Reed J, et al: Neuroretinitis associated with

Rochalimaea henselae bacteremia [Abstract no C-464]. In *Program and Abstracts of the 94th American Society for Microbiology General Meeting*. Washington, DC, American Society for Microbiology, 1994.

57. Golnik KC, Marotto ME, Fanous MM, et al: Ophthalmic manifestations of *Rochalimaea* species. *Am J Ophthalmol* 118:145–151, 1994.
58. Encephalitis associated with cat scratch disease—Broward and Palm Beach Counties, Florida, 1994. *MMWR* 43:909, 915–916, 1994.
59. Golden SE: Hepatosplenic cat-scratch disease associated with elevated anti-*Rochalimaea* antibody titers. *Pediatr Infect Dis J* 12:868–871, 1993.
60. Tappero J, Regnery R, Koehler J, et al: Detection of serologic response to *Rochalimaea henselae* in patients with bacillary angiomatosis (BA) by immunofluorescent antibody (IFA) testing [abstract no 674]. In *Program and Abstracts of the 32nd Interscience Conference on Antimicrobial Agents and Chemotherapy*. Washington, DC, American Society for Microbiology, 1992, p 223.
61. Kemper CA, Lombard CM, Deresinski SC, et al: Visceral bacillary epithelioid angiomatosis: Possible manifestations of disseminated cat scratch disease in the immunocompromised host: A report of two cases. *Am J Med* 89:216–222, 1990.
62. Tappero JW, Koehler JE: Cat-scratch disease and bacillary angiomatosis [letter]. *JAMA* 266:1938–1939, 1991.
63. Margileth AM: Antibiotic therapy for cat-scratch disease: Clinical study of therapeutic outcome in 268 patients and a review of the literature. *Pediatr Infect Dis J* 11:474–478, 1992.
64. Childs JE, Rooney JA, Cooper JL, et al: Epidemiologic observations on infection with *Rochalimaea* species among cats living in Baltimore, Md. *J Am Vet Med Assoc* 204:1775–1778, 1994.
65. Veterinary Service Market for Companion Animals, 1992. *J Am Vet Med Assoc* 201:990–992, 1992.
66. Glaser CA, Angulo FJ, Rooney JA: AIDS commentary: Animal-associated opportunistic infections among persons infected with the human immunodeficiency virus. *Clin Infect Dis* 18:14–24, 1994.
67. Regnery RL, Childs JE, Koehler JE: *Bartonella* (formerly *Rochalimaea*)–associated infections. USPHS/IDSA recommendations for prevention of opportunistic infections in HIV-infected persons, Joint Task Force (IDSA, NIH, CDC) on the Prevention of Opportunistic Infections. *Clin Infect Dis* (in press).

Cerebrospinal Fluid Shunt Infections

Willem A. Hanekom, M.B.Ch.B., D.C.H.(S.A.), F.C.P.(S.A.)
Instructor of Pediatrics, Northwestern University Medical School,
Fellow, Division of Infectious Diseases, The Children's Memorial
Hospital, Chicago, Illinois

Ram Yogev, M.D.
Professor of Pediatrics, Northwestern University Medical School,
Director, Section of Pediatric and Maternal HIV Infection, The
Children's Memorial Hospital, Chicago, Illinois

CEREBROSPINAL FLUID SHUNTS AND COMPLICATIONS

Prosthetic implants are used commonly in neurosurgery when normal homeostasis of cerebrospinal fluid (CSF) production or resorption is interrupted. The most common indication for CSF shunt insertion in pediatrics is hydrocephalus, caused by conditions such as congenital malformations of the central nervous system (e.g., myelomeningocele), intraventricular hemorrhage, central nervous system (CNS) infection, tumors, or trauma.[1, 2]

The proximal end of the shunt is usually placed in a lateral ventricle, but the catheter may also be placed in an intracranial cyst or in the subarachnoid space, should this be indicated. Some shunts—for example, those used for benign intracranial hypertension—use the lumbar CSF space as the proximal source for drainage or diversion.[3] The distal end drains to an extracranial reservoir such as the peritoneal or pleural cavity or to a vascular space such as the right atrium or jugular vein. A one-way flow valve, either pressure regulated or flow controlled, forms part of most systems and is placed just outside the skull under the skin. A reservoir may be added to the system or included in the valve assembly for percutaneous access to CSF for sampling, testing of shunt patency, or introduction of medication or contrast. Ventriculoperitoneal shunts are used most frequently because their placement is relatively easy and associated morbidity is less.[3, 4] A closed external drainage system (extraventricular drain, or EVD) is used in the treatment of shunt malfunctions or infections or for temporary diversion of CSF flow. Any shunt lends itself to complications, most of which occur in children younger than 2 years old.[1, 5] The majority of complications are functional or mechanical in nature.[1, 6, 7] Functional complications include inadequate drainage or overdrainage; the former may result in recrudescence of hydrocephalus whereas craniosynostosis or slit ventricle syndrome result from the latter. Mechanical shunt problems include obstruction, migration of the shunt, disconnection, fracture, or malposition. In addition, ventriculoperitoneal shunts may result in abdominal complications, including small bowel obstruction, abdominal abscess or cyst, intestinal or bladder perforation, and rarely pancreatitis. Only about one fourth of complications of CSF shunts relate to infection.[1] These infections cause morbidity and affect the long-term outcome of the patient[8, 9]; thus, major efforts should be taken to prevent and to treat shunt infections effectively.

EPIDEMIOLOGY

Incidence rates reported up to 1989 have been summarized by Kaufman and McLone.[10] The case incidence (i.e., infection rate per number of patients) has ranged from 8% to 40%, and the operative incidence (i.e., infection rate per number of procedures) has ranged from 4.5% to 14%. Lower rates have been reported since 1990 with case incidence of 0.3% to 15.6% and operative incidence of 0.17% to 12.9% (Table 1).[1, 4, 5, 11–17] Although the reliability of incidence rates reported in some smaller series has been questioned because of poor statistical power, the suboptimal retrospective design of the studies, and differences in duration of follow-up, an operative incidence of less than 5% is considered acceptable.[18]

The majority (up to 69%) of shunt infections occur within 1 month of the operative procedure and up to 86% of infections present within 6 months.[10, 12, 13, 15, 16] However, infections may manifest as long as 4 years or more after the shunting procedure.[12]

Some circumstances are associated with higher rates of shunt infection: age, revision of the shunt, the type of shunt, and perioperative preparation.

AGE

An increased operative infection rate has been reported in infants younger than 6 months, especially in preterm neonates. The majority of patients who have shunt infections are younger than 2 years old.[1, 5, 13, 14, 19]

REVISION OF SHUNT

Some studies report that revision of an infected shunt is associated with a higher subsequent operative infection rate of 12% to

TABLE 1.
Selected Reported Incidence of Shunt Infections Since 1989

Reference	No. of Procedures	Case Infection Rate (%)	Operative Infection Rate (%)
Ersahin et al.[11]	2,538	10.1	5
Cotton et al.[12]	372	—	10.5
Choux et al.[13]	606*	15.6*	7.8*
	1,197†	0.33†	0.17†
Pople et al.[14]	466	—	10.0
Kotney et al.[15]	350	9.8	8.0
Vernet et al.[4]	373‡	4.2	1.8
Morissette et al.[16]	1,061	—	2.6
Kestle et al.[17]	581*	—	12.9*
	576†	—	3.8†
Piatt and Carlson[5]	727	9.4	—
Di Rocco et al.[1]	764	—	6.7

*Retrospectively, without perioperative protocol (see discussion of prophylaxis in text).
†Prospectively, with perioperative protocol (see discussion of prophylaxis in text).
‡Ventriculoatrial shunts.

20%, often involving the same organism, and probably indicating inadequate initial treatment.[11, 18, 20] More recent studies do not confirm this observation.[5, 15]

TYPE OF SHUNT

There is no significant difference in the rates of infection between patients with ventriculoperitoneal shunts and those with ventriculoatrial shunts.[4, 21-24] Compared with ventriculoperitoneal shunts, there is a significantly lower incidence of infection of lumboperitoneal shunts, which are technically much more difficult to perform.[3] External shunts have an infection rate of less than 10% except when an EVD is used in preterm infants for treatment of posthemorrhagic hydrocephalus, which is associated with an infection rate of 40%.[10, 25] Reservoirs, internal devices that may be punctured percutaneously repeatedly, are the preferred treatment in this group of patients and have reported infection rates of 3% to 15%.[26]

PERIOPERATIVE PREPARATION

The administration of prophylactic antibiotics may have a significant effect in reducing the number of subsequent shunt infections.[27-30] The same applies to operative technique, especially attention to strict asepsis, duration of surgery, and experience of the surgeon.[13, 17] In fact, the lowest rates reported in Table 1 are from institutions that have applied various prophylactic measures, which will be discussed later.

ETIOLOGY

The most common organisms isolated from the CSF or shunt catheters during infective episodes are staphylococci (61%–85% of cases; Fig 1).* In virtually all studies the majority of these organisms were coagulase negative. *Staphylococcus epidermidis* is by far the most commonly reported, but other species such as *Staphylococcus capitis* and *Staphylococcus hominis* can also cause infection. *Staphylococcus aureus* is reported as the etiologic agent in as few as 4% and as many as 47% of the cases. Limited data are available regarding the proportion of staphylococcal species that are methicillin resistant, but the proportion is expected to increase because many of the infections are acquired in a hospital setting and because increasing proportions of community acquired coagulase-negative staphylococci are methicillin resistant.

The next most common group of organisms responsible for shunt infections are gram-negative bacilli, causing 6% to 25% of infections.* *Escherichia coli* is the most frequently isolated, responsible for more than 50% of the gram-negative infections. *Klebsiella* and *Proteus* species (responsible for 15% to 20% and 10% to 15% of all gram-negative infections, respectively), and *Acinetobacter* and *Pseudomonas* species also are reported.[38] An association between gram-negative infections and a primary diagnosis of myelomeningocele has been shown,[12] as well as when the distal catheter of a ventriculoperitoneal shunt has perforated a hollow viscus.[39] Streptococcal species, including *Streptococcus pyogenes*, viridans streptococci, and group C streptococci, cause 7% to 16% of infections.* Many other organisms have been isolated. These include anaerobes such as *Propionibacterium* species and *Corynebacterium* species (diphtheroids)[16, 40–42]; the incidence of the latter group of organisms may be underreported because not all laboratories routinely institute special diagnostic procedures necessary for the isolation of these organisms. Other etiologic agents described include *Candida albicans* and other fungal species,[43–46] *Neisseria* species,[47] *Haemophilus influenzae,*[48] *Streptococcus pneumoniae,*[49] nontuberculous mycobacteria,[50] *Pasteurella multo-*

---

*References 1, 4, 11–13, 15–17, 23, 31–37.

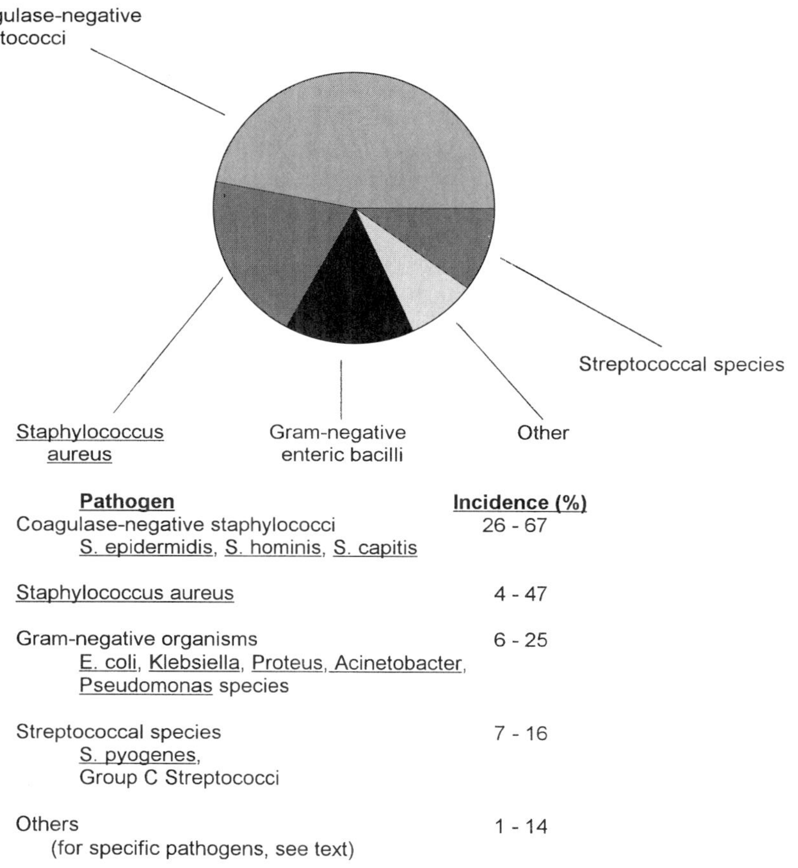

Pathogen	Incidence (%)
Coagulase-negative staphylococci	26 - 67
S. epidermidis, S. hominis, S. capitis	
Staphylococcus aureus	4 - 47
Gram-negative organisms	6 - 25
E. coli, Klebsiella, Proteus, Acinetobacter, Pseudomonas species	
Streptococcal species	7 - 16
S. pyogenes, Group C Streptococci	
Others	1 - 14
(for specific pathogens, see text)	

FIGURE 1.

Pathogens implicated in cerebrospinal fluid shunt infections (compiled from literature referred to in the chapter).

cida,[51] and even *Ascaris lumbrocoides*[52] (the latter after perforation of bowel by the distal portion of the shunt). Opportunistic infections such as *Candida* shunt infections occur in immunocompromised hosts such as neutropenic patients, patients with long-term intravenous catheters, and patients receiving chemotherapy. The prolonged use of broad-spectrum antibiotics also promotes infections with these pathogens. In up to 18% of cases of shunt infections more than one organism is isolated.[10, 26]

The spectrum of organisms in infected reservoirs and external shunts is similar, with slightly larger proportions of staphylococcal isolates in the former and slightly larger proportions of gram-negative isolates in the latter.[10, 26]

PATHOGENESIS

The operative procedure of shunt placement is the inciting event in the pathogenesis of most CSF shunt infections.[14, 53, 54] Bacteria contaminating the wound or shunt may originate from the skin of the patient, the air in the vicinity of the wound, or the surgical team's apparel, cloths, or instruments. The latter route of contamination has been shown to be less important than the first two. Evidence supporting that perioperative colonization may lead to shunt infection include the spectrum of organisms that are most frequently associated with shunt infections (normal skin commensals) and the observation that the majority of infections follow within 1 month of the procedure.

It has been documented that more than 50% of the pathogens isolated in CSF shunt infections are identical to organisms cultured from the patient's own skin, ear, or nose.[8] Density of bacterial contamination of the skin seems to be an important factor in the pathogenesis of infection. Increased infection rates result from higher densities of skin colonization. It is of interest that density of bacterial colonization with staphylococci and *Corynebacterium* species decreases with age.[14] This is analogous to the observation that shunt infections occur more frequently in premature infants or infants younger than 6 months old. This quantitative difference in density of colonization is not the only explanation for the increased infection rate in this age group. Qualitative characteristics of the infecting organism (e.g., increased adhesion of *S. epidermidis* to foreign material in this population) may also contribute to this observation.[14, 55]

Other studies of intraoperative wound contamination have indicated that up to 68% of organisms isolated from contaminated wounds originate from the air in the vicinity of the wound.[54, 56] These organisms are also mostly coagulase-negative staphylococci. It has been demonstrated that 35,000 to 60,000 organisms fall into a wound from the air every hour during surgery. The length of surgery may therefore be an important variable in determining whether infection will occur (100,000 organisms per gram of tissue is necessary to cause a surgical wound infection).[57]

The mechanisms just discussed apply largely to staphylococci (both coagulase negative and the more virulent coagulase positive) and to other skin contaminants such as *Micrococcus*. Three other mechanisms in addition to colonization of the operative site may be involved in the pathogenesis of shunt infection: "retrograde" infection, wound or skin breakdown, and direct hematogenous spread.

"Retrograde" infection may occur from the distal end of the catheter, such as gram-negative infections after perforation of bowel by the distal end of the shunt during ventriculoperitoneal shunt insertion. These gram-negative organisms usually produce low-grade infections, unlike the common scenario in systemic gram-negative sepsis.[38] We also have observed higher rates of EVD infection with gram-negative organisms related to frequent manipulation of the hardware. *Wound or skin breakdown* may occur in immunocompromised individuals, as a result of scratching infants, or as a result of minor trauma along the shunt tract. *Direct hematogenous spread* of organisms such as *H. influenzae, S. pneumoniae,* and *Neisseria meningitidis* is associated with bacteremia.

In recurrent shunt infections an abnormal communication with the CSF space may be present. There may be a defect in the cribriform plate, a sinus tract from the skin, or a fistula from the gut. The latter possibility should be excluded when a patient has recurrent gram-negative shunt infections (a rare occurrence).

It is unlikely that the immature humoral immune system can explain the increased incidence of shunt infections in patients younger than 6 months, because these infants develop antistaphylococcal antibody responses that are comparable with older children.[14] Although levels of opsonins such as immunoglobulins and complement proteins are lower in this young group, the levels of these proteins are normally very low in the CSF of older individuals (CSF levels of IgG and IgA are between 0.25% and 0.5% those in serum). In addition, the types of bacterium causing shunt infections are not commonly associated with humoral immunodeficiency states; little is known about the possible role of reduced tissue immunity in these infections.

The foreign body nature of the shunt apparatus introduces a localized defect in host defense.[10, 58, 59] Electron microscopic findings demonstrate irregularities of catheters in the form of pits and lumps, resulting in areas where micro-organisms can be buried. The function of neutrophils in the vicinity of foreign bodies is suboptimal, because phagocytic and bactericidal activities are reduced due to loss of lysosomal contents. Therefore, even when pathogens are phagocytized, they may not be killed if the intracellular environment provides a safe haven for the organisms, remote from antibiotics that do not penetrate the cell membrane. In addition, it has been shown that the virulence of *S. epidermidis* is increased when associated with a foreign body. Staphylococci can adhere to shunt hardware through various interactions that become even more potent when proteinaceous material, such as fibrin or collagen from the vicinity, is associated with the hardware. Some staphylococci are able to produce slime (consisting of high- and low-molecular weight polysaccharides), which irreversibly binds the bacteria to each other and to the shunt apparatus. The organisms are then protected from leukocyte enzymes while the slime at the same time provides an ion exchange resin for enhanced nutrition of the organisms. Some subtypes of *Corynebacterium* also produce slime.[60]

Other mechanisms that may contribute to shunt infections include abnormal CSF flow (not being absorbed by venous sinuses, thought to be important for infection prevention in the CNS) and interruption of the blood-brain barrier by the shunt catheter with the creation of a direct tract between the subcutaneous tissues and the ventricles, resulting in significant compromise of host defense.[53]

CLINICAL FEATURES AND DIAGNOSIS

Cerebrospinal fluid shunt infections may manifest as an overt disease process that incorporates all the classical signs of CNS inflammation. However, it is important to recognize that in up to 50% of patients, CSF shunt infections do not manifest in this manner; the infection is more subtle, and the symptoms and signs may be indicative of other shunt complications (i.e., malfunction) or of non-shunt-related systemic disease. The clue to diagnosis of CSF shunt infection is a high index of suspicion; if another disease process (e.g., upper respiratory tract or gastrointestinal infection) is not obvious, evaluation should proceed to exclude shunt problems.[53]

Most patients with shunt infections have signs of CNS inflammation, shunt malfunction, or both (Table 2).* Fever has been reported in up to 95% of cases of CSF shunt infection, but the rate may be as low as 14%. In most reviews, fever has been present in more than 50% of cases. Shunt dysfunction has been reported in 10% to 80% of cases and may manifest with nonspecific symptoms of increased intracranial pressure such as headache, nausea, vomiting, altered intellectual performance, ataxia, and altered level of consciousness. Intermittent or variable symptoms may be present when obstruction of the shunt system is intermittent. Parents may describe their children as "just not being themselves."

Signs of proximal involvement in the infective process may be those of ventriculitis or meningitis; headache and fever may be the

---

*References 12, 15, 17, 23, 26, 31, 33, 35, 38.

only symptoms. In addition to the symptoms of raised intracranial pressure described earlier, there may be overt signs such as a bulging fontanelle, raised blood pressure and bradycardia, paralysis of upward gaze, or cranial nerve palsies, although the latter are relatively rare. Papilloedema and frank signs of brain herniation are also rare and late findings. Meningismus occurs in 15% to 25% of cases. This sign is probably rare because of diversion of infected CSF away from the nuchal area. Empyema and brain abscess are rare complications that may manifest similarly with raised intracranial pressure or with focal neurologic signs.[61] Because shunt infections classically appear in the first postoperative month, careful inspection of the wound for evidence of cellulitis or dishiscence is essential. The shunt tract itself may be inflamed with resulting tenderness, erythema, and swelling. This may progress to an abscess with fluctuation. Signs of distal involvement of ventriculoperitoneal shunts may include peritoneal signs such as abdominal tenderness with or without guarding, encystment of the catheter (Fig 2) with a palpable abdominal mass, or decreased absorption with ascites. It is important to note that the majority of abdominal cysts are not infected. Signs of pleuritis or pleural fluid collection may be the presenting feature of a ventriculopleural shunt infection. Bacteremia with signs of systemic sepsis is unusual unless the distal end of the shunt had been placed in a venous space; other complications such as infective endocarditis and an immune complex—mediated glomerulonephritis ("shunt nephritis") may then occur.[62]

TABLE 2.

Signs and Symptoms of Shunt Infections*

	Etiology (%)	
Signs and Symptoms	**Gram-positive**	**Gram-negative**
Temperature (>38°C)	14–95	65
Change of mental status	35–85	65
Irritability	25–80	50
Nausea/vomiting	30–60	30
Abdominal pain	4–15	15
Headache	10–20	15
Meningismus	15–25	25

*Compiled from literature referred to in the text.

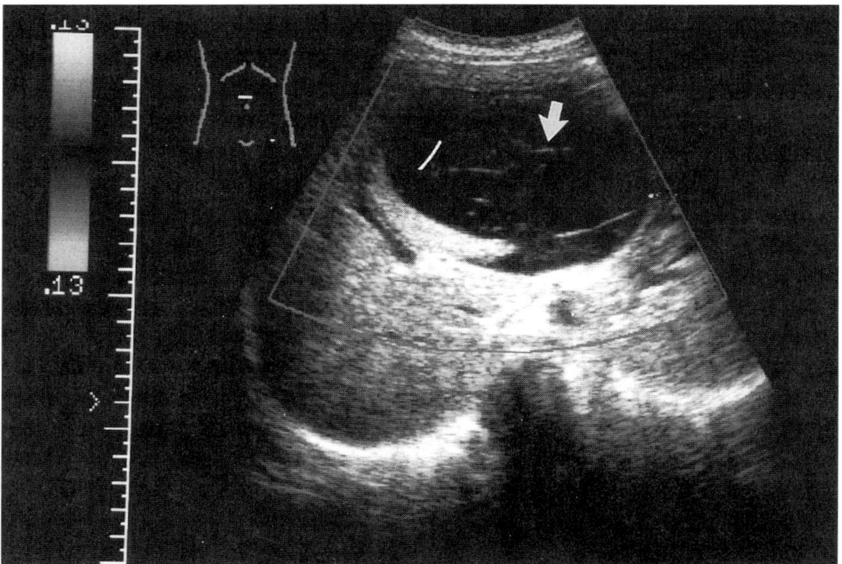

FIGURE 2.

Characteristic loculated appearance of a ventriculoperitoneal shunt pseudocyst in the epigastrium. *Arrow* indicates ventriculoperitoneal shunt pseudocyst. (Courtesy of A. Shkolnik, M.D.)

Differentiating clinical features according to infecting organism may be a difficult task (see Table 2). For example, although it has been stated that patients with gram-negative shunt infections characteristically appear more ill and "toxic," a recent review of such infections indicated that only about 20% of these patients manifested as such.[38] The majority (65%) had fever and an altered level of consciousness, but in some the presentation was insidious. Some reports suggest that patients with *S. aureus* infections appear more ill than those with coagulase-negative staphylococcal infections. Of interest, *S. aureus* infections have a high rate of inflammation along the shunt tract.[12] Infections with diphtheroids may present insidiously.[63]

CLINICAL AND LABORATORY EVALUATION

When CNS shunt dysfunction is suspected, the patient evaluation should include manual palpation of the shunt catheter and testing of the shunt chamber to identify whether obstruction is present proximally or distally.[6] A computed tomography scan of the head is usually required to document a proximal obstruction by observing enlarged ventricles and to exclude increased intracranial pressure or a mass. When distal obstruction or another complication such as a cyst related to a ventriculoperitoneal shunt is suspected, an imaging study of the abdomen such as an ultrasound is indicated. Radiographic studies of the rest of the shunt tract may also be indicated to identify potential "kinks," disconnections, or migration of the device. When infection is suspected, tapping fluid from a shunt or fluid in direct contact with the shunt is essential for accurate diagnosis. Because an underlying CNS abnormality may compromise communication between the CSF at the site of the shunt and the lumbar space, sampling of lumbar CSF may not reflect the state of the ventricular fluid and should not be done when CSF shunt infection is suspected. Cerebrospinal fluid Gram stain, culture, differential cell counts, and glucose level estimation should be requested. Although a CSF protein level is usually requested, it is of no use in evaluating the presence or absence of a shunt infection or response to treatment. The CSF may appear entirely normal in many cases, with less than 10 white blood cells per high-power field. The majority of leukocytes observed in patients with shunt infections are usually polymorphonuclear, although a mononuclear cell predominance is not uncommon.[12, 15, 23, 35, 38] The amount of leukocytes in the CSF is influenced by a number of factors, for example, blood contamination of the CSF, recent antibiotic therapy, and the type of infecting organism. Interestingly, it has been reported that up to 52% of leukocytes present in the CSF during shunt infection are eosinophils.[64, 65] The eosinophilia correlated with the evolution of infections, resolving with successful treatment, whereas persistence predicted later complications, including unresolved infections or obstructive complications. Cerebrospinal fluid eosinophilia may also be caused by antibiotics such as vancomycin introduced intraventricularly or by allergy to ethylene oxide used to sterilize shunt apparatus.[66, 67] A syndrome of allergy to the silicone of shunt hardware, associated with CSF eosinophilia, has also been described; in these patients characteristically the skin breaks down over the tract, which then leads to fungating granulomas with subsequent infection.[68] The early manifestation is therefore very similar to shunt infections, and a change to polyurethrane hardware (with or without immunomodulatory suppression) is indicated.

Compared with other organisms, gram-negative infections usually induce higher CSF cell counts with neutrophil predominance, lower CSF glucose and protein levels, and higher proportions of positive CSF Gram stains.[18] Low CSF glucose levels and a positive

Gram stain may have prognostic relevance in gram-negative infections; an association with persistence of positive CSF cultures requiring additional therapy has been shown.[38]

When CSF is sent for culture, the laboratory should also be requested to institute special culture procedures for organisms such as diphtheroids. Removed shunt catheters should also be sent for culture. Any positive culture should be viewed seriously and not merely assumed to represent contamination. Careful interpretation of laboratory findings in conjunction with positive clinical findings is important. The number of positive cultures and the original site of positive cultures are important considerations in treatment of patients (see later discussion).

Other laboratory investigations that may be employed include serum or shunt fluid C-reactive protein level and serum antistaphylococcal antibody titers. Serum or shunt fluid C-reactive protein levels may be raised in cases of shunt infection. This test may be helpful when a patient has shunt malfunction and an infection needs to be excluded.[53] Serum antistaphylococcal antibody titers of greater than 1/320 have been reported to have sensitivity, specificity, and positive and negative predictive values of 100% in diagnosing staphylococcal ventriculoatrial shunt infections only.[69] This test is of no use in ventriculoperitoneal or ventriculopleural shunts.

Distal shunt infections (without involvement of the cephalad portion) may be more difficult to diagnose. The shunt tap fluid may be completely normal, and the cultures may remain negative if no retrograde progression of the infection has occurred.[70] Diagnosis can usually be made by removal of the distal part of the shunt, with culture of the catheter and fluid aspirated from the vicinity of the catheter.

THERAPY

There is controversy regarding optimal therapy of patients with CSF shunt infections, especially concerning the optimal time of surgical intervention in management.[10, 53] The published literature is of limited help in deciding on the optimal treatment, because it is difficult to interpret many studies of various therapeutic modalities. Study design is often inadequate; in fact, studies are virtually invariably not prospective or randomized. In addition, sample sizes are often small, and subtle differences exist in definitions of shunt infection, timing of shunt catheter removal or replacement, and duration of antibiotic therapy.

The optimal therapy should achieve eradication of the infection in a manner that would result in lowest morbidity and mortality while maintaining adequate treatment of the underlying condition, such as drainage of hydrocephalus. Antibiotics are the mainstay of shunt infection therapy, and therefore pharmacokinetic, pharmacodynamic, and toxicity considerations are important in the selection and use of various antimicrobial agents.

Regarding pharmacokinetics, the route of antibiotic administration may be intravenous, directly into the CSF via the shunt apparatus, or via transcortical injection. The major justification for the occasional addition of antibiotics intraventricularly is failure to achieve adequate CSF concentrations by the parenteral route alone. The chosen parenteral antibiotic must be active both in the brain parenchyma and in the CSF, because a degree of cerebritis is present in addition to ventriculitis in most CSF shunt infections.[10] This would require penetration of the unfenestrated capillary layer of the blood-brain barrier, which is a function of antibiotic structure, serum protein binding, lipid solubility, transport mechanisms in the blood-brain barrier, and the degree to which inflammation influences these parameters.[71] It should be noted that first-generation cephalosporins and aminoglycosides, agents commonly used in the treatment of staphylococcal and gram-negative infections, respectively, penetrate the blood-brain barrier poorly.[72] Other agents with better CNS penetration (e.g., nafcillin for staphylococci and third-generation cepholosporins for gram-negative bacteria) may constitute better treatment choices for infections caused by these organisms.

Clearance of antimicrobials from the CSF may be influenced by many factors in a patient with a shunt infection. For example, when infection is caused by gram-negative bacteria or by multiple organisms, a reduced turnover of CSF occurs.[73–75] Extraventricular drains, commonly used as part of the management of shunt infections, influence CSF turnover and therefore antibiotic clearance.[75] The amount of drainage from an EVD is not only a function of age and weight (a mean drainage rate for a 1-year-old is about 5 mL/hr and for a 15-year-old is about 10 mL/hr) but also of patient position and activity, as well as the effect of the inflammatory process. Patients with EVDs should be managed in the supine position, because drainage from an EVD in this position equals that of implanted CSF shunts with standard valves. Elevation of the collecting bag reduces the amount of drainage and therefore systemic absorption of CSF. Careful management of the drainage rate of an EVD may be critical for efficacy of therapy in an individual patient.

In addition, although very little destruction of antibiotics occurs in the CSF, there are active transport mechanisms that remove antibiotics from the CSF, and these mechanisms may be affected differently by the various bacteria.[71]

Thus, dosage and dosing interval considerations are important, both when parenteral antibiotics are used and when antibiotics are introduced directly into the CSF. "Meningitic" (i.e., high) dosages of antibiotics should always be used parenterally. Most parenteral β-lactam antibiotics require frequent dosing intervals (every 4–6 hours) because of active removal via transport pumps in the choroid plexus; this is not the case with aminoglycosides, which can be administered less frequently. The dosage for intraventricular introduction of antibiotics is empiric (Table 3). Once daily regimens have been used commonly, based on studies of kinetics of intraventricular antibiotics in nonshunt and shunt systems.[76-78] When an antibiotic is given directly into the CSF, the EVD is often closed for 30 to 60 minutes after installation of the antibiotic to prevent outflow of the antibiotic. If closure of the EVD is not possible, the dosing interval is increased to more frequent than once daily. The adverse effects of intraventricular antibiotics limit their use. Aminoglycosides can be directly neurotoxic in dosages much lower than those commonly recommended.[79, 80] This class of agents has also been shown to cause CSF pleocytosis, which may relate to the preservative used.[10] There are no data on the potentially devastating ototoxicity that intraventricular aminoglycosides may produce. Cerebrospinal fluid irrigation with cephalothin and penicillin G

TABLE 3.

Suggested Dosages for Intraventricular Administration

	Dosage (mg/day)	
Antibiotic	**Per Kg**	**Total Dose**
Methicillin	1–2	50–100
Nafcillin	1–4	50–100
Vancomycin		4–10
Gentamicin		1–8
Chloramphenicol		25–50
Ampicillin		25–50
Cephalothin		25–100

has been shown to cause ventriculitis, transient neurologic deficits, and perivascular infiltration.[80] Preservative-containing vancomycin can also cause CSF pleocytosis.[10, 66]

Pharmacodynamic parameters such as the absolute amount of antibiotic in the CSF and the minimal inhibitory concentrations (MICs) of antibiotics against the etiologic agent are essential for devising effective therapy. Patients who do not clear the infecting organisms within 2 to 3 days of the onset of therapy may warrant further studies such as ventricular fluid bactericidal titer and antibiotic synergism studies to design more effective therapy. A practical parameter termed the "inhibitory quotient" has been used to evaluate the potential efficacy of an antibiotic by relating the MIC to the CSF antibiotic levels.[81] This is the measured CSF antibiotic level divided by the MIC of this antibiotic against the etiologic bacterium. An optimal inhibitory quotient is at least 10 and should ensure more consistent and efficient killing of bacteria.

A further important pharmacodynamic consideration is the degree of intracellular penetration of antibiotics, especially when one considers relatively incompetent neutrophils associated with slime around shunt hardware. Rifampin is the prototype agent for efficacy in these situations; it penetrates cells well and is bactericidal.[82] It is important to note that rifampin should never be given as a single agent because bacterial resistance develops almost immediately.[83] Recommendations for intravenous antibiotic use for CSF shunt infections (Table 4) should be adjusted for each institution's bacterial sensitivity patterns.

The use of antibiotics is one of several therapeutic tools available for the management of shunt infections. These include intravenous antibiotics only, combination of intravenous antibiotics with intraventricular antibiotics, or the combination of either or both of these with surgical management. Surgical management includes removal of the shunt hardware with either immediate or delayed replacement. An EVD may be used as a temporary drainage system. Review of the literature suggests that treatment with intravenous antibiotics only without removal of the shunt is associated with a high failure rate; only 20% of cases are cured. When intravenous and intraventricular antibiotics are given together but without surgical management, the cure rate is only 35% to 40%, and treatment must be given for an extended period. Combining removal of the infected shunt with immediate internal shunt replacement insertion and antibiotic therapy increases the cure rate to 60% to 70%. The optimal and most successful approach is removal of the shunt with temporary externalization (i.e., EVD) and antibiotic

TABLE 4.

Recommended Antibiotic Therapy for Shunt Infection According
to the Etiologic Agent

Etiologic Agent	Antibiotic	Dose (mg/kg/day)	Frequency
Coagulase-negative staphylococci or *Staphylococcus aureus* (oxacillin sensitive)	Oxacillin or Nafcillin	200–300 200	q6h q6h
Coagulase-negative staphylococci or *S. aureus* (oxacillin-resistant)	Vancomycin	60	q6h
Escherichia coli *Klebsiella* *Enterobacter* *Proteus*	Cefotaxime or Ceftriaxone or Gentamicin Amikacin Tobramycin	200 100 7.5 22.5 7.5	q6h q12h q8h q8h q8h
Pseudomonas	Ceftazidime or Aminoglycosides (as above) or Aminoglycosides and ticarcillin	200 As above + 300	q8h q8h + q6h
Anaerobes	Chloramphenicol or Penicillin or Metronidazole	100 400,000 units 30	q6h q6h q8h

therapy. A success rate of more than 85% is documented in this
group of patients.[10, 16]

Thus, the management of shunt infection should include removal of all components of an infected shunt at the beginning of
treatment and placing an EVD. The propensity for the entire shunt
to become colonized (or infected) when one portion becomes infected argues against partial shunt revisions. All culture-positive

shunts should be treated as infections, with hardware removal and externalization. The few cases with only distal shunt involvement should receive intravenous antibiotics with externalization of only the distal part of the shunt. Complete removal of the shunt hardware is still the recommended procedure. In addition, antibiotic therapy alone without removal of the shunt could be considered for shunt patients who have meningitis caused by *S. pneumoniae*, *N. meningitidis*, or *H. influenzae* type B. This approach has proved successful for *H. influenzae* meningitis, but treatment failures in pneumococcal meningitis have been reported.[2, 49]

In mildly sick children with mild CSF pleocytosis (100–200 white blood cells [WBCs]/mm^3) and negative gram stain, it is reasonable to initiate antibiotic therapy with antistaphylococcal agents only. The drug of choice depends on the proportion of staphylococci resistant to semisynthetic penicillins (e.g., oxacillin) at that institution. If the resistance rate is less than 15% to 20%, oxacillin or nafcillin should be used. If the resistance rate is higher, vancomycin should be administered until culture results and antibiotic sensitivities are available. Every effort should be made to discontinue vancomycin as soon as possible to reduce the probability of developing resistance to this agent. If the patient seems to be moderately to severely sick, a third-generation cephalosporin is added to the antistaphylococcal therapy. Positive gram stain may serve as a good indicator for the choice of the initial antibiotic. Table 4 represents some antibiotic choices according to the etiologic agent.

Duration of therapy depends on the etiologic agent and the time it takes to clear the organism from the CSF. For coagulase-negative staphylococci that grow only from the first culture (i.e., preexternalization or during removal of the shunt) while the CSF parameters (i.e., WBC and glucose levels) are close to the normal range, the duration of therapy should not exceed 3 to 4 days. The reason for such a short course of antibiotics is that in the majority of such cases the one positive culture represents colonization of the shunt or contamination of the culture. If, on the other hand, the first (and only) positive culture was from a CSF sample that shows signs of infection (pleocytosis, abnormal chemistry, or both), therapy should be given for 7 days. When cultures are positive for more than 1 day after externalization, treatment should continue until 10 days of negative culture are achieved. It has been suggested that after 10 days of negative cultures and completion of therapy, the patient's CSF should be cultured for 3 more days to assure sterility before reshunting is performed.[10] Although such an approach seems to be logical, in almost all cases it is unnecessary, and further cultures are not helpful. Thus, reshunting can occur at the end of 10 days of sterile cultures. *Staphylococcus aureus* and gram-negative bacteria are less likely to merely colonize the shunt and more likely to cause greater morbidity than the coagulase-negative staphylococci.[18] For these reasons a longer course of therapy (i.e., until 10 days of negative cultures are achieved) is recommended. Once again, there is no need to follow the patient's CSF cultures for an extra period without antibiotics to verify sterilization. Immediate reshunting is recommended.

The majority of infected shunts treated as suggested here will have sterile CSF cultures within 2 to 3 days. If CSF cultures remain positive for a longer period, two options should be considered. If the CSF parameters are improving or resolving, it is highly probable that the continued positive cultures represent colonization of the EVD, and therefore the EVD system should be replaced. If, on the other hand, the CSF parameters continue to show signs of infection, the therapy may be inadequate or the clearance of the infection is slower (often seen with gram-negative bacteria). To distinguish between the two possibilities, one should obtain bactericidal titers of the CSF. The test is done as follows: 2 to 3 hours after the administration of the antibiotic is complete, a CSF sample is drawn and tested in varying dilutions against the bacteria. If CSF dilutions equal or greater than 1:8 inhibit the growth of the bacteria, the continued positive CSF cultures probably represent slow clearance of the bacteria, and further follow-up without change in therapy is recommended. In contrast, if CSF dilutions of 1:8 or less do not inhibit the growth of the bacteria, the therapy is inadequate. Depending on the circumstances, therapy can be adjusted by either increasing the dose or changing the antibiotic or adding another antibiotic for synergistic effect (e.g., rifampin for gram-positive bacteria). In vitro studies for synergy should be performed before a second drug is added to ensure the optimal synergistic combination.

The additional use of intraventricular antibiotics should be reserved for cases that remain culture positive despite changes in the systemic antibiotics. As mentioned earlier, it should be remembered that the wide dose ranges have been determined empirically (see Table 3) and that their use and potential toxicity when administered intraventricularly have not been well studied. It is of interest that some dosages have been recommended as per weight (mg/ kg), which is not directly correlated to the CSF volume. Thus, it is not surprising that the CSF levels have been unpredictable and have often exceeded the recommended safe levels in the blood. For these reasons, irrigation of the ventricular system with an antibiotic solution (using two extraventricular drains) in which the antibiotic concentration is within the recommended safety range is more appropriate. Thus, for difficult gram-negative infections, an amikacin solution (30 mg/1 L of saline solution) or gentamicin (12–15 mg of special intrathecal preparation in 1 L of fluid) should be used to irrigate the ventricles. A continuous flow of 10 to 20 mL/h will remove debris and pus from the system and will ensure a continuous high concentration of antibiotic that will not accumulate or cause toxicity. Once sterility of the CSF is achieved, therapy should be continued as just described.

In some cases it may be possible to predict which patients will clear the CSF more slowly. For example, in patients with gram-negative infections in which an initial Gram stain was positive and CSF glucose level was low, CSF cultures remain positive longer, and more aggressive measures as described previously may then be instituted earlier.[38] Low CSF glucose levels or a mildly elevated CSF WBC count or protein level at the end of therapy are not contraindications for reshunting, because such findings are relatively common for a long period after CSF sterilization.

Neuroendoscopic third ventriculostomy without reshunting is a recently described definitive procedure for the treatment of recurrent or intractable shunt infections in children with noncommunicating hydrocephalus.[84] The few patients described have survived the procedure with no morbidity, and all remained shunt free after 21 to 46 months.

PROPHYLACTIC MEASURES

Prophylaxis includes the use of prophylactic antibiotics, either systemically or topically, and the implementation of perioperative measures, primarily concerning surgical technique, to reduce the incidence of shunt infections.

Numerous studies have investigated the effect of antibiotic prophylaxis on the incidence of shunt infections. Once again problems with study design and sample size preclude definitive conclusions. Most well-designed studies have not shown that prophylactic antibiotics reduce the incidence of shunt infections. Three meta-analyses have appeared in an attempt to overcome the problems of insufficient statistical power of individual studies.[28, 29, 85] Reider et al.[85] did not find a statistically significant reduction in infection rate associated with use of prophylactic antibiotics. However, two subsequent meta-analyses did find a significant difference. Although only 1 of 12 trials included in the investigation of Langley et al.[28] achieved statistical significance favoring prophylaxis, in the aggregate the use of prophylactic antibiotics was associated with a significant reduction of about 50% in the incidence of subsequent shunt infection. The same figure was the result of Haines and Walters'[29] analysis, but they also found that if the baseline operative infection rate was at or less than 5%, the protective effect of antibiotics disappeared. Therefore, they suggested that prophylactic antibiotics should be used only if the infection rate is higher than 5% at a given institution. The Infection in Neurosurgery Working Party of the British Society for Antimicrobial Chemotherapy has pointed out some weaknesses of these meta-analyses.[30] They were "unable to make recommendations either for or against the use of prophylaxis in shunt surgery on the basis of existing evidence."[30]

If prophylaxis is planned, it should be recognized that a wide range of antibiotics have been used, most commonly methicillin or oxacillin, a cephalosporin, or trimethoprim-sulfamethoxazole.[28, 29, 85] Therefore, no specific antibiotic can be recommended. The choice for a particular institution should be based on local epidemiology of potential pathogens, local patterns of antimicrobial susceptibility, cost, and expected toxicity in the particular population. Because the prophylactic antibiotic is given to prevent infection during the operation, antibiotics should be given shortly before the start of the operation and continued for no longer than 12 to 24 hours after the operation.

Another attempt at prophylaxis has involved impregnating shunt catheters with antibiotics.[86, 87] This approach, although seemingly promising, has not yet been established. It is noteworthy that impregnating catheters with bacitracin A can cause a dramatic increase in bacterial binding, most likely due to receptor-ligand binding of the bacteria with the incorporated bacitracin molecule.[88] Soaking shunt material in antimicrobial solutions such as bacitracin A, gentamicin, oxacillin, or vancomycin before implantation has also been suggested, proposing that this would reduce electrostatic properties of the silicone tubing, which favors adherence of bacteria.[10, 13]

Perioperative measures are important for the prevention of shunt infection.* The main focus has been the reduction of bacterial contamination at the time of surgery. Choux et al.[13] have developed a protocol of perioperative measures with astounding success in reducing the infection rates from 7.75% to 0.177% per pro-

---

*References 10, 13–15, 17, 54, 89, 90.

cedure over 7 years. Another group[17] was able to reduce its case infection rate from 12.9% to 3.8% with the introduction of measures similar to those of Choux et al.[13] Although these results are very impressive, other studies have failed to show that all of the factors deemed important by Choux et al.[13] influence the infection rates.[5, 14]

The following are suggested perioperative measures that may contribute to a reduction in shunt infections. Skin preparation should include a whole body wash and hair shampoo with an antiseptic solution such as chlorhexidine. This should be done the night before surgery and 1 hour before surgery. If possible, this should also be done 1 hour before an emergency procedure. Shaving of hair is not necessary. A first-generation cephalosporin (e.g., 25 mg of cephapirin/kg) or semisynthetic penicillin (e.g., 50 mg of oxacillin/kg) should be administered just before the patient is transported to the operating room. Patients who have had severe allergic reactions to penicillins (e.g., anaphylaxis or angioedema) or who have manifested allergic reactions to cephalosporins should receive clindamycin (25 mg/kg) intravenously.

During the operation an absolute minimum of personnel should be present, and people traffic should be limited during the procedure (i.e., nobody should be allowed to enter or leave the operating room). The procedure should be completed in the shortest time frame possible. Intraoperative skin preparation should include cleaning with a fat solvent, followed by preparation with soap and antibiotic solution. The skin should be draped with an adherent plastic drape. Shunt equipment should be kept in a bath of bacitracin solution, and sterile packaging should be opened at the last moment before use. Skin closure should be of high quality. Early morning scheduling of shunt procedures and experienced surgeons performing the procedure may possibly be of additional benefit.

In the postoperative period dressings should be changed within 24 hours to rule out local wound infection. Wet dressings should be examined even earlier. The use of postoperative antibiotics for prophylaxis should be restricted to one or two more dosages.

REFERENCES

1. Di Rocco C, Marchese E, Velardi F: A survey of the first complication of newly implanted CSF shunt devices for the treatment of nontumoral hydrocephalus. *Childs Nerv Syst* 10:321–327, 1994.
2. Kanev PM, Park TS: The treatment of hydrocephalus. *Neurosurg Clin North Am* 4:611–619, 1993.
3. Aoki N: Lumboperitoneal shunt: Clinical applications, complications,

and comparison with ventriculoperitoneal shunt. *Neurosurgery* 26:998–1004, 1990.

4. Vernet O, Campiche R, de Tribolet N: Long-term results after ventriculoatrial shunting in children. *Childs Nerv Syst* 9:253–255, 1993.
5. Piatt JH Jr, Carlson CV: A search for determinants of cerebrospinal fluid shunt survival: Retrospective analysis of a 14-year institutional experience. *Pediatr Neurosurg* 19:223–242, 1993.
6. Jordan KT: Cerebrospinal fluid shunts. *Emerg Med Clin North Am* 12:779–786, 1994.
7. Serlo W, Heikkinen E, Von Wendt L: The changing panorama of shunt complications: Twenty-five years' experience. *J Neurosurg Sci* 36:207–210, 1992.
8. McLone DG, Czyzewski D, Raimondi AJ, et al: Central nervous system infections as a limiting factor in the intelligence of children with myelomeningocoele. *Pediatrics* 70:338–342, 1982.
9. Storrs BB: Ventricular size and intelligence in myelodysplastic children. *Concepts Pediatr Neurosurg* 8:51–56, 1988.
10. Kaufman BA, McLone DG: Infections of cerebrospinal fluid shunts. In Scheld WM, Whitley RJ, Durack DT (eds): *Infections of the Central Nervous System.* New York, Raven Press, 1991, pp 561–585.
11. Ersahin Y, McLone DG, Storrs BB, et al: Review of 3,017 procedures for the management of hydrocephalus in children. *Concepts Pediatr Neurosurg* 9:21–28, 1989.
12. Cotton MF, Hartzenberg B, Donald PR, et al: Ventriculoperitoneal shunt infections in children: A 6-year study. *S Afr Med J* 79:139–142, 1991.
13. Choux M, Genitori L, Lang D, et al: Shunt implantation: Reducing the incidence of shunt infection. *J Neurosurg* 77:875–880, 1992.
14. Pople IK, Bayston R, Hayward R: Infection of cerebrospinal fluid shunts in infants: A study of etiological factors. *J Neurosurg* 77:29–36, 1992.
15. Kontny U, Höfling B, Gutjahr P, et al: CSF shunt infections in children. *Infection* 21:89–92, 1993.
16. Morissette I, Gourdeau M, Francoeur J: CSF shunt infections: A fifteen-year experience with emphasis on management and outcome. *Can J Neurol Sci* 20:118–122, 1993.
17. Kestle JRW, Hoffman HJ, Soloniuk D, et al: A concerted effort to prevent shunt infection. *Childs Nerv Syst* 9:163–165, 1993.
18. Yogev R: Cerebrospinal fluid shunt infections: A personal view. *Pediatr Infect Dis J* 4:113–118, 1985.
19. Resch B, Muller W, Oberbauer R: Precipitating factors for shunt insufficiency in post-hemorrhagic hydrocephalus in the premature infant. *Z Kinderchir* 45:203–208, 1990.
20. Meirovitch J, Kitai-Cohen Y, Keren G, et al: Cerebrospinal fluid shunt infections in children. *Pediatr Infect Dis J* 6:921–924, 1987.
21. Keucher TR, Mealey J: Long term results after ventriculoatrial and ven-

triculoperitoneal shunting for infantile hydrocephalus. *J Neurosurg* 50:179–186, 1979.

22. Olsen L, Frykberg T: Complications in the treatment of hydrocephalus in children. *Acta Paediatr Scand* 72:385–390, 1983.
23. Schoenbaum SC, Gardner P, Shillito J: Infections of cerebrospinal fluid shunts: Epidemiology, clinical manifestations, and therapy. *J Infect Dis* 131:543–552, 1975.
24. Shurtleff DB, Stuntz JT, Hayden PW: Experience with 1201 cerebrospinal fluid shunt procedures. *Pediatr Neurosci* 12:49–57, 1985–1986.
25. Hahn YS, McLone DG, Raimondi AJ, et al: Surgical outcome of preterm newborns with severe peri-ventricular-intraventricular hemorrhage and post-hemorrhagic hydrocephalus. *Concepts Pediatr Neurosurg* 4:66–80, 1983.
26. Siegel T, Pfeffer R, Steiner I: Antibiotic therapy for infected Ommaya reservoir systems. *Neurosurgery* 22:97–100, 1988.
27. Brown EM: Antimicrobial prophylaxis in neurosurgery. *J Antimicrob Chemother* 31(suppl B):49–63, 1993.
28. Langley JM, LeBlanc JC, Drake J, et al: Efficacy of antimicrobial prophylaxis in placement of cerebrospinal fluid shunts: Meta-analysis. *Clin Infect Dis* 17:98–103, 1993.
29. Haines SJ, Walters BC: Antibiotic prophylaxis for cerebrospinal fluid shunts: A meta-analysis. *Neurosurgery* 34:87–92, 1994.
30. Brown EM, de Louvois J, Bayston R, et al: Antimicrobial prophylaxis in neurosurgery and after head injury. *J Antimicrob Chemother* 344:1547–1551, 1994.
31. Odio C, McCracken GH, Nelson JD: CSF shunt infections in pediatrics. *Am J Dis Child* 138:1103–1108, 1984.
32. Shapiro S, Boaz J, Kleiman M, et al: Origin of organisms infecting ventricular shunts. *Neurosurgery* 22:868–872, 1988.
33. Walters BC, Hoffman HJ, Hendrick EB, et al: Cerebrospinal fluid shunt infection: Influences on initial management and subsequent outcome. *J Neurosurg* 60:1014–1021, 1984.
34. Meirovitch J, Kitai-Cohen Y, Keren G, et al: Cerebrospinal fluid shunt infections in children. *Pediatr Infect Dis J* 6:921–924, 1987.
35. Forward KR, Fewer HD, Stiver HG: Cerebrospinal fluid shunt infections—A review of 35 infections in 32 patients. *J Neurosurg* 59:389–394, 1983.
36. Raimondi AJ, Robinson JS, Kuwamura K: Complications of ventriculoperitoneal shunting and a critical comparison of the three-piece and one-piece systems. *Childs Nerv Syst* 3:321–342, 1977.
37. James HE, Walsh JW, Wilson HD, et al: Prospective randomized study of therapy in cerebrospinal fluid shunt infection. *Neurosurgery* 7:459–463, 1980.
38. Stamos JK, Kaufman BA, Yogev R: Ventriculoperitoneal shunt infections with gram-negative bacteria. *Neurosurgery* 33:858–862, 1993.

39. Rubin RC, Ghatak NR, Kisudhipan P: Asymptomatic perforated viscus and gram-negative ventriculitis as a complication of valve-regulated ventriculoperitoneal shunts. *J Neurosurg* 37:616–618, 1972.

40. Arisoy ES, Demmler GJ, Dunne WM Jr: *Corynebacterium xerosis* ventriculoperitoneal shunt infection in an infant: Report of a case and review of the literature. *Pediatr Infect Dis J* 12:536–538, 1993.

41. Gaskin PR, St John MA, Cave CT, et al: Cerebrospinal fluid shunt infection due to *Corynebacterium xerosis*. *J Infect* 28:323–325, 1994.

42. Knudsen JD, Nielsen CJ, Espersen F: Treatment of shunt-related cerebral ventriculitis due to *Corynebacterium jeikeium* with vancomycin administered intraventricularly. Case report. *APMIS* 102:317–320, 1994.

43. Cruciani M, Di Perri G, Molesini M, et al: Use of fluconazole in the treatment of *Candida albicans* hydrocephalus shunt infection. *Eur J Clin Microbiol Infect Dis* 11:957, 1992.

44. Tirahoschi T, Casas Parera T, Pikielny R, et al: Chronic *Histoplasma capsulatum* infection of the central nervous system successfully treated with fluconazole. *Eur Neurol* 32:70–73, 1992.

45. Walter EB Jr, Gingras JL, McKinney RE Jr: Systemic *Torulopsis glabrate* infection in a neonate. *South Med J* 83:837–838, 1990.

46. Ingram CW, Haywood HB III, Morris VM, et al: Cryptococcal ventricular-peritoneal shunt infection: Clinical and epidemiological evaluation of two closely associated cases. *Infect Control Hosp Epidemiol* 14:719–722, 1993.

47. Stotka JL, Rupp ME, Meier FA, et al: Meningitis due to *Neisseria mucosa*: Case report and review. *Rev Infect Dis* 13:837–841, 1991.

48. Brandstetter Y, Melzer-Lange M, Chusid MJ: *Haemophilus influenzae* type B meningitis in a patient with a ventriculoperitoneal shunt and meningomyelocele. *Wis Med J* 89:461–463, 1990.

49. O'Keeffe PT, Bayston R: Pneumococcal meningitis in a child with a ventriculoperitoneal shunt. *J Infect* 22:77–79, 1991.

50. Chan KH, Mann KS, Seto WH: Infection of a shunt by *Mycobacterium fortuitum*: Case report. *Neurosurgery* 29:472–474, 1991.

51. Lee T, Kerr RS, Adams CB: *Pasteurella multocida*: A rare case of shunt infection. *Br J Neurosurg* 4:237–238, 1990.

52. Peter JC, Lamprecht J, Rode H: *Ascaris lumbricoides*: An unusual cause of shunt infection. *Childs Nerv Syst* 8:294–296, 1992.

53. Walters BC: Cerebrospinal fluid shunt infection. *Neurosurg Clin North Am* 3:387–401, 1992.

54. Duhaime AC, Bonner K, McGowan KL, et al: Distribution of bacteria in the operating room environment and its relation to ventricular shunt infections: A prospective study. *Childs Nerv Syst* 7:211–214, 1991.

55. D'Angio CT, McGowan KL, Baumgart S, et al: Surface colonization with coagulase-negative staphylococci in premature neonates. *J Pediatr* 114:1029–1034, 1989.

56. Burke JF: Identification of the sources of staphylococci contaminating the surgical wound during operation. *Ann Surg* 158:898, 1963.
57. Heggens JP, Robson MC: *Quantitative Bacteriology: Its Role in the Armamentarium of the Surgeon.* Boston, CRC Press, 1991, pp 1–8.
58. Borges LF: Host defenses. *Neurosurg Clin North Am* 3:275–278, 1992.
59. Borges LF: Cerebrospinal fluid shunts interfere with most defenses. *Neurosurgery* 10:55–60, 1982.
60. Compton C, Bayston R, Richards K: Slime-producing coryneforms in hydrocephalus shunt infections. *Eur J Pediatr Surg* 2:37–38, 1992.
61. Gower DJ, Horton D, Pollay M: Shunt-related brain abscess and ascending shunt infection. *J Child Neurol* 5:318–320, 1990.
62. Samtleben W, Bauriedel G, Bosch T, et al: Renal complications of infected ventriculoatrial shunts. *Artif Organs* 17:695–701, 1993.
63. Rekate HL, Ruch T, Nulsen FE: Diphtheroid infections of cerebrospinal fluid shunts—the changing pattern of shunt infection in Cleveland. *J Neurosurg* 52:553–556, 1980.
64. Vinchon M, Vallee L, Prin L, et al: Cerebro-spinal fluid eosinophilia in shunt infections. *Neuropediatrics* 23:235–240, 1992.
65. Tung H, Raffel C, McComb JG: Ventricular cerebrospinal fluid eosinophilia in children with ventriculoperitoneal shunts. *J Neurosurg* 75:541–544, 1991.
66. Grabb PA, Albright AI: Intraventricular vancomycin-induced cerebrospinal fluid eosinophilia: Report of two patients. *Neurosurgery* 30:630–634, 1992.
67. Pittman T, Williams D, Rathore M, et al: The role of ethylene oxide allergy in sterile shunt malfunctions. *Br J Neurosurg* 8:41–45, 1994.
68. Jimenez DF, Keating R, Goodrich JT: Silicone allergy in ventriculoperitoneal shunts. *Childs Nerv Syst* 10:59–63, 1994.
69. Bayston R: Serological indication of *Staphylococcus albus* infection in children with colonized shunts. *Dev Med Child Neurol* 13(suppl 25):135–136, 1971.
70. Younger JJ, Simmons JCH, Barrett FF: Occult distal ventriculoperitoneal shunt infections. *Pediatr Infect Dis J* 23:372–373, 1988.
71. Barza M: Pharmacologic principles. In Gorbach SL, Bartlett JG, Blacklow NR (eds): *Infectious Diseases.* Philadelphia, WB Saunders, 1992, pp 147–153.
72. Neu HC: General therapeutic principles. In Gorbach SL, Bartlett JG, Blacklow NR (eds): *Infectious Diseases.* Philadelphia, WB Saunders, 1992, pp 153–160.
73. Breeze RE, McComb JG, Hyman S, et al: CSF production in acute ventriculitis. *J Neurosurg* 70:619–622, 1989.
74. Scheld WM, Dacey RG, Winn HR, et al: Cerebrospinal fluid outflow resistance in rabbits with experimental meningitis. *J Clin Invest* 66:243–253, 1980.
75. Drake JM, Sainte-Rose C, DaSilva M, et al: Cerebrospinal fluid flow dynamics in children with external ventricular drains. *Neurosurgery* 28:242–250, 1991.

76. James HE, Wilson HD, Connor JD, et al: Intraventricular cerebrospinal fluid antibiotic concentrations in patients with intraventricular infections. *Neurosurgery* 10:50–54, 1982.

77. Salmon JH: Intraventricular chloramphenicol. *Childs Nerv Syst* 4:114–119, 1978.

78. Reesor C, Chow AW, Kureishi A, et al: Kinetics of intraventricular vancomycin in infections of cerebrospinal fluid shunts. *J Infect Dis* 158:1142–1143, 1988.

79. Watanabe I, Hodges GR, Dworzack DL, et al: Neurotoxicity of intrathecal gentamicin: a case report and experimental study. *Ann Neurol* 4:564–572, 1978.

80. Weiss MH, Kurze T, Nulsen FE: Antibiotic neurotoxicity: laboratory and clinical study. *J Neurosurg* 41:486–489, 1974.

81. Yogev R: A strategy for evaluating which of the new cephalosporins to use. *Pediatr Ann* 15:470–477, 1986.

82. Tshefu K, Zimmerli W, Waldvogel FA: Short term administration of rifampin in the prevention or eradication of infection due to foreign bodies. *Rev Infect Dis* 5(suppl 3):S474–S480, 1983.

83. Craig WA: Rifampin and related drugs. In Gorbach SL, Bartlett JG, Blacklow NR (eds): *Infectious Diseases.* Philadelphia, WB Saunders, 1992, pp 265–271.

84. Jones RFC, Stening WA, Kwok BCT: Third ventriculostomy for shunt infections in children. *Neurosurgery* 32:855–860, 1993.

85. Rieder MJ, Frewen TC, Del Maestro RF, et al: The effect of cephalothin prophylaxis on postoperative ventriculoperitoneal shunt infections. *Can Med Assoc J* 136:935–938, 1987.

86. Bayston R, Milner RDG: Antimicrobial activity of silicone rubber used in hydrocephalic shunts, after impregnation with antimicrobial substances. *J Clin Pathol* 34:1057–1062, 1981.

87. Bayston R, Grove N, Siegel J, et al: Prevention of hydrocephalus shunt catheter colonization in vitro by impregnation with antimicrobials. *J Neurol Neurosurg Psychiatry* 52:605–609, 1989.

88. Gower DJ, Gower VC, Richardson SH, et al: Reduced bacterial adherence to silicone plastic neurosurgical prosthesis. *Pediat Neurosci* 12:127–133, 1985–1986.

89. Winston KR: Hair and neurosurgery. *Neurosurgery* 31:320–329, 1992.

90. Savitz SI, Bottone EJ, Savitz MH, et al: Investigations of the bacteriological factors in clean neurosurgical wounds. *Neurosurgery* 34:417–421, 1994.

Pneumococcal Infections in an Era of Multiple Antibiotic Resistance

Barry M. Gray, M.D.
Professor of Pediatrics and Microbiology, University of Alabama at Birmingham, Birmingham, Alabama

The pneumococcus has evolved with its human host over thousands of generations. Its name derives from the Greek *pneuma*—the subtle vital force, air, breath, spirit. Although recognized by Hippocrates and other physicians of antiquity, pneumonia did not become a clinical diagnosis until after Laënec's invention of the stethoscope in 1819. Diplococci were seen by Klebs in 1875 in bronchial secretions of patients with pneumonia, but credit for discovery of the organism goes to both Pasteur and Sternberg in 1881. Pasteur isolated it incidentally in a rabbit inoculated with the saliva of a child with rabies; Sternberg recovered the organisms from his own saliva and later from some of his medical students in Philadelphia, providing the first description of the carrier state. Within a few years, the organism was clearly identified as a major cause of pneumonia and named *Diplococcus pneumoniae* by Weichselbaum. Sternberg contended that it was really a streptococcus because of its tendency to form chains under certain growth conditions, but the name was not formally changed to *Streptococcus pneumoniae* until 20 years ago.[1-3]

"The captain of the men of death," according to Osler, pneumonia and other pneumococcal infections have continued to be a challenge, despite the advent of antibiotic therapy. The identification of capsular serotypes led to the development of effective serum therapy for a limited number of important types. Passive immunotherapy may yet find a place in prevention or adjunctive treatment in certain patient populations.[4, 5] The discovery in 1923 by Heidelberger and Avery[6] of the "soluble specific substance," now known as the capsular polysaccharide, led directly to the development of the first purified polysaccharide vaccines,[7, 8] and to the currently licensed vaccine containing polysaccharides of the 23 most common serotypes.[9] Along the way, scientific studies of

Advances in Pediatric Infectious Diseases®, vol. 11
© 1996, Mosby–Year Book, Inc.

pneumococcal genetics opened the door to the discovery of DNA as the "transforming principle" by Avery et al.[10] in 1946 and to the beginnings of molecular biology. Our quest to understand the pneumococcus and to cure or prevent pneumococcal disease has continued to be a prime factor motivating research in genetics, antibiotics, immunology, and host defense.[11]

A great turning point in the history of medicine was the therapeutic use of penicillin.[12] But having learned lessons from pneumococcal resistance to optochin and the sulfonamides, microbiologists in the early 1940s looked for and found resistance induced by exposure to penicillin in the laboratory.[13] It is quite amazing that penicillin resistance in the clinical setting took about 20 years to develop, after the introduction and widespread use of penicillin after World War II. Yet in the intervening years progress was slow in elucidating the epidemiology and pathogenesis of pneumococcal infections. The biology of bacterial cell wall synthesis, which underlies the mechanisms of action of penicillin, has been clarified only in recent years. According to MacLeod (in a 1970 text, as quoted by Johnston[14]) these difficult and unpopular areas of research "were virtually abandoned in the rush from serum therapy to the sulfonamides and thence to penicillins and other antibiotics, and the result was popular but relatively superficial research. It should be apparent that what we are most in need of at the present time is a return to the study of the obscure biological phenomena that dictate the behavior of this common disease of man."

It was not until 1965 that Wise and Park[15] and Tipper and Strominger[16] proposed that penicillin acted as a substrate analog to inhibit peptidoglycan cross linking, specifically by mimicking the structure of the acyl-D-alanyl-D-alanine tail of the muramic acid stem peptides. Details of the cross-linking enzymes, called penicillin-binding proteins (PBPs), began to emerge a few years later, as the first clinically important penicillin-resistant strains made their appearance. Pneumococci with increased resistance to penicillin were isolated in Australia and New Guinea in 1967.[17] One strain was from a patient with hypogammaglobulinemia who had received many courses of antibiotic therapy. Other strains were found during an investigation of prophylactic administration of penicillin to prevent pneumonia in a rural district of New Guinea where pneumococcal disease was especially prevalent. The first such isolate in the United States actually appeared several years earlier, without comment, in a collection of pneumococci used for susceptibility studies.[18] Another came from a child who had received multiple courses of methicillin and oxacillin over an extended period.[19] Within a few years, there were several reports of children with meningitis due to pneumococci with increased resistance to penicillin.[20–22] All of these strains were of "intermediate" susceptibility to penicillin by the current definition of minimum inhibitory concentration (MIC) of 0.1 to 1.0 μg/mL. Clinical cures were accomplished by increasing the dose of penicillin or adding chloramphenicol.

Before long highly resistant strains (penicillin MIC ≥ 2 μg/mL) began to emerge, first in South Africa,[23] then in the United States,[24] Spain, and elsewhere.[25] These strains brought added dimensions to the problem of antibiotic therapy; their MICs exceeded readily attainable cerebrospinal fluid (CSF) levels, and many strains were resistant to alternative antibiotics as well. A temporary respite was afforded by the introduction of several "third-generation" cephalosporins, especially cefotaxime and ceftriaxone. However, reports of resistance to these antibiotics have begun to appear, and therapeutic approaches to pneumococcal meningitis and other infections are currently undergoing a difficult reevaluation.[26–31]

Meanwhile, the pneumococcus continues to be the most common cause of invasive bacterial infection in the United States.[32] There is clearly a need for a better understanding of its pathogenesis and mechanisms of antibiotic resistance. During the coming years it will be more important than ever to monitor susceptibility patterns and serotype distributions, find rational approaches to antibiotic therapy, and improve vaccines and other preventive measures.

VIRULENCE FACTORS AND PATHOGENESIS

The pneumococci are considered part of the "normal" human respiratory flora in the sense that they are frequently carried in the nasopharynx for long periods without causing disease. Yet the serotypes often carried by healthy children are the same as those associated with common infections, including otitis media, pneumonia, and meningitis.[33] The close association between recent acquisition of a new serotype, noted by Hodges and MacLeod[34] in their studies of pneumonia and in our prospective study of young children,[35] suggests that pneumococci are not simply opportunistic invaders. It is evident that there is an intricate interplay between their human hosts and these pathogens, neither of which is created equal. Differences in pathogenicity occur among serotypes and among strains of the same serotype, and pathologic effects may be modified by characteristics of a particular host. Important aspects of pneumococcal pathogenesis have been reviewed recently, including pneumococcal virulence factors,[36, 37] pneumonia,[14] meningitis,[38, 39] and otitis media.[40] Certain groups of patients are at significantly higher risk for infection because of alterations in their host defenses. Some otherwise normal hosts, such as native Americans in the Southwest and in Alaska, are also at considerable risk due to genetic, social, or environmental factors that remain to be clearly defined. The pneumococci have so far yielded no easy answers to the question of why some people are infected while others are spared, and they are only beginning to give up their secrets of pathogenesis at the molecular level.

BACTERIAL FACTORS

ADHERENCE TO EPITHELIAL AND ENDOTHELIAL CELLS

Many respiratory bacteria, including pneumococci, adhere to epithelial cells by specific mechanisms, some involving attachment directly to β-GalNAc-(1$\rightarrow$3)-β-Gal or β-GalNAc-(1$\rightarrow$4)-β-Gal on respiratory glycolipids,[41, 42] or indirectly via a "sandwich" adhesion.[43] Attachment is regarded as the essential first step in bacterial infection, but the process of invasion is exceedingly complex and is modified by many bacterial and host factors. There is some indication that isolates from middle ear infections are more adherent than those from blood cultures.[44] In contrast, our investigation of adherence of pneumococci from prospectively studied children revealed no evidence to support the hypothesis that pneumococci associated with acute otitis media were more adherent than isolates associated with asymptomatic carriage in the same or different children.[45] We suggested that the ability to adhere was a property of a subset of the pneumococcal population and that adherence was necessary for the establishment and maintenance of colonization. Adherence may contribute to the disease process by ensuring a certain number of bacteria at the mucosal site, but adherence in vitro does not discriminate between carriage strains and those causing disease.

Once pneumococci broach the mucosal epithelial barriers, attachment to endothelial cells is apparently mediated by cell wall components. These contribute directly to cytopathic effects, at least as demonstrated in human endothelial cell cultures.[46] Blood-borne infection involves endothelial adherence and cytokine activity, which may play a role in tissue damage and in seeding of tissues during infection.

POLYSACCHARIDE CAPSULES AND SURFACE PROTEINS

The pneumococci are the prototype of encapsulated bacteria. The capsule is essential for virulence, probably by protecting the organism from a multitude of nonspecific host defenses, including direct phagocytosis by neutrophils and macrophages, complement components, C-reactive protein (CRP), and naturally occurring antibodies that bind to phosphorylcholine and other cell wall antigens. Despite the depiction of pneumococci as a small sphere surrounded by an impervious sugar coating (the candy-coated peanut theory), the capsule is actually a huge tangle of capsular polysaccharide polymers, C-polysaccharides, strands of peptidoglycan and teichoic acids, and surface proteins (Fig 1). The capsular polysaccharides shield other components from outside attack and hold water to form a mucoid barrier protecting the cell. Because the com-

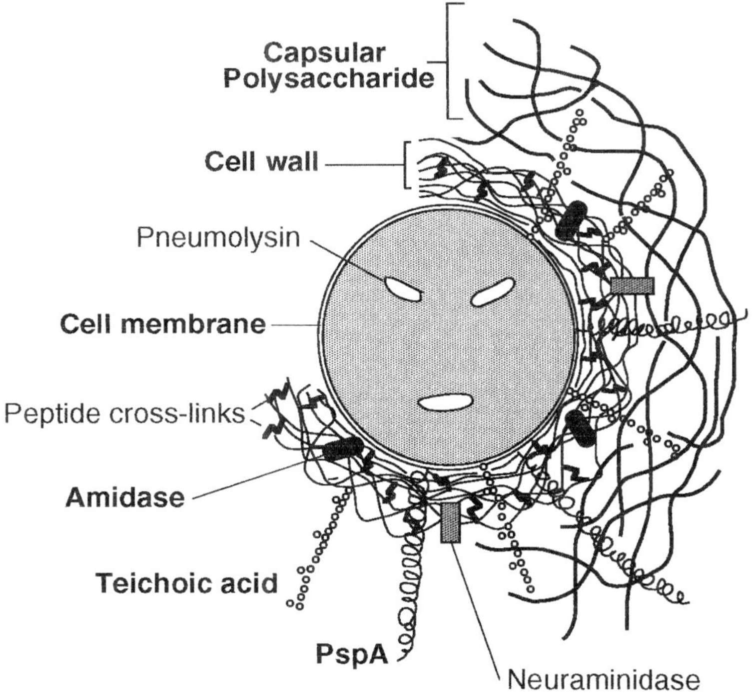

FIGURE 1.

Schematic representation of the structural anatomy and location of surface components of an encapsulated pneumococcus. (Courtesy of David E. Briles, University of Alabama, Birmingham.)

bined effects of surface components vary enormously by capsular serotype and by strain within types, the capsule might be better conceptualized in functional rather than morphologic terms. Figure 2 (part A), for example, shows a capsulelike area around an avirulent strain that produces no capsular polysaccharide. Such strains usually produce small "rough" colonies on blood agar compared with the large "smooth" colonies typical of strains that make capsular polysaccharide.

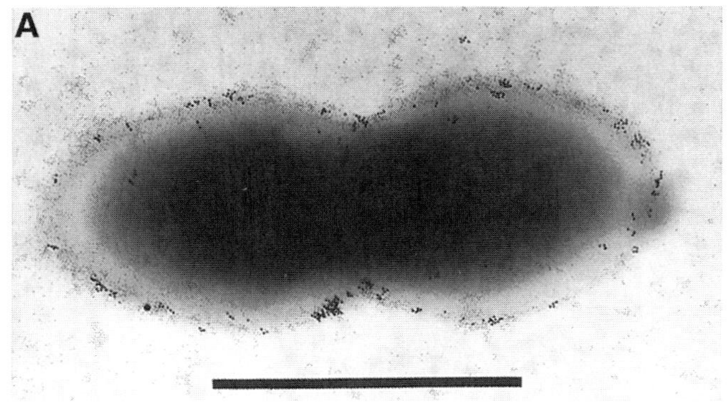

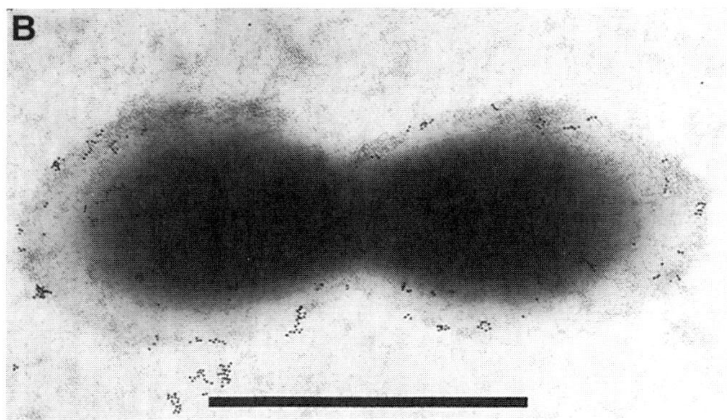

FIGURE 2.

Electron micrographs of whole cell mounts of *Streptococcus pneumoniae* showing the surface location of PspA. **A,** the rough strain Rx1, which produces no capsular polysaccharide. **B,** the type 3 strain WU2. PspA was identified by monoclonal antibody Xi-126[55] and tagged with anti-mouse immune globulin 10-nm gold beads (*large dark beads*); the capsular area was made visible with cationized ferritin (*fine grainy beads*), as previously described.[56] (Courtesy of Barry M. Gray and Elizabeth W. Cooney, EMLabs, Inc., Birmingham, Ala.)

TABLE 1.

Polysaccharide Repeating Units of Common Pneumococcal Types*

Type 3:   →3)-β-D-Glc-(1→4)-β-D-GlcpA-(1→

Type 6A: →2)-α-D-Galp-(1→3)-α-D-Glcp-(1→3)-α-L-Rhap-(1→3)-D-ribitol-5-PO$_4$→

Type 6B: →2)-α-D-Galp-(1→3)-α-D-Glcp-(1→3)-α-L-Rhap-(1→4)-D-ribitol-5-PO$_4$→

Type 14:   →6)-β-D-GlcNAc-(1→3)-β-D-Gal-(1→4)-β-D-Glc-(1→
$\qquad\qquad$ β|4
$\qquad\qquad$ Gal

Type 19F: →4)-β-N-ManpNAc-(1→4)-β-D-Glcp-(1→3)-α-L-Rhap-(1→PO$_4$→
$\qquad\qquad\qquad$ |2
$\qquad\qquad\qquad$ PO$_4$
$\qquad\qquad\qquad$ |1
$\qquad\qquad\qquad$ β-D-Gal
$\qquad\qquad\qquad$ |3
$\qquad\qquad\qquad$ β-D-GlcNAc

Type 23F: →3)-β-D-Glcp-(1→4)-β-D-Galp-(1→4)-α-L-Rhap-(1→
$\qquad\qquad$ | $\qquad\qquad$ |2
$\qquad\qquad$ PO$_4$ $\qquad$ α-L-Rhap

*p = pyranose form (five-carbon ring); Glc = glucose; GlcpA = glucuronic acid; GlcNAc = N-acetylglucosamine; Gal = galactose; Rha = rhamnose; ManNAc = N-acetylmannosamine.

Members of the species *S. pneumoniae* are quite heterogeneous, including more than 80 serotypes. Many of the capsular polysaccharides have been biochemically defined[8]; some are linear polymers, whereas some have branched chains, and others resemble teichoic acids with phosphodiester linkages. As shown in Table 1, a variety of secondary structures occur among the common pneumococcal capsular polysaccharides. Type 3 is a linear chain of glucose-glucuronic acid. Types 6A and 6B are more like teichoic acids in that they contain ribitol-phosphate linkages; types 6A and 6B differ only at the rhamnose-ribitol linkage. Type 14 has a galactose side chain linked to the N-acetylglucosamine (Glc-NAc) in the backbone of the repeating unit. Type 19F has phosphodiester linkages in both the side chain and the backbone of the repeating unit, and type 19A (not shown) has an additional fucose-phosphate side chain linked to the rhamnose. Type 23F has two single unit side chains of phosphate and rhamnose, respectively.

Serotyping is now generally done using Danish antisera, developed by Lund in the 1940s.[47, 48] This system includes some pneumococci that exist as single types, such as types 1 through 5, 8, and 14 (Table 2). It combines others into groups of two or more cross-reactive types. For example, group 6 includes types 6A and 6B, which are antigenically similar and differ by only one sugar linkage; group 9 has two common members, types 9N and 9V, as well as the rare types 9A and 9L. This system thus reduces the myriad of types to a more manageable 48 but has led to the invention of the unfortunate generic term "groups/types." Danish group/type antisera from the Statens Seruminstitut in Copenhagen are available through Dako Corporation, Carpinteria, California. The types within groups, such as 6A and 6B (sometimes called subtypes), may be distinguished for epidemiologic purposes by the use of "factor sera" that have been cross absorbed with the heterologous types (done only at the Centers for Disease Control and a few reference and research laboratories). The factor sera are then used in the Neufeld reaction to demonstrate "capsular swelling," actually a refractive artifact seen on microscopy. With these simple but powerful methods it was possible to track serotype distributions according to disease states and patient populations to select the most important types for inclusion in the original 14-valent vaccine introduced in 1977. For example, type 19F is predominant within group 19, type 23F is more common than 23A, and immunization with type 6B appeared to give adequate cross-protection against type 6A. Nine more types were added to the current for-

TABLE 2.

Common Pneumococcal Groups or Types, as Represented
in the Current 23-Valent Vaccine*†‡

Group/Type	Cross-Reactive Types in This Group	Most Common Type(s) in Group (% Occurrence of Disease Caused by Type(s) in Group)
1	None	—
2	None	—
3	None	—
4	None	—
5	None	—
6	**6A, 6B**	**6B** (61)
7	7F, 7A, 7B, 7C	7F (96)
8	None	—
9	**9V, 9N,** 9A, 9L	**9V** (57), **9N** (34)
10	10A, 10F	10A (89)
11	11A, 11B, 11C	11A (78)
12	12A, 12F	12F (84)
14	None	—
15	15F, 15A, 15B, 15C	15B (22), 15C (39)
17	17A, 17F	17F (88)
18	18F, 18A, 18B, **18C**	**18C** (83)
19	**19F, 19A,** 19B	**19F** (65), **19A** (34)
20	None	—
22	22F, 22A	22F (99)
23	**23F,** 23A, 23B	**23F** (90)
33	33F, 33A, 33B, 33C	33F (79)

*Adapted from Robbins JB, Austrian R, Lee C-J, et al: *J Infect Dis* 148:1136–1159, 1983, which used data from CDC and WHO surveys that included mainly blood and CSF isolates.
†The current 23-valent polysaccharide vaccine includes types 1, 2, 3, 4, 5, 6B, 7F, 8, 9N, 9V, 10A, 11A, 12F, 14, 15B, 17F, 18C, 19F, 19A, 20, 22F, 23F, and 33F. The types included in candidate protein-conjugated vaccines for children are types 4, 6B, 9V, 14, 18C, 19F, and 23F. Types 3 and 23A are also quite common in childhood otitis media, and type 18C is especially common in meningitis.
‡The most common groups or types in childhood infections are indicated in bold.

mulation of the 23-valent pneumococcal vaccine (licensed in 1983) including both types 9V and 9N, and both 19F and 19A, because all of these were common; their polysaccharides differed immunologically, however, and did not confer adequate cross-protection within respective groups.[8, 9]

Most adults respond fairly well to the majority of the capsular antigens included in the 23-valent vaccine, and the overall protective efficacy has been estimated to be about 60%.[49, 50] The major problem with pneumococcal vaccines in adults is underutilization. Unfortunately, the vaccines are not suitable for young children, because those younger than about 2 years old respond poorly or not at all to the most important types. This is consistent with the observation that infants do not respond to most bacterial polysaccharides. These antigens are considered "T-independent" because they do not directly involve the T-helper cells of the immune system. Conjugation of polysaccharides to proteins enhances their immunogenicity by activating T-helper cells engaged in responses to the carrier protein. Buoyed by the success of protein conjugate vaccines against *Haemophilus influenzae* type b, several polyvalent pneumococcal conjugate vaccines have been developed and are currently in phase 2 trials. The vaccines for infants include the types most commonly seen in otitis media (types 6B, 14, 19F, and 23F) and several less common types also seen in otitis media or meningitis (types 4, 9V, and 18C).[51]

Serotypes vary widely in their frequency and pathogenicity,[33] but virulence cannot be attributed solely to capsular type. Although we have shown a strong association between type and mouse virulence, only about 30% of fresh human disease isolates were lethal for mice, and there was no relationship between clinical diagnosis or tissue source of the isolates.[52] The effect of genetic switching of capsular type has recently been examined by Kelly et al.[53] by comparing the mouse virulence of parent strains of types 2, 6B, and 5 with isogenic derivatives that were constructed to express the type 3 capsule from a normally virulent strain. The highly virulent type 5 was essentially avirulent when expressing type 3 capsule, whereas the virulence of the 6B strain was about 100 times greater with the type 3 capsule. This showed that the capsular type expressed had a major effect but that lethality was dependent on other factors in the genetic background of the recipient strain.

One way that pneumococcal strains differ is in how complement is deposited and activated on the cell surface. This has been shown to vary considerably among serotypes.[54] Unencapsulated strains are easily killed, even though they bind comparatively less

C3 (converted to the active form C3b) than do encapsulated strains. This results, in part, because they have a smaller surface area and C3 may bind directly to "activator" surface structures, such as teichoic acids, via the alternative complement pathway.[14] Encapsulated pneumococci bind C3 in nonimmune sera, but they bind two to four times more C3 when antibody is present. Effective opsonization requires covalent binding of C3 via ester or amide linkages to cell surface structures or to antigen-bound antibodies. Also important is the pattern of C3 degradation that occurs on different pneumococcal serotypes. Hostetter[54] showed that types 6A and 14, which are less resistant to phagocytosis and also less immunogenic, had mostly iC3b (inactivated form) on their surface after opsonization. Types 3 and 4, which are more resistant to phagocytosis and more immunogenic, had more C3b and C3d. The presence of C3d may facilitate the immune response by engaging a specific receptor on B lymphocytes and promote the antibody response.

In addition to the capsular polysaccharide, pneumococcal surface protein A (PspA) is expressed by essentially all clinically important isolates.[55] The surface location of PspA has been demonstrated by its accessibility to antibodies and by immunogold electron microscopy (Fig 2).[56] This antigen is a coiled-coil protein that is highly variable among capsular serotypes with respect to antigenic epitopes and molecular size but is genetically stable for any given strain. More than 30 different PspA patterns have been identified using a panel of 7 monoclonal antibodies that each bind to a different epitope on the molecule. Several of the epitopes are quite common among strains of differing capsular serotypes, and antibodies elicited to a number of these epitopes protect mice from experimental infection. Candidate PspA vaccines are currently under development and may eventually be useful, because infants would be expected to respond to these protein antigens. Meanwhile, PspA typing has been found to reliably distinguish strains within serotypes in epidemiologic studies.[57] It has also been useful in confirming the clonality of four distinct families of pneumococci characterized by electrophoretic profiles of their PBPs.[58]

CELL WALL SYNTHESIS, PENICILLIN-BINDING PROTEINS, AND THE ROLE OF AMIDASE

The pneumococcal cell wall components consist primarily of cross-linked layers of peptidoglycan.[59] The cell wall is interspersed with an unusual teichoic acid–like polymer called the C-polysaccharide (the "group" antigen of this streptococcal species) and with a lipoteichoic acid (Forssman antigen). The precursor units of the peptidoglycan are synthesized in the cytoplasm from GlcNAc and N-acetylmuramic acid (MurNAc) to which are added a "stem peptide" and an undecaprenolpyrophosphate (a 55-carbon lipid carrier). The disaccharide unit is temporarily anchored to the cell membrane via the undecaprenol, and 20 or more disaccharide units are linked together to form a chain. This polymerization step is thought to occur in the cytoplasm, with the growing chain extruded through the membrane to the outside, where it is cross-linked to other chains. The prototypic stem peptide is the pentapeptide, L-alanine-D-isoglutamine-L-lysine-D-alanine-D-alanine, but most pneumococci are capable of producing an array of varied stem peptides, some of which are important in conferring β-lactam resistance.[60] Stem peptides from different peptidoglycan chains are linked together by transpeptidases and transcarboxylases, better known as the PBPs. Although the precise mechanism has not been completely defined in the pneumococcus, these enzymes are thought to cleave the terminal alanine and attach a bridge of 5 glycine units, which is, in turn, coupled to the lysine of a stem peptide on another peptidoglycan chain. Only about 1 in 10 stem peptides are used in structural cross-linkages.

Pneumococci have six PBPs: 1a, 1b, 2a, 2b, 2x, and 3.[61, 62] Penicillin-binding proteins 1a and 1b are bifunctional. They catalyze the linkage of the disaccharide subunits at one enzymatic site and cross-link the stem peptides at another site. Penicillin-binding proteins 2b and 2x are essential to cell growth, especially in resistant strains. The low molecular weight PBP 3 plays an important role in cell division; it is not involved in the killing action of penicillin but may be a factor in resistance to cefotaxime.[63]

Bacteria spend most of their time growing and dividing, and cell wall materials are constantly being remodeled and recycled. The breakdown of peptidoglycan is usually accomplished in a highly controlled manner by the autolytic enzyme N-acetyl-muramoyl-L-alanine amidase, familiarly called amidase. Pneumococcal mutants with defective amidase activity fail to divide into normal diplococci, forming short chains instead, and they also fail to lyse when exposed to β-lactam antibiotics.[64] The occurrence of amidase-defective mutants has allowed the detection of a second autolytic enzyme, a glycosidase that breaks down the saccharide units of the peptidoglycan.[65] Both this enzyme and the amidase are inhibited by the presence of teichoic acids and of choline (breakdown products of the C-polysaccharide in the cell wall).

Naturally occurring alterations in amidase activity have been shown in penicillin-resistant strains, making them more tolerant to the antibiotic and less susceptible to lytic killing.[66] Defective lysis has been described among strains from several immunocompromised patients. Although these organisms may be killed by penicillin, they fail to lyse and release the cell wall muramyl peptides that are potent initiators of inflammation in early infection.[67] One amidase studied at the molecular level has been shown to have lower specific activity and higher sensitivity to inhibition by choline.[68] The rate of release and quantity of cell wall breakdown fragments plays an important role in the pathophysiology of experimental pneumococcal meningitis in rabbits.[69] An early inflammatory response was clearly favorable, whereas more severe disease occurred in animals challenged with strains that grew to a higher density before lysing and provoking fever, CSF pleocytosis, and brain edema. The highly inflammatory muramyl dipeptide (MurNAc-D-alanyl-D-isoglutamine) is only the minimal active unit among a tribe of peptidoglycan breakdown fragments. It is likely that clinical presentations and pathologic findings may vary according to the characteristics of the infecting strain, but this has not been confirmed in the clinical setting.

PNEUMOLYSIN

Another effect of pneumococcal autolysis is the release of intracellular products, especially pneumolysin.[36, 37] This enzyme is a thiol-activated toxin similar to group A streptolysin O and to listeriolysin. It binds to mammalian cells, has cytotoxic properties, and inhibits neutrophil function by reducing chemotactic activity, phagocytosis, and the respiratory burst. Pneumolysin can activate complement directly in the fluid phase and cause additional tissue damage when it activates complement on tissue surfaces. Animal experiments demonstrate a modest but important role in pathogenesis, but its effects in human disease have not been determined. Humans make antibodies to pneumolysin, which have been used diagnostically to detect prior pneumococcal infection, but their potential in reducing the effects of infection is not known.

IMMUNOGLOBULIN A1 PROTEASE

Pneumococci were among the first of the major respiratory bacteria found to secrete an immunoglobulin A1 (IgA1) protease.[70] This enzyme cleaves serum and secretory IgA1 at the hinge region, releasing Fc, Fab, and SC fragments. The Fab fragments retain antigen-binding activity but cannot induce microbial agglutination, inhibit bacterial adherence, or perform other effector functions dependent on the intact molecule. Neither IgA2 nor secretory IgA2 are affected. A role in disease at the mucosal level is suggested by the observation that virtually all clinical pneumococcal isolates and pathogenic strains of *H. influenzae* and *Neisseria meningitidis* have IgA1 protease activity, whereas closely related nonpathogenic species of *Haemophilus* and *Neisseria* do not. Both IgA1 protease activity and IgA1 breakdown products have been detected in the CSF of patients with pneumococcal meningitis (Mogens Killian, personal communication, 1994). Humans make antibodies that neutralize protease activity and may have a role in protection or in modulating colonization of the mucosal surfaces of the nasopharynx.[71]

HYALURONIDASE

The majority of clinical isolates of pneumococci produce hyaluronidase.[36, 72] Known as the "spreading factor" of group A streptococci, hyaluronidases are thought to facilitate colonization and promote translocation of organisms from tissues such as lung to the vascular system.

NEURAMINIDASE

Pneumococci produce at least two distinct enzymes with neuraminidase activity.[36, 37] These enzymes remove the terminal sialic acid from many glycoconjugates found on mammalian cell surfaces. This is thought to expose underlying GlcNAc-Gal determinants on the epithelial surface and facilitate bacterial adhesion, as described earlier. Neuraminidases may participate in the invasion of choroid plexus and brain surfaces, which are heavily covered with sialyl moieties, and contribute directly to meningeal inflammation.

The hemolytic uremic syndrome associated with neuraminidase-producing pneumococci is a relatively rare but devastating form of pneumococcal disease. More than 12 cases have been described, and nearly half of these have been fatal.[73-78] Circulating neuraminidase exposes the T (Thomsen-Friedenreich) antigen on platelets, red blood cells, and glomeruli. Naturally occurring IgM antibodies bind to the T antigen in the kidney, induce thrombocytopenia and hemolysis, and create circulating antigen-antibody complexes. This disease is not associated with any one pneumococcal serotype, and it is not known if a particular neuraminidase or propensity for increased production is required or if there are certain predisposing host factors. Occurring primarily in young children, it manifests with microangiopathic anemia, thrombocytopenia, and acute renal failure. Clinical clues include pneumococcal pneumonia or meningitis and a positive direct Coombs test result or difficulties in ABO blood typing. Neuraminidase damage to red blood cells can be rapidly determined with peanut agglutinin, a lectin that binds specifically to the β-D-Gal-(1→3)-GalNAc determinant of the T antigen. Transfusions of plasma, red blood cells, or platelets should be used with caution, because they may exacerbate the condition. Exchange transfusions have been tried in several patients to help eliminate circulating neuraminidase and replace blood components, but meticulous supportive care appears to remain the key to a favorable outcome.[77]

HOST FACTORS

INVASION OF THE NORMAL HOST

Little is actually known about how pneumococcal infections develop in the normal human host.[14] It is presumed that systemic invasion begins when organisms multiply in the nasopharynx and breach the mucus blanket. They attach to epithelial cells and then make their way up the eustachian tube to the middle ear, down the trachea to the lung, or through the submucosa to the circulation. Some blockage or dysfunction of the eustachian tube is probably required to trap organisms in the middle ear space, such as the inflammation caused by viral respiratory tract infections.[40, 79, 80] The lung is difficult to infect under experimental conditions, because nonimmune clearance of pneumococci is extremely efficient. Perturbation of ciliated epithelia induced by ethanol or suppression of the cough reflex are usually needed to establish experimental pneumonia. The meninges are protected by the tight junctions of the blood-brain barrier, and invasion probably requires specialized attachment to endothelia, as well as enzymes for degrading cell surfaces and intracellular matrix materials.[39]

Humans have a variety of specific and nonspecific defenses that act to stifle infection. From very early exposure to various organisms, humans make antibodies that cross-react with the cell wall components of many bacteria. Both antibody-mediated (classical pathway) and antibody-independent (alternative pathway) activation of complement occurs when a pneumococcus breaks down and loses its protective capsular material. This, in turn, releases inflammatory activators, such as C5a, which attract phagocytes and help initiate release of cytokines, especially interleukin-1 (IL-1) and tumor necrosis factor (TNF). The cytokines, recently reviewed by Lau,[81] act to signal inflammation and eliminate pathogens but may also contribute to the cellular damage when their activity gets out of control, as often occurs in sepsis and meningitis.

C-reactive protein binds to the phosphorylcholine determinant of pneumococcal C-carbohydrate, fixes complement, and can protect mice from experimental infection.[82, 83] The degree of protection afforded by CRP in humans is unknown but is certainly not complete.[84] Its teleological function was probably not related to the pneumococcus but probably directed to detection of the phosphorylcholine moieties exposed by injury to tissue cell surfaces.[85] Humans, including children, also make antibodies to phosphorylcholine,[86] but it is far from clear what their function may be. Antiphosphorylcholine antibodies protect mice from experimental infections,[87] but recent studies confirm that human antibodies to cell wall components fail to opsonize encapsulated pneumococci.[88] Perhaps their function is to detect fragments of broken pneumococci and initiate an early inflammatory response and to help clean up the mess afterward.

The best defense against pneumococcal infections is, of course, type-specific anticapsular antibody. Most young children do not have antibodies to common serotypes and do not respond well to conventional vaccines. It will be a matter of time before we see if the new generation of conjugate vaccines afford the spectacular protection already apparent with similar vaccines against *H. influenzae* type b.[51]

IMMUNOCOMPROMISED HOST

Pneumococcal infections are more frequent among patients with sickle cell disease and functional or traumatic asplenia. The spleen (and to some extent the lung and liver) acts as a filter for clearing organisms in the presence of phagocytes that can readily dispose of the invaders. As a lymphoid organ, the spleen is also important in the development of the immune response to pneumococcal polysaccharides, such that patients with Hodgkin's disease or severe idiopathic thrombocytopenia respond better when the pneumococcal vaccine is administered several weeks before, rather than after, splenectomy.[9]

Patients with hypogammaglobulinemia and some with isolated IgG subclass deficiencies, especially the lack of IgG2, are also at considerable risk for infection. Passive immunization with γ-globulin is helpful in these patients, but the levels of specific antibodies vary widely and are not always protective. A special γ-globulin (bacterial polysaccharide immune globulin [BPIG]) has been prepared from serum donors immunized with vaccines against pneumococcus (23 types), *H. influenzae* type b, and meningococcus groups A and C. This product has been successful in preventing pneumococcal infections in Apache children and may be useful in selected immunocompromised patients as well.[5]

Complement defects are not a common factor in pneumococcal susceptibility, although pneumococcal infections have been seen with increased frequency in a few patients with C2 or C3 deficiency or consumption of C3 secondary to absence of factor I (C3b/C4b inactivator).[14] Phagocyte defects and disorders of neutrophil adhesion molecules are rare causes of increased susceptibility to pneumococcal and other bacterial infections.[14, 89]

Human immunodeficiency virus (HIV) infection is now the most rapidly expanding acquired immunodeficiency, and pneumococci are the leading cause of invasive bacterial respiratory tract infection in children and adults with this disease.[90] In two prospective studies HIV-positive infants younger than 1 year had the same or slightly greater risk of pneumococcal bacteremia as their HIV-negative peers. But risk among the HIV-positive groups increased 3-fold[91] to 12-fold[92] compared with HIV-negative children over the ensuing 2 years, possibly as the result of their declining immune status. Few of these children were receiving intravenous γ-globulin (IVIG) or antimicrobial prophylaxis, but there were two episodes of invasive pneumococcal disease in children who were taking trimethoprim-sulfamethoxazole (TMP-SMZ) on a regimen of 3 days/week. Otitis media is also a problem in HIV-infected children, and it appears to increase with age and with severity of the underlying condition.[93]

The bacterial and host factors described here do not begin to explain the diversity and complexity of pneumococcal disease. This was recently underscored by the report of septic shock and purpura fulminans with hemorrhage into skin or internal organs in four previously healthy young children in New Mexico.[94] Two of these cases were probably epidemiologically related, despite attempts at various preventive measures. The two others were not related and were caused by different serotypes. This is not a new phenomenon, but it serves as a reminder that our goal should be prevention rather than cure.

DEVELOPMENT OF ANTIBIOTIC RESISTANCE

Genetic analyses have revealed that penicillin resistance in pneumococci has developed by several independent routes in different parts of the world.[25, 62] Sequence analysis of PBP 2b clearly divides resistant strains into "class A," which probably arose in New Guinea in the early 1950s, and "class B," which was originally found in Europe and is usually associated with resistance to chloramphenicol and tetracyline.[95] Molecular epidemiologic methods have made it possible to track the spread of a multiresistant clone from Spain to Iceland in the late 1980s.[96] Spain has been a favorite vacationing place for families from Iceland and other parts of northern Europe. International travel and the environmental pressures of antibiotic use in different countries have contributed to the worldwide spread of penicillin-resistant clones.[25, 97] Similarly, the multiresistant isolates now prevalent in the United States almost certainly originated in Spain and South Africa.[98]

Antibiotic use and misuse are prime determining factors both in geographic dissemination of resistant strains and in selection of resistant organisms colonizing or infecting individual patients. In Spain, Baquero et al.[99] found a striking linear relationship between the prevalence of resistant or intermediate strains in a given region and the annual consumption of aminopenicillins (ampicillin and amoxicillin) in those localities. The widespread or indiscriminate use of penicillin has been recognized from the beginning as a major problem.[17, 23, 100] At the level of the individual, the literature is replete with cases in which the infected patient had prior, often long-term, exposure to penicillins.* Although some reports have not found an association with prior antibiotic therapy, most population-based and case-controlled studies have clearly identified this as a major risk factor.[102, 103] Immunocompromised individuals are at especially high risk because of their underlying conditions and also because they are more likely to receive antibiotics.

Age and serotype distribution appear to go hand in hand with penicillin resistance. Children younger than 2 years comprise the largest group receiving empirical antibiotic treatment for otitis media and other presumed infections. The serotypes most commonly carried by these children are type 6, 14, 19, and 23.[35] These four "childhood" groups/types account for about two thirds of all pediatric infections.[33, 104] In our past experience,[101] and in unpublished data completing the period through 1994, 95% of strains with intermediate or full resistance to penicillin were type 6, 14, 19, or 23. In other localities these types account for 75% to 93% of intermediate and resistant strains.[105–107]

---

*References 17, 19, 20, 22, 24, 101.

Resistance to other antibiotics, except to vancomycin, tends to parallel clinical practices and antibiotic use in given localities. Resistance to TMP-SMZ, macrolides, tetracyclines, chloramphenicol, and fluorquinolones has been reported throughout Europe and the United States.[98, 99] Often this relates not to treatment of suspected pneumococcal infections but to therapy of other unrelated diseases. For example, a high prevalence of pneumococcal resistance to rifampin was observed in areas of South Africa where many children were being treated for tuberculosis.[25]

MECHANISMS OF RESISTANCE

Penicillin resistance in pneumococci is a very complex phenomenon arising from multiple transformation and recombination events affecting PBPs, muramyl stem peptides, and other proteins involved in metabolism and cell division. Unlike many gram-negative bacteria, the pneumococci do not elaborate β-lactamases, which are plasmid-mediated enzymes that inactivate penicillins and cephalosporins by hydrolyzing the β-lactam ring of the antibiotic. Rifampin and quinolone resistance occurs under selective pressure after relatively simple mutations.[25, 62] Resistance to kanamycin, erythromycin, and tetracycline is transferred by a conjugative transposon.[108] Pneumococci are resourceful organisms that have proved to be survivors in an increasingly antibiotic-laden environment.

ALTERATIONS IN PENICILLIN-BINDING PROTEINS AND STEM PEPTIDES

The pneumococci have been slow to develop resistance to the β-lactam antibiotics for several reasons.[62] First, these antibiotics act on multiple killing targets, namely, the various PBPs required for cell wall synthesis. Second, β-lactams function as substrate analogs of the muramyl stem peptides, and resistance requires both subtle alterations in the enzymatic sites of the PBPs and complementary changes in the preferred structure of the stem peptides.[60] The development of resistance thus involves the restructuring of multiple metabolic processes in a stepwise fashion. It seems likely but not certain that altered PBPs evolved first or were borrowed from other species; the pneumococci then learned to change or regulate the expression of different stem peptides. This process has involved the development and conservation of numerous small mutations acquired by S. *pneumoniae* and its relatives over many years, probably in response to both naturally occurring and synthetic penicillins. These genetic changes have been altered and passed on by multiple transformation and recombination events.

The examination of several hundred clinical isolates revealed a large number of PBP electrophoretic profiles with polymorphisms of various PBPs. These have now been resolved into four distinct PBP families, each of which is clonally associated with a particular multilocus enzyme genotype, surface protein (PspA) type, and capsular serotype.[58] Within these groups considerable heterogeneity is still evident from studies using multilocus enzyme and ribosomal RNA typing.[98, 109]

The mechanism of penicillin action is simplistically depicted in Figure 3. The β-lactam ring mimics the structure of the muramyl stem peptide, forming an essentially irreversible complex with the PBP analogous to the acyl-D-alanyl-D-alanine transition state in the normal transpeptidation reaction. This prevents the enzymatic cross-linking of stem peptides, via a bridge of 5 glycine units, to other peptidoglycan chains. In reality penicillin must compete with structurally varied substrates having a range of binding affinities to the 5 different PBPs. Inhibition of peptidoglycan cross-linking may depend on which PBPs have the highest affinities for penicillin, because the different PBPs play metabolic roles that differ in importance in the maintenance of cellular integrity or in cell division. Different β-lactams also appear to exert differing influences in the development of resistance. Amoxicillin and cefixime effectively select for low-level but not high-level resistance in vitro, whereas cefuroxime and cefotaxime tend to select for high-level resistance to penicillin.[110] This effect was apparently seen in a recent case of a child with meningitis whose organism changed from intermediate to fully resistant during therapy with cefotaxime plus penicillin.[111]

The mechanism of penicillin resistance is depicted in Figure 4 to show the two changes that must occur for pneumococci to be able to cross-link peptidoglycan chain in the presence of penicillin. First, the strain must produce structurally different stem peptides that do not resemble the structure of penicillin. Most strains have this capability, but the regulation of production and preference for branched peptides are affected by the strain's genetic resources, as well as by the selective pressures of antibiotics.[60] Second, the enzymatic site of the PBP has been changed to accommodate the more complex stem peptides; the altered PBPs have lower affinity for penicillin, so that the stem peptides compete successfully for access to the PBP. Resistance to the various cephalospo-

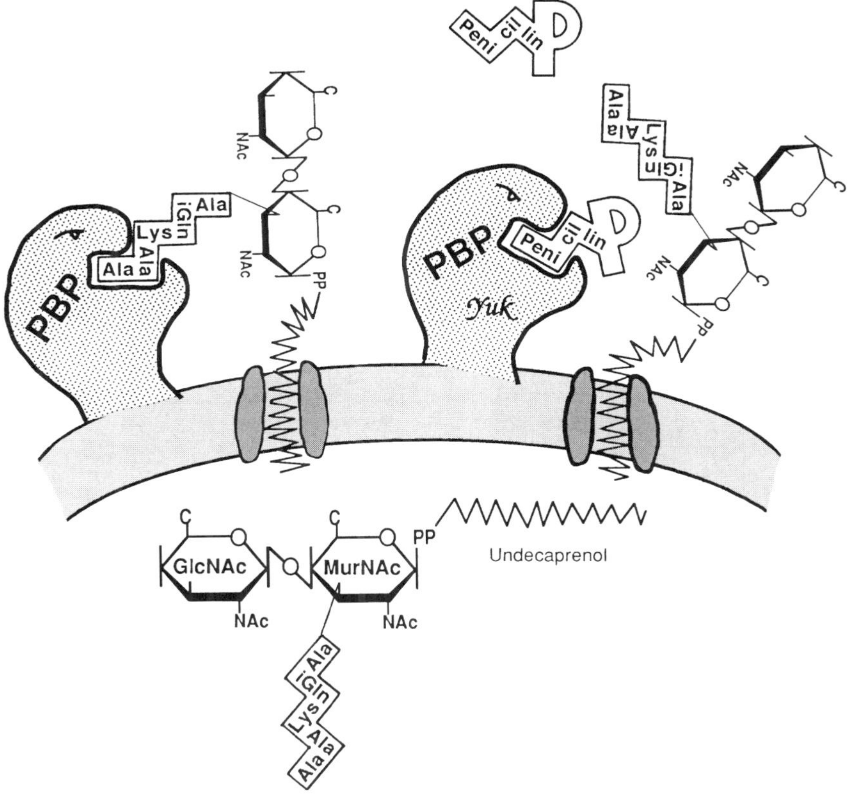

FIGURE 3.

Penicillin inhibits cell wall synthesis, as described in the text. The β-lactam ring mimics the structure of the acyl-D-alanyl-D-alanine tail of the muramyl stem peptide and prevents the penicillin-binding protein from cross-linking stem peptide of an emerging chain to other peptidoglycan chains.

rins occurs in a similar manner but with differences in affinities for different PBPs.[63, 110]

In addition to interfering with cell wall integrity, penicillins and most other β-lactams also act by independently triggering amidase activity.[112] This effect is quantitatively about 3-fold less than direct cell wall inhibition. Pneumococci do not have to undergo lysis to be killed by penicillins, but as noted earlier, lysis releases intracellular contents, including pneumolysin, and highly inflammatory cell wall breakdown products that provoke a strong inflam-

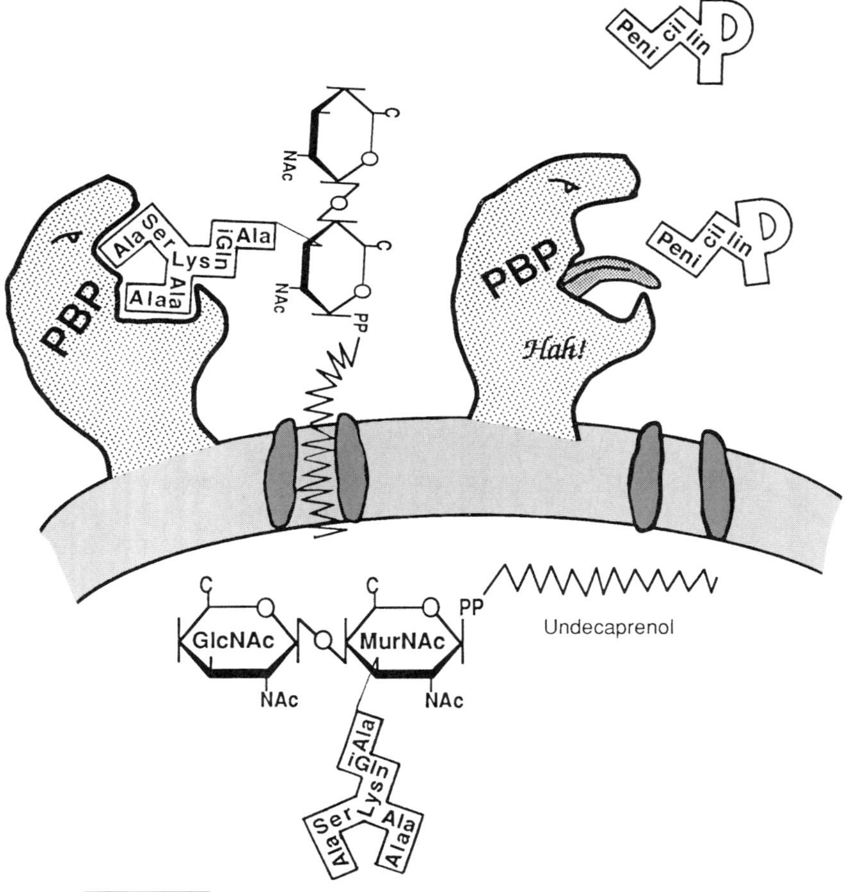

FIGURE 4.

In a penicillin-resistant strain, two separate changes must occur: the strain produces predominantly branched stem peptides that do not resemble the structure of penicillin, and the enzymatic site of the PBP, which has been altered to accommodate the more complex stem peptides, has much lower affinity for penicillin.

matory response in the host. Tolerance to penicillin is largely but not completely mediated by amidase activity. It has been suggested that cyclic antibiotic exposure, such as the intermittent dosing schedules used clinically, may provide two kinds of selective pressure on pneumococci.[113] Suppression of amidase activity, which paradoxically occurs at peak penicillin concentrations, dampens the effect of lytic killing and enhances the survival of some lysis-resistant members of the population. Meanwhile, the marginally inhibitory or trough levels tend to select for penicillin resistance. These mechanisms may act in concert to aid the selection of resistant strains or to abet the development of resistance during therapy.[111]

SENSITIVITY TO VANCOMYCIN

Pneumococci have remained sensitive to vancomycin, teicoplanin, and related glycopeptides because they act by at least two completely separate mechanisms, as illustrated in Figure 5, drawn after models described by Reynolds.[114] Vancomycin binds reversibly but with high affinity to the L-lysyl-D-alanyl-D-alanine tail of the muramyl stem peptide. It inhibits cell wall synthesis at two critical stages: by creating steric hindrance around the stem peptides to inhibit the transglycolsylase that normally links the disaccharide precursors (GlcNAc coupled to MurNAc pentapeptide), thus preventing the formation of larger peptidoglycan units; and sterically hindering the binding of stem peptides to the PBPs, which are prevented from performing the transpeptidase reaction in the formation of cross-linkages between peptidoglycan chains. Vancomycin must be present in high enough concentrations to saturate available stem peptide–binding sites, many of which are not involved in structural cross-linkages. Several *Enterococcus* species have reduced binding of vancomycin by cleavage or alterations of the terminal D-alanyl-D-alanine of their stem peptides. Resistance has also been reported in a few strains of coagulase-negative staphylococci.[115]

RESISTANCE TO OTHER ANTIBIOTICS

Pneumococci are frequently resistant to TMP-SMZ by yet undetermined mechanisms involving alterations in folate and dehydrofolate metabolism.[25] Chloramphenicol resistance seems to occur independently because of an inducible chloramphenicol acetyltransferase present alone[116] or in association with multiple resistance factors.[23, 25, 117] Resistance to some antibiotics is readily achieved by simple mutations, often involving as few as one nucleotide or one to several amino acids. These include rifampin, which interferes with RNA polymerase; quinolones, which act on DNA gyrase; and streptomycin, which has high affinity for ribosomes.[62, 100] Resistance to kanamycin, along with resistance to erythromycin and tetracycline, results from a phosphotransferase encoded in a transposon.[108] Some of the newer quinolones have enhanced activity against pneumococci, when compared with ciprofloxacin,[118] and

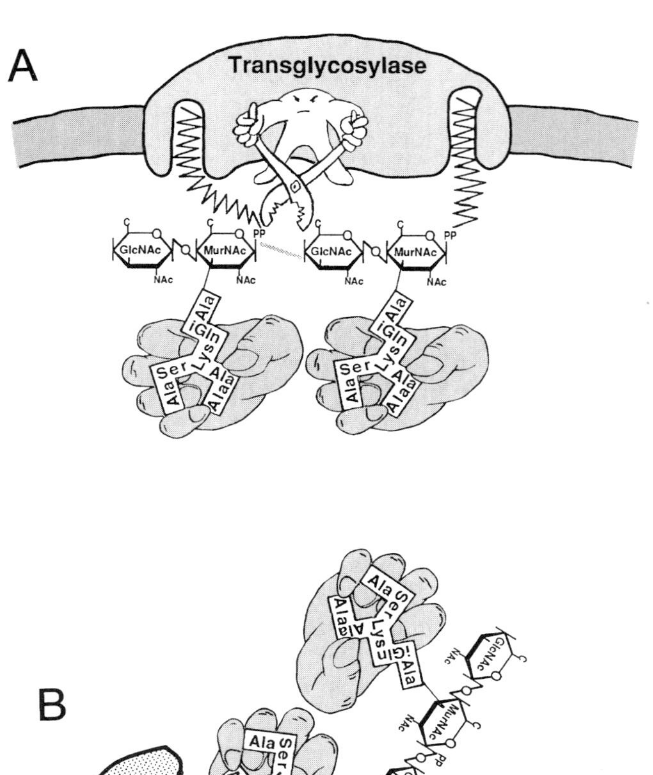
A
Transglycosylase
GlcNAc
MurNAc
NAc
NAc
PP
Ala
iGln
Lys
Ala
Ala
Ser
Ala

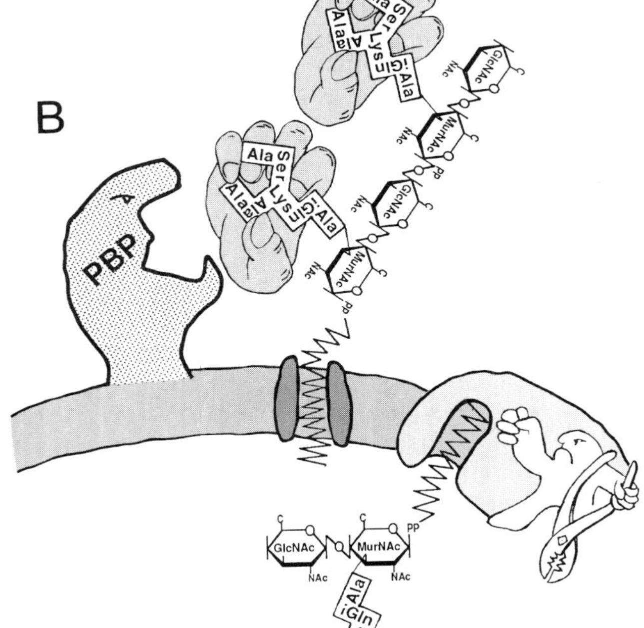
B
PBP
Ala
Ser
Ala
Lys
iGln
Ala
GlcNAc
MurNAc
NAc
PP
GlcNAc
MurNAc
NAc
PP
GlcNAc
MurNAc
NAc
NAc
PP
iAla
iGln
s

may eventually prove useful until the organisms take evasive action. Resistance to clindamycin and clarithromycin is currently rare in the United States,[107, 119] but experience suggests that conservative use and careful surveillance for resistance are needed to maintain the usefulness of these and other antibiotics.

SUSCEPTIBILITY TESTING

Prior to the coming of penicillin- and multiresistant strains, most clinical laboratories did not perform susceptibility tests of any kind for pneumococci, assuming them to be sensitive, unless a patient failed to improve on conventional therapy (the in vivo susceptibility test[120]). Quantitative dilution tests revealed little change in MICs before the mid-1970s.[121] A collection of pneumococci from 1975 to 1978 in our own community were uniformly susceptible at MICs less than 0.015 μg/mL, but by the early 1980s the median MIC for susceptible strains had crept up to 0.03 μg/mL,[101] and this trend has been observed throughout the world. One of the major difficulties with these fastidious organisms has been the lack of standardized methods for testing, which is overseen by the National Committee for Clinical Laboratory Standards. Progress is now being made in this area,[122, 123] and both disk screening methods and the E-test are proving to be reliable methods that can be easily performed by any competent laboratory.[27] The current breakpoints for penicillin G are susceptible (MIC < 0.1 μg/mL), intermediate (MIC 0.1–1.0 μg/mL), and resistant (MIC ≥ 2.0 μg/mL).

OXACILLIN DISK SCREENING TESTS

It was apparent early on that the conventional 10-μg penicillin disk failed to detect penicillin resistance by the Kirby-Bauer disk diffu-

---

FIGURE 5.

The mechanisms of action of vancomycin were drawn after models described by Reynolds.[114] Vancomycin, represented by hands, binds with high affinity to the L-lysyl-D-alanyl-D-alanine tail of the muramyl stem peptide and inhibits cell wall synthesis at two critical stages. **A,** within the cell, steric hindrance created by vancomycin bound to the stem peptides frustrates the transglycosylase that is normally able to link the disaccharide precursors (N-acetyl-glucosamine [GlcNAc] coupled to N-acetyl-muramic acid [MurNAc] pentapeptide), preventing the formation of larger peptidoglycan units. **B,** vancomycin bound to stem peptides sterically hinders the activity of the penicillin binding proteins (PBP), which are prevented from performing their duties as transpeptidases in the formation of cross-linkages between peptidoglycan chains of the cell wall.

sion method. This was soon supplanted by the 1-μg oxacillin disk, introduced by Dixon et al. in 1977 and further evaluated by Swenson et al.[124] Although about 40% of strains that appear to be resistant (zones ≤19 mm) proved to be susceptible (usually at a borderline MIC of 0.06 μg/mL), the oxacillin disk rarely fails to detect intermediate or resistant organisms.[101, 119] Most of the problems with this method involve careless errors,[25] such as failing to adjust the inoculum to the 0.5 McFarland density standard, using a loop instead of a swab to inoculate the plate, not allowing the inoculum to dry sufficiently before applying the disks, using out-of-date disks, or failing to check disks with control strains.

Properly done, the oxacillin disk test is not only simple and reliable but has the advantage of being more sensitive than the MIC tests in detecting small stepwise alterations in PBPs that may indicate potential for β-lactam resistance.[27] It is of considerable interest in this regard that the disk test has identified some pneumococci with resistance to oxacillin (MIC = 1.0 μg/mL) that have nevertheless remained sensitive to penicillin (MIC = 0.06 μg/mL).[125] These oxacillin-resistant strains often have increased MICs to cefotaxime, probably due to changes in PBP 2x. Because this situation is of possible clinical significance, it may be worthwhile to continue to use the oxicillin screening test, even for laboratories that rely primarily on MIC or E-test methods specific for penicillin or cephalosporins.

Disk susceptibility zone size criteria have been evaluated for some other antibiotics and found to be quite adequate for testing chloramphenicol (but see later discussion), erythromycin, orfloxacin, tetracycline, and vancomycin.[122] Disk testing standards have not been approved for cefotaxime, ceftriaxone, cefapime, imipenem, or TMP-SMZ, because of excessive, though mostly minor, interpretive errors. Cefuroxime, which was not included in the latter study, has been evaluated by Friedland et al.[126] The cefuroxime disk was found to be a reliable screening method for susceptibility to most cephalosporins and is certainly worth further consideration because it is simple, easily available, and much cheaper than the E-test. Thornsberry et al.[27] have extensively reviewed the testing of oral cephalosporins. Their general conclusions suggest that for penicillin-susceptible pneumococci, cefuroxime and cefprozil are the most active, cefaclor and loracarbef somewhat less so, and cefixime the least active. Cefuroxime and cefprozil were the only oral cephalosporins with activity at all against resistant strains. The authors also remind us that susceptibility breakpoints are by nature rather arbitrary and not always supported by data on clinical efficacy.

E-TEST

The E-test (AB Biodisk, Solna, Sweden, and Culver City, Calif.) is an ingenious extension of the disk diffusion idea in which a plastic strip is coated with an antibiotic gradient from low to high concentration.[127] The strip is applied to an agar plate that has been inoculated in the same fashion as the Kirby-Bauer method. As shown in Figure 6, inhibition of growth along the gradient results in an elliptical zone that intersects the strip at the point where inhibition occurs with the least amount of antibiotic. This point is read visually, and the approximate MIC is indicated by calibrations along the strip. Although the correlation with reference MICs may not be exact, the E-test for penicillin G discriminates between susceptible and intermediate strains as well as or better than the oxacillin disk.[127-129] It does not readily distinguish intermediate from resistant strains. E-tests have been developed for several other commonly used antibiotics, including cefotaxime, cefuroxime, ceftriaxone, choramphenicol, erythromycin, and tetracycline.[127, 130] Although many laboratories accept E-test results, most authorities recommend performing MICs on all strains to confirm resistance detected by either the E-test or disk diffusion methods.

QUANTITATIVE METHODS: MINIMUM INHIBITORY CONCENTRATION

Quantitative measurement of antibiotic susceptibilities is usually done by either broth microdilution or agar dilution methods.[123] In both methods antibiotics are added to specially supplemented media in a series of twofold dilutions covering the relevant range of concentrations for testing. Some laboratories, including our own, consider the agar method the more reliable for reference purposes.[101, 127, 128] The broth microdilution methods, however, are now mostly automated and are much more convenient for either small or large batches of strains. Commercially available broth dilution systems vary in their reliability, and some are not recommended for testing pneumococci.[128, 130]

Chloramphenicol is a special case, because some strains that appear susceptible by MIC or disk diffusion tests are actually quite tolerant to the drug. This is especially true of penicillin-resistant and multiresistant strains, which often have minimum bactericidal concentrations (MBCs) well above acceptable limits.[31, 131] An al-

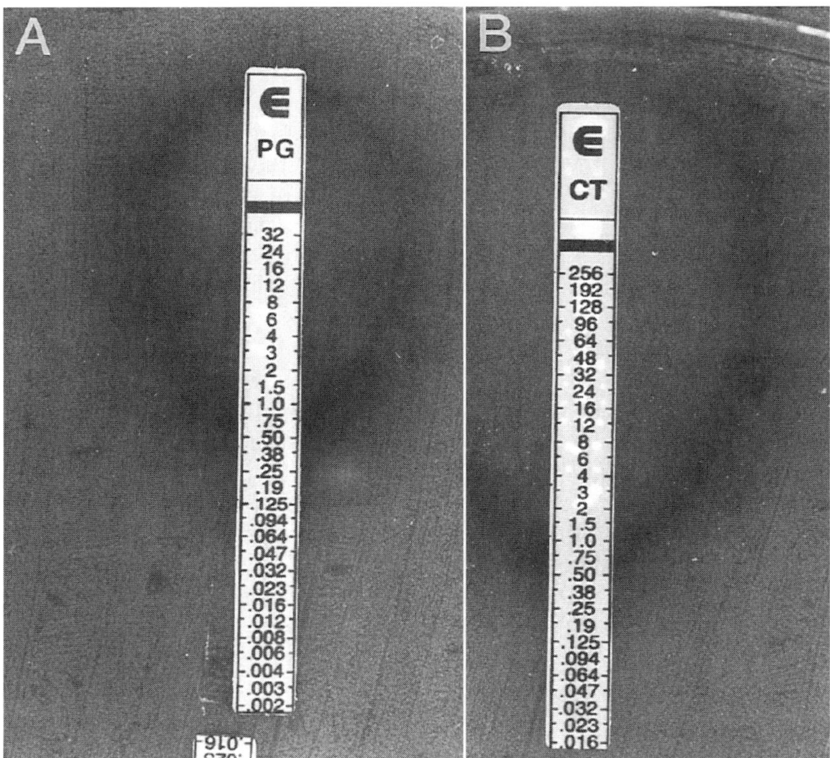

FIGURE 6.

The E-test is an extension of the disk diffusion idea, in which a plastic strip is coated with an antibiotic gradient from low to high concentration.[127] The strip is applied to an agar plate that has been inoculated in the same fashion as the Kirby-Bauer method. Inhibition of growth along the gradient results in an elliptical zone that intersects the strip at the point where inhibition occurs with the least amount of antibiotic. This point is read visually, and the approximate minimum inhibitory concentration is indicated by calibrations along the strip. The isolate pictured here was intermediate to penicillin at an MIC of approximately 0.5 μg/mL **(A)** and also intermediate to cefotaxime at about 0.5 μg/mL **(B).** The calibration of the strips is noticably different. The E-test is quite accurate for detecting *sensitive* strains (penicillin MIC < 0.1 μg/mL; cefotaxime or ceftriaxone MIC < 0.5 μg/mL); however, it is not as accurate at distinguishing intermediate (penicillin MIC 0.1–1.0 μg/mL; cephalosporin MIC 0.5–1.0 μg/mL) from resistant strains (penicillin or cephalosporin MIC ≥ 2.0 μg/mL). (Courtesy of Elizabeth W. Cooney, EMLabs, Inc., Birmingham, Ala.)

ternative is to assay for the chloramphenicol acetyltransferase directly using a simple 90-minute colorimetric method.[132]

ANTIBIOTIC MANAGEMENT OF PNEUMOCOCCAL INFECTIONS

The majority of pneumococcal infections are likely to be caused by penicillin-sensitive strains, even in localities with a high prevalence of penicillin resistance. The clinician's nightmare is the patient begun on empirically chosen antibiotic therapy who then develops severe disease due to resistant organisms. Some comfort may be afforded to physicians whose hospital or community surveillance can give assurance that resistance to the empirical choices remains less than 10% or so, as currently reported from Philadelphia and Houston.[119, 133] But laboratories in St. Louis, Memphis, and Kentucky are reporting penicillin resistance rates of 26% to 29%, and many of these strains are also resistant to cefotaxime and other antibiotics.[105, 107]

The major concern falls in the twilight zone between empiric antibiotics and definitive treatment based on culture results and known susceptibilities of the offending organism. Initial therapy is based on the clinician's best guess, taking into account the patient's age, medical history and prior antibiotics, the prevalance of resistant organisms in the community, and the site or apparent seriousness of infection. Appropriate, hopefully definitive, therapy generally depends on the ability to obtain culture material and prompt, accurate sensitivity results. Empirical antibiotic regimens must adequately cover the majority of likely pathogens, often including bacteria other than pneumococci. This is most often the case with pneumonia, otitis media, and sinusitis. At the same time treatment regimens must not squander valuable drugs such as vancomycin merely to treat a few patients who might harbor an otherwise resistant organism. Sooner or later there is an environmental price to pay for excessive antibiotic use in terms of the development of resistance either in the targeted species or in other pathogens that become inadvertently exposed to the selective pressures imposed by clinical practice.

MENINGITIS

Antibiotic therapies for meningitis are of greatest concern, because pneumococci have already developed some degree of resistance to many antibiotics in common use, and alternative choices are limited, as discussed in recent reviews.[26, 31] Initial therapy must also take into account the possibility of other pathogens, especially meningococci and *H. influenzae,* although the latter has become less common with the advent of effective vaccines. Definitive therapy remains complicated by the poor penetration of most agents into the CSF.[134]

Penicillin and ampicillin are still the mainstays of treatment for sensitive pneumococci. Recommended doses of penicillin G have been historically low, in part because they are measured in international units (1,595 units = 1 mg). Thus, 100,000 units/kg daily, commonly recommended for meningitis up until 10 years ago or so, is equivalent to 63 mg/kg daily—pitifully low compared with usual ampicillin doses of 200 to 400 mg/kg daily. We have often recommended ampicillin instead of penicillin simply because many physicians were reluctant to use penicillin at doses of 500,000 to 600,000 units/kg daily. Higher doses have been given in some cases, but it should be noted that potassium penicillin has 1.7 mEq K^+ per 1 million units, which may have to be figured into fluid and electrolyte orders. In a number of case reports high doses of penicillin (>500,000 units/kg daily) have been effective in meningitis due to penicillin-intermediate pneumococci,[20, 101] but we currently recommend penicillin only for unequivocally susceptible strains.

Cefotaxime and ceftriaxone have been effective against nearly all strains for many years, but at least a dozen treatment failures have been reported with third-generation cephalosporins.[135] Pneumococci with MICs 1.0 µg/mL or more are now considered to be resistant and have been isolated with increasing frequency.[105, 107] Meningitis due to such strains should probably be treated with the addition of another antibiotic, but experience to date has been too sparse to make firm recommendations. Particularly troublesome is the recent report of meningitis in a child with an isolate initially intermediate to penicillin (MIC = 0.12 µg/mL) and susceptible to cefotaxime (MIC = 0.06 µg/mL). He was treated with adequate doses of both drugs but relapsed on the tenth day, at which time the CSF isolate was resistant to both penicillin (MIC >1 µg/mL) and cefotaxime (MIC = 1 µg/mL).[111] This case shows that intermediate strains have the potential to develop resistance during treatment and should probably be considered clinically resistant. It also underscores the need for repeating CSF examinations at 24 to 36 hours to be sure of clinical efficacy, as recommended by these and other investigators.[31, 136]

Chloramphenicol has been used for treatment of meningitis for more than 40 years. It may be given intravenously or by the oral route with equal effectiveness and has good penetration into the CSF.[134] Resistance is uncommon in the United States,[117] but treatment failures have occurred here and elsewhere, especially in parts of the world where use of the drug is widespread.[23, 25, 31] As noted earlier, one of the chief disadvantages is that some strains have an inducable acetyltransferase that inactivates chloramphenicol, and these strains often appear to be sensitive by disk diffusion or MIC even though they are clearly resistant when the MBC is tested.[131] Chloramphenicol virtually always causes a reversible depression in red blood cell precursors in the bone marrow,[137] but idiopathic aplastic anemia is fortunately rare and should not deter use of the drug in appropriate situations.

Vancomycin has long been the rear guard of antibiotics for treating penicillin-resistant pneumococci. Although all strains remain susceptible, vancomycin penetrates poorly and unpredictably into the CSF, even when meninges are inflamed.[138] The only data on CSF penetration in children are from patients treated for ventriculoperitoneal shunt infections, revealing CSF concentrations from 1 to 12 μg/mL after conventional doses of up to 60 mg/kg daily.[134] Current vancomycin preparations do not appear to have significant ototoxicity or nephrotoxicity. A common problem, however, is the "red man syndrome," characterized by erythema and pruitis, thought to be associated with histamine release provoked by administration of the drug.[139] The value of monitoring serum concentrations has recently been challenged, because vancomycin levels have never been shown to correlate with either clinical efficacy or reduction in possible toxic side effects.[140] Vancomycin has found increasing use in the treatment of staphylococcal infections, but there are no data other than case reports to assess its efficacy in childhood meningitis due to pneumococci.

Combination therapies and other antibiotics have been used or recommended on the basis of individual cases or animal experiments. Vancomycin plus rifampin has been used in several cases,[135] although this combination has no synergistic or additive effect in vitro.[138] Vancomycin plus ceftriaxone was more effective than either drug alone in an animal model. Vancomycin penetration was impaired by treatment with dexamethasone, but ceftriaxone plus rifampin was effective in the presence of dexamethasone.[31] Teicoplanin is more active than vancomycin against multiresistant pneumococci, but CSF penetration is less than that with vancomycin, and there are no clinical data to support its use in the treatment of meningitis.[138] Although imipenem-cilastatin also penetrates poorly into CSF,[134] several patients have been successfully treated with doses up to 400 mg/kg daily.[141] The major problem with imipenem is the increased frequency of seizures,[142] but it may sometimes be difficult to distinguish drug-induced seizures from those associated with the underlying meningitis.[141] Several newer carbapenems are on the horizon (e.g., meropenem) that may avoid this disturbing side effect.

Clearly there is as yet inadequate data on which to guide either empirical or definitive treatment of meningitis due to multiresistant pneumococci. Despite some increased frequency of resistance, ceftriaxone or cefotaxime is currently the preferred empirical antibiotic choice.[31] Some authorities would use a cephalosporin in combination with chloramphenicol, rifampin, or vancomycin. In localities where cephalosporin resistance has become common, vancomycin would be an obvious choice; chloramphenicol might be an equally rational alternative, given the caveats just mentioned and accurate susceptibility and surveillance data.

To avoid unnecessary use of vancomycin, this drug should probably be reserved for patients who are considered septic or suspected of having meningitis on the basis of CSF pleocytosis and bacteria seen on the Gram stain. Microscopic examination of the CSF is likely to reveal gram-positive diplococci in about 80% of cases of pneumococcal meningitis. Latex agglutination generally yields fewer positives and rarely affects clinical decisions.[143, 144] Nevertheless, because of their specificity, antigen detection tests are sometimes helpful when results are positive in patients who have received prior antibiotic therapy. Polymerase chain reaction (PCR) tests have now been developed for detection of pneumococcal amidase and pneumolysin genes but have not been evaluated for the diagnosis of meningitis.[94, 145]

BACTEREMIA, PNEUMONIA, AND OTITIS MEDIA

Many of the same problems in choosing empirical therapy for meningitis also apply to children who appear critically ill or have sickle cell disease, asplenia, or immunodeficiency and who are suspected of having pneumococcal infection. Pneumococcal bacteremia without multiorgan involvement or other evidence of sepsis is surprisingly well tolerated in children. Half or more of children with bacteremia have a discrete focus of infection, such as pneumonia or otitis media.[33, 104] Conversely, about 10% of children with pneumonia or otitis media have positive blood cultures, most of whom do quite well as outpatients on oral antibiotics or ceftriaxone.[146, 147]

The clinician has a wider choice of antibiotics for pneumococcal infections other than meningitis.[27, 28, 31] These include penicillin and amoxicillin; numerous parenteral and oral cephalosporins; erythromycin, clarithromycin and azithromycin; clindamycin; TMP-SMZ; ciprofloxacin and ofloxacin; and teicoplanin. Chloramphenicol can also be given orally. The selection of an appropriate drug should take into account the age and condition of the patient, site and severity of infection, the ability to obtain cultures and sensitivity results, and known susceptibility patterns of organisms currently isolated in the community.

The pneumococcus is the leading cause of bacterial pneumonia in children, but there are other etiologies that may have to be considered in any given patient. A properly obtained sputum sample and carefully examined Gram's stain is still of considerable diagnostic utility and may help the clinician decide the proper course from among a number of empirical antibiotic regimens.[28, 148] Nasopharyngeal cultures are much less useful, but a resistant isolate from this site would at least alert the physician that such a strain is present and possibly involved. In localities where penicillin resistance is common or when a penicillin-resistant strain is recovered, the best oral antibiotic choices appear to be cefprozil or cefuroxime axetil, erythromycin or clarithromycin, and clindamycin. Loracarbef, cefpodoxime, and cefixime have less activity against penicillin-resistant strains.[27] Ciprofloxacin is not generally used in children, and resistance has developed quickly in areas where it is frequently used for whatever purposes. For susceptible strains TMP-SMZ may also be adequate. Patients who do not respond well should be carefully reevaluated, with cultures of blood and plural fluid, if present, and parenteral antibiotics should be given as indicated by clinical severity.

Pneumococci are the most frequent cause of otitis media in all age groups, although nontypeable *H. influenzae* and *Moroxella (Branhamella) catarrhalis* are also common in children.[29, 40] As in pneumonia and sinusitis, an etiologic diagnosis is seldom obtained, and therapy is begun empirically. Evaluation of therapeutic regimens is confounded by the observation that as many as 70% of cases resolve clinically, regardless of what antibiotic is prescribed. Marchant et al.[149] described this as the "Pollyanna effect," when clinical trials show apparent efficacy of marginally effective antibiotics. Most authorities continue to recommend amoxicillin for initial empirical treatment of otitis media.[29, 31, 40] This is based on the relative infrequency of encountering penicillin-resistant pneumococci or β-lactamase-producing *Haemophilus* or *Moraxella* (currently about 8% for each species)[40] but varying by locality. Therapy should be monitored clinically, with changes made as indicated. For most practitioners this means that patients showing poor clinical response will be given an alternative antibiotic. The antibiotic choices are essentially the same as for pneumonia. Other treatment modalities may include intramuscular injection of ceftriaxone,[150] but this is costly and painful, and widespread use may result in development of resistance in the community at large. Cefixime should not be used because of its poor efficacy against pneumococcal otitis media.[151] Tympanocentesis is a simple and underutilized procedure that is particularly useful when a child continues to have a purulent middle ear effusion. Ill-appearing children, as well as those with immunodeficiencies, should be approached in much the same fashion as those with meningitis, obtaining blood cultures, tympanocentesis, and lumbar puncture, as indicated, especially if a change to parenteral antibiotics is clinically warranted.

PREVENTION AND THE FUTURE

Penicillin- and multiresistant pneumococci are likely to be with us for many years into the future. It seems unlikely that resistant strains will become predominant, given the observation that the organisms must pay a biologic price to live in the presence of antibiotics.[60] Resistant strains expend additional energy in altering the peptidoglycan structure of their cell walls, and experience has shown that the frequency of resistant strains fluctuates with rates of consumption of specific antibiotics in the community. With rational, conservative use, our antibiotic armamentarium should remain adequate to cope with most clinical situations in normal hosts. Fortunately, the frequency of pneumococcal meningitis, the disease entity most difficult to treat, is relatively low. High-risk patients, such as those with sickle cell disease or immunodeficiencies, present difficult management problems because of the current practice of giving penicillin prophylaxis to prevent pneumococcal infection. These individuals can and do develop the further risk of becoming colonized by a penicillin-resistant strain. It may be argued that the short-term benefits of this practice still outweigh the long-term risks, but this question must obviously be reevaluated in light of the increasing frequency of isolating resistant organisms from colonized and infected patients. One alternative may be the use of the topical antibiotic murpirocin administered intranasally to eradicate colonization.[152]

Another situation that is probably associated with increased risk of pneumococcal infection is attendance at a day-care center. Although the spread of pneumococci appears to be much less than was seen with *H. influenzae* type b, several clusters of invasive pneumococcal infections have recently been reported in such settings.[94, 153, 154] Children frequently continue to carry pneumococci even after a course of conventional antibiotics,[35, 36] and rifampin has not proved to be effective in eliminating colonization or spread.[94, 153, 154] One of the outbreaks was caused by pneumococcus type 12F,[153] a serotype that is uncommon in children and unlikely to be included in future pneumococcal conjugate vaccines. Vigilance remains the order of the day.

In some high-risk populations, perhaps including day-care settings, passive immunization is a possible approach that deserves further consideration. As mentioned earlier, a specially prepared γ-globulin (BPIG) has been used with some success in Apache children[5] and also had some efficacy against recurrent pneumococcal otitis media in a middle-class suburban population.[155] It may also be an improvement over the conventional γ-globulins frequently given to immunodeficient patients and those with HIV infection. This modality will nevertheless require further study and analysis of costs and effectiveness.[156]

Considerable progress is currently being made in development of pneumococcal conjugate vaccines.[51] Although nearly all serotypes are capable of causing disease, only a few account for the majority of childhood infections, as indicated in Table 2. The addition of one or two more types (e.g., types 1 and 3) might also yield a vaccine appropriate for elderly individuals, who, like infants, often fail to generate protective responses to some types in the licensed 23-valent formulation. Protection, however, would be expected only against the serotypes chosen for the vaccine. A vaccine made from surface protein components, such as PspA epitopes common to many strains, could help fill the gap against other capsular types.

In the long term it is unlikely that any of these measures will completely solve the problem of pneumococcal infections any more than penicillin did half a century ago. We must maintain a broad view of antibiotic resistance to include the organisms we inadvertently expose to drugs in the course of treating a known infection. We must continue to teach and practice conservative use of antibiotics. And we must continue the search for answers to the mysteries of pathogenesis and host response.

REFERENCES

1. Heffron R: *Pneumonia With Special Reference to Pneumococcus Lobar Pneumonia.* New York, Commonwealth Fund, 1939; reprinted by Harvard University Press, Cambridge, Mass, 1979.
2. White B (with the collaboration of Robinson ES, Barnes LA): *The Biology of the Pneumococcus: The Bacteriological, Biochemical and Immunological Characters and Activities of* Diplococcus pneumoniae. New York, Commonwealth Fund, 1938; reprinted by Harvard University Press, Cambridge, Mass, 1979.
3. Austrian R: Pneumococcus: The first one hundred years. *Rev Infect Dis* 3:183–189, 1981.
4. Casadevall A, Scharff MD: Serum therapy revisited: Animal models of infection and development of passive antibody therapy. *Antimicrob Agent Chemother* 38:1695–1702, 1994.
5. Siber GR, Thompson C, Reid GR, et al: Evaluation of bacterial polysaccharide immune globulin for the treatment of prevention of *Haemophilus influenzae* type b and pneumococcal disease. *J Infect Dis* 165(suppl 1):S129–S133, 1992.
6. Heidelberger M, Avery OT: The soluble specific substance of pneumococcus. *J Exp Med* 38:73–79, 1923.
7. MacLeod CM, Hodges RG, Heidelberger M, et al: Prevention of pneumococcal pneumonia by immunization with specific capsular polysaccharides. *J Exp Med* 82:445–465, 1945.
8. Robbins JB, Austrian R, Lee C-J, et al: Considerations for formulating the second-generation pneumococcal capsular polysaccharide vaccine with emphasis on the cross-reactive type within groups. *J Infect Dis* 148:1136–1159, 1983.
9. Centers for Disease Control: Pneumococcal polysaccharide vaccine. *MMWR* 38:64–76, 1989.
10. Avery OT, MacLeod CM, McCarty M: Studies on the chemical nature of the substance inducing transformation of pneumococcal types: Induction of transformation by a desoxyribonucleic acid fraction isolated from pneumococcus type III. *J Exp Med* 79:137–157, 1944.
11. Watson DA, Musher DM, Jacobson JW, et al: A brief history of the pneumococcus in biomedical research: A panoply of scientific discovery. *Clin Infect Dis* 17:913–924, 1993.
12. Abraham EP, Gardner AD, Chain E, et al: Further observations on penicillin. *Lancet* 2:177–189, 1941.
13. Eriksen KR: Studies on induced resistance to penicillin in a pneumococcus type I. *Acta Pathol Microbiol Scand* 22:398–405, 1945.
14. Johnston RB Jr: Pathogenesis of pneumococcal pneumonia. *Rev Infect Dis* 13:S509–S517, 1991.
15. Wise EM Jr, Park JT: Penicillin: Its basic site of action as an inhibitor of a peptide cross-linking reaction in cell wall mucopeptide synthesis. *Proc Natl Acad Sci U S A* 54:75–81, 1965.
16. Tipper DJ, Strominger JL: Mechanism of action of penicillins: a pro-

posal based on their structural similarity to acyl-D-alanyl-D-alanine. *Proc Natl Acad Sci U S A* 54:1133–1141, 1965.

17. Hansman D, Glasgow H, Sturt J, et al: Increased resistance to penicillin of pneumococci isolated from man. *N Engl J Med* 284:175–177, 1971.
18. Kislak JW, Ravazi LMB, Daly AK, et al: Susceptibility of pneumococci to nine antibiotics. *Am J Med Sci* 250:261–268, 1965.
19. Shope TC, Quie PG: *D. pneumoniae:* Increased resistance to oxacillin and cloxacillin. *Minn Med* 51:37–38, 1968.
20. Naraqi S, Kirkpatrick GP, Kabins S: Relapsing pneumococcal meningitis: isolation of an organism with decreased susceptibility to penicillin G. *J Pediatr* 85:671–673, 1974.
21. Parades A, Taber LH, Yow MD, et al: Prolonged pneumococcal meningitis due to an organism with increased resistance to penicillin. *Pediatrics* 58:378–381, 1976.
22. Mace JW, Janik DS, Sauer RL, et al: Penicillin-resistant pneumococcal meningitis in an immunocompromised infant. *J Pediatr* 91:506–507, 1977.
23. Jacobs MR, Koornhof HJ, Robins-Brown RM, et al: Emergence of multiply resistant pneumococci. *N Engl J Med* 299:735–740, 1978.
24. Cates KL, Gerrard JM, Giebink GS, et al: A penicillin-resistant pneumococcus. *J Pediatr* 93:624–626, 1978.
25. Klugman KP: Pneumococcal resistance to antibiotics. *Clin Microbiol Rev* 34:171–196, 1990.
26. Chesney PJ: The escalating problem of antimicrobial resistance in *Streptococcus pneumoniae. Am J Dis Child* 146:912–916, 1992.
27. Thornsberry C, Brown SD, Yee YC, et al: Increasing penicillin resistance in Streptococcus pneumoniae in the U.S.: Effect on susceptibility to oral cephalosporins. *Infect Med* 10(suppl D):15–24, 1993.
28. Neu HC, Sabath LD: Criteria for selecting oral antibiotic therapy for community-acquired pneumonia. *Infect Med* 10(suppl D):33–40, 1993.
29. Stutman HR: Penicillin-resistant Streptococcus pneumoniae: Focus on otitis media. *Infect Med* 10(suppl D):51–55, 1993.
30. Baquero F, Loza E: Antibiotic resistance of microorganisms involved in ear, nose and throat infections. *Pediatr Infect Dis J* 13:S9–S14, 1994.
31. Friedland LR, McCracken GH Jr: Management of infections caused by antibiotic-resistant *Streptococcus pneumoniae. N Engl J Med* 331:377–382, 1994.
32. Wenger JD, Hightower AW, Facklam RR, et al: Bacterial meningitis in the United States, 1986: Report of a multistate surveillance study. *J Infect Dis* 162:1316–1323, 1990.
33. Gray BM, Dillon HC Jr: Clinical and epidemiologic studies of pneumococcal infection in children. *Pediatr Infect Dis J* 5:201–207, 1986.
34. Hodges RG, MacLeod CM: Epidemic pneumococcal pneumonia. *Am J Hyg* 44:183–243, 1946.

35. Gray BM, Converse GM III, Dillon HC Jr: Epidemiologic studies of *Streptococcus pneumoniae* in infants: Acquisition, carriage, and infection during the first 24 months of life. *J Infect Dis* 142:923–933, 1980.
36. Boulnois GJ: Pneumococcal proteins and the pathogenesis of disease caused by *Streptococcus pneumoniae*. *J Gen Microbiol* 138:249–259, 1992.
37. Paton JC, Andrew PW, Boulnois GJ, et al: Molecular analysis of the pathogenicity of *Streptococcus pneumoniae:* The role of pneumococcal proteins. *Ann Rev Microbiol* 47:89–115, 1993.
38. Guerra-Romero L, Tureen JH, Täuber MG: Pathogenesis of central nervous system injury in bacterial meningitis. *Antibiot Chemother* 45:18–29, 1992.
39. Tuomanen E: Breaching the blood-brain barrier. *Sci Am* 268:80–84, 1993.
40. Klein JO: Otitis media. *Clin Infect Dis* 19:823–833, 1994.
41. Andersson B, Dahmén J, Frejd T, et al: Identification of an active disaccharide unit of a glycoconjugate receptor for pneumococci attaching to human pharyngeal epithelial cells. *J Exp Med* 158:559–570, 1983.
42. Krivan HC, Roberts DD, Ginsberg V: Many pulmonary pathogenic bacteria bind specifically to the carbohydrate sequence GalNAcβ1–4Gal found in some glycolipids. *Proc Natl Acad Sci U S A* 85:6157–6161, 1988.
43. Andersson B, Beachy EH, Tomaz A, et al: A sandwich adhesion on *Streptococcus pneumoniae* attaching to human oropharyngeal epithelial cells in vitro. *Microb Pathog* 4:267–278, 1988.
44. Andersson B, Eriksson B, Falsen E, et al: Adhesion of *Streptococcus pneumoniae* to human pharyngeal epithelial cells in vitro: Differences in adhesive capacity among strains isolated from subjects with otitis media, septicemia, or meningitis or from healthy carriers. *Infect Immun* 32:311–317, 1981.
45. Andersson B, Gray BM, Dillon HC Jr, et al: Role of adherence of *Streptococcus pneumoniae* in acute otitis media. *Pediatr Infect Dis J* 7:476–480, 1988.
46. Geelen S, Bhattacharyya C, Tuomanen E: The cell wall mediates pneumococcal attachment to and cytopathology in human endothelial cells. *Infect Immun* 61:1538–1543, 1993.
47. Lund E: Laboratory diagnosis of *Pneumococcus* infections. *Bull WHO* 23:5–13, 1960.
48. Lund E, Henrichsen J: Laboratory diagnosis, serology and epidemiology of *Streptococcus pneumoniae*. *Methods Microbiol* 12:242–262, 1978.
49. Bolan G, Broome CV, Facklam RR, et al: Pneumococcal vaccine efficacy in selected populations in the United States. *Ann Intern Med* 104:1–6, 1986.

50. Shapiro ED, Berg AT, Austrian R, et al: The protective efficacy of polyvalent pneumococcal polysaccharide vaccine. *N Engl J Med* 325:1453–1460, 1991.
51. Giebink GS: Immunology: Promise of new vaccine. *Pediatr Infect Dis J* 13:1064–1068, 1994.
52. Briles DE, Crain MJ, Gray BM, et al: Strong association between capsular type and virulence for mice among human isolates of *Streptococcus pneumoniae*. *Infect Immun* 60:111–116, 1992.
53. Kelly T, Dillard JP, Yother J: Effect of genetic switching of capsular type on virulence of *Streptococcus pneumoniae*. *Infect Immun* 62:1813–1819, 1994.
54. Hostetter MK: Serotypic variation among virulent pneumococci in deposition and degradation of covalently bound C3b: Implications for phagocytosis and antibody production. *J Infect Dis* 153:682–693, 1986.
55. Crain MJ, Waltman WD II, Turner JS, et al: Pneumococcal surface protein A (PspA) is serologically highly variable and is expressed by all clinically important capsular serotypes of *Streptococcus pneumoniae*. *Infect Immun* 58:3293–3299, 1990.
56. Gray BM, Cooney EW: Electron microscopic visualization of polysaccharide capsules on whole cell mounts of group B streptococci. *Microscopy Res Tech* 24:455–456, 1993.
57. Waltman WD, Gray BM, Svanborg C, et al: Epidemiologic studies of Group 9 Pneumococci in terms of protein type and 9N versus 9V capsular type. *J Infect Dis* 163:812–818, 1991.
58. Munoz R, Musser JM, Crain M, et al: Geographic distribution of penicillin-resistant clones of *Streptococcus pneumoniae*: Characterization by penicillin-binding protein profile, surface protein A typing, and multilocus enzyme analysis. *Clin Infect Dis* 15:112–118, 1992.
59. Shockman GD, Barrett JF: Structure, function and assembly of gram-positive bacteria. *Ann Rev Microbiol* 37:501–527, 1983.
60. Garcia-Bustos J, Tomasz A: A biological price of antibiotic resistance: Major changes in the peptidoglycan structure of penicillin-resistant pneumococci. *Proc Natl Acad Sci U S A* 87:5415–5419, 1990.
61. Ghuysen JM: Serine β-lactamases and penicillin-binding proteins. *Ann Rev Microbiol* 45:37–67, 1991.
62. Spratt BG: Resistance to antibiotics mediated by target alterations. *Science* 264:388–393, 1994.
63. Selakovitch-Chenu L, Seroude L, Sicard MA: The role of penicillin-binding protein 3 (PBP 3) in cefotaxime resistance in *Streptococcus pneumoniae*. *Mol Gen Genet* 239:77–80, 1993.
64. Ronda C, García JL, García E, et al: Biological role of the pneumococcal amidase. *Eur J Biochem* 164:621–624, 1987.
65. García P, García JL, García E, et al: Purification of the autolytic glycosidase of *Streptococcus pneumoniae*. *Biochem Biophys Res Comm* 158:251–256, 1989.

66. Tomasz A: Penicillin-binding proteins and the antibacterial effectiveness of β-lactam antibiotics. *Rev Infect Dis* 8(suppl 3):S260–S278, 1986.
67. Tuomanen E, Pollack H, Parkinson A, et al: Microbiological and clinical significance of a new property of defective lysis in clinical strains of pneumococci. *J Infect Dis* 158:36, 1988.
68. Díaz E, López R, García JL: Role of the major pneumococcal autolysin in the atypical response of a clinical isolate of *Streptococcus pneumoniae*. *J Bacteriol* 174:5508–5515, 1992.
69. Täuber MG, Burroughs M, Neimöller UM, et al: Differences of pathology in experimental meningitis caused by three strains of Streptococcus pneumoniae. *J Infect Dis* 163:806–811, 1991.
70. Killian M, Mestecky J, Schrohenloher RE: Pathogenic species of the genus *Hemophilus* and *Streptococcus pneumoniae* produce immunoglobulin A1 protease. *Infect Immun* 26:143–149, 1979.
71. Killian M, Mestecky J, Russell MW: Defense mechanisms involving Fc-dependent functions of immunoglobulin A and their subversion by bacterial immunoglobulin A proteases. *Microbiol Rev* 52:296–303, 1988.
72. Berry AM, Lock RA, Thomas SM, et al: Cloning and nucleotide sequence of the *Streptococcus pneumoniae* Hyaluronidase gene and purification of the enzyme from recombinant *Escherichia coli*. *Infect Immun* 62:1101–1108, 1994.
73. Klein PJ, Bulla M, Newman RA, et al: Thomsen-Friedenreich antigen in haemolytic-uremic syndrome. *Lancet* 2:1024–1025, 1977.
74. Seger R, Joller P, Baerlocher K, et al: Hemolytic-uremic syndrome associated with neuraminidase-producing microorganisms: Treatment by exchange transfusion. *Helv Paediat Acta* 35:359–367, 1980.
75. Novak RW, Martin CR: Hemolytic-uremic syndrome and T-cryptantigen exposure by neuraminidase-producing pneumococci: An emerging problem? *Pediatr Pathol* 1:409–413, 1983.
76. Alon U, Adler SP, Chan JCM: Hemolytic-uremic syndrome associated with *Streptococcus pneumoniae*. *Am J Dis Child* 138:496, 1984.
77. Feld LG, Springate JE Jr, Darraugh R, et al: Pneumococcal pneumonia and hemolytic uremic syndrome. *Pediatr Infect Dis J* 6:693–695, 1987.
78. Martinot A, Hue V, Leclerc F, et al: Haemolytic-uraemic syndrome associated with *Streptococcus pneumoniae* meningitis. *Eur J Pediatr* 148:648–649, 1989.
79. Ruuskanen O, Heikkinen T: Viral-bacterial interaction in acute otitis media. *Pediatr Infect Dis J* 13:1047–1049, 1994.
80. Chonmaitree T, Patel JA, Lett-Brown MA, et al: Virus and bacteria enhance histamine production in middle ear fluids of children with otitis media. *J Infect Dis* 169:1265–1270, 1994.
81. Lau AS: Cytokines in the pathogenesis and treatment of infectious diseases. *Adv Pediatr Infect Dis* 9:211–236, 1994.
82. Volanakis JE, Kaplan HM: Specificity of C-reactive protein for choline

phosphate residues of pneumococcal C-polysaccharide. *Proc Natl Acad Sci U S A* 136:612, 1971.

83. Yother J, Volanakis JE, Briles DE: Human C-reactive protein is protective against fatal *Streptococcus pneumoniae* infection in mice. *J Immunol* 128:2374–2376, 1982.

84. Tillett WS, Francis T Jr: Serological reactions in pneumonia with a non-protein somatic fraction of pneumococcus. *J Exp Med* 52:561–571, 1930.

85. Gray BM, Simmons DR, Mason H, et al: Quantitative levels of C-reactive protein in cerebrospinal fluid in patients with bacterial meningitis and other conditions. *J Pediatr* 108:665–670, 1986.

86. Gray BM, Dillon HC Jr, Briles DE: Epidemiological studies of *Streptococcus pneumoniae* in infants: Development of antibody to phosphocholine. *J Clin Microbiol* 18:1102–1107, 1983.

87. Yother J, Forman C, Gray BM, et al: Protection of mice from infection with *Streptococcus pneumoniae* by anti-phosphocholine antibody. *Infect Immun* 36:184–188, 1982.

88. Vitharsson G, Jónsdóttir I, Jónsson S, et al: Opsonization and antibodies to capsular and cell wall polysaccharides of *Streptococcus pneumoniae*. *J Infect Dis* 170:592–599, 1994.

89. Watts RG, Howard TH: Functional disorders of granulocytes and monocytes. In Bick RL (ed): *Hematology: Clinical and Laboratory Practice*. St Louis, Mosby, 1993, pp 1099–1121.

90. Janoff AN, Breiman RF, Daley CL, et al: Pneumococcal disease during HIV infection. *Ann Intern Med* 117:314–324, 1992.

91. Andiman WA, Mezger J, Shapiro E: Invasive bacterial infections in children born to women infected with human immunodeficiency virus type 1. *J Pediatr* 124:846–852, 1994.

92. Farley JJ, King JC, Nair P, et al: Invasive pneumococcal disease among infected and uninfected children of mothers with human immunodeficiency virus infection. *J Pediatr* 124:853–858, 1994.

93. Barnett ED, Klein JO, Pelton SI, et al: Otitis media in children born to human immunodeficiency virus-infected mothers. *Pediatr Infect Dis J* 11:360–364, 1992.

94. Nims L, Hatch K, Gallaher M, et al: Hemorrhage and shock associated with invasive pneumococcal infection in healthy infants and children—New Mexico, 1993–1994. *MMWR* 43:949–952, 1995.

95. Dowson CG, Hutchinson A, Brannifan JA, et al: Horizontal transfer of penicillin-binding protein genes in penicillin-resistant clinical isolates of *Streptococcus pneumoniae*. *Proc Natl Acad Sci U S A* 86:8842–8846, 1989.

96. Soares S, Kristinsson KG, Musser JM, et al: Evidence for the introduction of a multiresistant clone of serotype 6B *Streptococcus pneumoniae* from Spain to Iceland in the late 1980's. *J Infect Dis* 168:158–163, 1993.

97. Sibold C, Wang J, Henrichsen J, et al: Genetic relationships of

penicillin-susceptible and -resistant *Streptococcus pneumoniae* strains isolated on different continents. *Infect Immun* 60:4119–4126, 1992.

98. McDougal LK, Facklam R, Reeves M, et al: Analysis of multiply antimicrobial-resistant isolates of *Streptococcus pneumoniae* from the United States. *Antimicrob Agents Chemother* 36:2176–2184, 1992.

99. Baquero F, Martínez-Beltrán J, Loza E: A review of antibiotic resistance patterns of *Streptococcus pneumoniae* in Europe. *J Antimicrob Chemother* 28:31–38, 1991.

100. Spanjaard L, Westra M, Caron HN, et al: Meningitis due to a multiply resistant *Streptococcus pneumoniae* in a child in the Netherlands. *Scand J Infect Dis* 24:117–118, 1992.

101. Willett LD, Dillon HC Jr, Gray BM: Penicillin-intermediate pneumococci in a children's hospital. *Am J Dis Child* 139:1054–1057, 1985.

102. Tan TQ, Mason EO, Kaplan SL: Penicillin-resistant systemic pneumococcal infections in children: A retrospective case-controlled study. *Pediatrics* 92:761–767, 1993.

103. Nava JM, Bella F, Garau J, et al: Predictive factors for invasive disease due to penicillin-resistant *Streptococcus pneumoniae*: A population-based study. *Clin Infect Dis* 19:884–890, 1994.

104. Orange M, Gray BM: Pneumococcal serotypes causing disease in children in Alabama. *Pediatr Infect Dis J* 12:244–246, 1993.

105. Block S, Hedrick J, Wright P, et al: Drug-resistant *Streptococcus pneumoniae* Kentucky and Tennessee, 1993. *MMWR* 43:23–25, 31, 1994.

106. Haglund LA, Istre GR, Pickett DA, et al: Invasive pneumococcal disease in Central Oklahoma: Emergence of high-level penicillin resistance and multiple antibiotic resistance. *J Infect Dis* 168:1532–1536, 1993.

107. Welby PL, Keller DS, Cromien JL, et al: Resistance to penicillin and non-beta-lactam antibiotics of *Streptococcus pneumoniae* at a children's hospital. *Pediatr Infect Dis J* 13:281–287, 1994.

108. Caillaud F, Trieu-Cuot P, Carlier C, et al: Nucleotide sequence of the kanamycin resistance determinant of the pneumococcal transposon Tn545: Evolutionary relationships and transcriptional analysis of *aphA-3* genes. *Mol Gen Genet* 207:509–513, 1987.

109. Harakeh H, Bosley GS, Keihlbaugh JA, et al: Heterogeneity of rRNA gene restriction patterns of multiresistant serotype 6B *Streptococcus pneumoniae* Strains. *J Clin Microbiol* 32:3046–3048, 1994.

110. Negri MC, Morosini MI, Loza E, et al: In vitro selective concentrations of β-lactams for penicillin-resistant *Streptococcus pneumoniae*. *Antimicrob Agents Chemother* 38:122–125, 1994.

111. Muñoz M, Valderrabanos ES, Diaz E, et al: Appearance of resistance to beta-lactam antibiotics during the treatment in *Streptococcus pneumoniae* meningitis. *J Pediatr* 127:98–99, 1995.

112. Moreillon P, Markiewicz Z, Nachman S, et al: Two bacterial targets for penicillin in pneumococci: Autolysis-dependent and autolysis-

independent killing mechanisms. *Antimicrob Agents Chemother* 34:33–39, 1990.

113. Moreillon P, Tomasz A: Penicillin resistance and defective lysis in clinical isolates of pneumococci: Evidence for two kinds of antibiotic pressure operating in the clinical environment. *J Infect Dis* 157:1150, 1988.

114. Reynolds PE: Structure, biochemistry and mechanism of action of glycopeptide antibiotics. *Eur J Clin Microbiol Infect Dis* 8:943–950, 1989.

115. Billot-Klein D, Gutmann L, Collatz E, et al: Analysis of peptidoglycan precursors in vancomycin-resistant Enterococci. *Antimicrob Agents Chemother* 36:1487–1490, 1992.

116. Robins-Brown RM, Gaspar MN, Ward JI, et al: Resistance mechanisms of multiply resistant pneumococci: Antibiotic degradation patterns. *Antimicrob Agents Chemother* 15:470–474, 1979.

117. Istre GR, Humphreys JT, Albrecht KD, et al: Chloramphenicol and penicillin resistance in pneumococci isolated from blood and cerebrospinal fluid: A prevalence study in metropolitan Denver. *J Clin Microbiol* 17:472–475, 1983.

118. Piddock LJV: New Quinolones and gram-positive bacteria. *Antimicrob Agents Chemother* 38:163–169, 1994.

119. Mason EO, Kaplan SL, Lamberth LB, et al: Increased rate of isolation of penicillin-resistant *Streptococcus pneumoniae* in a children's hospital and in vitro susceptibilities to antibiotics of potential therapeutic use. *Antimicrob Agents Chemother* 36:1703–1707, 1992.

120. Howie VM: The "in vivo susceptibility test"—bacteriology of middle ear exudate, during antimicrobial therapy in otitis media. *Pediatrics* 44:940–944, 1969.

121. Cooksey RC, Facklam RR, Thornsberry C: Antimicrobial susceptibility patterns of *Streptococcus pneumoniae*. *Antimicrob Agents Chemother* 13:654–648, 1978.

122. Jorgensen JH, Swenson JM, Tenover FC, et al: Development of interpretive criteria and quality control limits for broth microdilution and disk diffusion antimicrobial susceptibility testing of *Streptococcus pneumoniae*. *J Clin Microbiol* 32:2448–2459, 1994.

123. National Committee for Clinical Laboratory Standards: Performance standards for antimicrobial susceptibility testing. Fifth informational supplement M100–S5. Villanova, Penn, National Committee for Clinical Laboratory Standards, 1994.

124. Swenson JM, Hill BC, Thornsberry C: Screening pneumococci for penicillin resistance. *J Clin Microbiol* 24:749–752, 1986.

125. Dowson CG, Johnson AP, Cercenado E, et al: Genetics of oxacillin resistance in clinical isolates of *Streptococcus pneumoniae* that are oxacillin resistant and penicillin susceptible. *Antimicrob Agents Chemother* 38:49–53, 1994.

126. Friedland IR, Shelton S, McCracken GH Jr: Screening for

cephalosporin-resistant *Streptococcus pneumoniae* with the Kirby-Bauer disk susceptibility test. *J Clin Microbiol* 31:1619–1621, 1993.

127. Jacobs MR, Bajaksouzian S, Appelbaum PC, et al: Evaluation of the E-test for susceptibility testing of pneumococci. *Diagn Microbiol Infect Dis* 15:473–478, 1992.

128. Clark RB, Giger O, Mortensen JE: Comparison of susceptibility test methods to detect penicillin-resistant *Streptococcus pneumoniae*. *Diagn Microbiol Infect Dis* 17:213–217, 1993.

129. Macias EA, Mason EO, Ocera HY, et al: Comparison of E test with standard broth microdilution for determining antibiotic susceptibilities of penicillin-resistant strains of *Streptococcus pneumoniae*. *J Clin Microbiol* 32:430–432, 1994.

130. Krisher KK, Linscott A: Comparison of three commercial MIC systems, E test, fastidious antimicrobial susceptibility panel, and FOX fastidious panel, for confirmation of penicillin and cephalosporin resistance in *Streptococcus pneumoniae*. *J Clin Microbiol* 32:2242–2245, 1994.

131. Friedland IR, Shelton S, McCracken GH Jr: Chloramphenicol in penicillin-resistant pneumococcal meningitis. *Lancet* 324:240–241, 1993.

132. Walker CW, Brown DFJ: A rapid technique for detection of resistance to chloramphenicol in *Streptococcus pneumoniae* and comparison with minimum inhibitory concentration and disk diffusion methods. *J Med Microbiol* 31:133–136, 1990.

133. Foster JA, McGowen KL: Rising rate of pneumococcal bacteremia at the Children's Hospital of Philadelphia. *Pediatr Infect Dis J* 13:1143–1144, 1994.

134. Ristuccia AM, LeFrock JL: Cerebrospinal fluid penetration of antimicrobials. *Antibiot Chemother* 45:118–152, 1992.

135. John CC: Treatment failure with use of a third-generation cephalosporin for penicillin-resistant pneumococcal meningitis: Case report and review. *Clin Infect Dis* 18:188–193, 1994.

136. Kleiman MB, Weinberg GA, Reynolds JK, et al: Meningitis with beta-lactam-resistant *Streptococcus pneumoniae*: The need for early repeat lumbar puncture. *Pediatr Infect Dis J* 12:782–784, 1993.

137. Dillon HC Jr, Bridges RA, Null WA, et al: Erythropoietic changes associated with chloramphenicol therapy. *Ala J Med Sci* 1:368–375, 1964.

138. Klugman KP: Activity of teicoplanin and vancomycin against penicillin-resistant pneumococci. *Eur J Clin Microbiol Infect Dis* 13:1–2, 1994.

139. Wallace MR, Mascola JR, Oldfield EC: Red man syndrome: incidence, etiology and prophylaxis. *J Infect Dis* 164:1180–1185, 1991.

140. Cartú TG, Yamanak-Yuen NA, Lietman PS: Serum vancomycin concentrations: Reappraisal of their clinical value. *Clin Infect Dis* 19:533–543, 1180–1182 (correspondence), 1994.

141. Asensi F, Otero MC, Pérez-Tamarit D: Risk/benefit in the treatment of

children with imipenem-cilastatin for meningitis caused by penicillin-resistant pneumococcus. *J Chemother* 5:133–134, 1993.

142. Wong VK, Wright HTJ, Ross LA, et al: Imipenem/cilastatin treatment of bacterial meningitis in children. *Pediatr Infect Dis J* 10:122–125, 1991.

143. Ballard TL, Roe MH, Wheeler RC, et al: Comparison of three latex agglutination kits and counterimmunoelectrophoresis for the detection of bacterial antigens in a pediatric population. *Pediatr Infect Dis J* 6:630–634, 1987.

144. Maxson S, Lewno MJ, Schutze GE: Clinical usefulness of cerebrospinal fluid bacterial antigen studies. *J Pediatr* 125:235–238, 1994.

145. Virolainen A, Salo O, Jero J, et al: Comparison of PCR assay with bacterial culture for detecting *Streptococcus pneumoniae* in middle ear fluid of children with otitis media. *J Clin Microbiol* 32:2667–2670, 1994.

146. Leggiadro RJ, Davis Y, Tenover FC: Outpatient drug-resistant pneumococcal bacteremia. *Pediatr Infect Dis J* 13:1144–1146, 1994.

147. Tan TQ, Mason EO Jr, Kaplan SL: Systemic infections due to *Streptococcus pneumoniae* relatively resistant to penicillin in a Children's Hospital: Clinical management and outcome. *Pediatrics* 90:928–933, 1992.

148. Musher DM: Pneumococcal pneumonia including diagnosis and therapy of infections caused by penicillin resistant strains. *Infect Dis Clin North Am* 5:509–521, 1991.

149. Marchant CD, Carlin SA, Johnson CE, et al: Measuring the comparative efficacy of antibacterial agents for acute otitis media: The "Pollyanna phenomenon." *J Pediatr* 120:72–77, 1992.

150. Green SM, Rothrock SG: Single-dose intramuscular ceftriaxone for acute otitis media in children. *Pediatrics* 91:23–30, 1993.

151. Friedland IA: Cefixime therapy for otitis media. *Pediatr Infect Dis J* 12:544–545, 1993.

152. Workman MR, Layton M, Hussein M, et al: Nasal carriage of penicillin-resistant pneumococcus in sickle-cell patients. *Lancet* 342:746–747, 1993.

153. Cherian T, Steinhoff MC, Harrison LH, et al: A cluster of invasive pneumococcal disease in young children in child care. *JAMA* 271:695–697, 1994.

154. Reichler MR, Allphin AA, Breiman RF, et al: The spread of resistant *Streptococcus pneumoniae* at a day care center in Ohio. *J Infect Dis* 166:1346–1353, 1992.

155. Shurin PA, Rehmus JM, Johnson CA, et al: Bacterial polysaccharide immune globulin for prophylaxis of acute otitis media in high risk children. *J Pediatr* 123:801–810, 1993.

156. Gray BM: Immune globulin administration as an approach to prevention of acute otitis media. *J Pediatr* 123:739–741, 1993.

Foodborne and Waterborne Illness in Children

Idalia R. Rivera-Matos, M.D.
Fellow, Pediatric Infectious Diseases, University of Texas–Houston Health Science Center, Department of Pediatrics, Infectious Disease Division, Houston, Texas

Thomas G. Cleary, M.D.
Professor of Pediatrics, Director, Pediatric Infectious Diseases, University of Texas–Houston Health Science Center, Department of Pediatrics, Infectious Diseases Division, Houston, Texas

R egulations for the control of foodborne and waterborne illness have been in place since the beginning of the century in the United States.[1] Since 1961, the Center for Disease Control (CDC) has been responsible for investigation, control, and prevention of diseases spread by food and water. Reports are submitted to the CDC voluntarily; it is thought that the reported outbreaks are a small fraction of the outbreaks that occur.

Between 1986 and 1992, 202 outbreaks with 52,105 cases due to contaminated water were reported.[2–4] During the period 1983 to 1987, the CDC reported 2,397 foodborne outbreaks with 91,678 cases and 137 fatalities.[5] Waterborne and foodborne gastrointestinal illness worldwide accounts for much of the mortality due to diarrheal illness, estimated at 6 million deaths per year in children living in Asia, Africa, and Latin America.[6]

The economic impact of foodborne and waterborne outbreaks is severe. It is estimated that $1 to $10 billion is spent in the United States every year for treatment, diagnosis, and epidemiologic investigations of foodborne diseases.[1, 7]

EPIDEMIOLOGY

An outbreak of a foodborne or waterborne disease can be defined by the occurrence of illness in at least two persons with similar clinical symptoms after consumption of contaminated food or water.[3, 5] Factors contributing to outbreaks of foodborne illness include improper storage (ambient temperature), inadequate cooling or reheating, poor personal hygiene of the food handler, undercook-

TABLE 1.

Vehicles Associated With Foodborne Outbreaks Reported by the Centers for Disease Control During 1983–1987*†

Agent	Beef	Ham	Pork	Chicken	Turkey	Sausage	Milk	Cheese
Salmonella spp	+++	+	+	+++	+++	+	+	+
Staphylococcus aureus	+	++	+	0	+	0	0	0
Shigella spp	0	0	0	++	0	0	0	0
Clostridium botulinum	+	0	0	0	+	0	0	0
Bacillus cereus	+	+	+	0	0	0	0	0
Campylobacter spp	0	0	0	+	0	0	+++	0
Clostridium perfringes	+	0	0	+	+	0	0	0
Escherichia coli	+	0	0	0	0	0	0	0
Brucella spp	0	0	0	0	0	0	0	+
Streptococcus (Group A)	0	0	0	0	0	0	0	0
Other streptococci	0	0	0	0	0	0	0	+
Vibrio parahemolyticus	0	0	0	0	0	0	0	0
Trichinella	+	0	+++	0	0	0	0	0
Giardia	0	0	0	0	0	0	0	0
Hepatitis A	0	+	0	0	0	0	0	0
Norwalk virus	0	0	0	0	0	0	0	0

ing, raw food consumption, cross contamination, and contaminated processing or packaging of food.[8] Certain foods are associated with specific pathogens (Table 1). For example, fried rice is the leading cause of *Bacillus cereus* food poisoning in the United States.[9] Ham was the most frequently incriminated vehicle for *Staphylococcus* food poisoning during 1977 to 1981.[10] Outbreaks of *Escherichia coli* 0157:H7 have been associated with consumption of undercooked hamburger and raw milk. Ciguatera poisoning has been associated with ingestion of snappers, amber jacks,

Eggs	Ice Cream	Shell-fish	Fruits/ Veg.	Potato Salad	Chinese Food	Mexican Food	Baked Foods	Fried Rice
+++	+	+	++	+	0	+	+	0
+	0	+	+	+	0	0	+	0
+	0	+	+	+	0	+	0	+
0	0	0	+++	+	0	+	0	0
0	0	+	+	0	+	0	0	+
0	0	0	+	0	+	0	0	0
0	0	0	0	0	0	++	0	0
+	0	0	0	0	0	+	0	0
0	0	0	+	0	0	0	0	0
0	0	0	0	+	0	0	0	0
0	0	0	0	0	0	0	0	0
0	0	+	0	0	0	0	0	0
0	0	0	0	0	0	0	0	0
0	0	0	+	0	0	0	0	0
0	0	0	+	0	0	0	0	0
+	0	+	0	0	0	0	0	0

*Data from Bean NH, Griffin PM, Goulding JS, et al: *MMWR* 39:SS–1; 1–57, 1990.
†0 = no outbreaks;
+ = occasional (between 1 and 4 outbreaks);
++ = frequent (between 5 and 8 outbreaks);
+++ = common (>9 outbreaks).

TABLE 2.
Clinical Characteristics of Foodborne and Waterborne Infectious Agents*

Usual Incubation Period	Diarrhea		Vomiting	Fever	Causative Agent	Laboratory Diagnostic Test
	Watery	Bloody				
1–6 hr	++	—	+++	—	Staphylococcus aureus	Detection of 10^5 S. aureus or B. cereus enterotoxin in food
	+	—	+++	—	Bacillus cereus (emetic)	
	+++	—	+	—	B. cereus (diarrheal)	
7–14 hr	+++	—	+	+	Clostridium perfringes	Detection of 10^5 organism/g in food or stools in ill persons
16–36 hr	+++	+++	++	+++	Shigella spp.	Isolation of the organism in food or stools of ill persons
	+++	+++	++	+++	Salmonella spp.	
	+++	+++	++	+++	EIEC	
	+++	+++	++	+++	Yersinia enterocolitica	
12–36 hr	—	—	—	—	Clostridium botulinum	Confirmation of botulism toxin in serum, gastric or feces or isolation of Clostridium botulinum in stools of ill persons
	(Diploplia, dry mouth, dysarthria, disturbance in vision)					

16–72 hr	+++	—	+++	++	ETEC	Isolation of the organism in food or stools of ill persons
	+++	++	++	+	*Vibrio parahaemolyticus*	
	+++	—	++	+	*Vibrio cholerae*	
24–48 hr	+++	—	+++	+	Norwalk virus	Immune electron microscopy; fourfold increase in serum antibody; viral antigen detection; RT-PCR (investigational)
3–5 days	+++	+++	++	+	EHEC (e.g., *E. coli* 0157:H7)	Isolation of the organism in food or stools
1–7 days	+	+++	++	++	*Campylobacter jejuni*	Isolation of the organism in food or stools of ill persons
2–14 days	+++	—	+++	+	*Cryptosporidium parvum*	Detection of organism in the stools of ill persons by modified acid-fast stains

(continued)

TABLE 2 (continued).
Clinical Characteristics of Foodborne and Waterborne Infectious Agents*

Usual Incubation Period	Diarrhea		Vomiting	Fever	Causative Agent	Laboratory Diagnostic Test
	Watery	Bloody				
	+++	—	—	—	*Giardia lamblia*	Detection of trophozoite or cyst in the stools or duodenal aspirates, or detection of *Giardia* antigens in these specimens by enzyme immunoassay
	+++	—	++	+	*Trichinella spiralis*	Muscle biopsy; fourfold increase in serum antibody
1–70 days	+	—	+	+++	*Listeria monocytogenes*	Isolation of the organisms from normally sterile body fluids
3–6 wk	— (Jaundice, malaise, anorexia)	—	++	+++	Hepatitis A	Serologic tests

*— = rarely or never reported; + = occasionally reported; ++ = common finding; +++ = typical feature; EIEC = enteroinvasive *Escherichia coli*; ETEC = enterotoxigenic *E. coli*; RT-PCR = reverse transcription–polymerase chain reaction; EHEC = enterohemmorlogic *E. coli*.

TABLE 3.
Foodborne Disease Outbreaks With Confirmed Etiology*

	No. of Outbreaks	% of Outbreaks	Cases	Deaths
Bacteria				
Salmonella spp.	342	57.3	31,245	39
Shigella spp.	44	18.3	9,971	2
Staphylococcus aureus	47	5.8	3,181	0
Clostridium perfringens	24	5.0	2,743	2
Group A *Streptococcus*	7	1.8	1,001	0
Campylobacter spp.	28	1.3	727	1
Escherichia coli	7	1.1	640	4
Bacillus cereus	16	0.5	261	0
Listeria monocytogenes	2	0.4	201	70
Clostridium botulinum	74	0.2	140	10
Other streptococci	2	0.1	85	3
Brucella spp.	2	0.1	38	1
Vibrio parahaemolyticus	3	<0.1	11	0
Vibrio cholerae	1	<0.1	2	0
Other bacteria	1	0.1	58	0
Parasites				
Giardia lamblia	3	<0.1	41	0
Trichinella spiralis	33	0.3	162	1
Viruses				
Hepatitis A	29	1.9	1,067	1
Norwalk	10	2.1	1,164	0
Other viruses	2	1.0	558	0
Chemicals/toxins				
Ciguatoxin	87	1.0	332	0
Scombrotoxin	83	0.5	306	0
Heavy metal	13	0.3	176	0
Mushrooms	14	<0.1	49	2
Monosodium glutamate	2	<0.1	7	0
Paralytic shellfish poisoning	2	<0.1	3	0
Other poisoning syndromes	31	0.7	371	1
TOTAL	909	100	54,540	137

*Data from Bean NH, Griffin PM, Gonlding JS, et al: *MMWR* 39:SS−1; 1−57, 1990.

barracuda, grouper, and parrot fish species.[11] Eggs and eggs-containing food have been the most important cause of *Salmonella enteritidis* outbreaks in the United States.[12] Contaminated goat cheese has been related to infection with *Brucella* spp.[5] Chitterlings are frequently the source of *Yersinia enterocolitica* infections.

The causes for waterborne outbreaks differ for community and noncommunity water systems.[13] Community public water systems include public and investor-owned water systems that serve mu-

TABLE 4.

Waterborne Disease Outbreaks With Confirmed Cause Associated With Water Intended for Drinking*†

	No. of Outbreaks	Cases	% of Outbreaks
Bacteria			
Salmonella spp.	2	70	4.1
Shigella spp.	5	2,883	10.2
Campylobacter spp.	1	250	2.0
Escherichia coli (EHEC)	1	243	2.0
Cyanobacteria‡	1	21	2.0
Parasites			
Giardia lamblia	20	1,989	40.8
Cryptosporidium parvum	3	16,551	8.2
Viruses			
Norwalk	1	135	2.0
Norwalk-like	3	6,239	6.0
Hepatitis A	3	35	6.0
Chemicals			
Sodium hydroxide	1	11	2.0
Fluoride	2	314	4.0
Nitrate	2	2	4.0
Ethylene glycol	1	29	2.0
Alkaline water	2	11	4.0
CGI	1	72	2.0

*Adapted from Levine WC, Stephenson WT, Craun GF: *MMWR* 39:SS–1; 1–13, 1990; Herwaldt BL, Craun GF, Stokes SL, et al: *MMWR* 40:SS–3; 1–22, 1991; Moore AC, Herwaldt BL, Craun GF, et al: *MMWR* 42:SS–5; 1–22, 1993.

†EHEC = Enterohemorrhagic *E. coli*; CGI = chronic gastrointestinal illness of unknown cause.

‡It has been suggested that these organisms belong to the genus *Cyclospora*.

nicipalities. Inadequate disinfection of surface water, contamination of water in the distribution system due to cross connections, repairs of mains, and failure of filtration systems have been associated with outbreaks in community systems. Noncommunity public water systems are generally wells and springs used by one or several residences or by persons traveling outside populated areas, including parks or camps.[2] Contaminated, untreated, and inadequately disinfected groundwater have been the major factors responsible for these outbreaks. Outbreaks of disease due to recreational water occur after unintentional ingestion or contamination of skin and mucous membranes. Wound or skin infection caused by water-related organisms are usually excluded from the reports of outbreaks.

Geographic considerations are also relevant to food poisoning syndromes. Coastal regions have been associated with *Vibrio* infections (including *Vibrio parahemolyticus*), scombroid fish poisoning, and paralytic shellfish poisoning.[14] *Yersinia enterocolitica* is most prevalent in cooler areas, including Finland, Canada, and the north-central United States.

The inoculum size of the pathogen required to cause infection is an important element in the development of disease. Ten to 1,000 oocysts are needed to cause *Cryptosporidium* infection.[6] Less than 10 cysts of *Giardia* spp. are thought to be the infectious dose. Shigella species can cause illness with ingestion of as few as 10 viable organisms.[15] However, many other pathogens require higher inocula to produce foodborne or waterborne illness. *Vibrio cholerae* requires ingestion of approximately 10 million organisms to cause disease. In healthy adults *Salmonella* spp. require an infective dose of at least 1 million organisms; in very young children and elderly persons fewer organisms (between 10 and 100 bacteria) probably can cause illness.[7]

The interval between exposure and symptoms sometimes suggest a cause. The appearance of symptoms in less than 1 hour after ingestion of contaminated food or water is typically caused by a chemical intoxication. Symptoms occurring after an incubation period of 1 to 7 hours are most often caused by *Staphylococcus* poisoning. Those between 8 and 14 hours are likely to be caused by *Clostridium perfringens* food poisoning. After 14 hours, other agents are more likely (Table 2). Many illnesses occur in which the cause is not defined.

Surveillance summaries for foodborne and waterborne illness with known etiologic agents reported by the CDC are summarized in Tables 3 and 4.

ETIOLOGIC AGENTS AND RELATED CLINICAL FEATURES

Summary of the major agents follow.

BACTERIAL PATHOGENS OR TOXINS

Salmonella

Salmonella spp. have been a leading cause of bacterial foodborne disease worldwide. There were 342 outbreaks of salmonellosis foodborne with 31,245 cases during 1983 to 1987 in the United States (see Table 3). Animals (cows, pigs, sheep, cats, dogs, hamsters, mice, turtles, snakes, ducks, geese, chickens, turkeys, doves, pigeons, and parrots) provide the natural reservoir for nontyphoidal salmonella. Contaminated milk, pork, poultry, and eggs have been implicated in many outbreaks. Although *Salmonella* spp. have been transmitted in waterborne outbreaks,[16] through contact with infected animals[17, 18] via person-to-person transmission[19] and by contact with contaminated medications or medical instruments,[20, 21] the main mode of transmission has been ingestion of contaminated food, so-called *Salmonella* food poisoning.

There are three species of *Salmonella*: *Salmonella typhi*, *Salmonella cholerae-suis*, and *S. enteritidis*. Most of the 2,000 serotypes belong to the *S. enteritidis* species. *Salmonella typhimurium* was the most common *Salmonella* serotype isolated from outbreaks during the early 1980s in the United States; however, it has declined, and presently *S. enteritidis* is the most frequent serotype. This change has been attributed to contamination of shell eggs with *S. enteritidis*.[12]

Five clinical syndromes have been recognized in persons with *Salmonella* infection: asymptomatic infection (including the carrier state), enteric fever, gastroenteritis, bacteremia, and focal infections. The gastrointestinal illness is the most common of these syndromes. The symptoms of *Salmonella* gastroenteritis are caused by mucosal invasion and inflammation.[22] Nausea, vomiting, crampy abdominal pain, myalgia, headaches, and fever usually occur. The stools often contain white blood cells and blood.[15] The illness is often self-limited with resolution in 5 to 7 days in the absence of antibiotic therapy. Persons in certain high-risk groups can have a more severe and prolonged illness. Blood cultures can be positive in up to 10% of such cases. High-risk persons include infants less than 3 months of age, human immunodeficiency virus (HIV)–infected individuals, and other immunocompromised hosts. Antimicrobial therapy is not required for uncomplicated gastroenteritis. Therapy causes no clinical improvement and can prolong the excretion of the organisms. Antimicrobial therapy is usually recommended for high-risk patients, although it is of unproven efficacy and benefit. Ampicillin, trimethoprim-sulfamethoxazole (TMP-SMX), ceftriaxone, or cefotaxime can be used in high-risk hosts, those for whom therapy is recommended. Susceptibility testing should guide therapy. *Salmonella* spp. are susceptible to the fluoroquinolones, but these agents are rarely used in pediatric populations because of concerns about damage to growing cartilage. Multiple resistant *Salmonella* spp. have been a major problem in developing countries due to widespread use of over-the-counter antimicrobials.

Shigella

Shigella spp. were the second most common cause of bacterial foodborne illnesses reported by the CDC from 1983 to 1987 and the leading cause in bacterial waterborne outbreaks during 1986 to 1992 in the United States (see Tables 3 and 4). There are four species: *Shigella dysenteriae* (serogroup A), *Shigella flexneri* (serogroup B), *Shigella boydii* (serogroup C), and *Shigella sonnei* (serogroup D).

Although this pathogen has been reported in contaminated food and water, the principal mode of transmission is person-to-person contact. There is no known animal reservoir. *Shigella* is capable of surviving in foods such as milk, whole eggs, flour, and shrimp for up to 30 days.[23] Foods incriminated in *Shigella* outbreaks in the United States include shellfish, fruits, vegetables, chicken, potato salad, fried rice, and Mexican food.[5]

Outbreaks of shigellosis have been reported in summer camps for the mentally handicapped, among institutionalized persons, and on cruise ships where overcrowded conditions exist.[24-26] Waterborne outbreaks have been related to ingestion of water contaminated with human waste during swimming or bathing.[27]

Clinical manifestations include an abrupt onset with high fever, toxic appearance, and crampy abdominal pain. Profuse watery diarrhea may be followed by small amount of mucous and bloody stools whose passage is associated with urgency and tenesmus. Antimicrobial therapy of susceptible *Shigella* strains dramatically shortens the duration of diarrhea, fever, and period of communicability. The choice of antimicrobial therapy can be difficult due to the frequency of antibiotic-resistant strains. Nalidixic acid, TMP-SMX, oxyquinolones, ceftriaxone, and cefixime are considered adequate empirical therapy, but susceptibility testing is recommended for all isolates; antimicrobial therapy is usually modified based on susceptibility and clinical response. Complications of shigellosis include rectal prolapse, seizures, leukemoid reaction, hemolytic uremic syndrome, and Reiter's syndrome. Strict attention to hand washing and personal hygiene is necessary to prevent spread of shigellosis.

Staphylococcus aureus

Preformed enterotoxins A to E have been related to enteric disease. Type A has been responsible for more than half of the reported outbreaks of staphylococcal food poisoning in the United States.[10] Forty-seven *Staphylococcus* outbreaks with 3,181 cases were reported to the CDC during a recent 5-year period. However, because the symptoms are self-limited and of short duration, the disease is probably underreported.

The growth of *Staphylococcus* is favored by the high-sugar, -salt, and -protein contents found in dairy products, egg salads, fish, poultry, and cream-filled foods.[28] Asymtomatic individuals carrying *Staphylococcus* on skin or nose can contaminate foods during preparation.

The illness is characterized by vomiting, diarrhea, and abdominal pain without fever lasting less than 24 hours. A minimum of 1 ng of toxin/g of food is thought to be required to cause clinical symptoms.

Staphylococcal illness can be prevented by good hygiene (to avoid contamination during preparation and handling) and by keeping high-risk foods refrigerated until served.[28]

Clostridium perfringes

Clostridium perfringes was the fourth most common cause of foodborne outbreaks in the United States during 1983 to 1987. *Clostridium perfringes* is a gram-positive, anaerobic, spore-forming bacillus. The spores can survive high temperatures during initial cooking and can germinate during the cooling process. The organism can multiply if food is held at temperatures between 15.6° C and 51.7° C.[29] If the food is ingested without appropriate reheating, the enterotoxin is not destroyed.

In Europe and the United States meat and meat products are the principal foods associated with outbreaks.[5, 30] There are five strains of *C. perfringes* (A–E). Type A has been responsible for all cases of foodborne illness.[30] *Clostridium perfringes* type C causes necrotic enteritis ("pig bel") in malnourished children living in New Guinea who ingest undercooked pig meat.[31]

The onset of symptoms begins with watery diarrhea and severe crampy abdominal pain. Fever, nausea, and vomiting are unusual. *Clostridium* "food poisoning" is a self-limited disease and requires no therapy. Mortality has been commonly associated with *C. perfringes* type C in Papua New Guinea.

Clostridium botulinum

There are seven toxin types (A–G) and three syndromes described with *Clostridium botulinum:* foodborne botulism, wound botulism, and infant botulism. *Clostridium botulinum* type E, the most common toxin type, is usually associated with fish consumption, especially in Alaska and Canada, where fishborne botulism is common.[11] Improper preparation of home-preserved canned vegetables has been the main cause of intoxication in the rest of North America.[30]

Honey has been implicated in cases of infant botulism in California.[32] As little as 0.1 g of a food contaminated with the organism contains enough neurotoxin to produce illness. The incubation period is usually between 12 and 36 hours but can be as long as 8 days, depending on the dose of toxin ingested.[30]

Initial symptoms include acute symmetric descending flaccid paralysis with initial involvement of the cranial nerves but without sensory involvement. Common symptoms include diplopia, dry mouth, dysarthria, and disturbances in vision. Infant botulism occurs in children younger than 6 months old and is accompanied by lethargy, weak cry, poor feeding, constipation, generalized weakness, subtle ocular palsies, and hypotonia.[33]

For foodborne botulism, emetic and gastric lavage can be beneficial in reducing the amount of toxin absorbed. The trivalent antitoxin (types A, B, and E) is considered part of therapy for foodborne and wound botulism and needs to be given as soon as possible. The antitoxin is of equine origin, so hypersensitivity reactions occur in up to 20% of the cases.[33] Infant botulism is managed with supportive care only.

Escherichia coli

There are five categories of diarrheogenic *E. coli* that cause foodborne and waterborne diseases and are defined by specific virulence properties: enteropathogenic *E. coli* (EPEC), enteroinvasive *E. coli* (EIEC), enterotoxigenic *E. coli* (ETEC), enterohemorrhagic *E. coli* (EHEC), and enteroaggregative *E. coli* (EAggEC).

The EPEC has been associated with outbreaks of infantile diarrhea, which often have occurred in hospital nurseries and in communities.[34] Although an uncommon cause of diarrhea in areas with good hygiene such as the United States, EPEC has been an important cause of acute and chronic diarrhea in the first 2 years of life in developing countries. Contaminated food and water have been the cause of outbreaks.[34] The disease usually peaks in the summer months. The mechanism of disease relates to specific "attaching and effacing" adherence of the organisms to intestinal epithelial cells and damage to the microvilli.[35]

The most common cause of travelers' diarrhea, ETEC,[36, 37] produces two types of enterotoxins: a low molecular weight heat-stable toxin and a high molecular weight heat-labile toxin (which resembles cholera toxin). Diarrhea is caused by ingestion of contaminated food or water rather than person-to-person spread. Illness in the United States may occur after the travelers return from high-risk areas, including southern Asia, the Middle East, Africa, and Latin America.[36] The microorganisms have been isolated from tap water and ice.[36] The diarrhea is watery and associated with crampy abdominal pain, nausea, vomiting, and malaise. High fever is uncommon. Antimicrobial prophylaxis is not recommended for pediatric patients.[38] Although antimicrobial use has been demonstrated to shorten the duration of the illness,[37] the diarrhea is self-limited, and oral rehydration is considered the treatment of choice. A 5-day course of TMP-SMX or furazolidone has been shown to shorten the duration of illness in pediatrics cases.[35] Ciprofloxacin is effective in adolescents and young adults.

The EIEC produces an invasive, dysenteric illness. It shares identical (or nearly identical) virulence genes with *Shigella*. Although person-to-person transmission can occur, EIEC is 10,000-fold less infectious than *Shigella*, so foodborne and waterborne disease rather than person-to-person spread is more common.[35] A major outbreak (involving 387 people) was described in 1971 in the United States related to the consumption of contaminated Brie and Camembert cheeses.[34] The typical symptoms include watery diarrhea, followed by bloody, mucousy stools, high fever, severe abdominal pain, vomiting, and a toxic appearance. If EIEC is suspected, TMP-SMX can be used. An oral third-generation cephalosporin is an alternative to TMP-SMX.[39] However, multiresistant EIEC is common.[35]

The EHEC produces *Shiga*-like toxins (also called verotoxins). More than 50 different EHEC serotypes have been described.[40] Serotype *E. coli* 0157:H7 has been the cause of major foodborne outbreaks of hemorrhagic colitis and hemolytic uremic syndrome in the United States.[41] A multistate foodborne outbreak of *E. coli* 0157:H7 occurred in the western United States from Nov. 15, 1992 through Feb. 28, 1993 and involved 583 cases with 171 patients requiring hospitalization and 4 fatalities.[42] Clusters of the illness occurred in Washington, Idaho, Nevada, and California. The illness was traced to hamburger from a fast-food restaurant chain. Illness due to home-cooked hamburger has also been reported.[43] Other food vehicles associated with outbreaks of *E. coli* 0157:H7 include roast beef, unpasteurized milk, and apple cider.[42, 44, 45] The first waterborne outbreak associated with this pathogen was reported in a Missouri community during 1989 to 1990.[46] In this outbreak 243 persons were affected and there were 4 deaths. A failure in disinfection of the water system occurred after repair of two broken pipes with secondary contamination by unchlorinated well water. Other waterborne outbreaks have also been associated with untreated municipal water and swimming in lakes contaminated with fecal materials.[27, 46] Person-to-person transmission in child day-care centers has been documented.[47, 48]

Enterohemorrhagic *E. coli* illness usually begins with a nonbloody diarrhea that may progress to bloody diarrhea with severe abdominal cramps, with little or no fever (hemorrhagic colitis). The major complications of EHEC infection are hemolytic uremic syndrome (which occurs in approximately 8% of children with hemorrhagic colitis) and postdiarrhea thrombocytopenic purpura (in a few adults). When *E. coli* 0157:H7 is suspected, the stool should be cultured on MacConkey's sorbitol media and the diagnosis confirmed by latex agglutination of nonsorbitol-fermenting *E. coli*.[35] Fecal leukocytes can be present in up to one third of the cases. Currently EHEC other than 0157:H7 cannot be detected by procedures available in hospital laboratories. The role of antimicrobial therapy in hemorrhagic colitis is unclear; some studies have suggested an increase risk of hemolytic uremic syndrome with their use. Antimotility agents are contraindicated.

The EAggEC has been the least studied of the diarrheagenic *E. coli*. The mechanism of diarrhea is thought to involve cell adherence. Clinical manifestations include low-grade fever, abdominal cramps, and prolonged watery diarrhea (>2 weeks).[49] Adequate fluid replacement and nutritional support are the main therapies.

Vibrio parahemolyticus

Vibrio parahemolyticus accounts for less than 1% of foodborne outbreaks in the United States. However, in Japan it is the principal cause of foodborne diarrhea. This organism occurs wherever consumption of contaminated seafood and shellfish is common.[34] *Vibrio parahemolyticus* is usually a marine isolate, but it also can be found in freshwater or nonmarine environments.[50]

Clinical manifestations include self-limited watery diarrhea, abdominal pain, nausea, and vomiting. The organism can be isolated by culture of the stool on thiosulfate citrate bile salt sucrose (TCBS) agar.

Vibrio cholerae

Vibrio cholerae has long been endemic in Asia and Africa. The Americas had been free of cholera until epidemic cholera arrived in Lima, Peru in 1991. Since that time more than 500,000 individuals have been ill; there have been more than 4,700 deaths.[51] In the United States, 128 cases have been reported in travelers returning from endemic areas of Central and South America.[52]

Vibrio cholerae has been separated into serogroups. Epidemic cholera has in the past always been caused by serogroup 01. Classic cholera tends to produce symptomatic severe cases.[52, 53] The E1 Tor biotype tends to produce asymptomatic cases in up to 75% of the infections.[54] In 1993, epidemic cholera due to a non-01 strain emerged for the first time in Southeast Asia. This *V. cholerae* was classified as serogroup 0139 Bengal. It has been associated with up to 5% mortality.[55]

There are two main reservoirs for cholera: humans and water. Most of the infections have been associated with ingestion of contaminated water. However exposure to contaminated shellfish, including oysters, shrimp, mussels, and conch,[53] and spread through household contacts[56] also play a role in transmission. Food imported into the United States has been associated with three recent outbreaks. The contaminated foods were crabmeat from Ecuador and commercially imported frozen coconut milk from Thailand.

The spectrum of clinical manifestations range from asymptomatic infection to severe watery diarrhea with up to 50 stools/day leading to hypovolemic shock and death. Patients also can experience vomiting, muscle spasms, abdominal pain, and abdominal distention.[52] The gold standard for diagnosis is isolation of the organism from a stool sample on a selective medium (TCBS).

The most effective therapy is prompt fluid and electrolytes replacement. Antimicrobial therapy has been effective in reducing duration of symptoms. Tetracycline or doxycycline are the drugs of choice (for use in children older than 9 years). Erythromycin, TMP-SMX, furazolidone, and chloramphenicol have been effective alternative therapies for sensitive isolates; however, multiresistant strains have been reported.[57]

Campylobacter

Campylobacter species are carried by a wide variety of domestic and wild animals, including birds, cattle, sheep, pigs, dogs, and cats.[58] Transmission has been associated with handling, preparation, and consumption of contaminated, raw, or undercooked animal meat and poultry.[59] Outbreaks due to raw or unpasteurized milk have been described.[60] Twenty-eight foodborne outbreaks of campylobacteriosis were documented by the CDC between 1983 and 1987.[5] Several waterborne outbreaks of *Campylobacter* gastroenteritis have been associated with drinking contaminated water.[61, 62] The disease has a bimodal age distribution with peaks in those younger than 5 years and between 15 to 29 years old.[59] Illness can be seen year round in tropical climates, but in temperate climates, it occurs most often during the summer.[58]

The spectrum of clinical manifestations is broad and depends on the species involved and characteristics of the host; *Campylobacter jejuni* causes watery, secretory, and inflammatory diarrhea. Diarrhea subsides without therapy within the first week in up to 60% to 70% of the cases.[58] *Campylobacter* bacteremia is rare (except with *Campylobacter fetus*). Antibiotic therapy of gastroenteritis is controversial but is usually recommended for patients with severe diarrhea and those who are immunocompromised. Erythromycin can shorten the duration of excretion.[63] Strains are usually susceptible to tetracycline, chloramphenicol, aminoglycosides, and quinolones.

Yersinia enterocolitica

Yersinia enterocolitica is a cause of foodborne outbreaks in Europe and cooler regions of North America.[34] In the United States, serotype 0:8 has been responsible for the majority of infections, whereas in Europe serotypes 0:3 and 0:9 have been found most commonly.[64] The illness occurs mainly during autumn and winter months. The major reservoir for this pathogen is pigs, although birds, dogs, cats, cows, and rabbits can also carry the organism.[65] Ingestion of contaminated pork is the major source of *Y. enterocolitica*.[34] Contaminated pork chitterlings have been commonly implicated as a source of infection.[66] Some outbreaks of yersiniosis have been caused by contaminated milk.[67] Waterborne outbreaks due to contaminated spring and stream water have also been reported.[34]

The pathogenesis of yersiniosis is thought to involve invasion of the ileal mucosa (causing bloody, mucosy diarrhea) and production of heat-stable toxin–like enterotoxin (causing watery diarrhea).

Clinical manifestations depend on the age of the persons involved, with children younger than 5 years having a self-limited gastroenteritis.[65] Fever, abdominal pain, and vomiting can occur. In older children, mesenteric adenitis mimicking acute appendicitis can occur. Complications in adults include reactive polyarthritis, arthralgia, and erythema nodosum.[15] The specific diagnosis is made by isolation of the organism from stool in standard media or on the selective medium cefsulodin-Irgasan (triclosan)-novobiocin (CIN). *Yersinia enterocolitica* is usually susceptible to TMP-SMX, aminoglycosides, chloramphenicol, tetracycline, quinolones, and third-generation cephalosporins.[64]

Bacillus cereus

Bacillus cereus is reported to cause 2% of foodborne outbreaks.[9] Two syndromes are cause by *B. cereus*.[9, 68] The emetic syndrome is associated with the ingestion of farinaceous foods, especially fried rice. The syndrome is manifested by an acute onset of nausea, vomiting, and malaise after ingestion of a preformed heat-stable toxin. Symptoms last 6 to 24 hours. The less common *B. cereus* diarrhea syndrome is associated with the ingestion of high-protein foods, vegetables, sauces, and puddings. It is manifested by abdominal pain, watery diarrhea, and tenesmus. Nausea and vomiting are uncommon. The symptoms last 12 to 24 hours. Treatment is supportive.

Listeria monocytogenes

Listeria is an important bacterial foodborne pathogen that causes invasive infections in newborns, pregnant women, and immuno-compromised hosts.[69] Although there are seven species of *Listeria*, only *Listeria monocytogenes* is commonly associated with human diseases.[70] *Listeria monocytogenes* is carried by many wild and domestic animals and occurs in the environment.[70] Large outbreaks of human listeriosis have been reported in Europe and North America.[71] The foods implicated in these outbreaks included coleslaw, Mexican-style soft cheese, milk, Swiss cheese, shrimp, and salted mushrooms.[69]

Clinical manifestations vary from a mild influenza-like illness to severe meningoencephalitis. In newborns, *L. monocytogenes* can manifest as pneumonia, septicemia, or meningitis.[72] Gastrointestinal symptoms are uncommon.[69] Mortality rates up to 30% are reported especially in elderly or immunocompromised patients. The treatment of choice is ampicillin, usually combined with an aminoglycoside such as gentamicin. Vancomycin, erythromycin, chloramphenicol, and TMP-SMX (alone or in combination) have been used for penicillin allergic patients.

Aeromonas Species

Aeromonas are gram-negative rods found in fresh and brackish water and cold-blooded animals worldwide.[50] There are four species: *Aeromonas hydrophila, Aeromonas sobria, Aeromonas caviae,* and *Aeromonas salmonicida*. Because *Aeromonas* is not a reportable disease, the incidence is unknown. An epidemiologic study in the United States demonstrated the association of outbreaks of *Aeromonas* gastroenteritis with drinking untreated water.[73] A broad spectrum of clinical manifestations have been documented, including gastroenteritis, skin and wound infection, osteomyelitis, sepsis, and meningitis in normal and immunocompromised hosts. Gastrointestinal illness is the most common manifestation of *Aeromonas* infection. It lasts up to 12 days, with fever and vomiting seen in up to one third of the patients.[74] In adults, the gastrointestinal illness tends to be chronic, whereas in children it may be acute and severe.[73] *Aeromonas* can grow in routine culture media but is best isolated with the use of selective media such as ampicillin-blood agar, CIN agar, and peptone broth. The strains are usually susceptible in vitro to aminoglycosides, TMP-SMX, and quinolones, but the benefit of antibiotic therapy for gastroenteritis has not been well documented.[75]

Pleisiomonas shigelloides

Pleisiomonas shigelloides is a gram-negative rod found in surface water, intestines of freshwater fish, and sometimes other animals, including dogs and cats, particularly in tropical and subtropical habitats.[76] This pathogen has been the cause of sporadic and epidemic diarrheal illness in the United States.[77] Infection is caused by consumption of seafood (including raw shellfish and shrimp) or untreated water. Travel to Southeast Asia, Central America, Africa, and the Caribbean is also a risk.[78, 79] Secretory or invasive diarrhea is the most common manifestation. Fever, abdominal pain, vomiting, and dehydration are seen commonly. Extraintestinal manifestation, including cellulitis, sepsis, and meningitis, is rare.[80] The illness is usually self-limited in healthy individuals; however, it can be prolonged in immunocompromised hosts.[76] Oral agents (TMP-SMX or quinolones) have been used for treatment of gastroenteritis. Intravenous antibiotics such as third-generation cephalosporins, chloramphenicol, and quinolones (for older adolescents and adults) have been used to treat extraintestinal manifestations.[81]

PARASITIC INFECTIONS

Giardia

Giardia lamblia (duodenalis) is the most frequent agent causing waterborne outbreaks of gastroenteritis in the United States.[13] It has a worldwide distribution. The life cycle consists of trophozoite and cyst forms. Drinking contaminated water has been the most common cause of epidemics, but person-to-person transmission occurs, especially in day-care centers (in which *Giardia* can be detected in up to 20% of asymptomatic children.[82] Ground water contaminated with feces accounted for 65% of the cases in waterborne outbreaks in the United States in last decade.[13] Foodborne transmission of giardiasis in rare; however, there have been small outbreaks.[83–86] Infection occurs after ingestion of as few as 10 viable cysts, with an incubation period between 1 and 45 days and a mean of 1 to 2 weeks.[82]

Clinical manifestations include watery or mushy diarrhea, which is foul smelling and associated with abdominal distention and cramps. Fever and vomiting are rare.[87] Acute illness can be self-limited, lasting between 3 and 4 days. Chronic infections develop mainly in infants and immunocompromised patients, particularly those with HIV infection or agammaglobulinemia, and are characterized by recurrent episodes of malabsorption diarrhea, bloating, abdominal distention, weight loss, and anorexia. Children may develop failure to thrive. Treatment is recommended for symptomatic cases. Quinacrine hydrochloride is effective for treatment of giardiasis, although its bitter taste compromises compliance.[88] Metronidazole and furazolidone are often better tolerated in children.

Cryptosporidium parvum

Cryptosporidium parvum, a coccidian intracellular protozoan, has been well recognized as a cause of gastroenteritis in immunocompetent and immunocompromised patients worldwide.[89] Although the true prevalence is unknown, the estimated overall frequency has been reported to be 2.1% in developed countries and 8.5% in developing countries.[90]

The most important mode of transmission is through contaminated water, although person-to-person transmission also occurs in day-care centers.[91, 92] The occurrence of *Cryptoporidium* is widespread in water supplies in the United States.[13] This parasite is resistant to common disinfectants and can be found even in adequately treated water supplies.[3] A massive outbreak of disease was reported in Milwaukee in the spring of 1993 due to contaminated municipal drinking water.[93] More than 400,000 persons developed gastroenteritis. The severity and duration of the illness depend of the host's immune status. For immunocompetent patients, the illness is self-limited, manifesting with acute watery diarrhea, abdominal cramps and distention, nausea, and vomiting. Fatigue, myalgia, headache, and low-grade fever occur.[93] The duration of the illness is between 1 and 2 weeks. For immunocompromised patients, the symptoms are chronic and insidiously increase in severity. Acquired immunodeficiency syndrome (AIDS) patients can develop profuse watery diarrhea with weight loss and dehydration. There is no proven effective therapy for cryptoporidiosis. Azithromycin, paromomycin, and bovine milk globulin have been beneficial in some reported cases.

Trichinella spiralis

Thirty-three foodborne outbreaks of *Trichinella spiralis* were reported to the CDC during 1983 to 1987, with 162 cases accounting for 0.3% of total reported foodborne outbreak cases. The northeast area of the United States and Alaska had the highest incidence of trichinosis during 1975 to 1986.[94] Trichinosis has traditionally been associated with ingestion of pork. With improvement in commercially available pork products, ingestion of wild swine, bear, and other wild animals is now the most common source.[94]

Diarrhea and abdominal pain occur during the first week after ingestion when the worms mature and release larvae; edema of eyelids and face, myositis, fever, and eosinophilia occur during tissue invasion. The symptoms may be self-limited. Mebendazole is the treatment of choice for the acute enteric syndrome. Thiabendazole is an alternative therapy. Corticosteroid are indicated for severe extraintestinal disease.

Entamoeba histolytica

Entamoeba histolytica is one of the most common parasites causing gastroenteritis worldwide. The main mode of transmission in endemic areas, including India, South and Central America, and West and South Africa, is through ingestion of contaminated water.[95] Person-to-person transmission occurs. Standard water disinfection techniques do not kill this parasite; the only completely effective method is to boil the water. Many infections are asymptomatic or associated with mild nonspecific diarrhea. Invasive disease typically has two major manifestations. Amebic dysentery manifests with bloody diarrhea and fever. In adults, amebic liver abscess manifests with fever, upper abdominal pain, and hepatomegaly; in children, the clinical manifestation includes high fever, abdominal distention, and irritability. Abdominal pain is uncommon. Examination of stools for ova and parasites, as well as amoebic serologic tests, are required for diagnosis. Serologic test results are positive most often with invasive disease. Metronidazole is considered the treatment of choice for invasive disease; it is given in conjunction with an intraluminal agent such as iodoquinol or paronomycin.

VIRAL ETIOLOGIES

Norwalk Virus and Norwalk-like Viruses

The Norwalk and Norwalk-like calici viruses have been the most commonly recognized viral agents causing foodborne and waterborne illness in the United States, the United Kingdom, Japan, and Australia.[96] The CDC reported 10 outbreaks of foodborne viral gastroenteritis with 1,164 cases during 1983 to 1987; these accounted for 2.1% of all outbreaks during this period. There has been no clear-cut seasonal pattern. Unlike rotavirus gastroenteritis, which occurs primarily among younger children, Norwalk viruses cause illness in older children and adults.

Foodborne transmission has been associated with ingestion of contaminated (or raw) oysters, clams, cockles, and mussels.[97-99] Infected food handlers have been implicated in both foodborne and waterborne outbreaks.[100] Waterborne illness has also been associated with swimming and contamination of groundwater supplies. Children and adolescents usually experience more vomiting than diarrhea, whereas adults experience more diarrhea than vomiting.[101] Other manifestations include nausea, abdominal cramps, fever, headache, and myalgia. The illness is self-limited, lasting between 12 and 60 hours, with a mean duration of 48 hours.[96] The treatment is supportive care.

Hepatitis A

Hepatitis A is mainly transmitted by direct person-to-person contact. However, 3% to 8% of reported hepatitis A cases have been associated with foodborne or waterborne outbreaks.[102] The most common cause of outbreaks is contamination of food during preparation by an anicteric infected food handler. Shellfish have often been a source of infection.[102] Twenty-nine outbreaks of hepatitis A were reported to the CDC during 1983 to 1987, with 1,067 cases. These outbreaks accounted for 2% of all outbreaks reported during that period.[5] Due to the long incubation period (3–6 weeks), it is thought that foodborne hepatitis is underrecognized.

Hepatitis is characterized by an acute illness with jaundice, malaise, and anorexia. The treatment is supportive.

ROTAVIRUS

Rotavirus has been shown to be a major cause of infantile gastroenteritis worldwide.[103] In children person-to-person fecal-oral spread is the most common route of transmission. However, in adults, contaminated environmental sources including water and inanimate surfaces, contact with pediatric cases, and travel, play important roles in acquisition.[104, 105] Waterborne outbreaks of ro-

TABLE 5.
Clinical Manifestations of Mushroom Poisoning*

Chemical	Species	Clinical Symptoms	Onset of Symptoms
Coprine	*Coprinus atramentarius*	Disulfiram-like effect (if alcohol is consumed): flushing, tingling in the fingers, sweating, nausea, and vomiting	30 min after alcohol consumption
Cyclopeptides	Many *Amanita* spp. and a few *Galerina* spp.	Nausea, vomiting, painful colic, severe watery diarrhea, followed by liver and/or renal necrosis	12–24 hr
Ibonetic acid	*Amanita muscaria, Amanita pantherine* and others	Dizziness, incoordination, and visual disturbances	30 min–2 hr
Monomethyl-hydrazine	*Gyromitra esculenta* and others	Bloating, nausea, vomiting, diarrhea (watery or bloody), muscle cramps, faintness, and loss of coordination	6–12 hr
Muscarine	Many *Clitocybe* spp. and *Inocybe* spp.	Perspiration, salivation, lacrimation, decrease blood pressure, abdominal cramps, watery diarrhea	30 min–2 hr
Psilocybin and other indoles	Many *Psilocybe* spp.	Muscle weakness, drowsiness, and hallucinations	30–60 min

*Data from Rumack BH, Salzman E: *Mushroom Poisoning: Diagnosis and Treatment.* West Palm Beach, Fla, CRC Press, 1978, pp 171–179.

TABLE 6.
Clinical Manifestations Associated With Fish Toxins*

Toxin	Fish	Clinical Symptoms	Onset of Symptoms
Ciguatoxin	Snappers, jacks, barracuda, grouper and parrot fish species	Neurologic: heat-cold reversal, dental pain (symptoms can last up to 6 mo) Gastrointestinal: diarrhea, vomiting, abdominal pain	1–3 hr (90% of the cases within 12 hr)
Domoic acid	Mussels	Initial gastrointestinal symptoms with nausea, vomiting, cramps and diarrhea, followed by neurologic symptoms with headache, confusion, and memory loss (anterograde)	15 min–38 hr (mean 5.5 hr)
Paralytic compounds	Shellfish (mussels, oysters, scallops, clamps and other mollusks)	Paresthesia, followed by incoordination, weakness, dysphonia, dysphagia, ataxia and paralysis; minimal gastrointestinal symptoms	30 min

Neurotoxins	Shellfish (mussels, oyster, scallops, clamps, and other mollusks)	Neurologic: vertigo, ataxia, and incoordination Gastrointestinal: nausea, vomiting, abdominal pain, and diarrhea	30 min–3 hr
Scombrotoxin	Tuna, bonito, skipjack, wahoo, and mackerel	Histamine reaction: flushing, headache, dizziness, urticaria, pruritis, cramps, and diarrhea	1 hr
Tetrodotoxin	Puffer fish	Oral, followed by general paresthesia, with severe nausea and vomiting; respiratory failure and shock in severe cases	10 min–4 hr

*Data from Underman AE, Leedom JM: *Curr Clin Topics Infect Dis* 13:203–225, 1993.

tavirus gastroenteritis due to sewage contamination have been reported in Sweden, Australia, China, Brazil, and the United States.[105]

Clinical manifestations include vomiting and fever followed by watery diarrhea.[50] The illness is self-limited in normal hosts. Diagnosis is made by antigen detection using commercially available kits. Therapy is fluid and electrolyte replacement; usually oral rehydration is preferred. Intravenous hydration is recommended for those patients in shock, those who are deeply obtunded, and those with an ileus.

TABLE 7.

Clinical Manifestations of Foodborne and Waterborne Chemical Poisoning*

Chemicals	Vehicle of Transmission	Clinical Manifestations	Onset of Symptoms
Arsenic	Contaminated water (well water) and occasional foods	Dysphagia, epigastric pain, vomiting, and diarrhea (watery and/or bloody)	30 min–4 hr
Cadmium	Contaminated water (environmental pollution) and occasional foods	Increased salivation, vomiting, abdominal pain, diarrhea, and urgency	15–30 min
Copper	Contaminated water (environmental pollution) and occasional foods	Nausea, vomiting, abdominal pain, hemorrhagic gastritis, and diarrhea	Within 1 hr
Lead	Contaminated water (lead solder in pipes) and food (primarily from canned foods)	Large ingestion: seizures, coma, and death Chronic exposure: fatigue, sleep disturbance, headache, aching bones, anemia, constipation, abdominal pain, decreased appetite	Acute: hours Chronic: weeks to months

Mercury	Contaminated water (environmental pollution) and foods (especially fish)	Headache, dizziness, restlessness, irritability, sleepiness, tremors, loss of appetite, nausea, vomiting, diarrhea, and loss of memory	Symptoms appear after chronic exposure
Monosodium glutamate	Chinese food	Neurologic: somnolence, hallucinations, headache, dyspnea Gastrointestinal: nausea and vomiting	Within 1 hr

*Data from Sitting M: *Handbook of Toxic and Hazardous Chemicals and Carcinogens*, ed 3. Park Ridge, NJ, Noyes Publications, 1991.

CHEMICAL OR TOXIN ETIOLOGIES

Chemical agents caused 26% of foodborne outbreaks and 2% of the cases during 1983 to 1987, with ciguatoxin and scombrotoxin accounting for 73% of cases. Waterborne outbreaks of disease due to chemical agents accounted for 16% of the outbreaks and 1.3% of the cases reported to the CDC during 1986 to 1992.

An outbreak of methemoglobinemia, due to soup contaminated with nitrites in a broiler additive, was reported.[106] Contaminated water, meat preservatives, and vegetables (including carrots and spinach) have been associated with methemoglobinemia. Acute onset of cyanosis in a patient without underlying cardiovascular or pulmonary disease should alert the physician to the possibility of methemoglobinemia. Other symptoms include abdominal pain, nausea, vomiting, and dizziness. The diagnosis is made by measurement of the methemoglobin levels in blood. Moderate to severe cases (level >20%) require administration of 100% oxygen and methylene blue (1–2 mg/kg given over 10–15 minutes). Methylene blue is contraindicated in patients with glucose-6-phosphate dehydrogenase deficiency (G6PD). For patients who fail to respond to the initial therapy with methylene blue or have G6PD deficiency, exchange transfusion and hyperbaric oxygen are options.

Toxins synthesized by fungi occur in food stored at high temperature and humidity.[107] *Claviceps* spp. has caused outbreaks of

TABLE 8.
Clinical Manifestations of Poisoning Associated With Edible Plants*

Plant	Clinical Manifestations	Toxic Product	Onset of Symptoms
Cassava (peel)	Dyspnea, gasping, paralysis, coma, and death	Cyanide	Hours
Fava beans	Initial symptoms: headache, nausea, vomiting, lumbar pain, and fever, followed by hemoglobinuria, jaundice, and death	Hazard for individuals with glucose-6-phosphate dehydrogenase deficiency, which cannot reduce endogenous oxidants	24 hr–8 days after consumption of the bean
Potatoes (sun-greened skin)	Neurologic: apathy, restlessness, drowsiness, and visual disturbances Gastrointestinal: diarrhea, vomiting, abdominal pain, and fever (severe in children)	Solanine glycoalkaloids	4–19 hr

*Adapted from Lampe KF, McCann MA: *AMA Handbook of Poisonous and Injurious Plants* [cassava]. Chicago, Chicago Review Press, 1985, pp 114–115; Frohne D, Pfander HJ: *A Colour Atlas of Poisonous Plants. A Handbook for Pharmacists, Doctors, Toxicologists, and Biologists*, (translated by Bisset NG). London, Wolfe, 1984, p 214.

ergotism due to contaminated rye or wheat. Aflatoxins synthesized by *Aspergillus flavus* and *Aspergillus parasiticus* have been found in cereals and peanuts. The association between aflatoxins and cancer in humans is controversial. Alimentary toxic aleukia, produced by consumption of cereal contaminated with *Fusaria* spp., was described in early 1940 in the Soviet Union.[108] The illness was very serious, and most cases were fatal, accompanied by severe leukopenia, hemorrhages, sepsis, and bone marrow suppression.

Chemical and toxin poisonings and their clinical manifestations are summarized in Tables 5 to 8. Mushroom poisoning is related to multiple toxins produced by various species; symptoms occur after a short incubation period (see Table 5). Fish toxins and heavy metals cause both acute and chronic symptoms (see Tables 6 and 7). A few plants that are normally safe to eat are dangerous under special circumstances or in hosts with an underlying condition (e.g., G6PD deficiency) (see Table 8).

REFERENCES

1. Thompson P, Salsbury PA, Adams C, et al: US food legislation. *Lancet* 336:1557–1562, 1990.
2. Levine WC, Stephenson WT, Craun GF: Waterborne disease outbreaks, 1986–1988. *MMWR* 39:SS–1; 1–13, 1990.
3. Herwaldt BL, Craun GF, Stokes SL, et al: Waterborne-disease outbreaks, 1989–1990. *MMWR* 40:SS–3; 1–22, 1991.
4. Moore AC, Herwaldt BL, Craun GF, et al: Surveillance for waterborne disease outbreaks—United States, 1991–1992. *MMWR* 42:SS–5; 1–22, 1993.
5. Bean NH, Griffin PM, Goulding JS, et al: Foodborne disease outbreaks, 5-year summary, 1983–1987. *MMWR* 39:SS–1; 1–57, 1990.
6. Guerrant RL, Bobak DA: Bacterial and protozoal gastroenteritis. *N Engl J Med* 325:327–340, 1991.
7. Baird-Parker AC: Foodborne salmonellosis. *Lancet* 336:1231–1235, 1990.
8. Diane R: Sources of infection: Food. *Lancet* 336:859–861, 1990.
9. Khodr M, Hill S, Perkins L: *Bacillus cereus* food poisoning associated with fried rice at two child day care centers—Virginia, 1993. *MMWR* 43:177–178, 1994.
10. Holmerg SD, Blake PA: Staphylococcal food poisoning in the United States. *JAMA* 251:487–489, 1984.
11. Underman AE, Leedom JM: Fish and shellfish poisoning. *Curr Clin Topics Infect Dis* 13:203–225, 1993.
12. Mishu B, Koehler J, Lee LA, et al: Outbreaks of *Salmonella enteritidis* infections in the United States, 1985–1991. *J Infect Dis* 169:547–552, 1994.
13. Craun GF: Waterborne disease outbreaks in the United States of America: Causes and prevention. *World Health Stat Q* 45:192–199, 1992.
14. Bishai WR, Sears C: Food poisoning syndromes. *Gastroenterol Clin North Am* 22:579–608, 1993.
15. Dupont HL, Levine MM, Hornick RB, et al: Inoculum size in shigellosis and implications for expected mode of transmission. *J Infect Dis* 159:1126–1127, 1989.

16. Haley CE, Gunn RA, Hughes JM, et al: Outbreaks of waterborne disease in the United States, 1978. *J Infect Dis* 141:794–797, 1980.

17. Rubin BK, Delisle G: Transfer of *Typhimurium* from tigers to a toddler. *Pediatr Infect Dis* 5:589–590, 1986.

18. Cohen ML, Potter M, Pollard R, et al: Turtle-associated salmonellosis in the United States. Effect of public health action, 1970–1976. *JAMA* 243:1247–1249, 1980.

19. Lyons RW, Samples CL, DeSilva HN, et al: An epidemic of resistant *Salmonella* in a nursery. Animal to human spread. *JAMA* 243:546–547, 1980.

20. McAllister TA, Roud JA, Marshall A, et al: Outbreak of *Salmonella eimsbuettel* in newborn infants spread by rectal thermometers. *Lancet* 1:1262–1264, 1986.

21. Riley KB, Antoniskis D, Maris R, et al: Rattlesnake capsule–associated *Salmonella arizona* infections. *Arch Intern Med* 148:1207–1210, 1988.

22. Hayani KC, Pickering LK: Salmonella *Infections*, ed 3. Philadelphia, WB Saunders, 1992, pp 620–636.

23. Ashkenazi S, Cleary T: Shigella *infections*, ed 3. Philadelphia, WB Saunders, 1992, pp 637–646.

24. Coles FB, Kondracki SF, Gallo RJ, et al: Shigellosis outbreaks at summer camps for the mentally retarded in New York State. *Am J Epidemiol* 130:966–975, 1989.

25. Mahoney FJ, Farley TA, Burbank DF, et al: Evaluation of an intervention program for the control of an outbreak of shigellosis among institutionalized persons. *J Infect Dis* 168:1177–1780, 1993.

26. Centers for Disease Control: Outbreak of *Shigella flexneri* 2a infections on a cruise ship. *MMWR* 43:657, 1994.

27. Keene WE, McAnulty JM, Hoesly FC, et al: A swimming-associated outbreak of hemorrhagic colitis caused by *Escherichia coli* 0157:H7 and *Shigella sonnei*. *N Engl J Med* 331:579–584, 1994.

28. Tranter HS: Foodborne staphylococcal illness. *Lancet* 336:1044–1046, 1990.

29. Zimomra J, Wenderoth T, Snyder, et al: *Clostridium perfringens* gastroenteritis associated with corned beef served at St. Patrick's day meals, 1993. *MMWR* 43:137–143, 1994.

30. Lund BM: Foodborne disease due to *Bacillus* and *Clostridium* species. *Lancet* 336:982–986, 1990.

31. Lawrence G, Walker PD: Pathogenesis of enteritis necroticans in Papua New Guinea. *Lancet* 1:125–126, 1976.

32. Midura TF, Snowden S, Wood RM, et al: Isolation of *Clostridium botulinum* from honey. *J Clin Microbiol* 9:282–283, 1979.

33. Clostridial Infections. In Peter G (ed): *1994 Red Book Report of the Committee on Infectious Diseases*. Elk Grove Village, Ill, American Academy of Pediatrics, 1994, pp 160–164.

34. Doyle MP: Pathogenic *Escherichia coli, Yersinia enterocolitica*, and *Vibrio parahaemolyticus*. *Lancet* 336:1111–1115, 1990.

35. Gomez HF, Cleary TG: *Escherichia coli* as a cause of diarrhea in children. *Semin Pediatr Infect Dis* 5:175–182, 1994.
36. Chak A, Banwell JG: Traveler's diarrhea. *Gastroenterol Clin North Am* 22:549–561, 1993.
37. Okhuysen PC, Ericsson CD: Travelers' diarrhea. *Med Clin North Am* 76:1357–1373, 1992.
38. *Escherichia coli* diarrhea. In Peter G (ed): *1994 Red Book Report of the Committee on Infectious Diseases.* Elk Grove Village, Ill, American Academy of Pediatrics, 1994, pp 187–191.
39. Prado D, Lopez E, Liu H, et al: Ceftibuten and trimethoprim-sulfamethoxazole for treatment of *Shigella* and enteroinvasive *Escherichia coli* disease. *Pediatr Infect Dis* 11:644–647, 1992.
40. Cleary TG: *Escherichial coli* that cause hemolytic uremic syndrome. *Infect Dis Clin North Am* 6:163–176, 1992.
41. Pickering LK, Obrig TG, Stapleton FB: Hemolytic-uremic syndrome and enterohemorrhagic *Escherichia coli. Pediatr Infect Dis* 13:459–476, 1994.
42. Davis M, Osak C, Gordon D, et al: Update: Multistate outbreak of *Escherichia coli* 0157:H7 infections from hamburgers—Western United States, 1992–1993. *MMWR* 42:258–262, 1993.
43. Turney C, Green-Smith M, Mordhorst C, et al: *Escherichia coli* 0157:H7 outbreak link to home-cooked hamburger—California, July 1993. *MMWR* 43:213–215, 1994.
44. McDonough S, Shireley L: Foodborne outbreak of gastroenteritis cause by *Escherichia coli* 0157:H7—North Dakota, 1990. *MMWR* 40:265–267, 1991.
45. MacDonald KL, Osterholm MT: The emergence of *Escherichia coli* 0157:H7 infection in the United States. *JAMA* 269:2264–2265, 1993.
46. Swerdlow DL, Woodruff BA, Brady RC, et al: A waterborne outbreak in Missouri of *Escherichia coli* 0157:H7 associated with bloody diarrhea and death. *Ann Intern Med* 117:812–819, 1992.
47. Ostroff SM, Kobayashi JM, Lewis JH: Infections with *Escherichia coli* 0157:H7 in Washington State. *JAMA* 262:355–359, 1989.
48. Belongia EA, Osterholm MT, Soler JT, et al: Transmission of *Escherichia coli* 0157:H7 infection in Minnesota child day-care facilities. *JAMA* 269:883–888, 1993.
49. Afghani B, Stutman HR: Toxin-related diarrheas. *Pediatr Ann* 23:549–555, 1994.
50. Pickering L, Cleary TG: *Approach to Patients with Gastrointestinal Tract Infections and Food Poisoning,* ed 3. Philadelphia, WB Saunders, 1992, pp 565–596.
51. Swerdlow DL, Mintz ED, Rodriguez M, et al: Waterborne transmission of epidemic cholera in Trujillo, Peru: Lessons for a continent at risk. *Lancet* 340:28–32, 1992.
52. Paya E, O'Ryan ML, Prado V: Resurgence of *Vibrio cholera* in the Americas. *Semin Pediatr Infect Dis* 5:168–174, 1994.

53. World Health Organization: Cholera in 1992. *Wkly Epidemiol Rec* 68:149–155, 1993.
54. Woodward WE, Mosley WH: The spectrum of cholera in rural Bangladesh. *Am J Epidemiol* 96:342–351, 1972.
55. World Health Organization: Epidemic diarrhoea due to *Vibrio cholera non-01*. *Wkly Epidemiol Rec* 68:141–148, 1993.
56. Mhalu FS, Mtango FDE, Msengi AE: Hospital outbreaks of cholera transmitted through close person-to-person contact. *Lancet* 64:378–387, 1984.
57. Weber JT, Mintz ED, Canizares R, et al: Epidemic cholera in Ecuador: Multidrug-resistance and transmissin by water and seafood. *Epidemiol Infect* 112:1–11, 1994.
58. Skirrow MD: *Campylobacter*. *Lancet* 336:921–923, 1990.
59. Ruiz-Palacios G, Pickering LK: Campylobacter *and Helicobacter Infections*, ed 3. Philadelphia, WB Saunders, 1992, pp 1072–1084.
60. Riley LW, Finch MJ: Results of the first year of national surveillance of *Campylobacter* infections in the United States. *J Infect Dis* 151:956–959, 1985.
61. Melby K, Petter Dahl O, et al: Clinical and serological manifestations in patients during a waterborne epidemic due to *Campylobacter jejuni*. *J Infect Dis* 21:309–316, 1990.
62. Palmer SR, Gully PR, White JM: Water-borne outbreak of *Campylobacter* gastroenteritis. *Lancet* 2:287–289, 1983.
63. *Campylobacter* infections. In Peter G (ed): *1994 Red Book Report of the Committee on Infectious Diseases*. Elk Grove Village, Ill, American Academy of Pediatrics, 1994, pp 146–147.
64. Cover TL, Aber RC: *Yersinia enterocolitica*. *N Engl J Med* 321:16–24, 1989.
65. Weinstein L: *Yersiniosis*, ed 3. Philadelphia, WB Saunders, 1992, pp 646–655.
66. Lee LA, Russell Gerber A, Lonsway DR, et al: *Yersinia enterocolitica* 0:3 infections in infants and children associated with the household preparation of chitterlings. *N Engl J Med* 332:984–987, 1990.
67. Black RE, Jackson RJ, Tsai T, et al: Epidemic *Yersinia enterocolitica* infection due to contaminated chocolate milk. *N Engl J Med* 298:76–79, 1978.
68. Terranova W, Blake PA: *Bacillus cereus* food poisoning. *N Engl J Med* 298:143–144, 1978.
69. Riedo FX, Pinner RW, Tosca ML, et al: A point-source foodborne listeriosis outbreak: Documented incubation period and possible mild illness. *J Infect Dis* 170:693–696, 1994.
70. Jones D: Foodborne listeriosis. *Lancet* 336:1171–1174, 1990.
71. Gellin BG, Broome CV: Listeriosis. *JAMA* 261:1313–1320, 1989.
72. Bortolussi R, Evans J: *Listeriosis*, ed 3. Philadelphia, WB Saunders, 1992, pp 1180–1185.
73. Holmberg SD, Schell WL, Fanning GR, et al: *Aeromonas* intestinal infections in the United States. *Ann Intern Med* 105:683–689, 1986.

74. San Joaquin VH, Pickett DA: *Aeromonas*-associated gastroenteritis in children. *Pediatr Infect Dis* 7:53–57, 1988.
75. San Joaquin VH: *Aeromonas, Yersinia*, and miscellaneous bacterial enteropathogens. *Pediatr Ann* 23:544–548, 1994.
76. Tippen PS, Meyer A, Blank EC, et al: Aquarium-associated *Plesiomonas shigelloides* infection–Missouri. *MMWR* 38:617–619, 1989.
77. Holmberg SD, Wachsmuth IK, Hickman-Brenner FW, et al: *Plesiomonas* enteric infections in the United States. *Ann Intern Med* 105:690–694, 1986.
78. Brenden RA, Miller MA, Janda JM: Clinical disease spectrum and pathogenic factors associated with *Plesiomonas shigelloides* infections in humans. *Rev Infect Dis* 10:303–316, 1988.
79. Kain KC, Kelly MT: Clinical features, epidemiology, and treatment of *Plesiomonas shigelloides* diarrhea. *J Clin Microbiol* 27:998–1001, 1989.
80. Billier J, Kuypers S, Lierde SV, et al: *Plesiomonas shigelloides* meningitis and septicemia in a neonate: Report of a case and review of the literature. *J Infect Dis* 19:267–271, 1989.
81. Kain KC, Kelly MT: Antimicrobial susceptibility of *Pleisiomonas shigelloides* from patients with diarrhea. *Antimicrob Agents Chemother* 33:1609–1610, 1989.
82. Grazioso CF, Mitchell DK: Parasitic causes of diarrhea in children. *Semin Pediatr Infect Dis* 5:191–201, 1994.
83. Petersen LR, Cartter ML, Hadler JL: A food-borne outbreak of *Giardia lamblia. J Infect Dis* 157:846–848, 1988.
84. Grabowsk DJ, Tiggs KJ, Hall JD, et al: Common-source outbreak of giardiasis. *MMWR* 38:405–407, 1989.
85. Osterholm MT, Forfan JC, Ristinen TL, et al: An outbreak of foodborne giardiasis. *N Engl J Med* 304:24–28, 1987.
86. Karabiber N, Aktas F: Foodborne giardiasis. *Lancet* 337:376–377, 1991.
87. Wolfe MS: Giardiasis. *Clin Microbiol Rev* 5:93–100, 1992.
88. *Giardia lamblia* infections. In Peter G (ed): *1994 Red Book Report of the Committee on Infectious Diseases*. Elk Grove Village, Ill, American Academy of Pediatrics, 1994, pp 193–195.
89. Casemore DP: Foodborne protozoal infection. *Lancet* 336:1427–1432, 1990.
90. Crawford FG, Vermund SH: Human cryptoporidiosis. *Crit Rev Microbiol* 16:113–158, 1988.
91. Alpert G, Bell LM, Kirkpatrick CE, et al: Outbreak of cryptosporidiosis in a day-care center. *Pediatrics* 77:152–157, 1986.
92. Addiss DG, Stewar JM, Finton RJ, et al: *Giardia lamblia* and *Cryptosporidium* infections in child day-care centers in Fulton County, Georgia. *Pediatr Infect Dis J* 10:907–911, 1991.
93. Mac Kenzie WR, Hoxie NJ, Proctor ME, et al: A massive outbreak in Milwaukee of *Cryptosporidium* infection transmitted through the public water supply. *N Engl J Med* 331:162–167, 1994.

94. Bailey TM, Schantz PM: Trends in the incidence and transmission patterns of trichinosis in humans in the United States: Comparison of the periods 1975–1981 and 1982–1986. *Rev Infect Dis* 12:5–11, 1990.

95. LaVia WV: Parasitic gastroenteritis. *Pediatr Ann* 23:556–560, 1994.

96. Hedberg CW, Osterholm MT: Outbreaks of food-borne and waterborne viral gastroenteritis. *Clin Microbiol Rev* 6:199–210, 1993.

97. Davis C, Smith A, Walden R: Viral gastroenteritis associated with consumption of raw oysters—Florida, 1993. *MMWR* 43:446–449, 1994.

98. Appleton H: Foodborne viruses. *Lancet* 336:1362–1364, 1990.

99. Conrad C, Hemphill K, Wilson S, et al: Multistate outbreak of viral gastroenteritis related to consumption of oysters—Louisiana, Maryland, Mississippi, and North Carolina, 1993. *MMWR* 42:945–948, 1993.

100. Kuritsky JN, Osterholm MT, Korlath JA, et al: A statewide assessment of the role of Norwalk virus in outbreaks of food-borne gastroenteritis. *J Infect Dis* 151:568, 1985.

101. Kaplan JE, Gary W, Baron RC, et al: Epidemiology of Norwalk gastroenteritis and the role of Norwalk virus in outbreaks of acute nonbacterial gastroenteritis. *Ann Intern Med* 96:756–761, 1982.

102. Skala M, Collier C, Hinkle CJ, et al: Foodborne hepatitis A—Missouri, Wisconsin, and Alaska, 1990–1992. *MMWR* 42:526–531, 1993.

103. Matson DO: New aspects of viral gastroenteritis. *Semin Pediatr Infect Dis* 5:183–190, 1994.

104. Hardy DB: Epidemiology of rotaviral infection in adults. *Rev Infect Dis* 9:461–469, 1987.

105. Ansari SA, Springthorpe S, Sattar SA: Survival and vehicular spread of human rotaviruses: Possible relation to seasonality of outbreaks. *Rev Infect Dis* 13:448–461, 1991.

106. Askew GL, Finelli L, Genese CA, et al: Boilerbaisse: An outbreak of methemoglobinemia in New Jersey in 1992. *Pediatrics* 94:381–384, 1994.

107. Morgan MRA, Fenwick GR: Natural foodborne toxicants. *Lancet* 336:1492–1495, 1990.

108. Wyllie TD, Morehouse LG: *Mycotoxic Fungi, Mycotoxins, Mycotoxicoses: An Encyclopedic Handbook,* vol 3. New York, Marcel Dekker, 1978, pp 21–86.

109. Rumack BH, Salzman E: *Mushroom Poisoning: Diagnosis and Treatment.* West Palm Beach, Fla, CRC Press, 1978, pp 171–179.

110. Sitting M: *Handbook of Toxic and Hazardous Chemical and Carcinogens,* ed 3. Park Ridge, NJ, Noyes Publications, 1991.

111. Lampe KF, McCann MA: *AMA Handbook of Poisonous and Injurious Plants* [cassava]. Chicago, Chicago Review Press, pp 114–115, 1985.

112. Frohne D, Pfander HJ: *A Colour Atlas of Poisonous Plants. A Handbook for Pharmacists, Doctors, Toxicologists, and Biologists,* (translated by Bisset NG). London, Wolfe Publishing, 1983, p 214.

Congenital Cytomegalovirus Infection and Disease

Gail J. Demmler, M.D.

Associate Professor of Pediatrics (Section of Infectious Diseases) and Pathology, Baylor College of Medicine; Director, Diagnostic Virology Laboratory, Texas Children's Hospital, Houston, Texas

Cytomegalovirus (CMV) was originally described in the late nineteenth and early twentieth centuries as a rare cause of "cytomegalic inclusion disease" of the fetus and newborn.[1] The virus was originally called the "salivary gland virus" when it was first cultivated in cell culture in 1956 by three independent investigators. The descriptive name, "cytomegalovirus," was designated by Weller in 1960.[2–5] Since 1971 CMV has been recognized as a common congenital infection with major public health implications.[6] Approximately 1% of all newborns are infected with CMV, and it is estimated to be the leading infectious cause of mental retardation and nonhereditary sensorineural deafness.[7]

DESCRIPTION

Cytomegalovirus is a member of the Herpesviridae (herpes = creeping) family of large DNA viruses, along with herpes simplex virus types 1 and 2, Epstein-Barr virus, varicella-zoster virus, and human herpesviruses 6 and 7. This family of viruses are enveloped, and they all contain a double-stranded DNA genome surrounded by a protein icosahedral capsid. They also share the important biologic properties of latency and reactivation. Despite certain similarities, however, infection with one member of the family does not confer protection against infection or disease with the other members of the herpes family. In addition, CMV is species specific because human CMV will infect only humans and animal viruses will infect only specific species of animals.

There are no distinct serotypes of CMV.[1] However, strain relatedness can be determined by molecular analysis of viral DNA. Restriction enzyme analysis of DNA extracted from CMV isolates that are epidemiologically linked (e.g., serial isolates from the same

Advances in Pediatric Infectious Diseases®, vol. 11
© 1996, Mosby–Year Book, Inc.

person, mother-infant pairs, family members, or sexual partners)
will show identical or very similar DNA fragment mapping patterns.[8–12] In one small study, no common pattern was associated
with CMV strains from eight congenitally infected infants with
neurologic sequelae when compared with each other or with
strains from healthy children in a day-care center, implying host
factors may be more important than viral factors in the pathogenesis of congenital CMV disease.[13] Newer modifications using polymerase chain reaction (PCR) methods also have been applied to
study the molecular epidemiology of CMV in a variety of settings,
including families and day-care centers, and may further our
knowledge of the pathogenesis of congenital disease.[11, 12, 14, 15]

EPIDEMIOLOGY

The epidemiology of CMV is complex, and many aspects are still
poorly understood. A knowledge of viral transmission to the pregnant women and her fetus will facilitate an understanding of congenital CMV infection and disease.

GENERAL POPULATION

Cytomegalovirus is spread (1) by close or intimate contact of either a sexual or nonsexual nature with another person who is shedding the virus in bodily secretions, (2) vertically from mother to
infant, or (3) by blood product transfusion or organ or marrow
transplantation from a CMV seropositive donor. Infection with
CMV can be classified as either primary or recurrent. Primary infection is the individual's first experience with the virus, whereas
recurrent infection may be either a reactivation of the individual's
original, previously latent strain of virus or a reinfection with a new
strain of CMV. The relative importance of primary vs. recurrent maternal infections in the transmission and disease expression of congenital CMV infection is important and will be discussed later in
the chapter. Naturally acquired CMV infection appears to confer
cross-reactive immunity to infection with new strains of CMV, but
this protection is not complete, because reinfection with a second
strain of CMV has been documented in transplant recipients,
women attending a clinic for sexually transmitted diseases, and
healthy children attending day-care centers.[9, 16, 17]

Seroepidemiologic studies have shown that infection with
CMV is very common worldwide, it is usually an inapparent infection, and it has no obvious seasonal predilection. However, the
prevalence of CMV-IgG antibody (as a marker of past or present
infection) is influenced by many factors, including the age, geo-

graphic location, cultural and socioeconomic status, and child-bearing practices of the group being studied. For example, in developed countries such as Great Britain and the United States, the prevalence of CMV IgG antibody is 40% to 60% in adult populations of middle to upper socioeconomic status and more than 80% in lower socioeconomic status groups.[18-20] In contrast, 80% of children in developing countries appear to acquire CMV by age 3 years, and almost all persons have been infected by adulthood.[21-23]

CHILDREN AND ADOLESCENTS

Studies on the age-related prevalence of infection with CMV in the United States suggest there may be three periods of increased acquisition of the virus: early childhood, adolescence, and the childbearing years.[21, 24, 25] Approximately 1% (range, 0.2%–2.4%) of all newborns are congenitally infected with CMV, making CMV the most common congenital infection.[7, 26] Infants also may be infected naturally during the perinatal period from CMV-infected maternal cervicovaginal secretions or breast milk.[27, 28] Children not congenitally or perinatally infected with CMV may be infected during the toddler or preschool years by contact with family members or other children.[6, 9, 29-33]

Teenage years are another period of rapid acquisition of CMV, presumably because of the intimate physical contact and sexual experimentation that is so common.[21, 25, 34] Vertical transmission of CMV acquired during the teenage years may result in congenital infection with CMV in infants born to teenaged mothers.[35] Epidemiologic data collected by the National Registry for Congenital Cytomegalovirus disease also have shown young maternal age to be associated with delivery of an infant with congenital CMV disease.[36] In the future, if a vaccine is used to prevent congenital CMV disease, it will have to be administered at an age that will protect the infants of adolescent mothers.

SEXUAL TRANSMISSION

Cytomegalovirus appears to be transmitted by sexual contact.[37] It has been cultured from the semen in 2% of apparently healthy men and from up to 21% of sexually active young women. The increased prevalence of CMV IgG antibody in women has been found to correlate with young age at the onset of sexual activity, recent sexual debut, multiple sexual partners, and a prior history of a sexually transmitted disease.[38-41] The strongest evidence to support the importance of sexual transmission of CMV is provided from molecular analyses of viral DNA that show the same CMV strain among sexual partners.[10, 42] Also of interest, multiple strains of CMV have been found in serially collected specimens from women attending a clinic for sexually transmitted diseases, implying sexually active individuals may be reinfected with multiple strains of CMV.[17] Whether this phenomenon reflects local infection of the cervix or systemic infection is unknown, but it may have implications if a CMV vaccine becomes available. It also is unclear whether reinfection with another strain of CMV can infect or cause disease in the fetus of a pregnant woman. Also, the role of CMV-infected semen in transmission of the virus to women or the embryo at the time of conception is unknown.

TRANSMISSION WITHIN FAMILIES

Cytomegalovirus also appears to be readily transmitted within the family setting, with attack rates up to 53%.[43–46] Young children between the ages of 12 and 24 months who are cared for in group settings such as day-care centers appear to be a common source of CMV for the family. Once the virus has entered the household, it appears to spread to susceptible siblings and parents within 1 year. Fourteen (21%) of 67 parents whose children attended three day-care centers in Alabama acquired CMV for the first time during a 1-year period compared with none of a comparison group of parents whose children were cared for at home.[43] Further support for the importance of intrafamilial transmission of CMV has been provided by several published studies in which molecular analysis showed that the same strain of CMV was spread within each family.[44, 45, 47–49]

OCCUPATIONAL RISKS

Most women of childbearing age are employed outside the home, and many work throughout their pregnancies. However, only two occupations have been studied sufficiently to assess risk: the day-care center worker and the health care professional. Despite intense efforts by many different investigators using serologic, virologic, and molecular techniques, in no instance has the transmission of CMV from patient to health care worker been documented.[50–57] Furthermore, several studies indicate health care workers caring for hospitalized patients who are excreting CMV have no greater incidence of CMV infection than the general population. It therefore appears that if CMV is transmitted in the hospital to health care workers, this occurrence is exceedingly rare, and the routine hygienic precautions practiced by health care professionals when caring for all patients are adequate to prevent transmission of the virus within the hospital setting. On the other hand, CMV-infected children in day care may transmit CMV to day-care center workers. Adler[58] showed that the annual rates of CMV antibody seroconversion were higher in day-care center workers than in hospital employees (11% vs. 2%; $P < 0.001$), and caring for children less than 2 years old was a risk factor for seroconversion in the day-care center workers. Furthermore, of nine day-care center workers who became infected with CMV and shed virus, seven were shown by molecular analysis to be shedding strains of CMV similar or identical to strains shed by the children in the day-care center. Day-care center workers who are pregnant or of childbearing age should be aware of this increased risk, and if they choose to continue to work during pregnancy should take precautions to try to prevent the acquisition of CMV from toddlers. Day-care workers are an ideal target population for vaccine administration if a CMV vaccine becomes available.

BLOOD TRANSFUSIONS

Blood products are a well-established source of CMV infection; donor-to-recipient transmission of CMV has been documented by restriction enzyme analysis of viral DNA.[59] Approximately 15% to 17% of CMV-seronegative neonates who receive blood products from CMV-seropositive donors become infected with the virus. Posttransfusion CMV infection in neonates, especially premature infants, can cause a syndrome of shock, lymphocytosis, and pneumonitis.[60] Cytomegalovirus also may be transmitted and produce a congenital infection if a pregnant woman or her fetus receives a blood product transfusion from a CMV-seropositive donor.[61, 62] Because transfusion-acquired CMV infection and disease is preventable, CMV-seronegative blood should be used, if available, when transfusions are given to a pregnant woman, her fetus, or her newborn infant.

IMMUNOSUPPRESSED MOTHERS AND THEIR INFANTS

With new advances in chemotherapy and transplantation medicine, women who are immunosuppressed may become pregnant and experience primary, reinfection or reactivation infections with CMV. Although the influence of maternal immunosuppression on congenital CMV infection and disease has not been studied in depth, there are reports of infants with symptomatic congenital CMV infection being born to women who experienced recurrent CMV infections while immunosuppressed from renal transplantation or corticosteroid administration.[63–65] Mothers who are human immunodeficiency virus (HIV) infected also may transmit CMV to their infants either congenitally or perinatally, and this infection may result in serious disease in the infant.[66-68] Extremely low birth weight infants with congenital CMV infection who receive corticosteroids for the treatment of bronchopulmonary dysplasia also may experience severe illness that may respond to antiviral therapy.[69] Specific defects in the host immune response, either cellular or humoral, may be responsible for transmission of the virus to the fetus or for disease expression in the neonate, and further investigation is needed to define these defects.[70]

CYTOMEGALOVIRUS IN PREGNANT WOMEN

Cytomegalovirus infections in pregnant women can be defined as either primary or recurrent.[71] Primary maternal CMV infections are the initial acquisition of virus during pregnancy and are best documented by a seroconversion of IgG antibodies to CMV during pregnancy. The presence of both IgG and IgM antibodies to CMV may be considered presumptive evidence of a primary maternal infection during pregnancy, although these findings also may indicate a primary infection having occurred in the weeks or months preceding conception. Recurrent infection usually is defined as the presence of maternal antibody to CMV before conception and congenital CMV infection in the offspring. Recurrent CMV infections in pregnancy include both reactivation of the woman's own strain of CMV acquired previously and possible reinfection with a new strain of virus.

Large-scale prospective seroepidemiologic studies have shown that primary CMV infection occurs in 0.7% to 4.1% of pregnancies and that the majority of these infections do not produce symptoms in the pregnant woman or her fetus.[7, 72] The average rate of transmission to the fetus in primary maternal CMV infection is 40%, with reported ranges of 24% to 75%.[73-76] In most studies, gestational age at the time of primary maternal infection has not been shown to significantly influence disease expression in the fetus or newborn. However, in one study, infection in the first half of pregnancy was more likely, although not significantly so, to produce serious handicaps in infants than those infections that occurred in the second half of pregnancy.[75] Infants born to mothers who are infected early in pregnancy may be more likely to be small for gestational age and to have microcephaly and intracranial calcifications, whereas those infants who are born to mothers infected later in pregnancy are more likely to have acute visceral disease with hepatitis, pneumonia, purpura, and severe thrombocytopenia.[77]

In populations in which the majority of women of childbearing age have antibodies to CMV, there is a higher rate of congenital CMV infection but not of clinical disease than in populations with a lower prevalence of CMV antibodies. In seven published reports including more than 28,000 mother-infant pairs in which the CMV antibody prevalence was 25% to 60%, the average rate of congenital infection was 0.41% (range 0.24%–0.69%). In six reports including 4,307 mother-infant pairs in which the CMV antibody prevalence was 80% to 100%, the average rate of congenital infection was 1.52% (range 1.2%–2.2%).[72] These observations suggest that maternal antibody to CMV does not protect the fetus from infection. This finding is in contrast to congenital rubella and toxoplasmosis in which antibodies have been found to protect the fetus against infection. In populations with a high prevalence of antibodies to CMV, recurrent infections in the mother probably account for most of the congenital infections with CMV, although the relative role of reinfection with a new strain of virus has not been adequately studied.

Although maternal antibodies do not appear to prevent transmission of CMV to the fetus, they do prevent disease in the fetus, or alternatively, they may be markers for another host factor that protects the fetus.[71] Primary infection with CMV during pregnancy is much more likely than recurrent maternal infection to produce symptoms and sequelae in the infant. In fact, only a handful of symptomatic newborns are known to have been born to mothers who were seropositive before pregnancy, and most of those mothers were either immunosuppressed or experienced a primary CMV infection close to the time of conception.[7]

CLINICAL MANIFESTATIONS

SYMPTOMS IN THE NEWBORN

From an average prevalence of 1% of all newborns and an estimated annual birth rate in the United States of 4 million, it can be calculated that 40,000 infants are born each year congenitally infected with CMV (Fig 1). Up to 10% of these infants will have symptoms at birth that are commonly associated with congenital CMV disease, including intrauterine growth retardation, jaundice, hepatosplenomegaly, petechiae or purpura, thrombocytopenia, and pneumonia (Table 1). Hepatomegaly, splenomegaly, and petechiae are the most common abnormalities seen. The liver is usually smooth and nontender and commonly measures 5 cm or more below the right costal margin. Ascites may be present prenatally and persist

4 million births annually

↓

40,000 each year born congenitally infected with CMV

↙   ↘

4,000 born each year with CMV   36,000 each year born with

disease   "silent" CMV infection

↓   ↓

90% will have neurologic   15% will have sequelae,

sequelae, although spectrum is   mostly hearing problems

diverse

FIGURE 1.
Estimated annual public health impact of congenital cytomegalovirus infection in the United States. (Data from Demmler GJ: *Rev Infect Dis* 13:315−329, 1991.)

postnatally for 1 to 2 weeks. The hepatomegaly usually resolves by 3 months of age, and persistence beyond 1 year is highly unusual. A mild hepatitis is usually present, but the transaminase levels in neonatal hepatitis due to CMV rarely exceed 300 IU. Hyperbilirubinemia, on the other hand, may be quite striking, with conjugated (direct) bilirubin levels up to 30 mg/dL. The abnormal results of liver function tests gradually resolve over the first few weeks of life. Chronic hepatitis due to a congenital infection with CMV is unusual but can occur. Enlargement of the spleen is very common in congenital CMV infection, and in some infants it may be the only abnormality detectable at birth.

Petechiae observed in congenital CMV disease are usually pinpoint and generalized over the infant's trunk and extremities. Present at birth, they can be transient and resolve within 48 to 72 hours. Petechiae can be the only apparent manifestation of congenital CMV disease; however, more commonly, the triad of hepatomegaly, splenomegaly, and petechiae is seen. Petechiae are usually, but not always, accompanied by thrombocytopenia, and platelet counts in the first few weeks of life range from 2,000 cells/mm^3 to 125,000 cells/mm^3, with most counts between 20,000 cells/mm^3 and 60,000 cells/mm^3. Usually thrombocytopenia resolves during the second week of life, but occasionally it can persist for weeks after birth, requiring repeated platelet transfusions. Rarely it may produce intrauterine intracranial hemorrhage. Occasionally the in-

TABLE 1.

Estimated Frequency of Abnormalities Observed at Birth in Infants With Congenital Cytomegalovirus Disease*

Abnormality	Approximate % of Cases
Nonneurologic	
Small for gestational age	50
Petechiae/purpura†	50–75
Hepatosplenomegaly†	40–60
Jaundice at birth	40–65
Pneumonia	5–10
Neonatal death	10
Neurologic‡	
Microcephaly	35–50
Intracranial calcifications	40–80
Seizures	10
Chorioretinitis	10–20
Lethargy/hypotonia	30
Hearing impairment	25–50
Laboratory	
Hemolytic anemia	10–50
Platelet count $\leq 75,000/mm^3$	50
Direct hyperbilirubinemia ≥ 3 mg/dL	35–70
Elevated alanine aminotransferase level >100 IU/L	25–80
Elevated cerebrospinal fluid protein level >120 mg/dL	45–50

*Data from Istas A, Demmler GJ, Dobbins JG, et al: *Clin Infect Dis* 20:665–670, 1995.
†Occurs in about 75% of symptomatic patients.
‡Neurologic abnormalities are seen at birth in about 60% to 70% of symptomatic patients.

fant may have a generalized purpuric rash, with evidence of extramedullary hematopoiesis, similar to congenital rubella syndrome. Hemolytic anemia is an unusual but well-documented hematologic condition associated with congenital CMV infection.

Pneumonitis is unusual in infants with congenital CMV disease. It is usually a severe, interstitial pneumonitis occurring in the context of a diffuse, multisystem infection. Occasionally it can produce mild illness with tachypnea and a modest oxygen requirement for several weeks after birth.

Central nervous system manifestations are very common and include lethargy and poor feeding, hypertonia or hypotonia, microcephaly, intracranial calcifications, chorioretinitis, and sensorineural deafness. Ocular involvement with CMV occurs in 10% to 20% of symptomatic infants. Most commonly it produces a chorioretinitis that is usually old and inactive at birth. This retinitis is usually unilateral but can produce blindness if the macula is involved, as well as strabismus and optic atrophy. Congenital CMV and congenital toxoplasmosis produce similar lesions; however, congenital CMV characteristically does not produce microphthalmia or cataracts, and alternative diagnoses such as congenital rubella or toxoplasmosis or metabolic disorders should be sought if these eye findings are present. Occasionally it may be difficult to determine if a retinal lesion represents CMV or hemorrhage from thrombocytopenia, and repeat examinations may be necessary before a definitive diagnosis can be made. Generally CMV retinitis associated with congenital CMV disease does not progress postnatally, and it is rare in those infants who are asymptomatic at birth. However, a recent report by Boppana et al.[81] showed 23% of children with congenital CMV infection had either progression of an existing retinal lesion or delayed development of chorioretinitis between the ages of 1.5 and 10 years. Therefore, further studies may be needed to define the long-term risk of retinal disease in these infants.

Microcephaly, defined as a head circumference of less than the third percentile for gestational age, may be present at birth. It may be part of the overall small size of a growth-retarded infant or may be disproportionate and accompanied by normal weight, length, and chest circumferences measurements. Disproportionate microcephaly, especially if severe, is frequently accompanied by intracranial calcifications. However, even apparently asymptomatic infants may have intracranial calcifications detected by unenhanced computed tomography (CT) scan of the brain.[82] Characteristically the calcifications are distributed in a linear, periventricular pattern ranging from tiny, punctate lesions to large deposits of calcium that appear to line the entire ventricular system (Figs 2 and 3). Calcifications also may involve the cortical and subcortical regions or involve the basal ganglia.[83, 84] Other neuroradiographic abnormalities that have been observed in congenital CMV infection include periventricular leukomalacia, cortical atrophy, unilateral or bilateral ventricular enlargement (rarely causing clinical hydrocephalus), subdural effusions and hemorrhage, and polycystic encephalomalacia.[85, 86] Infants with intracranial calcifications are more likely to experience cognitive and audiologic deficits later in life than those infants who do not have detectable abnormalities, but their functional outcome varies widely, and further studies are needed to determine if the pattern or density of the calcifications are predictive of outcome.[86]

Approximately half of the infants with symptomatic and about 15% of infants with asymptomatic congenital CMV infection will have an associated hearing loss. This hearing loss is sensorineural, is variable in its severity at birth, can be unilateral or bilateral, and can progress in severity in approximately 30% of children.[87, 88] Congenital CMV infection also has been associated with abnormalities of higher level auditory functions that may be evident during the school-age years.[89]

A variety of congenital conditions have occurred in infants with congenital CMV infection. It is doubtful that a true cause and effect relationship is present, but these conditions reflect a coincidental occurrence. For example, infants with congenital CMV infection also may have cardiovascular abnormalities, such as septal defects, because both diseases are relatively common. Infants with biliary atresia, inguinal hernias, hip dislocation, and other musculoskeletal abnormalities also may be congenitally infected with

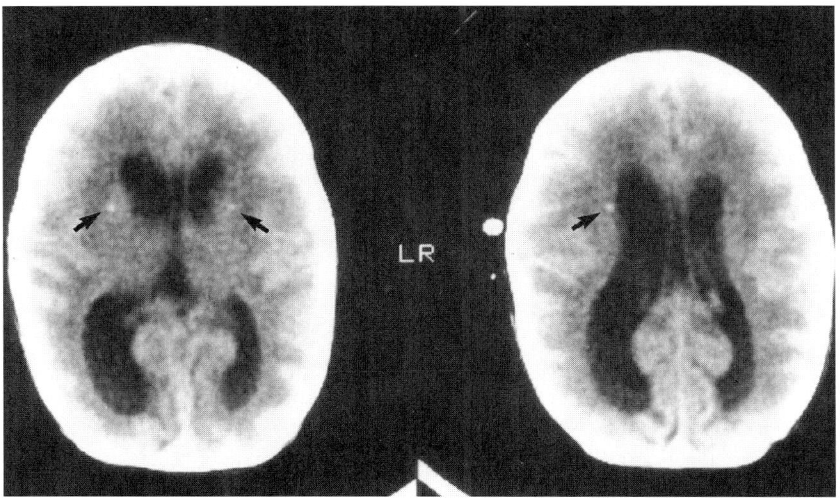

FIGURE 2.

Unenhanced computed tomography scans of the brain showing punctate calcifications and ventriculogemaly (right greater than left) in an infant with prematurity and virologically confirmed congenital cytomegalovirus disease manifested by ascites, hepatosplenomegaly, thrombocytopenia, and deafness. At 4 years, this patient had bilateral profound sensorineural hearing loss but had normal growth and development and cognitive assessments in the above-average ranges for age.

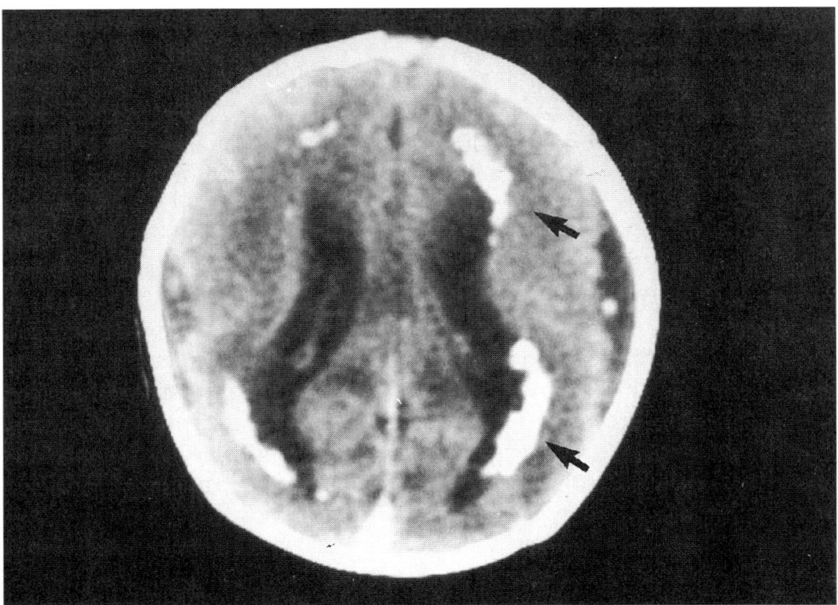

FIGURE 3.

Unenhanced computed tomography scan of the brain showing severe linear periventricular calcifications in a term infant with virologically confirmed congenital cytomegalovirus disease with microcephaly, petechiae, hepatosplenomegaly, and chorioretinitis. At 3½ years, this patient was severely impaired with microcephaly, poor growth, bilateral sensorineural hearing loss, visual impairment, cerebral palsy, and impaired development with cognitive assessments showing function at the 3-month level.

CMV. In addition, infants with toxoplasmosis, herpes simplex virus, syphilis, and HIV infections may be coinfected with CMV, and infants with congenital metabolic disorders, such as maple syrup urine disease, may have congenital CMV infection as well.[90] Therefore, it may be difficult to tell in these patients which symptoms and sequelae, if any, are caused by CMV and which are caused by the confounding condition. It should be noted that noninfectious disorders, especially genetic and metabolic diseases, can produce clinical findings similar to those found in infants with congenital CMV.[91]

The majority of infants who are congenitally infected with CMV are asymptomatic at birth. Yet even these well-appearing infants may have subtle differences in their birth measurements and have been found to be significantly smaller than uninfected infants.[79, 80] In addition, 15% to 17% of these "silently" infected infants will experience significant sensorineural deafness that can be unilateral, bilateral, and even progressive.[87]

SYMPTOMS IN THE FETUS

A fetus infected with CMV may be asymptomatic or have symptoms characteristic of congenital CMV disease, including growth retardation, hepatosplenomegaly, ascites or hydrops, microcephaly, intracranial calcifications, or ventriculomegaly.[92-95] Other manifestations such as lung hypoplasia, ileus, pericardial and pleural effusions, intrahepatic calcifications, and nephritis can occur as well.[96-100] The CMV-infected fetus may have abnormal hematologic indices, most commonly thrombocytopenia, but also anemia and an abnormal white blood cell count; abnormal liver function test results suggest hepatitis. The amniotic fluid often contains infectious virus detectable by viral cultural when fetal infection or disease is present.[93] The presence of signs and symptoms in the fetus does not always predict severe involvement at birth and does not necessarily predict an adverse long-term outcome. For example, fetal ascites and pericardial and pleural effusions may resolve in utero, and their presence does not necessarily mean the newborn will have serious disease or be destined to suffer serious sequelae.[90, 93, 96] The prenatal diagnosis of CMV and careful fetal monitoring will provide more information on the natural history of this infection in the fetus in utero.

Twin fetuses can respond differently when exposed to a maternal CMV infection.[90, 101] Either one or both members of the pair can be infected, and either one or both members of the pair can have disease. I have observed one set of triplets in whom only one of the set was congenitally infected with CMV. It is possible the placentas play a role in transmitting the infection, because in monozygotic twins with monochorionic placentas, both twins are usually infected, whereas in dizygotic twins with either dichorionic or fused placentas, usually only one twin will be infected.

DIAGNOSIS

DIAGNOSIS IN THE PREGNANT WOMAN

The diagnosis in a pregnant woman of a primary infection with CMV can be accomplished by demonstration of seroconversion of CMV-specific IgG antibodies from negative to positive. Unfortunately, such specimens are rarely available in routine clinical practice. The presence of CMV IgG antibodies indicates either a past or current infection, and the height of the titer is not helpful in determining the difference. A rise from a low titer to a very high titer on two serum samples obtained 2 to 3 weeks apart suggests a recent primary infection, but it is not diagnostic because recurrent CMV infection also can be accompanied by a boost in antibody titer. The presence of CMV IgM antibodies suggests a recent primary CMV infection has occurred.[102] However, caution should be exercised in interpreting this test because CMV IgM antibody may persist for 10 to 12 weeks on the average, with ranges between 2 weeks and 6 months observed, after a primary CMV infection in a healthy individual.[90, 103-105] Antibodies to certain viruses, such as Epstein-Barr virus and human herpesvirus type 6 may cross-react with CMV and produce false-positive results.[106, 107] Furthermore, an Epstein-Barr virus mononucleosis may produce a polyclonal B-cell activation and a false-positive CMV serologic test result. Cultures of the urine, saliva, or cervicovaginal secretions are not helpful in discerning whether an asymptomatic woman is experiencing a primary or recurrent CMV infection, nor are they helpful in predicting which women will transmit the virus to their offspring.[72]

DIAGNOSIS IN THE FETUS

The presence of oligohydramnios or polyhydramnios, fetal ascites, nonimmune hydrops, intrauterine growth retardation, hepatosplenomegaly, ileus, pleural or pericardial effusion, microcephaly, cerebral ventriculomegaly, or intracranial or intrahepatic calcifications suggests fetal disease due to intrauterine CMV infection.[93-97] Fetuses with CMV disease also may have anemia, thrombocytopenia, elevated liver function test results, and elevated total IgM levels.[97] Infection with CMV in the fetus can be established by isolation of the virus from amniotic fluid.[92, 93] Detection of CMV DNA by PCR amplification and product detection also has been used, but at the present time this test is considered a research tool. The presence of CMV-specific IgM antibody in fetal blood obtained by cordocentesis suggests the fetus may be infected with CMV. However, negative CMV culture and serologic test results at a particular point in the pregnancy do not eliminate intrauterine CMV infection as a possibility.[72] Although there are uncertainties regarding the diagnostic accuracy of some of these tests, the specific diagnosis of intrauterine CMV disease is important to assist in planning fetal intervention strategies and alerting the pediatrician or neonatologist to potential problems that may be present at birth. This information may be of value to the mother and her obstetrician if termination of pregnancy is a consideration. Specific medical treatment for intrauterine CMV disease also may be available in the future, similar to the therapeutic interventions now available for fetal toxoplasmosis.

Although the use of prenatal tests to establish the diagnosis of CMV-associated fetal disease is warranted, the value of such tests to determine the presence of fetal infection in the absence of fetal disease is uncertain.[108, 109] If a pregnant woman experiences a primary CMV infection, the gestational timing of the transplacental transmission and detection of CMV by culture of amniotic fluid or fetal blood are unknown. However, two small series suggest false-negative amniotic fluid cultures are not common and that amniocentesis can determine if fetal infection with CMV is present, even if the fetus appears normal.[93, 110] In contrast to the prenatal diagnosis of genetic diseases, for which the diagnosis and outcome can be established with reasonable certainty, most of the infants with congenital CMV infection are asymptomatic and do not suffer sequelae. Therefore, both obstetrician and the pregnant women should know the relative frequency of all the possible outcomes before an informed decision can be made regarding the pregnancy. If the woman decides to continue her pregnancy, it may be prudent, and many times reassuring, to monitor the growth and development of the fetus with serial ultrasound examinations.[93] Other experts argue that in the absence of fetal disease, the prenatal diagnosis of fetal infection is not warranted because the predictive value of positive and negative results are not clear and should not be used as a basis for management decisions.[109]

DIAGNOSIS IN THE NEWBORN

The diagnosis of congenital CMV infection is established by isolating the virus from urine, saliva, or tissue obtained during the first 3 weeks of life. All infants in whom the diagnosis is suspected should have a viral culture performed. The virus is usually present in a very high titer, and cultures are commonly positive within 2 or 3 days of incubation. It is important the test be performed early in life, because detection of the virus in bodily fluids or tissue after the age of 3 weeks can indicate either a congenital, perinatal, or postnatal infection.

Standard serologic tests, such as detection of CMV IgG and IgM antibodies used alone or as part of a TORCH (toxoplasmosis, rubella, CMV, and herpes simplex) titer panel are commonly used to diagnose congenital CMV infection, but this approach has several drawbacks and should be discouraged. Although the absence of IgG antibodies to CMV in cord or infant blood probably rules out congenital CMV infection in an immune-competent mother-infant pair, its presence has limited value because 50% to 80% of women of childbearing age will have CMV IgG antibodies that will be transplacentally transferred to their infant. A significantly higher titer of IgG antibodies to CMV in the infant than in the mother may imply an active congenital infection, but in practice this difference is usually difficult to ascertain. Serologic samples obtained serially at 1 month, 3 months, and 6 months may rule out congenital infection if the level of CMV antibodies gradually declines and disappears. However, if antibody persists, serologic test results alone cannot determine whether the infant was congenitally or perinatally infected. The presence of CMV IgM antibodies at birth, however, is highly suggestive of a congenital CMV infection, provided the test was performed properly, but a confirmatory urine culture for CMV is recommended to definitively establish the diagnosis. Furthermore, a negative CMV IgM antibody test result does not exclude the diagnosis of congenital CMV infection, because only between 30% and 89% of infants with virologically confirmed CMV infection will have a positive CMV IgM antibody determination.[7]

The diagnosis of congenital CMV is almost always suspected in symptomatic infants, and the proper diagnostic tests are ordered based on clinical suspicion. However, the presence of an asymptomatic congenital CMV infection can be established only if newborns are routinely screened. The concept of screening newborns for this congenital infection is not new. In fact, over the past 20 years, a variety of methods have been evaluated, including cell culture of urine and saliva, electron microscopy to directly visualize viral particles in urine, detection of viral antigens in urine by enzyme immunoassay, and detection of viral DNA by isotopic and enzyme hybridization.[7] Recently CMV DNA has been detected by PCR in urine from newborns and in urine that has been applied to glass filter paper.[111, 112] A rapid, centrifugation-enhanced culture assay for detection of CMV in saliva of newborns, based on monoclonal antibody detection of early antigen fluorescent foci, has been shown to be as sensitive as traditional cell culture on urine samples and may be useful as a screening test.[113] A method that provides a rapid and readily available diagnosis of congenital CMV disease will become increasingly important as antiviral therapy becomes available. Infants with asymptomatic congenital CMV infection also would benefit if a rapid, simple, cost-effective test were available that allowed the routine screening of newborns, because, if identified at birth, these infants could receive the proper anticipatory guidance, including early detection of hearing loss and neurodevelopmental problems.

Recently CMV DNA has been detected in the cerebrospinal fluid of neonates with congenital CMV disease, and its presence appears to be significantly associated with developmental delay.[114] It is possible this evaluation may be used in the future to identify infants who are at risk for neurodevelopmental problems and who may therefore benefit from antiviral therapy.

EVALUATION OF THE NEWBORN WITH CONGENITAL CYTOMEGALOVIRUS INFECTION

A newborn identified as having a congenital infection with CMV should be evaluated to determine the extent of the viral infection in various organ systems, especially the central nervous system (Table 2). A CT scan of the brain is particularly important to document the extent of central nervous system involvement. Skull radiographs are not recommended, and even cranial ultrasound examinations may be insensitive in visualizing intracranial calcifications. Furthermore, long-bone radiographs rarely provide useful

---

TABLE 2.
Suggested Evaluation of the Neonate With Congenital Cytomegalovirus Infection

---

Clinical
   Height, weight, and head circumference measurements
   Measure liver/spleen size
   Ophthalmologic examination
Laboratory
   Complete blood count and peripheral smear
   Platelet count
   Liver transaminase levels
   Bilirubin level, direct and indirect
   Urine cytomegalovirus culture
   Cerebrospinal fluid for cell count, protein level, glucose level,
     cytomegalovirus culture and DNA (if tests are available, patient
     is stable, and platelet count is adequate)
Other
   Unenhanced computed tomography scan of brain
   Hearing assessment by brain stem–evoked responses

clinical information and are similarly discouraged as part of the routine evaluation of a child with congenital CMV disease. An examination of the eyes and retina should be performed by an ophthalmologist experienced in examining infants and children, and retinal lesions should be carefully followed. If retinal lesions are not present at birth, consideration still should be given to periodic eye examinations, including the retina, to watch for late-onset retinitis.[81] A neurophysiologic assessment of the newborn's auditory status, usually obtained by performing auditory brain stem–evoked responses is indicated to determine if deafness is present. Regardless of the neonatal hearing evaluation, the child should be followed up at least annually, and more frequently if hearing loss is detected early, to monitor for late-onset or progressive hearing loss.[87] Careful longitudinal follow-up of the child's development also is needed to identify and manage developmental disabilities at the earliest possible age.[88] Congenitally infected infants who are symptomatic at birth are at high risk for long-term neurodevelopmental sequelae. However, some symptomatic infants, especially those who do not have significant intracranial calcifications or microcephaly at birth, may have normal growth and development.[86] Therefore, care should be taken not to generalize a poor outcome for all these children but to be cautiously optimistic when appropriate and to take a "wait and see" approach.

TREATMENT

Two antiviral chemotherapeutic agents, ganciclovir and foscarnet, are licensed specifically for treatment of serious, life-threatening, or sight-threatening CMV disease in immunocompromised patients. Currently a randomized, controlled multicenter clinical trial evaluating the use of ganciclovir for the treatment of infants with symptomatic congenital CMV infection and evidence of central nervous system involvement is in progress. In this trial sponsored by the National Institutes of Health–National Institute of Allergy and Infectious Diseases, ganciclovir, administered in a 6 mg/kg dose intravenously as a 1-hour infusion every 12 hours for up to 6 weeks, has been tolerated when cautiously administered to newborns and has decreased excretion of virus during its administration.[115] It is unknown whether this early and intensive administration of ganciclovir will hasten resolution of acute disease, beneficially influence growth and development, decrease auditory and visual impairments, or improve intellectual outcome in these infants. Reports suggest that ganciclovir is being used to treat selected infants with congenital CMV disease; however, because of the potential bone marrow suppression, as yet unforeseen long-term effects such as testicular atrophy and its as yet unproven benefit on long-term neurodevelopmental outcome, it is recommended that ganciclovir not be routinely used to treat infants with congenital CMV disease until the results of ongoing clinical trials establish its safety and efficacy.[115, 116] Anecdotal evidence does suggest, however, that critically ill newborns, especially those who are premature and have CMV pneumonia, may acutely benefit from ganciclovir treatment, and its use should be carefully considered in selected cases.[117, 118]

A CMV hyperimmune globulin has been licensed to prevent CMV disease in renal transplant patients, but its use in the treatment of newborns with congenital CMV disease or in the prevention of transmission of CMV infection to the fetus has not been evaluated.[119] A national collaborative trial is in progress to evaluate the safety, pharmacokinetics, and possible benefits of a new, human anti-CMV monoclonal antibody preparation administered to infants with symptomatic congenital CMV infection who do not have central nervous system involvement.

The treatment of newborns with asymptomatic congenital infection currently is not indicated, even though these infants are at some risk for hearing loss, because of the side effects of therapy with currently available antiviral agents. More research is needed to develop less toxic antiviral agents that are active against CMV and that can be administered orally for a prolonged period or that cross the placenta and can be administered to pregnant women.

PREVENTION

Prevention of congenital CMV disease is desirable and urgently needed. Not only does the disease cause individual pain and suffering, as well as grief and hardship for family, but caring for these children in the United States costs collectively almost $2 billion each year.[120, 121] Because the majority of symptomatic congenital CMV disease and its sequelae occur in women who have experienced primary CMV infection during pregnancy, pregnant women and their fetuses would benefit greatly if a safe, effective CMV vaccine were licensed.[71, 120] The use of a CMV vaccine to prevent congenital disease also appears to be cost effective. Porath et al.[122] used a decision analysis to consider three strategies (routine immunization of all healthy women aged 15 to 25 years, immunization of only nonimmune women in this age group, and no immunization).

Both routine immunization and selective immunization of seronegative women were found cost effective when compared with no immunization. Routine immunization of toddlers was not considered in this particular study but is another possible strategy that deserves consideration.

Currently no acceptable CMV vaccine is available for general use. An experimental, live-attenuated CMV vaccine, Towne 125, has been evaluated in more than 500 volunteers, including renal-transplant recipients and healthy adult male and female volunteers.[123] These studies showed Towne 125 to be safe, attenuated, and apparently capable of directing an immunologic response that results in synthesis of antibodies and priming of lymphocytes. In addition, the vaccine appeared protective in a randomized, placebo-controlled study of 91 immunosuppressed renal transplant recipients.[124] Clinical trials of this vaccine in women of childbearing age who are exposed daily to CMV-infected children in the home or workplace are needed.

Another vaccine alternative is to use a subunit or recombinant vaccine based on one of the surface glycoproteins of the virus. This approach is problematic because the CMV genome codes for more than 100 proteins, many of which are recognized by human convalescent sera and are targets of neutralizing antibodies. The surface glycoprotein important in maternal immunity and prevention of virus transmission to the fetus is unknown. Nonetheless, certain proteins, especially glycoprotein B (gp55-116 or gB), show promise and should be targets for recombinant vaccine development and clinical trials.[125–127]

While research continues on a potential CMV vaccine, alternative options for prevention of primary CMV infection in pregnant women should be considered and studied. Some experts think that because reliable, inexpensive serologic tests are now available for CMV, all women of childbearing age should know their CMV serostatus.[120] Those women who are CMV seronegative should be aware that young children are likely sources of CMV infection, and they should practice good hygiene when they are with young children in their home or in group child-care environments.[120, 128–130] A similar form of behavioral intervention is currently practiced by women who wish to avoid exposure to toxoplasmosis during pregnancy (avoidance of raw meat, cat litter boxes, and sandlots), and was also practiced during rubella epidemics before a vaccine was available (susceptible pregnant women avoided contact with children with suspected rubella). Because of the current complexities of antiviral therapy and vaccine development, it is the only available option at this time to a pregnant woman who wishes to try to reduce her risk and the risk to her fetus.

REFERENCES

1. Ho M: History of cytomegalovirus. In Ho M (ed): *Cytomegalovirus: Biology and Infection*, ed 2. pp 1–10, 57–60, 189–203, 1991.
2. Rowe WP, Hartley JW, Waterman S, et al: Cytopathogenic agent resembling human salivary gland virus recovered from tissue cultures of human adenoids. *Proc Soc Exp Biol Med* 92:418–424, 1956.
3. Smith MG: Propagation in tissue cultures of a cytopathogenic virus from human salivary gland virus (SGV) disease. *Proc Soc Exp Biol Med* 92:424–430, 1956.
4. Weller TH, Macauley JC, Craig JM, et al: Isolation of intranuclear inclusion-producing agents from infants with illnesses resembling cytomegalic inclusion disease. *Proc Soc Exp Biol Med* 94:4–12, 1957.
5. Weller TH, Hanshaw JB: Virological and clinical observation of cytomegalic inclusion disease. *N Engl J Med* 266:1233–1344, 1962.
6. Weller TH: The cytomegaloviruses: Ubiquitous agents with protean clinical manifestations. *N Engl J Med* 285:203–214, 1971.
7. Demmler GJ: Summary of a workshop on surveillance for congenital cytomegalovirus disease. *Rev Infect Dis* 13:315–329, 1991.
8. Adler SP: The molecular epidemiology of cytomegalovirus transmission among children attending a day care center. *J Infect Dis* 152:760–767, 1985.
9. Adler S: Molecular epidemiology of cytomegalovirus: A study of factors affecting transmission among children at three day-care centers. *Pediatr Infect Dis J* 10:585–594, 1991.
10. Demmler G, O'Neil G, O'Neil J, et al: Transmission of cytomegalovirus from husband to wife [letter]. *J Infect Dis* 154:545–546, 1986.
11. Sokol D, Demmler G, Buffone G: Rapid epidemiologic analysis of cytomegalovirus by using polymerase chain reaction amplification of the L-S junction region. *J Clin Microbiol* 30:839–844, 1993.
12. Bale J, O'Neil M, Fowler S, et al: Analysis of acquired human cytomegalovirus infections by polymerase chain reaction. *J Clin Microbiol* 31:2433–2438, 1993.
13. Grillner L, Ahlfors K, Ivarsson S, et al: *Pediatrics* 81:27–30, 1988.
14. Zaia J, Gallez-Hawkins G, Churchill M, et al: Comparative analysis of human cytomegalovirus α-sequence in multiple clinical isolates by using polymerase chain reaction and restriction fragment length polymorphism assays. *J Clin Microbiol* 28:2602–2607, 1990.
15. Chou S: Differentiation of cytomegalovirus strains by restriction analysis of DNA sequences amplified from clinical specimens. *J Infect Dis* 162:738–742, 1990.
16. Chou S: Acquisition of donor strains of cytomegalovirus by renal transplant recipients. *N Engl J Med* 22:1418–1423, 1986.
17. Chandler SH, Handsfield HH, McDougall JK: Isolation of multiple

strains of cytomegalovirus from women attending a clinic for sexually transmitted diseases. *J Infect Dis* 15:655–660, 1987.

18. Griffiths PD, Baboonian D: A prospective study of primary cytomegalovirus infection during pregnancy: Final report. *Br J Obstet Gynaecol* 92:307–315, 1984.

19. Stagno S, Pass RF, Dworsky ME, et al: Congenital cytomegalovirus infection: The relative importance of primary and recurrent maternal infection. *N Engl J Med* 306:945–949, 1982.

20. Yow MD, Williamson DW, Leeds LJ, et al: Epidemiologic characteristics of cytomegalovirus infection in mothers and their infants. *Am J Obstet Gynecol* 158:1189–1195, 1988.

21. Alford CA, Stagno S, Pass RF, et al: Epidemiology of cytomegalovirus infections. In Nahmias AJ, Dowdle WR, Schinazi RF (eds): *The Human Herpesviruses: An Interdisciplinary Perspective.* New York, Elsevier North Holland, 1987, pp 373–393.

22. Ashraf SJ, Parande CM, Arya SC: Cytomegalovirus antibodies of patients in the Gizen area of Saudi Arabia. *J Infect Dis* 152:1351, 1985.

23. Wang PS, Evans AS: Prevalence of antibodies to Epstein-Barr virus and cytomegalovirus in sera from a group of children in the People's Republic of China. *J Infect Dis* 153:150–152, 1986.

24. Yow MD, White NH, Taber LH, et al: Acquisition of cytomegalovirus infection from birth to 10 years: A longitudinal serologic study. *J Pediatr* 111:37–42, 1987.

25. White NH, Yow MD, Demmler GJ, et al: Prevalence of cytomegalovirus antibody in subjects between the ages of 6 and 22 years. *J Infect Dis* 159:1012–1017, 1989.

26. Saigal S, Luny KO, Larke R, et al: The outcome in children with congenital cytomegalovirus infection. *Am J Dis Child* 136:896–901, 1982.

27. Dworsky ME, Yow MD, Stagno S, et al: Cytomegalovirus infection of breast milk and transmission in infancy. *Pediatrics* 72:295–300, 1983.

28. Reynolds DW, Stagno S, Hosty TS, et al: Maternal CMV excretion and perinatal infection. *N Engl J Med* 289:4–7, 1973.

29. Pass RF, August AM, Dworsky M, et al: Cytomegalovirus infection in a day-care center. *N Engl J Med* 307:477–479, 1982.

30. Jones LA, Duke-Duncan PM, Yeager AS: Cytomegaloviral infections in infant-toddler centers: Centers for the developmentally delayed versus regular day care. *J Infect Dis* 151:953–955, 1985.

31. Murph JR, Bale JF: The natural history of acquired cytomegalovirus infection among children in group day care. *Am J Dis Child* 142:843–846, 1988.

32. Pass RF, Hutto C: Group day care and cytomegaloviral infections of mothers and children. *Rev Infect Dis* 8:599–605, 1986.

33. Pass RF, Hutto C, Reynolds DW, et al: Increased frequency of cytomegalovirus infection in children in group day care. *Pediatrics* 74:121–126, 1984.

34. Demmler GJ, Schydlower M, Lampe RM: Texas, teenagers, and CMV [letter]. *J Infect Dis* 152:1350, 1985.
35. Kumar ML, Gold E, Jacobs IB, et al: Primary cytomegalovirus infection in adolescent pregnancy. *Pediatrics* 74:493–500, 1984.
36. Istas A, Demmler GJ, Dobbins JG, et al: Surveillance for congenital cytomegalovirus disease: A report from the National Congenital Cytomegalovirus Disease Registry. *Clin Infect Dis* 20:665–670, 1995.
37. Chretien JH, McGinniss CG, Muller A: Venereal causes of cytomegalovirus mononucleosis. *JAMA* 238:1644–1645, 1977.
38. Lang DJ, Kummer JF, Hartley DP: Cytomegalovirus in semen: Persistence and demonstration in extracellular fluids. *N Engl J Med* 291:121–123, 1974.
39. Lang DJ, Kummer JF: Cytomegalovirus in semen: Observations in selected populations. *J Infect Dis* 132:472–473, 1975.
40. Jordan MC, Rousseau WE, Noble GR, et al: Association of cervical cytomegaloviruses with venereal disease. *N Engl J Med* 288:932–934, 1973.
41. Collier AC, Handsfield HH, Roberts PL, et al: Cytomegalovirus infection in women attending a sexually transmitted disease clinic. *J Infect Dis* 162:46–51, 1990.
42. Handsfield HH, Chandler SH, Caine VA, et al: Cytomegalovirus infection in sex partners; evidence for sexual transmission. *J Infect Dis* 151:344–348, 1985.
43. Pass RF, Hutto C, Ricks R, et al: Increased rate of cytomegalovirus infection among parents of children attending day-care centers. *N Engl J Med* 314:1414–1418, 1986.
44. Adler SP: Cytomegalovirus transmission among children in day care, their mothers and caretakers. *Pediatr Infect Dis* 7:279–285, 1988.
45. Adler SP: Molecular epidemiology of cytomegalovirus: Viral transmission among children attending a day care center, their parents, and caretakers. *J Pediatr* 112:366–372, 1988.
46. Yeager A: Transmission of cytomegalovirus to mothers by infected infants: Another reason to prevent transfusion-acquired infections. *Pediatr Infect Dis* 2:295–297, 1983.
47. Spector SA, Spector DH: Molecular epidemiology of cytomegalovirus infections in premature twin infants and their mother. *Pediatr Infect Dis* 1:405–409, 1982.
48. Dworsky M, Lakeman A, Stagno S: Cytomegalovirus transmission within a family. *Pediatr Infect Dis* 3:236–238, 1984.
49. Pass RF, Little EA, Stagno S, et al: Young children as a probable source of maternal and congenital cytomegalovirus infection. *N Engl J Med* 316:1366–1370, 1987.
50. Dworsky ME, Welch K, Cassady G, et al: Occupational risk for primary cytomegalovirus infection among pediatric healthcare workers. *N Engl J Med* 309:950–953, 1983.
51. Balfour CL, Balfour HH Jr: Cytomegalovirus is not an occupational risk

for nurses in renal transplant and neonatal units: Results of a prospective surveillance study. *JAMA* 256:1909–1914, 1986.

52. Demmler GJ, Yow MD, Spector SA, et al: Nosocomial cytomegalovirus infections within two hospitals caring for infants and children. *J Infect Dis* 156:9–16, 1987.

53. Adler SP, Baggett J, Wilson M, et al: Molecular epidemiology of cytomegalovirus in a nursery: Lack of evidence for nosocomial transmission. *J Pediatr* 108:117–123, 1986.

54. Balcarek KB, Bagley R, Cloud GA, et al: Cytomegalovirus infection among employees in a children's hospital: No evidence for increased risk associated with patient care. *JAMA* 263:840–844, 1990.

55. Yow MD, Lakeman AD, Stagno S, et al: Use of restriction enzymes to investigate the source of a primary cytomegalovirus infection in a pediatric nurse. *Pediatrics* 70:713–716, 1982.

56. Wilfert CM, Huang ES, Stagno S: Restriction endonuclease analysis of cytomegalovirus deoxyribonucleic acid an epidemiologic tool. *Pediatrics* 70:717–721, 1982.

57. Hokeberg I, Brillner L, Reisenfeld T: No evidence of hospital-acquired cytomegalovirus infection in a pregnant pediatric nurse using restriction endonuclease analysis. *Pediatr Infect Dis J* 7:812–814, 1988.

58. Adler SP: Cytomegalovirus and child day care: Evidence for an increased infection rate among day care workers. *N Engl J Med* 321:1290–1296, 1989.

59. Tolpin MD, Stewart JA, Warren D, et al: Transfusion transmission by restriction endonuclease analysis. *J Pediatr* 107:953–956, 1985.

60. Yeager AS, Grumet FC, Hafleigh EB, et al: Prevention of transfusion-acquired cytomegalovirus infections in newborn infants. *J Pediatr* 98:281–287, 1981.

61. McGregor JA, Rubright G, Ogle JW: Congenital cytomegalovirus infection as a preventable complication of maternal transfusion: A case report. *J Reprod Med* 35:61–64, 1990.

62. Evans DGR, Lyon AJ: Fatal congenital cytomegalovirus infection acquired by an intrauterine transfusion. *Eur J Pediatr* 780–781, 1991.

63. Jones MM, Lidsky MD, Brewer EJ, et al: Congenital cytomegalovirus infection and maternal systemic lupus erythematosus: A case report. *Arthritis Rheum* 29:1402–1404, 1986.

64. Hayes K, Symington G, Mackey IR: Maternal immunosuppression and cytomegalovirus infection of the fetus. *Aust N Z J Med* 9:430–433, 1979.

65. Evans TJ, McCollum JPK, Vladimarsson H: Congenital cytomegalovirus infection after maternal renal transplantation. *Lancet* 1:1359–1360, 1975.

66. Witzleben CL, Marshall GS, Wenner W, et al: HIV as a cause of giant cell hepatitis. *Hum Pathol* 19:603–605, 1988.

67. Belec L, Tayot J, Tron J, et al: Cytomegalovirus encephalopathy in an infant with congenital acquired immunodeficiency syndrome. *Neuropediatr* 21:124–129, 1990.

68. Cooper ER, Schwartz T, Brena A, et al: Cytomegalovirus as a cofactor in transmission and progression of perinatal HIV infection. *Pediatr AIDS HIV Inf Fet Adolesc* 3:302–307, 1992.
69. Vallejo JG, Englund JA, Garcia-Prats J, et al: Ganciclovir treatment of steroid-associated cytomegalovirus disease in a congenitally infected neonate. *Pediatr Infect Dis J* 13:239–241, 1994.
70. Britt WJ, Vugler LG: Antiviral antibody responses in mothers and their newborn infants with clinical and subclinical congenital cytomegalovirus infections. *J Infect Dis* 161:214–219, 1990.
71. Fowler K, Stagno S, Pass RF, et al: The outcome of congenital cytomegalovirus infection in relation to maternal antibody status. *N Engl J Med* 326:663–667, 1992.
72. Stagno S, Pass RF, Dworsky ME, et al: Maternal cytomegalovirus infection and perinatal transmission. *Clin Obstet Gynecol* 25:563–576, 1982.
73. Alford CA, Stagno S, Pass RF, et al: Congenital and perinatal cytomegalovirus infections. *Rev Infect Dis* 12S7:S745–S753, 1990.
74. Stagno S, Whitley R: Herpesvirus infections in pregnancy: I. Cytomegalovirus and Epstein-Barr virus infections. *N Engl J Med* 313:1270–1274, 1985.
75. Stagno S, Pass RF, Cloud G, et al: Primary cytomegalovirus infection in pregnancy: Incidence, transmission to fetus, and clinical outcome. *JAMA* 256:1904–1908, 1986.
76. Nankervis GA, Kumar ML, Cox FE, et al: A prospective study of maternal cytomegalovirus infection and its effect on the fetus. *Am J Obstet Gynecol* 149:435–440, 1984.
77. Yow MD: CMV infection in young women. *Hosp Pract (Off)* March 30:61–79, 1990.
78. Boppana SB, Pass RF, Britt WJ, et al: Symptomatic congenital cytomegalovirus infection: Neonatal morbidity and mortality. *Pediatr Infect Dis J* 11:93–99, 1992.
79. Berge P, Stagno S, Federer W, et al: Impact of asymptomatic congenital cytomegalovirus infection on size at birth and gestational duration. *Pediatr Infect Dis J* 9:170–175, 1990.
80. Demmler GJ, Istas AS, Griesser CM, et al: Risk factors for congenital cytomegalovirus infection. In *Final Program and Abstracts.* Infectious Diseases Society of America 32nd Annual Meeting, Abstract no 329, Oct 7–9, 1994.
81. Boppana S, Amos C, Britt W, et al: Late onset and reactivation of chorioretinitis in children with congenital cytomegalovirus infection. *Pediatr Infect Dis J* 13:1139–1142, 1994.
82. Williamson WD, Percy AK, Yow MD, et al: Asymptomatic congenital cytomegalovirus infection: Audiologic, neuroradiologic and neurodevelopmental abnormalities during the first year. *Am J Dis Child* 144:1365–1368, 1990.
83. Roach ES, Sumner T, Volbert F, et al: Radiologic case of the month:

Intracranial calcification with cytomegalovirus. *Am J Dis Child* 137:799−800, 1983.

84. Sowers J, Jaeckle K, Allen J, et al: Computed tomography in the diagnosis of congenital cytomegalic inclusion disease. *South Med J* 75:1421−1424, 1982.

85. Bale J, Bray P, Bell W: Neuroradiographic abnormalities in congenital cytomegalovirus infection. *Pediatr Neurol* 1:42−47, 1985.

86. Williamson WD, Demmler GJ, Bale J, et al: Symptomatic congenital CMV infection: Relationship of CT scans to neurodevelopmental and audiologic outcome [Abstract no 1106] *Pediatr Res* 33:187A, 1993.

87. Williamson WD, Demmler GJ, Percy AK, et al: Progressive hearing loss in infants with asymptomatic congenital cytomegalovirus infection. *Pediatrics* 90:862−866, 1992.

88. Williamson WD: The longitudinal assessment of congenitally infected infants. *Semin Pediatr Neurol* 1:58−62, 1994.

89. Connolly PK, Jerger S, Williamson DW, et al: Evaluation of higher-level auditory function in children with asymptomatic congenital cytomegalovirus infection. *Am J Otol* 13:185−193, 1992.

90. Demmler GJ: Unpublished data, 1994.

91. Bale J: Conditions mimicking congenital infections. *Semin Neurol* 1:63−70, 1994.

92. Grose C, Weiner CP: Prenatal diagnosis of congenital cytomegalovirus infection: Two decades later. *Am J Obstet Gynecol* 163:447−450, 1990.

93. Hohlfeld P, Vial Y, Maillard-Brignon C, et al: Cytomegalovirus fetal infection: Prenatal diagnosis. *Obstet Gynecol* 78:615−618, 1991.

94. Ghidini A, Sirtori M, Vergani P, et al: Fetal intracranial calcifications. *Am J Obstet Gynecol* 160:86−87, 1989.

95. Mittelmann-Handwerker A, Pardes JG, Post RC, et al: Ventriculomegaly and brain atrophy in a woman with intrauterine cytomegalovirus infection: A case report. *J Reprod Med* 31:1061−1064, 1986.

96. Binder ND, Buckmaster JW, Benda GI: Outcome for fetus with ascites and cytomegalovirus infection. *Pediatrics* 82:100−103, 1988.

97. Yamashita Y, Iwanaga R, Goto A, et al: Congenital cytomegalovirus infection associated with fetal ascites and intrahepatic calcifications. *Acta Pediatr Scand* 78:965−967, 1989.

98. Stocher JT: Congenital cytomegalovirus infection presenting as massive ascites with secondary pulmonary hypoplasia. *Hum Pathol* 16:1173−1175, 1985.

99. Cramer BC, Jequier S, Chen MF: Sonographic appearance of cytomegalovirus nephritis in a neonate. *Pediatr Radiol* 15:56−57, 1985.

100. Dechelotte PJ, Mulliez NM, Bouvier KJ, et al: Pseudomeconium ileus due to cytomegalovirus infection: A report of three cases. *Pediatr Pathol* 12:73−82, 1992.

101. Ahlfors K, Ivarsson SA, Nilsson H: On the unpredictable development of congenital cytomegalovirus infection: A study of twins. *Early Hum Dev* 18:125−135, 1988.

102. Griffiths PD, Stagno S, Pass RF, et al: Infection with cytomegalovirus during pregnancy: Specific IgM antibodies as a marker of recent primary infection. *J Infect Dis* 145:647–653, 1982.
103. Stagno S, Tinker MK, Elrod C, et al: Immunoglobulin M antibodies detected by enzyme-linked immunosorbent assay and radioimmunoassay in the diagnosis of cytomegalovirus infections in pregnant women and newborn infants. *J Clin Microbiol* 21:930–935, 1985.
104. Demmler GJ, Six HR, Hurst SM, et al: Enzyme-linked immunosorbent assay for the detection of IgM-class antibodies to cytomegalovirus. *J Infect Dis* 153:1152–1155, 1986.
105. Schaefer L, Cesario A, Demmler G, et al: Evaluation of Abbott CMV-M enzyme immunoassay for detection of cytomegalovirus immunoglobulin M antibody. *J Clin Microbiol* 26:2041–2043, 1988.
106. Sumaya CV: Endogenous reactivation of Epstein-Barr virus infections. *J Infect Dis* 135:374–379, 1977.
107. Chou S, Scott KM: Rises in antibody to human herpesvirus 6 detected by enzyme immunoassay in transplant recipients with primary cytomegalovirus infection. *J Clin Microbiol* 28:851–854, 1990.
108. Grose C, Meehan T, Weiner CP: Prenatal diagnosis of congenital cytomegalovirus infection by virus isolation after amniocentesis. *Pediatr Infect Dis J* 11:605–607, 1992.
109. Pass RF: Commentary: Is there a role for prenatal diagnosis of congenital cytomegalovirus infection? *Pediatr Infect Dis J* 11:608–609, 1992.
110. Skvorc-Ranko R, Lavoie H, St Denis P, et al: Intrauterine diagnosis of cytomegalovirus and rubella infections by amniocentesis. *Can Med Assoc J* 145:649–654, 1991.
111. Demmler G, Buffone G, Schimbor, et al: Detection of cytomegalovirus in urine from newborns by using polymerase chain reaction DNA amplification. *J Infect Dis* 158:1177–1184, 1988.
112. Sokol D, Demmler G, Troendle J, et al: Glass filter paper, polymerase chain reaction to screen newborns for congenital cytomegalovirus. *Pediatr Res* 31:282A, 1992.
113. Balcarek K, Warren W, Smith R, et al: Neonatal screening for congenital cytomegalovirus infection by detection of virus in saliva. *J Infect Dis* 67:1433–1436, 1993.
114. Troendle Atkins J, Demmler GJ, Williamson WD, et al: Polymerase chain reaction to detect cytomegalovirus DNA in the cerebrospinal fluid of neonates with congenital infection. *J Infect Dis* 169:1334–1337, 1994.
115. Trang J, Kidd L, Gruber W, et al: Linear single-dose pharmacokinetics of ganciclovir in newborns with congenital cytomegalovirus infections. *Clin Pharmacol Ther* 53:15–21, 1993.
116. Nigro G, Scholz H, Bartmann U: Ganciclovir therapy for symptomatic congenital cytomegalovirus infection in infants: A two-regimen experience. *Pediatrics* 124:318–322, 1994.

117. Hocker J, Cook L, Adams G, et al: Ganciclovir therapy of congenital cytomegalovirus pneumonia. *Pediatr Infect Dis J* 9:743–745, 1994.
118. Vallejo J, Englund J, Garcia-Prats J, et al: Ganciclovir treatment of steroid-associated cytomegalovirus disease in a congenitally infected neonate. *Pediatr Infect Dis J* 13:239–241, 1994.
119. Demmler G: Cytomegalovirus infections. In Kaplan S (ed): *Current Therapy in Pediatric Infectious Disease.* St Louis, Mosby, 1993, pp 191–197.
120. Yow MD, Demmler GJ: Congenital CMV disease: 20 years is long enough. *N Engl J Med* 326:702–703, 1992.
121. Dobbins JG, Stewart J, Demmler G, et al: *MMWR* 41(SS-2):35–44, 1991.
122. Porath A, McNutt RA, Smiley LM, et al: Effectiveness and cost benefit of a proposed live cytomegalovirus vaccine in the prevention of congenital disease. *Rev Infect Dis* 12:31–40, 1990.
123. Demmler G: Vaccines for cytomegalovirus. *Semin Pediatr Infect Dis* 2:186–190, 1991.
124. Plotkin S, Friedman H, Fleisher G, et al: Towne-vaccine induced prevention of cytomegalovirus disease after renal transplants. *Lancet* 1:528–530, 1984.
125. Boppana SB, Pass RF, Britt WJ: Virus-specific antibody responses in mothers and their newborn infants with asymptomatic congenital cytomegalovirus infections. *J Infect Dis* 167:72–77, 1993.
126. Rasmussen L, Matkin C, Spaete R, et al: Antibody response to human cytomegalovirus glycoproteins gb and gH after natural infection in humans. *J Infect Dis* 164:835–842, 1991.
127. Urban M, Winkler T, Landini M, et al: Epitope-specific distribution of IgG subclasses against antigenic domains on glycoproteins of human cytomegalovirus. *J Infect Dis* 169:83–90, 1993.
128. Murph J, Bale J, Murray J, et al: Cytomegalovirus transmission in a Midwest day care center: Possible relationship to child care practices. *J Pediatr* 109:35–39, 1986.
129. Demmler GJ: Congenital cytomegalovirus infection: Strategies for prevention. *Pediatr Virol* 4:1–4, 1989.
130. Yow MD: Congenital cytomegalovirus disease: A NOW problem. *J Infect Dis* 159:163–167, 1989.

Recent Advances in the Prevention of *Pneumocystis carinii* Pneumonia

Walter T. Hughes, M.D.
Chairman, Department of Infectious Disease, St. Jude Children's
Research Hospital, Memphis, Tennessee

W ithin recent years *Pneumocystis carinii* pneumonia (PCP) has gained prominence as a major infectious disease of humans. Currently more people die of PCP in the United States than the total deaths from all contagious infectious diseases reported to the Centers for Disease Control and Prevention (CDC), including meningitis, hepatitis, tuberculosis, encephalitis, polio, tetanus, measles, varicella, diphtheria, gonorrhea, syphlitis, and typhoid. This surge of cases is the result of the acquired immunodeficiency syndrome (AIDS) epidemic. Even as the epidemic began in 1980, PCP was clearly identified as the major opportunistic infection of the syndrome, occurring in about 75% of cases, and fatal in approximately 100% of cases, if untreated. Prior to the epidemic, PCP was known to occur in severely immunocompromised patients with cancer, congenital immunodeficiency syndromes, organ transplant recipients, and other entities affecting the immune system. A unique feature of PCP is its almost exclusive occurrence in the compromised host. Thus, a population of individuals at high risk for PCP can be easily identified. These factors provide a basis for prophylaxis. Only three general approaches have been effective in the prevention of an infectious disease: quarantine (isolation), immunization, and chemoprophylaxis. Although quarantine is inappropriate and not feasible and attempts at immunization were found ineffective, chemoprophylaxis has been shown to be highly effective and practical in the management of high-risk patients.

The purpose of this chapter is to review developments in PCP prophylaxis in recent years. Emphasis will be placed on studies reported during the past 3 years, after a brief review of earlier studies.

Advances in Pediatric Infectious Diseases®, vol. 11
© 1996, Mosby–Year Book, Inc.

EARLY STUDIES

The development of effective prophylactic and therapeutic drugs for PCP has been greatly aided by an excellent experimental animal model for the infection. Using the corticosteroid-treated rat, the drug combination trimethoprim-sulfamethoxazole (TMP-SMZ) was shown to be highly effective for the prevention of murine PCP.[1] A placebo-controlled clinical trial over a 2-year period in the mid-1970s found the occurrence of PCP to be 21% in 80 leukemic children receiving the placebo, whereas none of the 80 children receiving TMP-SMZ daily had PCP.[2] Later studies demonstrated TMP-SMZ administered only 3 consecutive days per week was as effective as 7 days per week.[3] A feasibility study proved the success of TMP-SMZ prophylaxis in clinical practice.[4] In subsequent studies the chemoprophylaxis was also found effective in children with cancer[5-8] and organ transplant recipients.[9]

It is noteworthy that in the controlled study rashes occurred in 28% of the 80 patients on TMP-SMZ, but this was also observed in 37% of the similar group given the placebo.[2,8] Thus, unexplained signs and symptoms in this study occurred with equal frequency between the treated and placebo groups, an item of importance in the consideration of current studies in AIDS. This study points out the difficulty in attributing adverse events to this and many other drugs. For almost 20 years TMP-SMZ has been used for PCP prophylaxis in non-AIDS patients, and the true rate of drug-related adverse effects has been considered relatively low at less than 6% of cases receiving the drug combination.

When the AIDS epidemic began, it became obvious that human immunodeficiency virus (HIV)–infected patients, a prime group for PCP prophylaxis, experienced a remarkably high rate of adverse effects of TMP-SMZ. Four studies reported that 44% to 83% of AIDS patients have adverse reactions, such as rash, fever, neutropenia, and liver dysfunction.[10-13]

Although TMP-SMZ is highly effective in the prevention of PCP in both AIDS and non-AIDS patients and its use is both simple and inexpensive, the high rate of adverse reactions demands alternate methods for prophylaxis. Within the last few years significant advances have occurred that already impact positively on the prevention of this life-threatening disease.

DEVELOPMENT OF NEW REGIMENS FOR PROPHYLAXIS

Several drugs other than TMP-SMZ have been identified and have undergone adequate clinical trials. Currently only one of these, aerosol pentamidine, is approved by the Food and Drug Administration for prophylactic use but the approval is limited to adults and adolescents. However, other drugs have undergone sufficient clinical trials to demonstrate efficacy and reasonable safety. These include dapsone, dapsone-trimethoprim, dapsone-pyrimethamine, and pyrimethamine-sulfadoxine (Fansidar).

Even more drugs have shown great promise in the corticosteroid-treated rat model, such as atovaquone, clindamycin plus primaquine, erythromycin-sulfisoxazole, and azithromycin or clarithromycin plus sulfamethoxazole.

Most of the clinical studies of PCP prophylaxis in AIDS have been done in adults. It is reasonable to believe efficacy demonstrated in adults will also apply to infants and children.

AEROSOL PENTAMIDINE

In the late 1980s several studies showed the delivery of pentamidine to the lung by aerosol was safe and effective in the prevention of PCP.[14, 15] The controlled study of Montaner et al.[16] was the most convincing of these clinical trials. Adults with AIDS, having recovered from one episode of PCP, were randomized to receive aerosol pentamidine or a placebo. Of the 78 patients receiving this placebo, 27 (35%) developed PCP, whereas only 5 (6%) of the 84 patients who received aerosolized pentamidine biweekly acquired pneumonitis. Lidman et al.[17] also studied prospectively 61 patients given aerosolized pentamidine monthly and 60 patients received no prophylaxis. *Pneumocystis carinii* pneumonia occurred in 8 (13%) of the pentamidine group and 19 (32%) of the untreated group.

Aerosolized pentamidine has been used in open label studies for bone marrow transplant patients.[18] No cases of PCP occurred in 31 allogeneic and 12 autologous bone marrow transplant case patients given aerosolized pentamidine during the 6-month posttransplantation period.

Mustafa et al.[19] administered aerosolized pentamidine, 200 mg/m^2 monthly, to 60 children with malignancy who were intolerant of TMP-SMZ. No patient developed PCP during the observation of 21,600 patient-days. The drug was well tolerated, with only 10% having possible adverse effects (bronchospasm, cough, nausea, and vomiting). Weinthal et al.[20] found similar results in 22 children with acute leukemia.

Twenty-two children (3–15 years old) with AIDS at the National Institutes of Health were given 300 mg of aerosolized pentamidine by Respirgard II nebulizer once monthly for a mean observation period of 9.8 months.[21] None of these patients developed PCP. Five (23%) patients had reversible bronchospasms requiring bronchodilators; 15 (68%) had coughing, and 16 (73%) had bitter taste associated with drug administration. Hand et al.[22] gave aerosolized pentamidine to seven HIV-infected infants 3.5 to 11 months old. The dose was based on an adult dose of 300 to 600 mg monthly but adjusted for minute ventilation and body weight. The infants tolerated this treatment well, and no cases of PCP were encountered. Of note, urinary concentrations of pentamidine were measured after aerosolized treatment, and the drug was detected in each sample tested. Using technetium 99m–labeled colloidal human serum albumin as an indirect marker for pentamidine deposition in the lungs of 12 children and 6 adults, O'Doherty et al.[23] found that children probably require lower nebulized doses to produce pentamidine concentrations in the lung equivalent to those found to be effective for preventing PCP in adults using the Respirgard II nebulizer. Conte and Wara[24] administered 300 mg of aerosolized pentamidine to children 2.8 to 11 years old and measured peak and trough plasma concentrations of pentamidine. The mean peak concentration of 3.9 M/mL did not differ from adult controls receiving the same dose.

Katz and Rosen[25] administered doses of 100 to 150 mg of aerosolized pentamidine to five infants and children from age 8 months to 5 years. The drug was delivered by a cushion face mask held by an attendant with the child sitting in the lap.

In a relatively large, uncontrolled study, 98 HIV-infected children received aerosolized pentamidine by the Fisoneb Ultrasonic nebulizer.[26] The dose was either 60 mg twice monthly or 120 mg monthly. Age ranged from 4 months to 14 years, and one half of the patients were less than 5 years old. The mean duration of observation was 5.9 months, and during this time one (1%) of the patients developed PCP.

DAPSONE

Dapsone was initially found to have anti–*P. carinii* activity in experimental animals, both as prophylaxis and therapy.[27] A synergistic effect between dapsone and trimethoprim was also demonstrated in these studies. Clinical trials in HIV-infected adults confirmed the anti–*P. carinii* effect and the synergistic effect of trimethoprim.[28, 29] Two prominent advantages of dapsone as a prophylactic agent for PCP are the long plasma half-life and low cost.

The earliest human studies showed dapsone to be effective in the prevention of PCP in HIV-infected adults when given daily or once per week. In an open label study in 1987, Metroka et al.[30] administered dapsone in the dose of 100 mg daily to 156 HIV-infected patients with CD4[+] lymphocyte counts less than 200 cells/mm³. Only one patient (0.6%) developed PCP, whereas 14 (74%) of 19 similar patients who refused prophylaxis developed PCP.

In 1990 Hughes et al.[31] reported that 61 HIV-infected adults given only one dose of 100 or 200 mg of dapsone once weekly effectively prevented PCP, with only 1 case occurring during the mean observation period of 9 months. Possible adverse effects occurred in 13% of cases. Many other studies have evaluated dapsone in HIV-infected adults with results generally showing efficacy and reasonable safety. The more recent studies reported from 1992 through 1994 have been summarized in Tables 1 and 2. Although these studies are not closely comparable, no obvious difference in dose, dose interval, or combination with pyrimethamine was noted for efficacy or safety.

The data on the use of dapsone prophylaxis in children are limited. Especially useful are pharmacokinetic studies of dapsone in infants and children. In six HIV-infected patients, aged 9 months

TABLE 1.
Dapsone Prophylaxis Studies, 1992–1994: Efficacy

| % PCP Breakthrough Rate (n) | Dose | | Interval | Author |
	Dapsone (mg)	Pyrimethamine (mg)		
18 (126)	100	—	2 × wk	Torres et al.[32]
18 (50)	100	—	2 × wk	Salvin et al.[33]
15 (85)	100	25	weekly	Podzamczer et al.[34]
14 (14)	100	—	3 × wk	Jorde et al.[35]
12.5 (56)	100	12.5	weekly	Dorrell et al.[36]
9.8 (21)	100	25	2 × wk	Gruenwald et al.[37]
8 (116)	100	25	weekly	Mallolas et al.[38]
6.5 (77)	50	—	Daily	Martin et al.[39]
5.8 (173)	50	50	Daily	Girard et al.[40]
2.0 (47)	100	—	Daily	Blum et al.[41]
2.0 (287)	200	75	weekly	Opravil et al.[42]
0 (79)	100	—	2 × wk	Hill et al.[43]

TABLE 2.

Dapsone Prophylaxis Studies, 1992–1994: Adverse Effects

	Dose			
% Adverse Event Rate (n)	**Dapsone (mg)**	**Pyrimethamine (mg)**	**Interval**	**Author**
55 (77)	50	—	Daily	Martin et al.[39]
42 (85)	100	25	Weekly	Podzamczer et al.[34]
39 (14)	100	—	3 × wk	Jorde et al.[35]
33 (54)	100	—	3 × wk	Hill et al.[43]*
30 (287)	200	75	Weekly	Opravil et al.[42]
24 (173)	50	50	Daily	Girard et al.[40]
16 (25)	100	25	3 × wk	Hill et al.[43]†
12 (50)	100	—	2 × wk	Salvin et al.[33]
11 (126)	100	—	2 × wk	Torres et al.[32]
10 (116)	100	25	Weekly	Mallolas et al.[38]
9.5 (21)	100	25	2 × wk	Gruenwald et al.[37]
8.2 (56)	100	12.5	Weekly	Dorrell et al.[36]

*Trimethoprim-sulfamethoxazole (TMP-SMZ) adverse effects.
†No prior TMP-SMZ adverse effects.

to 9 years, a single dose of dapsone, 2.0 mg/kg (suspension of pulverized tablets), was administered orally and plasma concentrations determined.[44] The maximum concentration (C_{max}) ranged from 0.4 to 1.7 μg/L (mean = 1.05 μg/L); time of maximum concentration (T_{max}) ranged from 2 to 4 hours (mean = 3.7 hours); half-life ($t_{1/2}$) ranged from 14 to 34 hours (mean = 24 hour). These findings suggest the dose of 2.0 mg/kg at intervals of less than daily is reasonable for prophylaxis. Pharmacokinetic studies of weekly doses of dapsone with or without pyrimethamine in adults suggest such an interval would provide effective prophylaxis.[45, 46]

Mirochnick et al.[47] studied dapsone pharmacokinetics in children ages 1.1 to 11.3 years (mean = 3.1 years). A tablet and two liquid formulations were administered orally. One liquid formulation was provided by the manufacturer (Jacobus Pharmaceuticals, Princeton, NJ), and the other was prepared by pulverizing the tablets, dissolving them in ethanol and suspending in cherry syrup to make 5.0 mg/mL. After a dose of 1.0 mg/kg, the C_{max} was less than 0.5 μg/mL for the extemporaneous liquid formulation but ranged from 0.72 to 1.33 µg/mL after the tablet and proprietary liquid preparation. With long-term administration of the proprietary liquid, C_{max} values of 1.48 to 3.28 µg/mL were obtained. The mean elimination $t_{1/2}$ was 15.1 hours, somewhat lower than that found in adults. The 1.0 mg/kg dose of dapsone provides plasma concentrations similar to those in adults given one 50-mg tablet.

Stavola and Noel[48] reported 20 HIV-infected children (2 months–13 years) given dapsone prophylaxis over an average of seven months. Two (12.5%) of the 16 high-risk patients developed PCP. Three of the 20 patients taking dapsone had adverse reactions: two cases with rash and one with methemaglobinemia. Barnett et al.[49] describe a child with breakthrough PCP who was receiving 1.0 mg/kg daily and steady-state dapsone plasma concentration of 0.95 µg/mL.

PYRIMETHAMINE-SULFADOXINE

The first evidence that PCP could be prevented was obtained from a study of epidemic infantile pneumocystosis in which the administration of pyrimethamine-sulfadoxine at least twice monthly aborted endemic PCP in an orphanage.[50] Subsequently several uncontrolled studies of small numbers of AIDS and non-AIDS patients indicated this drug combination was effective for the prevention of PCP. However, adverse reactions occur frequently, and rarely they may be fatal. Stevens-Johnson syndrome and hepatic necrosis have caused fatalities attributed to the drug. Some patients who have adverse reactions to TMP-SMZ will tolerate pyrimethamine-sulfadoxine.

A recent study of interest used pyrimethamine-sulfadoxine once per week for HIV-infected adults with $CD4^+$ lymphocyte counts less than 200 cells/mm^3.[51] Three (4%) of the 73 patients had PCP during the 3-month observation period. Only three patients had adverse reactions, and none was of significance.

INTRAVENOUS OR INTRAMUSCULAR PENTAMIDINE

The efficacy of widely spaced doses of intravenous or intramuscular pentamidine, similar to the scheme for aerosolized pentamidine, has not been firmly established. No controlled study has been reported. A retrospective analysis in 1993 of 96 HIV-infected patients at the Mount Sinai Medical Center treated with 4 mg of pentamidine isethionate/kg intramuscularly once per month showed only three patients (3%) had PCP breakthrough. The ages ranged from 21 to 60 years; one half of the 96 patients were receiving secondary prophylaxis for 426 months and one half received primary prophylaxis (CD4$^+$ lymphocyte count = < 200 cells/mm^3) over 350 patient-months.[52]

In 1994 Ena et al.[53] reported their retrospective review of 52 HIV-infected patients given 4 mg of pentamidine isethionate/kg intravenously once per month as PCP prophylaxis. No cases of PCP occurred in the 37 patients on primary prophylaxis during the 387 patient months of observation. Of the 15 patients receiving secondary prophylaxis, 1 case of PCP (7%) was diagnosed during the period of 200 patient-months. Side effects were mild.

COMPARISON OF CHEMOPROPHYLAXIS REGIMENS

In recent years all clinical trials comparing two or more drug regimens for the prevention of PCP have been in adults with HIV in-

TABLE 3.

Comparison of Trimethoprim-Sulfamethoxazole and Aerosolized Pentamidine for *Pneumocystis carinii* Pneumonia Prophylaxis in AIDS Patients, 1992–1994*

Author	Drugs	No. of Patients	No. With PCP Breakthroughs (%)	No. With Adverse Effects (%)
Carr et al.[54]	TMP-SMZ	60	1 (1.7)	3 (5)
	Aerosol pentamidine	73	31 (42.5)	4 (5)
	None	38	21 (55.3)	—
Hardy et al.[55]	TMP-SMZ	154	14 (9)	27 (17.5)
	Aerosol pentamidine	156	36 (23)	4 (3)
Schneider et al.[56]	TMP-SMZ	142	0 (0)	18 (12.7)
	Aerosol pentamidine	71	6 (8.5)	2 (2.8)
Rizzardi et al.[57]	TMP-SMZ	95	1 (1)	24 (25)
	Aerosol pentamidine	105	5 (5)	5 (5)
May et al.[58]	TMP-SMZ	108	2 (1.8)	33 (31)
	Aerosol pentamidine	106	5 (5)	5 (5)

*AIDS = acquired immunodeficiency syndrome; TMP-SMZ = trimethoprim-sulfamethoxazole.

TABLE 4.

Comparison of Dapsone With Other Regimens for *Pneumocystis carinii* Pneumonia Prophylaxis in AIDS Patients, 1992–1994*

Author	Drugs	No. of Patients	No. With Breakthrough (%)	No. With Adverse Effects (%)
Martin et al.[59]	Dapsone	77	5 (6.5)	42 (55)
	TMP-SMZ	133	0 (0)	75 (56)
	Aerosol pentamidine	125	17 (14)	3 (2)
Torres et al.[60]	Dapsone	126	13 (10)	14 (11)
	Aerosol pentamidine	152	15 (10)	3 (2)
Salvin et al.[33]	Dapsone	50	9 (18)	6 (12)
	Aerosol pentamidine	46	8 (17)	8 (17)
Opravil et al.[42]	Dapsone and pyrimethamine	287	6 (2)	9 (3)
	Aerosol pentamidine	241	13 (5.4)	10 (4)
Girard et al.[40]	Dapsone and pyrimethamine	173	10 (17)	42 (24)
	Aerosol pentamidine	176	10 (17)	3 (1.7)
Podzamczer et al.[34]	Dapsone and pyrimethamine	85	13 (15)	36 (42.4)
	TMP-SMZ	81	3 (3.7)	54 (66.7)
Mallolas et al.[38]	Dapsone and pyrimethamine	116	10 (8.3)	9 (7.8)
	TMP-SMZ	107	3 (3)	10 (11)
	Aerosol pentamidine	108	6 (5.6)	1 (0.9)

*AIDS = acquired immunodeficiency syndrome; PCP = *Pneumocystis carinii* pneumonia; TMP-SMZ = trimethoprim-sulfamethoxazole.

fection. However, these studies have established data useful in the management of immunosuppressed children. Tables 3 and 4 summarize comparative studies of TMP-SMZ, dapsone, dapsone plus pyrimethamine, and aerosol pentamidine. All of the studies show TMP-SMZ to be more effective in preventing PCP than aerosol pentamidine, and the adverse reactions are more frequent with TMP-SMZ. Either dapsone or dapsone plus pyrimethamine is as effective as aerosol pentamidine, but the rate of adverse effects is less with pentamidine. It should be pointed out that doses and frequency of doses varied from study to study, and the criteria for adverse events also differed between studies. Pyrimethamine is used in combination with dapsone to provide coverage for infections from *Toxoplasma gondii*. The combination is effective in the prevention of toxoplasmosis.[40]

Because it is not possible to test in a clinical trial all the drugs known to have anti–*P. carinii* activity, the experimental animal model, known to be highly representative of human disease, was

TABLE 5.

Relative Potency of Drugs in Preventing Experimental *Pneumocystis carinii* Pneumonitis*

	% Animals With Breakthrough PCP†		
Drug	**Basic Dose**	**⅒ of Basic Dose**	**¹⁄₁₀₀ of Basic Dose**
Untreated control	100	100	—
Trimethoprim-sulfamethoxazole	0	0	11
Azithromycin-sulfamethoxazole	0	0	89
Erythromycin-sulfisoxazole	0	33	—
Dapsone-trimethoprim	0	44	—
Atovaquone	0	50	—
Clarithromycin-sulfamethoxazole	11	0	—
Sulfadoxine-pyrimethamine	22	50	—
Clindamycin-primaquine	80	100	—
Pentamidine (intravenous)	100	100	—

*Adapted from Hughes WT, Killmar JT, Oz HS: *J Infect Dis* 170:906–911, 1994.
†PCP = *Pneumocystis carinii* pneumonia.

used for such comparisons.[61] The drugs with possible application to prophylaxis were administered in diminishing doses until PCP breakthrough occurred, thereby establishing the relative efficacy. As shown in Table 5, TMP-SMZ is the most effective, with azithromycin-sulfamethoxazole and clarithromycin-sulfamethoxazole the next most effective. Intravenous pentamidine and clindamycin-primaquine were the least effective. Atovaquone, sulfadoxine-pyrimethamine, erythromycin-sulfisoxazole, and dapsone-trimethoprim had intermediate activity. No clinical studies of the macrolide and sulfonamide combinations or atovaquone have been reported. Animal studies have shown azithromycin, erythromycin, and clarithromycin alone to have no anti–*P. carinii* effect but are synergistic with sulfonamides.[62, 63]

RECENT STUDIES RELATED TO THE MECHANISM OF ADVERSE REACTIONS TO TRIMETHOPRIM-SULFAMETHOXAZOLE

Except for the high rate of adverse reactions to TMP-SMZ, this drug combination would be close to the ideal prophylactic agent. It is highly effective, inexpensive, and available in tablet, parenteral, and oral liquid formulations, and it probably provides additional protection against toxoplasmosis and certain bacterial infections. However, since the onset of the AIDS epidemic, many reports have made obvious the exaggerated adverse reaction rate in AIDS patients compared with non-AIDS, normal, or immunosuppressed patients.

Recent studies shed some insight into the mechanisms of adverse responses to TMP-SMZ in AIDS, although a complete understanding is lacking. Carr et al.[64] examined the acetylation phenotype of AIDS patients with cutaneous hypersensitivity to TMP-SMZ. Genetically determined slow and fast acetylator phenotypes are distributed equally in whites. Non-AIDS individuals who acetylate slowly have an increased rate of rashes to certain drugs, including sulfamethoxazole and dapsone. These investigators determined the acetylation phenotype of 28 HIV-infected patients. Sixteen of these patients had experienced hypersensitivity reactions to TMP-SMZ, and 12 had received the drug without evidence of hypersensitivity. Of 29 healthy controls, 15 (52%) expressed a slow phenotype, whereas 20 (71%) of the 28 HIV-infected patients had this phenotype. Of the 16 AIDS patients with cutaneous hypersensitivity, 15 (94%) had a slow acetylation phenotype, and 5 (42%) of the 12 patients without cutaneous hypersensitivity had a slow phenotype (P = < 0.01). The investigators propose that sulfamethoxazole is metabolized by hepatic acetylation to a stable N-4-acetyl-sulfamethoxazole and by cytochrome P_{450} to 5-hydroxy-sulfamethoxazole or to an active hydroxylamine metabolite. The hydroxylamine is an oxidative radical that damages cellular proteins and may be inactivated by glutathione. Thus, HIV-infected patients might have relatively large amounts of sulfamethoxazole-hydroxylamine, increasing their risk for "hypersensitivity." Rieder et al.[65] found HIV-infected lymphoblasts (MOLT-III) to be exquisitely sensitive to sulfa-reactive metabolites and associated with greater cellular toxicity than uninfected cells. Lee et al.[66] measured the urine concentrations of sulfamethoxazole-hydroxylamine in 15 HIV-infected patients. The proportions of the sulfamethoxazole-hydroxylamine excreted from eight patients who discontinued TMP-SMZ because of toxicity were similar to those of the seven patients who did not have toxic effects. Although these data help clarify the mechanism at this time, correlation of hydroxylamine measurements or slow acetylation phenotype is insignificant to warrant the use of these measures as tests predictive of adverse reaction to TMP-SMZ.

Some of the adverse events associated with TMP-SMZ are those seen with folate deficiency, although quantitative methods have not demonstrated a consistent deficit in folinic acid. A recent study attempted to alleviate the toxicity, in part or whole, through the administration of folinic acid to patients with PCP.[67] Ninety-two AIDS patients with PCP received either folinic acid or a placebo in a double-blind study during treatment with TMP-SMZ. Although the frequency of dose-limiting toxicity was not significantly different between the groups, the unexpected finding was a higher rate of therapeutic failure ($P = 0.01$) and death ($P = 0.06$) in the group receiving folinic acid. The incidence of neutropenia was less in the folinic acid group than the placebo group ($P = 0.03$). Animal studies have indicated the administration of folinic acid does not adversely effect the use of TMP-SMZ.[68]

CURRENT RECOMMENDATIONS ON PROPHYLAXIS FOR *PNEUMOCYSTIS CARINII* PNEUMONIA

Although PCP occurs almost exclusively in immunosuppressed hosts, the disease is generally limited to those with *severe* immunocompromise, especially of cell-mediated immunity. Infection with HIV has provided an informative model for the pathogenesis of PCP, showing specifically the role of the CD4[+] T-lymphocyte (by its impairment) in the human's resistance to PCP. Individuals with specific defects of humoral immunity such as X-linked Bruton's agammaglobulinemia, are seemingly at a lower risk than those with T-lymphocyte defects. At very high risk are children with severe combined immunodeficiency syndrome where more than 40% of patients will acquire PCP[69] and those with AIDS in whom PCP will occur in more than one half the patients if no prophylaxis is given. At less risk are children with cancer or organ transplantation where PCP occurs in about 5% to 15% of cases.

No guidelines have been published for PCP prophylaxis in non-AIDS patients, but considerable attention by national task forces or committees have outlined strategic plans and recommendations, based on data available, for selection of AIDS patients to undergo chemoprophylaxis.

Recommendations for PCP prophylaxis from the U.S. Public Health Service were published in the *Morbidity and Mortality Weekly Report* in 1989 and 1992 for adults[70] and 1991 for children[71] with HIV infection. Since then more data have accumulated on risk factors and the efficacy and safety of drugs to allow revisions of these guidelines. New guidelines for both adults and adolescents[72] and infants and children[73] were published in 1995.

The current recommendations for HIV-infected pediatric patients are as follows.

INDIVIDUALS RECOMMENDED FOR *PNEUMOCYSTIS CARINII* PNEUMONIA PROPHYLAXIS

Previous Episode of *Pneumocystis carinii* Pneumonia

Because the likelihood of recurrence exceeds 50% after an episode of PCP, all patients who have had one or more episodes of PCP should be placed on prophylaxis regardless of $CD4^+$ lymphocyte count or any other factor.

$CD4^+$ Lymphocyte Count Less Than 200 Cells/μL

Any HIV-infected patient, regardless of age qualifies for prophylaxis if the $CD4^+$ lymphocyte count is less than 200 cells/μL or the $CD4^+$ lymphocyte percentage is less than 15%.

All Infants Born From HIV-Infected Mothers

All infants born of women known to be HIV-infected should be given chemoprophylaxis beginning at age 1 month. Both HIV-infected and HIV-indeterminate infants are included. During the first month of life, PCP has rarely been encountered, so no prophylaxis is recommended for this period. Prophylaxis is started at 1 month because most of the episodes of PCP in pediatric AIDS occur during the first year of life. In this age group the CD4$^+$ lymphocyte count is not a highly reliable risk indicator for PCP, so this parameter is not taken into consideration during the first year of life.

Because at birth, and often during the first few months of life, the presence or absence of HIV infection cannot be determined, PCP prophylaxis is administered to all offspring of HIV-infected mothers until this delineation can be made. Thus, during the course of this prophylaxis one of these events will eventually occur: (1) the absence of HIV infection is established; (2) the presence of HIV-infection is established, and the patient is in a high risk category for PCP; or (3) the presence of HIV-infection is established, and the patient is at low risk for PCP. The following recommendations apply to these events.

1. *The absence of HIV-infection is established.* The prophylaxis can be stopped when HIV infection can be excluded with reasonable assurance: two or more negative diagnostic test results (HIV-PCR or virus culture), both of which are obtained at age 1 month or older and one of which is done at age 4 months or older. If these test results are unavailable, the prophylaxis may be continued until age 1 year. If after age 6 months or older two separate blood samples are negative for HIV antibody and no other evidence of HIV infection exists, prophylaxis may be stopped.

2. *Presence of HIV infection is established and the infant is in a high-risk category for PCP.* All HIV-infected infants remain on PCP prophylaxis through the first year of life. At the end of the first year a decision is made to continue or stop the prophylactic drug. The following findings indicate sufficient high risk to *continue* the prophylaxis: (1) a CD4$^+$ lymphocyte count less than 750 cells/μL or CD4$^+$ cell percentage less than 15% on any measurement during the first year, (2) recent rapid decline in CD4$^+$ cell count, or (3) occurrence of severely symptomatic HIV disease.

3. *Presence of HIV infection is established, and the infant is in a low-risk category for PCP.* The prophylaxis may be stopped at age 1 if the CD4$^+$ lymphocyte count has remained greater than 750 cells/μL (or 15%) during the year and has had no clinical evidence of HIV disease. Evaluation at age 2 years should use the CD4$^+$ lymphocyte count to determine whether to continue, discontinue, or add PCP prophylaxis.

HIV-Infected Children Not on Prophylaxis

HIV-infected children not on prophylaxis should begin if the $CD4^+$ lymphocyte count indicates severe immunocompromise. The following guide may be used[73]:

	Extent of Immunocompromise	
Age	**Moderate** ($CD4^+$ **Lymphocyte Counts, Cells/μL**)	**Severe** ($CD4^+$ **Lymphocyte Counts, Cells/μL**)
≤11 mo	750–1,499	<750
1–5 yr	500–999	<500
6–12 yr	200–499	<200

For patients being monitored for possible entry into PCP prophylaxis, $CD4^+$ lymphocyte counts should be done about every 3 months.

Summary of Guidelines

Table 6 summarizes the new CDC recommendations.

Comment on Centers for Disease Control Recommendations

The CDC recommendations provide a useful guide for physicians in the management of infants and children with HIV infection. These guidelines are reasonable for medical centers and clinics where HIV-infected infants can be followed in an organized and comprehensive manner and where stipulated follow-up visits are honored by patients and parents and $CD4^+$ lymphocyte counts, HIV viral cultures, and PCR methods are available. Of concern, however, is the noncompliant patient or parent and the health care sites in communities that do not have the diagnostic tests needed available.

Although the majority of PCP episodes occur in patients with severely decreased $CD4^+$ cell counts, some do not. The physician should be attentive to this possibility in HIV-infected children with normal counts but who have early clinical evidence of HIV disease, such as oral candidiasis, generalized adenopathy, failure to thrive, and frequent infection. Because PCP is the most serious opportunistic infection in AIDS, with a fatality rate of close to 100% if untreated, and because PCP is often the first "AIDS-defining" illness, these patients may warrant prophylaxis with normal $CD4^+$ counts.

No data are available on the consequences of stopping PCP prophylaxis in HIV-infected patients who have received such drugs during the first year of life. The rationale for covering this period

TABLE 6.

Recommendations for *Pneumocystis carinii* Pneumonia Prophylaxis and CD4$^+$ Monitoring for HIV-Exposed Infants and HIV-Infected Children*†

Age	PCP Prophylaxis	CD4$^+$ Monitoring
Birth to 4–6 wk	No prophylaxis	Age 1 mo
4–6 wk to 4 mo	Prophylaxis	Age 3 mo
4–12 mo		
HIV-infected or indeterminate	Prophylaxis	Age 6, 9, and 12 mo
HIV infection reasonably excluded‡	No prophylaxis	None
1–5 yr	Prophylaxis if CD4$^+$ count <500 cells/μL or CD4$^+$ < 15%§‖	Every 3–4 mo
6–12 yr	Prophylaxis if CD4$^+$ count <200 cells/μL or CD4$^+$ < 15%‖	Every 3–4 mo¶

*From Centers for Disease Control and Prevention: *MMWR* 44(RR-4):1–11, 1995.

†HIV = human immunodeficiency virus; PCP = *Pneumocystis carinii* pneumonia.

‡≥2 negative HIV diagnostic test results (culture or polymerase chain reaction), both of which are performed at ≥1 mo and one of which is performed at ≥4 mo, or ≥2 negative HIV IgG antibody test results performed at >6 mo in a child who has no clinical evidence for HIV disease.

§Children 1–2 yr old who were on PCP prophylaxis and had a CD4$^+$ count <750 cells/μL in the first year of life should continue on prophylaxis.

‖Prophylaxis should be considered on a case-by-case basis for children with rapidly declining CD4$^+$ counts or percents and for children with category C conditions.[16]

¶More frequent monitoring (e.g., monthly) is recommended for children whose CD4$^+$ measurements are approaching the threshold for prophylaxis.

is the finding that the majority of cases of PCP diagnosed have been in the first year of life.[74] Certainly the recommendation is sound, and coverage of this key period is the major thrust of the prophylaxis program for infants. However, stopping prophylaxis at 1 year in HIV-infected children with CD4 lymphocyte counts in or near the range of normal raises some points of concern in the form of unanswered and, at this time, unanswerable questions. Will prophylaxis during the first year merely prevent the primary infection during this time and shift the period of risk to the second year? Because TMP-SMZ prophylaxis also provides prophylaxis against some bacterial infections[2] and toxoplasmosis,[40] will patients not be provided of these benefits? Outside ACTG centers and large medical centers, can adequate follow-up be achieved to reinstitute prophylaxis when recommended? Although drug resistance of *P. carinii* to TMP-SMZ and other drugs has not been recognized at this time, will the extensive use plus intermittent schedules of administration lead to the development of resistant strains of *P. carinii*? Will parents, as well as some health care workers, understand the rationale for stopping prophylaxis? Should informed consent be obtained to *discontinue* prophylaxis? Finally, in compliant patients on TMP-SMZ prophylaxis who develop lower respiratory tract infections, PCP is unlikely the cause of the illness, perhaps avoiding an invasive diagnostic study.

TABLE 7.

Drug Regimens for *Pneumocystis carinii* Pneumonia Prophylaxis for Children*

Recommended regimen (children ≥4–6 wk old):
  Trimethoprim-sulfamethoxazole (TMP-SMZ), 150 mg TMP/m²/daily with 750 mg SMX/m²/daily given orally in divided doses bid 3 × wk on consecutive days (e.g., Monday-Tuesday-Wednesday)
  Acceptable alternative TMP-SMX dosage schedules:
- 150 mg TMP/m²/day with 750 mg SMX/m²/daily given orally *as a single daily dose* 3 × wk on consecutive days (e.g., Monday-Tuesday-Wednesday)
- 150 mg TMP/m²/daily with 750 mg SMX/m²/daily orally divided bid and *given 7 days/wk*
- 150 mg TMP/m²/daily with 750 mg SMX/m²/daily given orally divided bid and given 3 × wk on *alternate days* (e.g., Monday-Wednesday-Friday)

Alternative regimens, if TMP-SMX is not tolerated:
  Dapsone (4–6 wk old), 2 mg/kg (not to exceed 100 mg) given orally once daily
  Aersolized pentamidine (≥5 yrs old), 300 mg given via Respirgard II inhaler monthly
  If neither dapsone nor aerosolized pentamidine is tolerated, some clinicians use *intravenous pentamidine* (4 mg/kg) given every 2 or 4 wk.

---

*From Centers for Disease Control and Prevention: *MMWR* 44(RR-4):1–11, 1995.

DRUG REGIMENS RECOMMENDED FOR *PNEUMOCYSTIS CARINII* PNEUMONIA PROPHYLAXIS IN PEDIATRIC HIV INFECTION

The CDC recommendations for drug use in PCP prophylaxis are summarized in Table 7. The drug of choice is TMP-SMZ and may be given 3 days per week or daily. Available data indicate one of these schemes is as effective as the other in the prevention of PCP.

For patients who cannot tolerate TMP-SMZ, dapsone may be used for infants and children less than age 5 years and aerosol pentamidine for those older than 5 years who are able to receive the nebulized drug. No comparative data for dapsone and pentamidine prophylaxis are available in infants and children. Data from adults would suggest dapsone might be as effective as pentamidine in the older patients. Most children less than 5 years may not be able to properly use the Respirgard II nebulizer.

A final point in PCP prophylaxis is the axiom that effective prophylaxis is provided only while the patient receives the drugs. None of the currently available drugs for prophylaxis eradicates *P. carinii*. If prophylaxis is withheld for more than 10 to 14 days, one may expect the risk for PCP to increase in the host at high risk.

REFERENCES

1. Hughes WT, McNabb PC, Makres TD, et al: Efficacy of trimethoprim and sulfamethoxazole in the prevention and treatment of *Pneumocystis carinii* pnumonitis. *Antimicrob Agents Chemother* 5:289–293, 1974.
2. Hughes WT, Kuhn S, Chandhary S, et al: Successful chemoprophylaxis for *Pneumocystis carinii* pneumonitis. *N Engl J Med* 297:1419–1426, 1977.
3. Hughes WT, Rivera GK, Schell MJ, et al: Successful intermittent chemoprophylaxis for *Pneumocystis carinii* pneumonia. *N Engl J Med* 316:1627–1632, 1987.
4. Wilbur RB, Feldman S, Malone WJ, et al: Chemoprophylaxis for *Pneumocystis carinii* pneumonitis: Outcome of unstructured delivery. *Am J Dis Child* 134:643–648, 1980.
5. Harris RE, McCallister JA, Allen SA, et al: Prevention of *Pneumocystis* pneumonia. *Am J Dis Child* 134:35–38, 1980.
6. Wolff LJ, Baehner RL: Delayed development of *Pneumocystis* pneumonia following administration of short-term high-dose trimethoprim-sulfamethoxazole. *Am J Dis Child* 132:525–526, 1978.
7. Chusid MJ, Heyrman KA: An outbreak of *Pneumocystis carinii* pneumonia at a pediatric hospital. *Pediatrics* 62:1031–1035, 1978.
8. Hughes WT: Five-year absence of *Pneumocystis carinii* pneumonitis in a pediatric oncology center. *J Infect Dis* 150:305–306, 1984.

9. Hardy AM, Wajszczuk CP, Suffredini AF, et al: *Pneumocystis carinii* pneumonia in renal-transplant recipients treated with cyclosporine and steroids. *J Infect Dis* 149:143–147, 1984.

10. Mitsuyasu R, Groopman J, Volderbing P: Cutaneous reaction to trimethoprim-sulfamethoxazole in patients with AIDS and Kaposi's sarcoma. *N Engl J Med* 308:1535–1536, 1983.

11. Small CB, Harris CA, Klein RS, et al: Trimethoprim-sulfamethoxazole treatment of *Pneumocystis carinii* pneumonia. [Abstract no 630] In *Proceedings of the Interscience Conference of Antimicrob Agents Chemotherapy*. Las Vegas, 1983.

12. Jaffe HS, Abrams DI, Ammann AJ, et al: Complications of cotrimoxazole in treatment of AIDS-associated *Pneumocystis carinii* pneumonia in homosexual men. *Lancet* 2:1109–1111, 1983.

13. Gordin FM, Simon GL, Wofsky CB, et al: Adverse reactions to trimethoprim-sulfamethoxazole in patients with the acquired immunodeficiency syndrome. *Ann Intern Med* 100:495–499, 1984.

14. Leoung GS, Feigal DW Jr, Montgomery AB, et al: Aerosolized pentamidine for prophylaxis against *Pneumocystis carinii* pneumonia: The San Francisco Community Prophylaxis Trial. *N Engl J Med* 323:769–775, 1990.

15. Girard P-M, Landman R, Ganderbout C, et al: Prevention of *Pneumocystis carinii* pneumonia relapse by pentamidine aerosol in zidovudine-treated AIDS patients. *Lancet* 1:1348–1352, 1989.

16. Montaner JSG, Lawson LM, Gervais A, et al: Aerosol pentamidine for secondary prophylaxis of AIDS-related *Pneumocystis carinii* pneumonia: A randomized, placebo-controlled study. *Ann Intern Med* 114:948–953, 1991.

17. Lidman C, Berglund O, Tynell E, et al: Aerosolized pentamidine as primary prophylaxis for *Pneumocystis carinii* pneumonia: Efficacy, mortality and morbidity. *AIDS* 8:935–939, 1994.

18. Link H, Vohriger HF, Wingen F, et al: Pentamidine aerosol for prophylaxis of *Pneumocystis carinii* pneumonia after BMT. *Bone Marrow Transplant* 11:403–406, 1993.

19. Mustafa MM, Pappo A, Cash J, et al: Aerosolized pentamidine for the prevention of *Pneumocystis carinii* in children with cancer intolerant or allergic to trimethoprim-sulfamethoxazole. *J Clin Oncol* 12:258–261, 1994.

20. Weinthal J, Frost JD, Briones G, et al: Successful *Pneumocystis carinii* pneumonia prophylaxis using aerosolized pentamidine in children with acute leukemia. *J Clin Oncol* 12:136–140, 1994.

21. Orcutt TA, Godwin CR, Pizzo PA, et al: Aerosolized pentamidine: A well-tolerated mode of prophylaxis against *Pneumocystis carinii* pneumonia in older children with human immunodeficiency virus infection. *Pediatr Infect Dis J* 11:290–294, 1992.

22. Hand IL, Wizuria AA, Porricolo M, et al: Aerosolized pentamidine for prophylaxis of *Pneumocystis carinii* pneumonia in infants with hu-

man immunodeficiency virus infection. *Pediatr Infect Dis J* 13:100–104, 1994.

23. O'Doherty MJ, Thomas SHL, Gibb D, et al: Lung deposition of nebulised pentamidine in children. *Thorax* 48:220–226, 1993.

24. Conte JE, Wara D: Pharmacokinetics of aerosolized pentamidine in children [Abstract no 1477]. In *Proceedings of the International Conference on AIDS*. Berlin, 1993.

25. Katz BZ, Rosen C: Aersolized pentamidine in young children. *Pediatr Infect Dis* 10:1991, 1991.

26. Onorato J: Primary prophylaxis against PCP by aerosolized pentamidine in children. The Italian Pediatric Collaborative Study on Pentamidine. *Int Conf AIDS* 8:B200, 1992.

27. Hughes WT, Smith BL: Efficacy of diaminodiphenyl-sulfone and other drugs in murine *Pneumocystis carinii* pneumonitis. *Antimicrob Agents Chemother* 26:436–440, 1984.

28. Leoung GS, Mill J, Hopewell PC, et al: Dapsone-trimethoprim in *Pneumocystis carinii* pneumonia in acquired immunodeficiency syndrome. *Ann Intern Med* 105:45–48, 1986.

29. Medina I, Mills J, Leoung G, et al: Oral therapy for *Pneumocystis carinii* pneumonia in the acquired immunodeficiency syndrome. A controlled trial of trimethoprim-sulfamethoxazole versus trimethoprim-dapsone. *N Engl J Med* 323:776–782, 1990.

30. Metroka CE, Jacobus D, Lewis N: Successful chemoprophylaxis for pneumocystis with dapsone or bactrim (Abstract no T.B.O.4). In *Proceedings of the Fifth International Conference on AIDS*. Montreal, June 1989.

31. Hughes WT, Kennedy W, Dugdale M, et al: Prevention of *Pneumocystis carinii* pneumonitis in AIDS patients with weekly dapsone. *Lancet* 336:1066, 1990.

32. Torres RA, Barr M, Thorn M, et al: Randomized trial of dapsone and aerosolized pentamidine for the prophylaxis of *Pneumocystis carinii* pneumonia and toxoplasmosic encephalitis. *Am J Med* 95:573–583, 1993.

33. Salvin MA, Hoy JF, Stewart K, et al: Oral dapsone versus nebulized pentamidine for *Pneumocystis carinii* pneumonia prophylaxis: An open randomized prospective trial to assess efficacy and haematological toxicity. *AIDS* 6:1169–1174, 1992.

34. Podzamczer D, Santin M, Jimencz J, et al: Thrice-weekly cotrimoxazole is better than weekly dapsone-pyrimethamine for the primary prevention of *Pneumocystis carinii* pneumonia in HIV-infected patients. *AIDS* 7:501–506, 1993.

35. Jorde VP, Horowitz HW, Wormser GP: Utility of dapsone for prohylaxis of *Pneumocystis carinii* pneumonia in trimethoprim-sulfamethoxazole-intolerant, HIV-infected individuals. *AIDS* 7:355–359, 1993.

36. Dorrell L, McCallum AK, Snow MH, et al: Dapsone-pyrimethamine

versus aerosolized pentamidine as prophylaxis against *Pneumocystis carinii* pneumonia in HIV infection [Abstract no PO-BIO-1420]. In *Proceedings of the International Conference on AIDS.* Berlin, 1993.

37. Gruenwald T, Bergmann F, Eljaschewitsch J, et al: Antiprotozoan prophylaxis in AIDS patients—results of a prospective randomized study comparing dapsone/pyrimethamine and sulfadoxine/pyrimethamine [Abstract no B13-3]. In *International Conference on AIDS.* Berlin, 1993.

38. Mallolas J, Zamora GL, Gatell JM, et al: Primary prophylaxis for *Pneumocystis carinii* pneumonia: A randomized trial comparing cotrimoxazole, aerosolized pentamidine and dapsone plus pyrimethamine. *AIDS* 7:59–64, 1993.

39. Martin MA, Cox PH, Beck K, et al: A comparison of the effectiveness of three regimens in the prevention of *Pneumocystis carinii* pneumonia in human immunodeficiency virus-infected patients. *Arch Intern Med* 152:523–528, 1992.

40. Girard P-M, Landman R, Gaudebout C, et al: Dapsone-pyrimethamine compared with aerosolized pentamidine as primary prophylaxis against *Pneumocystis carinii* pneumonia and toxoplasmosis in HIV infection. *N Engl J Med* 328:1514–1520, 1993.

41. Blum RN, Miller LA, Gaggini LC, et al: Comparative trial of dapsone versus trimethoprim-sulfamethoxazole for primary prophylaxis of *Pneumocystis carinii* pneumonia. *J Acquir Immune Defic Syndr* 5:341–347, 1992.

42. Opravil M, Heald A, Lazzarin A, et al: Dapsone-pyrimethamine vs. aerosolized pentamidine for combined prophylaxis of PCP and toxoplasmic encephalitis [Abstract no PO-BIO-1429]. In *Proceedings of the International Conference on AIDS.* Berlin, June 1993.

43. Hill HE, Wallace M, Kennedy C, et al: Prophylaxis of *Pneumocystis carinii* pneumonia (PCP) with dapsone: An evaluation of toxicity and cross-reactivity with trimethoprim-sulfamethoxazole [Abstract no B137]. In *International Conference on AIDS.* Amsterdam, 1992.

44. Cruciani M, Concia E, Gatti G, et al: Dapsone prophylaxis against *Pneumocystis carinii* pneumonia in human immunodeficiency virus-infected children [letter and comment]. *Pediatr Infect Dis J* 13:80–81, 1994.

45. Falloon J, Lavelle J, Ogata-Arakaki AB, et al: Pharmacokinetics and safety of weekly dapsone and dapsone plus pyrimethamine for prevention of *Pneumocystis* pneumonia. *Antimicrob Agents Chemother* 38:1580–1587, 1994.

46. Opravil M, Joos B, Luthy R: Levels of dapsone and pyrimethamine in serum during once-weekly dosing for prophylaxis of *Pneumocystis carinii* pneumonia and toxoplasmic encephalitis. *Antimicrob Agents Chemother* 38:1197–1199, 1994.

47. Mirochnick M, Michaels M, Clarke D, et al: Pharmacokinetics of dapsone in children. *J Pediatr* 122:806–809, 1993.

48. Stavola JJ, Noel GJ: Efficacy and safety of dapsone prophylaxis against *Pneumocystis carinii* pneumonia in human immunodeficiency virus-infected children. *Pediatr Infect Dis J* 12:644–647, 1993.
49. Barnett ED, Pelton SI, Mirochnick M, et al: Dapsone for prevention of pneumocystis pneumonia in children with acquired immunodeficiency syndrome. *Pediatr Infect Dis J* 13:72–73, 1994.
50. Post C, Fakouki T, Dutz W, et al: Prophylaxis of epidemic infantile pneumocystosis with a 20:1 sulfadoxine + pyrimethamine combination. *Curr Ther Res* 13:273–279, 1971.
51. Jurado R, Garcia-Herola A, Garcia-Lazaro M, et al: Pyrimethamine/sulfadoxine for prevention of *Pneumocystis carinii* pneumonia in patients infected with the human immunodeficiency virus. *Clin Infect Dis* 19:218–219, 1994.
52. Cheung TW, Matta R, Neibart E, et al: Intramuscular pentamidine for the prevention of *Pneumocystis carinii* pneumonia in patients infected with human immunodeficiency virus. *Clin Infect Dis* 16:22–25, 1993.
53. Ena J, Amador C, Pasquaw F, et al: Once-a-month administration of intravenous pentamidine to patients infected with human immunodeficiency virus as prophylaxis for *Pneumocystis carinii* pneumonia. *Clin Infect Dis* 18:901–904, 1994.
54. Carr A, Tindall B, Penny R, et al: Trimethoprim-sulfamethoxazole appears more effective than aerosolized pentamidine as secondary prophylaxis against *Pneumocystis carinii* pneumonia in patients with AIDS. *AIDS* 6:165–171, 1992.
55. Hardy WD, Feinberg J, Finkelstein DM, et al: A controlled trial of trimethoprim-sulfamethoxazole or aerosolized pentamidine for secondary prophylaxis of *Pneumocystis carinii* pneumonia in patients with the acquired immunodeficiency syndrome. *N Engl J Med* 327:1842–1848, 1992.
56. Schneider MM, Hoepelman AI, Eeftinck-Schattenkerk JK, et al: A controlled trial of aerosolized pentamidine or trimethoprim-sulfamethoxazole as primary prophylaxis against *Pneumocystis carinii* pneumonia in patients with human immunodeficiency virus infection. *N Engl J Med* 327:1836–1841, 1992.
57. Rizzardi GP, Frigerio D, Lazzarin A, et al: Prospective study on prophylaxis for PCP: A 1-yr. randomized trial comparing aerosolized pentamidine vs. daily cotrimazole. Italian PCP PP Study Group [Abstract no PO-388]. In *Proceedings of the International Conference on AIDS*. Berlin, 1993.
58. May T, Beuscart C, Reynes J, et al: Trimethoprim-sulfamethoxazole versus aerosolized pentamidine for primary prophylaxis of *Pneumocystis carinii* pneumonia: A prospective, randomized, controlled clinical trial. LEPMI Study Group. *J Acquir Immune Defic Syndr* 7:457–462, 1994.
59. Martin MA, Cox PH, Beck K, et al: A comparison of the effectiveness

of three regimens in the prevention of *Pneumocystis carinii* pneumonia in HIV-infected patients. *Arch Intern Med* 152:523–528, 1992.

60. Torres RA, Barr M, Thorn M, et al: Randomized trial of dapsone and aerosolized pentamidine for the prophylaxis of *Pneumocystis carinii* pneumonia and toxoplasmic encephalitis. *Am J Med* 95:573–583, 1993.

61. Hughes WT, Killmar JT, Oz HS: Relative potency of 10 drugs with anti–*Pneumocystis carinii* activity in an animal model. *J Infect Dis* 170:906–911, 1994.

62. Hughes WT: Macrolide-antifol synergism in anti–*Pneumocystis carinii* therapeutics. *J Protozool* 38:2S, 1991.

63. Hughes WT, Killmar JT: Synergistic anti–*Pneumocystis carinii* effects of erythromycin and sulfisoxazole. *J Acquir Immune Defic Syndr* 4:532–537, 1991.

64. Carr A, Gross AS, Hoskins JM, et al: Acetylation phenotype and cutaneous hypersensitivity to trimethoprim-sulfamethoxazole in HIV-infected patients. *AIDS* 8:333–337, 1994.

65. Rieder MJ, Krause R, Bird IA, et al: Effect of HIV-infection on toxicity of sulphonamide reactive derivatives [Abstract no 499]. In *First National Conference on Human Retroviruses.* Washington, DC, December 1993.

66. Lee BL, Delahunty T, Safrin S: The hydroxylamine of sulfamethoxazole and adverse reactions in patients with acquired immunodeficiency syndrome. *Clin Pharmacol Ther* 56:184–189, 1994.

67. Safrin S, Lee BL, Sande MA: Adjunctive folinic acid with trimethoprim-sulfamethoxazole for *Pneumocystis carinii* pneumonia in AIDS patients is associated with an increased risk of therapeutic failure and death. *J Infect Dis* 170:912–917, 1994.

68. D'Antonio RG, Johnson DB, Winn RE, et al: Effect of folinic acid on the capacity of trimethoprim-sulfamethoxazole to prevent and treat *Pneumocystis carinii* pneumonia in rats. *Antimicrob Agents Chemother* 29:327–329, 1986.

69. Leggiadro R, Winkelstein JA, Hughes WT: Prevalence of *Pneumocystis carinii* pneumonitis in severe combined immunodeficiency. *J Pediatr* 99:96–98, 1981.

70. Centers for Disease Control: Recommendations for prophylaxis against *Pneumocystis carinii* pneumonia for adults and adolescents infected with human immunodeficiency virus. *MMWR* 41(RR-4):1–10, 1992.

71. Centers for Disease Control: Guidelines for prophylaxis against *Pneumocystis carinii* pneumonia for children infected with human immunodeficiency virus. *MMWR* 49(RR-2):1–13, 1991.

72. Centers for Disease Control and Prevention: USPHS/IDSA guidelines for the prevention of opportunistic infections in persons infected with human immunodeficiency virus. *MMWR* 44(RR-8), 1995.

73. Centers for Disease Control and Prevention: 1995 revised guidelines for prophylaxis against *Pneumocystic carinii* pneumonia for children

infected with or perinatally exposed to human immunodeficiency virus. *MMWR* 44(RR-4):1–11, 1995.

74. Simonds RJ, Oxtoby MJ, Caldwell MB, et al: *Pneumocystis carinii* pneumonia among U.S. children with perinatally acquired HIV infection. *JAMA* 270:470–473, 1993.

Invasive Fungal Infections in Children: Recent Advances in Diagnosis and Treatment*

Thomas J. Walsh, M.D.
Head, Mycology Unit, Infectious Diseases Section, Pediatric Branch, National Cancer Institute, Bethesda, Maryland

Corina Gonzalez, M.D.
Infectious Diseases Section, Pediatric Branch, National Cancer Institute, Bethesda, Maryland

Caron A. Lyman, M.D.
Infectious Diseases Section, Pediatric Branch, National Cancer Institute, Bethesda, Maryland

Stephen J. Chanock, M.D.
Infectious Diseases Section, Pediatric Branch, National Cancer Institute, Bethesda, Maryland

Philip A. Pizzo, M.D.
Head, Infectious Diseases Section, Chief, Pediatric Branch, National Cancer Institute, Bethesda, Maryland

---

Invasive fungal infections have emerged as important causes of morbidity and mortality in immunocompromised children. During the past decade, *Candida* spp. have emerged as one of the most common causes of nosocomial infections, particularly in the setting of prolonged antibacterial therapy, chronic indwelling central venous catheters, granulocytopenia, complicated surgical procedures, and very low birth weight. Mucosal candidiasis is the most common opportunistic infection in human immunodeficiency virus (HIV)–infected patients. *Aspergillus* spp. often cause devastating respiratory tract infections in immunocompromised patients, including neutropenic hosts and recipients of organ and bone marrow transplants. Emerging opportunistic pathogens, including *Trichosporon* spp., *Fusarium* spp., and dematiaceous fungi, are often highly resistant to amphotericin B. At the same

---

*By permission of the Department of Health and Human Services/National Institutes of Health.

"

time, recent advances in diagnosis, treatment, and prevention of invasive fungal infections offer hope for children afflicted with these life-threatening infections. Increased awareness of the early patterns of fungal infection and new methods for blood culture detection have contributed to improved recognition of life-threatening mycoses. Detection of fungal-specific biochemical, antigenic, and molecular markers are providing new avenues for early detection and therapeutic monitoring. Therapeutic advances have improved understanding of existing antifungal drugs, particularly amphotericin B, and development of new compounds, especially antifungal triazoles. Novel biochemical targets for antifungal drug development offer hope for a more versatile therapeutic armamentarium. Because there are few recent comprehensive reviews of these advances as they pertain to pediatrics, we will discuss the recent advances in approaches to diagnosis, treatment, and prevention of invasive fungal infections in children.

CANDIDIASIS

Candidiasis is the most common mucosal and deeply invasive mycosis affecting children. *Candida albicans* is the most common species of the genus *Candida* causing infections. Other species such as *Candida tropicalis, Candida parapsilosis, Candida krusei, Torulopsis glabrata* (considered by some authorities to belong to genus *Candida*) are increasing in incidence and may cause serious infection. The genus *Candida* is characterized by yeasts forms (blastoconidia), which may also form pseudohyphae and hyphae in tissue. *Torulopsis glabrata* has no pseudohyphae or hyphae. The salient microbiologic features of *Candida* spp. and other selected medically important fungi in children are outlined in Table 1.

Candida albicans is a normal part of the flora of the alimentary tract. As an opportunistic pathogen, *Candida* spp. require compromised immunologic or mechanical host defenses to establish infection. *Candida* infections are classified as cutaneous candidiasis, mucosal candidiasis, and deeply invasive candidiasis. Mucosal candidiasis may be further classified as cutaneous, oropharyngeal, and esophageal infection. Deeply invasive candidiasis may be further classified as fungemia, acute disseminated candidiasis, chronic disseminated candidiasis, and single-organ candidiasis.

Invasive candidiasis has become recognized as one of the most common causes of positive blood cultures. Moreover, mucosal candidiasis is the most common opportunistic infection of HIV-infected children. Recent advances in the use of amphotericin B and in the development of antifungal triazoles have expanded the options for treatment of these debilitating and life-threatening infections (Table 2).

MUCOSAL CANDIDIASIS

Mucosal candidiasis may develop in the oropharynx, esophagus, gastrointestinal tract, urinary tract, vaginal mucosal, and tracheobronchial tree. The risk factors for developing mucosal candidiasis include broad-spectrum antibiotic therapy, impaired or immature cell-mediated immunity (e.g., HIV infection, chronic mucocutaneous candidiasis, very low birth weight), corticosteroid therapy, and diabetes mellitus.[1-3] Although most children with thrush who are seen in a general pediatric setting have no underlying immune impairment and are usually treated successfully, the management of mucosal candidiasis in immunocompromised patients may be more complicated. We will thus focus our attention on the management of mucosal candidiasis in the compromised host.

A diagnosis of mucosal candidiasis is best established by a combination of physical examination, direct microscopic examination, and culture confirmation. The principal treatment of mucosal candidiasis consists of reversal of known risk factors and administration of antifungal therapy. Depending on the severity of mucosal candidiasis and the underlying host defects, topical therapy is administered initially; systemic therapy is indicated if topical therapy is unsuccessful or contraindicated (e.g., severe, painful mucositis in a young child).

OROPHARYNGEAL CANDIDIASIS

The clinical manifestations of oral candidiasis are variable, including a punctate mucosal erythema, a diffuse mucosal erythema, and white-beige pseudomembranous plaques on the buccal mucosa, hard palate, oropharyngeal mucosa, and gingivae.[1] These lesions may become confluent plaques, involving extensive regions of the mucosa of the oral cavity. These plaques can be removed with difficulty to reveal a granular base that bleeds easily. A more chronic form of oropharyngeal candidiasis, known as atrophic *Candida* glossitis, may develop on the dorsum of the tongue, appearing as an erythematous lesion associated with the loss of papillae. The lesions may become sufficiently severe as to impair alimentation. Oral candidiasis in immunocompromised patients also may be complicated by extension to esophageal candidiasis,[2-4] laryngeal candidiasis, or *Candida* epiglottis, which may cause hoarseness or threaten patency of the airway.[2, 5-9]

TABLE 1.
Essential Microbiologic Characteristics of Fungi Infecting Immunocompromised Children

Organism	Morphologic Features	Biochemical, Immunologic, or Molecular Diagnostic Characteristics	Comments
Candida spp.	Budding yeasts (blastoconidia) with pseudohyphae and hyphae; *Candida albicans* identified by germ-tube production; morphology on corn meal agar with Tween-80 identifies different *Candida* spp.	Assimilation and fermentation patterns are utilized to distinguish non-*albicans* spp. of *Candida*	Different species of *Candida* have different virulence potentials and susceptibility to antifungal agents
Torulopsis glabrata	Small budding yeast that does not produce germ tubes, pseudohyphae, or hyphae	Assimilation and fermentation patterns	Needs to be distinguished from other yeastlike fungi
Cryptococcus neoformans	Encapsulated yeast	Urease activity and phenol oxidase activity distinguish *C. neoformans*; assimilation pattern identifies non-neoformans spp. of *Cryptococcus*	Presumptive diagnosis can be made on direct examination of india ink preparation of cerebrospinal fluid

Histoplasma capsulatum	Dimorphic fungus*: yeast form at 37° C (including tissue) and filamentous form at 20° C–30° C	RNA hybridization studies or exoantigen identification of isolated organism by immunodiffusion	H. capsulatum grows slowly (4–6 wk) in conventional media but may be recovered within 1–3 weeks from lysis centrifugation or mycobacterial radiometric blood culture systems
Coccidioides immitis	Dimorphic fungus*: spherule in tissue (37° C) and filamentous form (arthroconidia and hyphae) at 20° C–30° C in culture	RNA hybridization studies or exoantigen identification of isolated organism by immunodiffusion	Caution for clinical laboratory workers in handling organisms
Sporothrix schenckii	Dimorphic fungus* growing within 3–5 days at 25° C as a hyaline mould and can be converted to a cigar-shaped yeast at 37° C	Not routinely used	Biopsy results of infected tissue is often negative; culture is preferred means of microbiologic diagnosis
Aspergillus spp.	Angular branching hyphae in tissue and characteristic vesicle, phialides, and conidia	Not routinely used	Conidia, vesicles, and phialides are not produced in tissue
Malassezia furfur	Identified by skin scrapings as a characteristic cluster of blastoconidia and hyphae; flask-shaped blastoconidia are found in culture	Supplementation of the agar plate with olive oil or other oil that has 12–24 length carbon chains is necessary to promote growth of this lipophilic yeast	Distinguish from other yeastlike fungi if recovered from blood

*The living filamentous forms of these dimorphic fungi (H. capsulatum, C. immitis, and S. schenckii) are highly infectious and are examined only within a biosafety cabinet.

TABLE 2.

Approaches to Treatment of Mucosal and Invasive Candidiasis in Children

Patterns of Candidiasis	Treatment	Comments
Mucosal		
Oropharyngeal candidiasis	Nystatin suspension Clotrimazole troches Ketoconazole, PO* Fluconazole, PO/IV Itraconazole, PO Amphotericin B	Selection depends on severity of infection, host status, and *Candida* spp. involved
Esophageal candidiasis	Fluconazole, PO/IV Ketoconazole Amphotericin, B, IV	Selection depends on severity of infection, host status, *Candida* spp. involved, and probability of concomitant dissemination†
Vaginal candidiasis	Nystatin suspension Clotrimazole troches or cream Miconazole cream Ketoconazole, PO Fluconazole, PO	Selection depends on severity of infection, host status, and *Candida* spp. involved
Candida cystitis	Fluconazole, PO/IV Amphotericin B, IV Amphotericin B, bladder washout	Selection depends on severity of infection, host status, *Candida* spp. involved
Nonmucosal deep tissue		
Fungemia	Amphotericin B, IV ± flucytosine (5-FC) Fluconazole, PO/IV	Removal of vascular catheter; selection of compound depends on severity of infection, host status, *Candida* spp. involved
Acute disseminated candidiasis	Amphotericin B, IV ± 5-FC	Removal of vascular catheter
Chronic disseminated candidiasis	Amphotericin B, IV ± 5-FC Fluconazole, PO/IV	Protracted therapy usually required
Single-organ candidiasis	Amphotericin B, IV ± 5-FC Fluconazole, PO/IV	Removal of vascular catheter; possible surgical intervention, depending on site
Candida peritonitis	Amphotericin B, IV ± 5-FC Fluconazole, PO/IV	Removal of peritoneal catheter

*PO = by mouth; IV = intravenously; ± = with or without.

Management of oropharyngeal candidiasis consists initially of establishing an accurate diagnosis. Many cases of apparent thrush, particularly in granulocytopenic patients, may have other causes including herpes simplex or mixed oral bacterial flora. Because white mucosal plaques are not necessarily pathognomonic of oropharyngeal candidiasis, direct microscopic examination of scrapings of lesions and culture confirmation are the most reliable means of establishing this diagnosis. Such a diagnostic approach becomes even more important when a child does not respond to topical or systemic antifungal therapy.

Recovery of host defense is an integral part of managing oropharyngeal and other forms of mucosal candidiasis. For example, treatment of underlying HIV infection with antiretroviral therapy and discontinuation of corticosteroids may lead to partial recovery of cell-mediated immunity, mucosal host defense, and oropharyngeal candidiasis. Topical antifungal treatment is usually effective in controlling most cases of oropharyngeal candidiasis and is recommended as the initial therapeutic intervention. Nystatin has limited activity in moderate to advanced forms of oropharyngeal candidiasis in severely immunocompromised hosts. Nystatin is also limited by its somewhat bitter taste, which may be a major impediment to compliance. In this regard, clotrimazole, administered four to five times daily, appears to be more active than nystatin in treatment of oropharyngeal candidiasis, possibly due to improved compliance. The more prolonged exposure of the oral cavity to clotrimazole also may substantially contribute to its antifungal activity. Nevertheless, administration of clotrimazole troches requiring retention of the troche in the oral cavity until it is completely dissolved may be difficult in younger children. In cases where the child is not able to maintain a clotrimazole troche under the tongue or under buccal mucosal for a sustained period, the clotrimazole troches may be pulverized and formulated into a suspension to be given by syringe.

Children with oropharyngeal candidiasis refractory to topical therapy are candidates for systemic therapy using ketoconazole or, when approved, fluconazole. Ketoconazole and fluconazole for oropharyngeal candidiasis may be administered at 3.0 mg/kg in two divided doses.[10, 11] Recent reports of itraconazole also suggest a potential role for this agent in treatment of oropharyngeal candidiasis in children, including those with chronic mucocutaneous candidiasis.[12, 13] For smaller children, a tablet may be divided and pulverized into a suspension and administered as a fraction of that suspension twice daily. The optimal use of the antifungal azoles, however, in HIV-associated oropharyngeal candidiasis has at this point not been clearly elucidated. Children with particularly depressed cell-mediated immunity may have oropharyngeal and esophageal candidiasis that becomes completely refractory to topical and oral therapy.[14] Such patients may respond well to intermittent courses of amphotericin B at 0.5 mg/kg/daily for approximately 7 to 14 days, depending on therapeutic response. Lower doses of amphotericin B for refractory mucosal candidiasis may not be successful in eradicating the infection. In addition to treating the oropharyngeal candidiasis, one should treat any concomitant infections such as those due to herpes simplex virus that may occur concomitantly with invasive candidiasis. Advanced stages of oropharyngeal candidiasis in HIV-infected children and granulocytopenic children may often be accompanied by esophageal candidiasis. Recent findings indicate that azole-resistant *C. albicans* may emerge in HIV-infected children as a cause of esophageal candidiasis.[15]

ESOPHAGEAL CANDIDIASIS

Esophageal candidiasis is associated with risk factors similar to those of oropharyngeal candidiasis but may occur in the absence of conspicuous oropharyngeal *Candida* infection.[2–4, 16] Radiation to the mediastinum and gastroesophageal reflux are additional risk factors for esophageal candidiasis.[17] Concomitant infections due to herpes simplex, cytomegalovirus, and bacteria may coincide with or precede esophageal candidiasis.

Esophagoscopy with mucosal biopsy is the most definitive method for establishing a diagnosis of esophageal candidiasis. Although biopsy of the esophageal mucosa is the gold standard for diagnosis of esophageal candidiasis, this may not be feasible in many children. Accordingly, an empirical approach is often warranted in children with suspected esophageal candidiasis. Such an empirical approach in children with granulocytopenia may consist of initial clotrimazole, systemic azole, or both. However, because the esophagus may be the portal of entry for candidiasis, failure to symptomatically respond promptly is an indication for empirical amphotericin B. One must also be aware that the resolution of symptoms does not necessarily signify the eradication of esophageal candidiasis in granulocytopenic patients. Thus, a persistently febrile patient with proven esophageal candidiasis may still require empirical amphotericin B therapy, despite resolution of esophageal symptoms. Children with HIV infection, who are also highly susceptible to development of esophageal candidiasis, may initially receive therapy, depending on severity of symptoms and level of immunosuppression, with ketoconazole, fluconazole, or amphotericin B. Nystatin appears to have little or no effect in management of esophageal candidiasis. Initial studies in children indicate that fluconazole is effective in the treatment of esophageal candidiasis. Appropriate dosages of fluconazole for treatment of esophageal candidiasis have yet to be defined, but 3 mg/kg in nonneutropenic patients is active.

GENITOURINARY CANDIDIASIS

Urinary candidiasis should be evaluated as either involvement of the upper or lower urinary tract. The management of urinary candidiasis is controversial and depends on the state of the host and the location of infection. Removal of urinary catheters and other foreign bodies (e.g., urinary stents), when possible, is a basic principle for the management of urinary catheter infections. The diagnostic significance of candiduria depends on the host. Candiduria proved through a reliable clean-catch specimen or a straight catheterized specimen in a low birth weight infant or granulocytopenic child should be considered significant and treated as evidence for disseminated candidiasis until proved otherwise. By comparison, the nonimmunocompromised child with candiduria and temporary placement of a urinary catheter or congenital ureteral and bladder anatomic abnormalities, probably does not have disseminated candidiasis. Instead, such patients more likely have infection restricted to the mucosa. Thus, treatment of *Candida* cystitis with systemic antifungal therapy depends on the probability of concomitant deeply invasive candidiasis.

The medical management of uncomplicated *Candida* cystitis may include fluconazole (3 mg/kg/daily), intravenous (IV) amphotericin B (0.3–0.5 mg/kg/daily), oral flucytosine (5-fluorocytosine, or 5-FC; 150 mg/kg/daily in three to four divided doses), or amphotericin B bladder washout (concentration of 5 μg/mL in sterile 5% aqueous dextrose solution [D_5W] with closed continuous irrigation of 15 mL/kg/daily in three to four divided doses). Bladder irrigations with amphotericin B may not permanently eradicate *Candida* cystitis in patients who remain catheterized. Oral 5-FC, which achieves high urinary concentrations, is not used alone in view of the potential of emergence of resistance. Single doses or short courses of intravenous amphotericin B achieve sufficiently high fungicidal concentrations in the urine to eradicate *Candida*. Nevertheless, candiduria may recur as long as the patient remains catheterized. Given its high urinary concentrations, fluconazole may be highly effective in the treatment of urinary tract infections due to

C. albicans, C. tropicalis, and possibly *C. parapsilosis.*[17] Other yeastlike fungi, such as *C. parapsilosis, T. glabrata, C. krusei,* and *Hansenula anomala,* however, may emerge as resistant superinfecting pathogens when fluconazole is used as therapy.[18–21]

Vaginal candidiasis is another manifestation of genitourinary candidiasis. The management of vaginal candidiasis includes establishing a direct microscopic and microbiologic diagnosis, ruling out other causes of vaginal discharge, and administering appropriate antifungal chemotherapy. Recurrent vulvovaginal candidiasis in an adolescent may be the first manifestation of HIV infection. Most cases of vaginal candidiasis may be treated by topical therapy such as clotrimazole or miconazole cream or clotrimazole troches. Ketoconazole may be used for treatment of recurrent vaginal candidiasis. Fluconazole recently has been approved for treatment of vaginal candidiasis in adults but also is likely to be effective for this infection in children and adolescents.

TRACHEOBRONCHIAL CANDIDIASIS

Tracheobronchial candidiasis, particularly in HIV-infected patients, is yet another manifestation of impaired mucosal immunity. This process is generally an asymptomatic infection that does not require antifungal treatment. Diagnosis and treatment of pulmonary candidiasis are described in greater detail in a subsequent section. Notably, pulmonary candidiasis reflecting deep tissue parenchymal invasion, although well described as a complication of neutropenia and very low birth weight infancy,[22–25] is seldom a complication of tracheobronchial candidiasis in HIV-infected patients.

CANDIDEMIA

The risk factors for hospital-acquired candidemia include the simultaneous use of more than two antibiotics, the use of chronic Silastic indwelling catheters (e.g., Hickman-Broviac catheters), granulocytopenia, and abdominal surgery.[26] These risk factors for candidemia are frequently encountered in very low birth weight infants and children with neutropenia, as well as HIV infection. Diagnosis of suspected fungemia is highly dependent on the blood culture detection system.[27] The lysis centrifugation system is as sensitive or more sensitive than other systems and is especially valuable in conveying a semiquantitative determination of the number of yeast cells per quantity of blood. Despite these technologic merits, lysis centrifugation blood cultures, similar to other blood cultures systems, may not detect patients with deeply invasive candidiasis early in the course of infection. For example, a recent study comparing the frequency of detection of fungemia by lysis centrifugation vs. the frequency of autopsy-proven invasive candidiasis demonstrated that lysis centrifugation blood cultures may not detect as much as 50% of patients with deep tissue candidiasis.[28]

Detection of *Candida* in blood cultures in virtually all cases should be considered evidence of invasive candidiasis, thereby warranting a course of antifungal therapy. Untreated candidemia may be followed in nongranulocytopenic patients by approximately 10% to 20% frequency of late complications, including *Candida* endophthalmitis, meningitis, osteomyelitis, arthritis, endocarditis, and renal candidiasis.[29-34] Disseminated candidiasis in neonates and granulocytopenic patients is often reflected by fungemia and carries a high mortality if treatment is delayed.[35-47] Fungemia may be followed in granulocytopenic patients by the complication of hepatosplenic candidiasis.[48-51] Candidemia may be a reflection of clinical occult deep tissue seeding. Indeed, candidemia should be considered with the same clinical significance as that of a positive blood culture for *Staphylococcus aureus*, whose complications after bacteremia are as dangerous as those of candidemia.

Management of candidemia depends on the host and the organism isolated. Although the optimal dosage and duration for treatment of fungemia with amphotericin B have not been well defined, sufficient experience exists to suggest some general principles. Uncomplicated candidemia can be treated by a 2-week course of amphotericin B at 0.5 mg/kg/daily, particularly if the fungemia is caused by *C. albicans* in a nongranulocytopenic patient and is accompanied by removal of the intravascular catheter. Given the higher level of resistance of *C. tropicalis* and *C. parapsilosis*, fungemia due to these organisms may require higher doses of amphotericin B (e.g., 0.75–1.0 mg/kg/daily) and more protracted courses (e.g., 3–4 weeks). Fluconazole was equivalent to amphotericin B in treatment of uncomplicated catheter-associated fungemia in non-neutropenic, nonimmunosuppressed adults.[52] Whether these findings can be extended to children, particularly immunosuppressed children and low birth weight infants, warrants further study. Persistent fungemia, despite amphotericin B, is treated by increasing the dosage of amphotericin B, the addition of 5-FC, and removal of any intravascular foreign bodies. Fungemia due to *C. parapsilosis* is highly associated with intravascular catheters.[32, 42, 53, 54]

The gastrointestinal tract is an important portal of entry for *Candida* spp. in immunocompromised hosts.[55, 56] However, intravascular catheters also may be a source of fungemia, as well as a target for attachment of circulating *Candida* spp. from a different portal of entry (e.g., the gastrointestinal tract). Intravascular catheters in either circumstance serve as a source for continued seeding of the bloodstream. Thus intravascular catheters should be removed, whenever feasible, in patients with fungemia. Lecciones et al,[41] in a study of 155 episodes of vascular catheter-associated fungemia, found that the longer the central venous catheter remained in place, the greater the frequency of persistent fungemia and complications of disseminated candidiasis. Eppes et al.[32] found that among all pediatric patients with fungemia and central venous or arterial catheters, there was a significant reduction of persistent fungemia and a trend toward reduction of complications of disseminated candidiasis in those whose vascular catheter was removed. Dato and Dajani[31] also concluded from their study that catheter removal for candidemia was an important determinant of outcome. Prompt removal of catheters was significantly associated with improved survival in 31 children with candidemia from their center. Moreover, a literature review conducted by the same authors revealed a significantly improved survival rate among patients treated with amphotericin B whose catheters were removed vs. those in whom the catheter was retained.

Peripheral IV catheters clearly can be a portal of entry and a focus for *Candida* suppurative thrombophlebitis.[56, 57] In addition to IV amphotericin B therapy, removal of peripheral vascular catheters and segmental resection of the infected vein are important for complete therapeutic response. Delay in resecting the infected venous segment can result in persistent fungemia, progressive thrombophlebitis, or relapse of infection after discontinuation of antifungal chemotherapy.

Fungemia seldom occurs as a direct complication of mucosal candidiasis in HIV-infected patients. Instead, fungemia in HIV-infected hosts classically has been considered as a nosocomial infection after the typical previously described risk factors.[58] These children have a high mortality due to invasive candidiasis.

More recently we found that fungemia among our HIV-infected children was seen most frequently in the ambulatory clinic as a vascular catheter-associated community-acquired infection.[59] Fungemia was detected in the outpatient clinic by blood cultures in the process of evaluating patients for new onset of fever. There was a strong association between the presence of chronic indwelling central venous catheters and the development of fungemia. Vascular catheters appeared to be the portal of entry for fungemia in these patients. All patients with fungemia had vascular catheters, but no patient without catheters had fungemia. The organisms causing fungemia in more than half of all cases consisted of non-*albicans Candida* spp. or other species of fungi. These patients were managed consistently with an approach using (1) early detection of fungemia by blood cultures at the new onset of fever in patients seen in the outpatient clinic, (2) prompt initiation of amphotericin B at 0.5 to 1 mg/kg/daily on recovery of fungus from blood, and (3) removal of the central venous catheter within 2 days of initiating antifungal therapy. This strategy resulted in a 95% survival rate and no posttherapeutic infectious sequelae. These findings contrast with the high mortality of nosocomial invasive candidiasis in HIV-infected children observed by Leibovitz et al.[58] Such differences may be related to concomitant underlying diseases and timing of detection of *Candida* as the cause of fever in these seriously ill children.

Central venous catheters associated with candidemia in neonates may cause severe complications of superior or inferior vena caval thrombosis.[34, 60] Early recognition, initiation of amphotericin B, catheter removal, and administration of heparin are important elements of management. Diagnosis may be facilitated by echocardiography and ultrasonography. Long durations of high-dose amphotericin B (1.0 mg/kg/daily) appear to be a critical element in assuring clearance of this endovascular infection.

Fungemia may develop because of yeastlike organisms resistant to conventional antifungal compounds. These organisms include *Candida lusitaniae*,[61–63] *Candida guilliermondii*,[64, 65] *C. krusei*,[19, 66] *T. glabrata*,[18, 67–69] *Candida lipolytica*,[70] and *Trichosporon beigelii*.[71] *Candida lusitaniae, C. guilliermondii,* and *C. lipolytica* may have high minimum inhibitory concentrations (MICs) in vitro and may be the cause of fungemia refractory to amphotericin B. *Candida krusei* and *T. glabrata* may emerge as superinfecting causes of fungemia in neutropenic patients receiving prophylactic antifungal azole therapy.[19, 66–69] Most isolates of *C. krusei* are intrinsically resistant to antifungal azoles, whereas some isolates of *T. glabrata* may be initially susceptible but become resistant during the course of antifungal azole therapy. *Torulopsis glabrata* infections have developed in our center and others in patients receiving fluconazole.

DISSEMINATED CANDIDIASIS

Tissue-proven disseminated candidiasis may be classified as acute disseminated or chronic disseminated candidiasis. The syndromes of acute and chronic disseminated candidiasis occupy two ends of a spectrum that is particularly well demonstrated in granulocytopenic patients. Acute disseminated candidiasis occurs typically in granulocytopenic children and manifests with persistent fungemia, hemodynamic instability, multiple cutaneous and visceral lesions, and high mortality despite antifungal therapy. By comparison, chronic disseminated candidiasis, otherwise known as hepatosplenic candidiasis, is characterized by an indolent process of disseminated candidiasis, often without detectable fungemia, in a hemodynamically stable patient and carries a relatively high survival rate when antifungal therapy is administered. Of course, there is a continuum of patterns of infection between these two distinctive syndromes of disseminated candidiasis. We treat acute disseminated candidiasis with high doses of amphotericin B ($\geq$1.0 mg/kg/ daily) plus 5-FC. Prompt initiation of aggressive antifungal therapy is necessary in such patients.

A similar syndrome of acute disseminated candidiasis may develop in low birth weight infants and may be manifest by apnea, hypotension, and fever or hypothermia.[71] Early recognition of disseminated candidiasis in this patient population and initiation of effective antifungal therapy are essential for optimal management and outcome.

Candida albicans is the most frequent cause of disseminated candidiasis in neutropenic children; however, *C. tropicalis* has been increasingly implicated as an important pathogen in neutropenic children. Flynn et al.[40] reported from St. Jude Children's Research Hospital 19 children treated for leukemia in whom *C. tropicalis* infections developed. Fungemia without meningitis in 11 children was treated successfully, whereas *C. tropicalis* meningitis in 7 children was uniformly fatal. An additional patient had clinically unsuspected, disseminated candidiasis found at autopsy. This study provides an important insight that meningitis is a critical factor for outcome in disseminated candidiasis due to *C. tropicalis* in neutropenic patients. A high index of suspicion and the early use of aggressive amphotericin B therapy are critical for the successful management of *C. tropicalis* infections in neutropenic children with leukemia.

Chronic disseminated candidiasis is a more indolent condition that develops during the course of granulocytopenia but usually becomes apparent only on recovery from granulocytopenia. A computed tomography (CT) scan or a magnetic resonance imaging (MRI) scan performed at this time often demonstrates multiple lesions in liver, spleen, and at times other organs such as kidneys and lungs. A biopsy of hepatic lesions is important in management of these patients for several reasons: (1) other infections (including other mycoses), neoplastic processes, and inflammatory lesions may simulate the conditions of hepatosplenic candidiasis; (2) the administration of long-term amphotericin B is justified only with definitive evidence of candidiasis; and (3) biopsy confirmation of candidiasis is necessary for the delivery of investigational agents (e.g., lipid preparations of amphotericin B), which are often required in refractory cases. Our initial approach in managing hepatosplenic candidiasis is administration of amphotericin B, usually with 5-FC, followed by long-term fluconazole (6–10 mg/kg/daily) therapy until resolution or calcification of lesions. Such a course of therapy may require 6 months to 1 year. Hepatosplenic candidiasis due to *C. tropicalis* may be particularly refractory to fluconazole therapy and may be amenable only to long-term amphotericin B for 6 to 12 months. Fluconazole also has been used in patients with hepatosplenic candidiasis refractory to amphotericin B or in patients with amphotericin B–associated nephrotoxicity.[72, 73] During therapy for chronic disseminated candidiasis, children requiring continued cycles of chemotherapy may receive such cycles without progression of hepatosplenic candidiasis or breakthrough fungemia, provided that the disseminated infection has stabilized or is resolving.[74] Clearly an infection not responding to antifungal therapy precludes concomitant administration of cytotoxic chemotherapy.

Over the past decade, *Candida* spp. have become increasingly common pathogens among infants requiring neonatal intensive care. Disseminated candidiasis occurs predominantly in premature infants with birth weights less than 1,500 g. Previous studies have estimated an incidence of disseminated *Candida* infections of 2% to 4% in these very low birth weight premature infants, a rate two to four times higher than the incidence of candidemia in the overall neonatal population.[24, 36, 71, 75–81] Very low birth weight infants have a high predilection for development of disseminated candidiasis due to tenuous cutaneous anatomic barrier and immunologic deficits. These deficits include low serum immunoglobulin and complements levels,[82] impaired opsonic ability, and defective neutrophil and monocytic functions, specifically chemotaxis, intracellular killing, and oxidative burst.[83]

Among the many risks factors reported, all are related to prolonged hospitalizations of usually more than 7 days under intensive care support. Antimicrobial therapy was the strongest risk factor associated with the development of fungemia in a case control study performed in this population of patients.[37] The protracted use of antibiotics increases the risk of gastrointestinal and cutaneous colonization by *Candida* spp.[54] Recently an outbreak of *C. tropicalis* fungemia in a neonatal intensive care unit due to cross-infection between medical staff and patients was described, underscoring *Candida* spp. as contact-transmissible nosocomial pathogens.[35]

Most neonates with systemic candidiasis are symptomatic at the onset of their disease. Signs and symptoms are virtually identical to those of the sepsis due to other etiologic agents. The affected infants may develop respiratory deterioration, bradycardia, abdominal distention, temperature instability, hypotension, and erythematous rash or skin pustules. The most frequent laboratory abnormalities associated with fungemia in preterm infants are elevated band count, thrombocytopenia, hyperglycemia, and glycosuria. Acute disseminated candidiasis in newborns may ensue as a postpartum, nosocomially acquired infection or may be acquired as a congenital infection.[75] These authors also emphasized that histopathologic examination of the umbilical cord vessels may be an effective means of early detection of congenital candidemia. Umbilical cords typically demonstrated pseudohyphae amid an acute necrotizing inflammation.

Candida has a well-documented predilection for the invasion of specific tissue sites in neonates. Analysis of 89 cases of systemic candidiasis reported in the literature reveled that central nervous system (CNS) (32%), eye (4%), kidneys (67%), and lungs (32%) are the most common sites involved in disseminated disease in infants.[42, 71, 76] Skin rash or pustules positive for *Candida* spp. are also associated findings in these patients (15%) as is osteoarthritis (1%). Catheter-related septic thrombosis and endocarditis associated with refractory candidemia is an uncommon but serious complication in these infants that may be further complicated by the development of intracardiac fungal masses.[34, 78, 84] *Candida* peritonitis in newborns is uncommon and occurs generally as a consequence of gastrointestinal disease such as necrotizing enterocolitis or gastrointestinal perforations.[85, 86] Morbidity due to the consequences of disseminated candidiasis is serious and includes poor vision or blindness attributable to macular or perimacular lesions, osteoarthritis, venous septic thrombosis, multiple cerebral abscesses and chronic neurologic deficits.

Antifungal therapy is recommended for all infants with at least one positive blood culture or those highly suspected of having an invasive fungal infection.[87, 88] Butler et al.[88] reviewed 38 neonates with invasive candidiasis, including 28 (74%) with disseminated candidiasis and 10 with catheter-associated candidemia. These investigators concluded that catheter-associated candidiasis could be treated effectively with removal of the vascular catheter and administration of amphotericin B alone for a total dosage of 10 to 15 mg/kg/daily. By comparison, higher total dosages of 25 to 30 mg/kg/daily were encouraged for treatment of disseminated candidiasis. For acute disseminated candidiasis, particularly when due to non-*albicans Candida* spp., we recommend amphotericin B (0.5−1 mg/kg) combined with 5-FC (50− 100 mg/kg/daily) as the treatment of choice. Most side effects of 5-FC can be prevented or managed by monitoring and adjusting dosage, as described later on. The relatively high frequency of CNS infection during proven disseminated candidiasis suggests that initial therapy of systemic candidiasis should include 5-FC, which readily penetrates the blood-brain barrier. Data concerning treatment with the antifungal triazole compounds itraconazole and fluconazole in very low birth weight infants are sparse; however current findings warrant further investigation of these agents in this high-risk population.[89−93]

Fluconazole was evaluated prospectively by Fasano et al.[94] in 40 neonates and infants with invasive candidiasis between the ages of 2 days and 3 months in whom conventional antifungal therapy was ineffective or contraindicated. The patients received therapy on an individual compassionate request basis for microbiologically documented or presumed fungal infection. The mean fluconazole dosage was 5.3 mg/kg/daily (range 1−16 mg/kg/daily), and the mean duration of therapy was 26 days (range 2−80 days). Efficacy was evaluated in neonates with proven fungal infection as documented by the presence of a pathogen at baseline. A positive clinical response was achieved in 97% (31/32) of the clinically evaluable patients; eradication of the fungal organism was achieved in 97% (30/ 31) of evaluable patients. Adverse events occurred in two patients (5%); therapy was not discontinued in either patient. These favorable safety and efficacy data are similar to results obtained with fluconazole in older children and adults. These findings warrant further investigation of fluconazole compared with amphotericin B for treatment of invasive candidiasis in a thoughtfully designed and carefully conducted randomized clinical trial in neonates and infants. Recently two cases of systemic candidiasis treated with liposomal amphotericin B (AmBisome) were reported showing good therapeutic response and lower toxicity than with conventional therapy.[95]

Candida albicans and other *Candida* spp. may be transferred by contact transmission from patient to patient on the hands of medical staff. Various outbreaks in pediatric intensive care units by strains of *Candida* spp. have been identified.[35, 64] As discussed by Betremieux et al.,[96] molecular epidemiologic studies demonstrate that a given strain of *Candida* spp. is transmissible to patients from medical personnel. Thus, handwashing becomes paramount in preventing this mode of nosocomial acquisition of pathogenic fungi.

DEEP CANDIDIASIS INVOLVING SINGLE NONMUCOSAL ORGAN SITES

Candida Peritonitis

Candida peritonitis in children is well described in three different clinical settings: gastrointestinal surgery, necrotizing colitis, and peritoneal dialysis.[79, 85, 86, 97–100] The first setting of gastrointestinal surgery usually follows leakage of lumenal contents into the peritoneum from an anastamotic site, particularly in children receiving broad-spectrum antibacterial antibiotics. Management of this condition requires reexploration of the abdominal cavity, drainage of the infection, and administration of IV amphotericin B. Perforation of necrotic bowel in infants who are receiving broad-spectrum antibiotics may result in *Candida* peritonitis. Surgical drainage, resection of necrotic bowel, and amphotericin B are the foundations of management in these critically ill patients. Peritoneal-dialysis-catheter-associated *Candida* peritonitis requires removal of the catheter and administration of IV amphotericin B therapy for optimal therapy. Failure to remove the peritoneal dialysis catheter often results in relapses after discontinuation of antifungal therapy. Direct intraperitoneal administration of amphotericin B is not recommended. Intraperitoneal instillation of Amphotericin B may cause abdominal pain and peritoneal adhesions, which may compromise subsequent courses of peritoneal dialysis. Intravenously administered amphotericin B obtains levels within peritoneal fluid that are fungicidal against most susceptible strains of *Candida* spp. Oral antifungal azoles, specifically ketoconazole and fluconazole, have been reported to be useful in the selected children with *Candida* peritonitis related to chronic ambulatory peritoneal dialysis.[101, 102]

Candida Meningitis

Candida meningitis in children is most frequently encountered in low birth weight infants and older immunosuppressed patients.[29, 40, 103–105] *Candida* meningitis also is increasingly recognized as a complication of ventricular shunts and drains.[106] Chiou et al. recently reported that fungi accounted for 8 (17%) of 48 shunt infections. All babies were born prematurely and required a ventriculoperitoneal shunt for hydrocephalus. Diagnosis of *Candida* meningitis may be elusive due to subtle clinical findings and the inherent difficulty in culturing the organism from the cerebrospinal fluid (CSF). Elevated protein levels, hypoglycorrhachia, and pleocytosis may be present but are not characteristic.

Amphotericin B plus 5-FC in combination is the most appropriate regimen for treatment of *Candida* meningitis. Despite this aggressive therapy, *Candida* meningitis is notorious for relapses of infection, particularly in patients in whom immunosuppression persists. Cultures of CSF may be initially negative despite symptomatic relapse. As a general guideline, antifungal therapy will require continuation as long as pharmacologic or intrinsic immunosuppression persists. In patients with *Candida* meningitis and ventricular shunts or drains, removal of any ventricular prosthetic device is required for successful eradication of *Candida* from the CSF.[106, 107] Because intraventricular administration of amphotericin B can cause chemical ventriculitis, arachnoiditis, severe headache, and seizures, all of the aforementioned interventions should be exhausted before pursuing this approach. Although fluconazole penetrates CSF well and has some reported efficacy in *Candida* meningitis,[108] cases of pediatric *Candida* meningitis not responding to this agent warrant caution in the use of antifungal triazoles.[93, 109]

Candida Osteomyelitis

Candida osteomylitis may develop as a complication of fungemia in low birth weight infants, older immunosuppressed children, and immunocompetent patients. Multiple bony lesions may evolve in immunocompromised hosts.[110, 111] *Candida* osteomyelitis requires surgical debridement of the bone for both diagnostic and therapeutic effects and parenteral amphotericin B. Monitoring of bone scans or MRI scans, as well as erythrocyte sedimentation rate, aids in determining therapeutic end points.

Candida Endocarditis

Candida endocarditis requires a timely diagnosis of fungemia with valvular involvement. Diagnosis may be difficult to establish and may be heralded by the abrupt onset of an embolic event to a major artery. The recent introduction of transesophageal echocardiography may substantially improve detection of valvular vegetations in suspected cases with negative transthoracic echocardiograms.[112] Definitive treatment requires resection of the valve and administration of amphotericin B, 5-FC, or both. Rare cases of *Candida* endocarditis treated with medical therapy alone[53, 113] do not justify this approach as a standard of care. Given the risk and unpredictability of lethal or neurologically catastrophic embolization, surgical resection should be promptly pursued in fungal endocarditis.

Candida Endophthalmitis

The presence of characteristic white vitreal opacities in a patient with candidemia signifies the development of *Candida* endophthalmitis.[114] Management is conducted in concert with pediatric ophthalmologic consultation.[115] Amphotericin B plus 5-FC is recommended for this infection; however, timely use of vitrectomy may be critical to saving vision. The role of intravitreal amphotericin B in children is not well defined.

Pulmonary Candidiasis

Pulmonary candidiasis may be a primary bronchopneumonia or secondary process arising from hematogenous dissemination.[116] Primary *Candida* bronchopneumonia may be found in neutropenic patients with extensive chemotherapy-induced oral mucositis, very low birth weight infants, and low birth weight deliveries associated with *Candida* chorioamnionitis.[22–25] Aspiration of infected oral secretions into the tracheobronchial tree with extension into pulmonary parenchyma is the primary route of infection for *Candida* bronchopneumonia. True pulmonary candidiasis develops most frequently as hematogenous infection of the lungs in granulocytopenic children or *Candida* bronchopneumonia in low birth weight infants.

Fever and pulmonary infiltrates in an immunocompromised patient should not be ascribed solely to *Candida* unless proved by biopsy. Biopsy of lung tissue is the only reliable means of establishing a diagnosis in patients with pulmonary candidiasis. Lung biopsy may also demonstrate other unsuspected causes of infiltrates in such patients. The presence of *Candida* spp. in bronchioalveolar lavage (BAL) fluid from a patient with pulmonary infiltrates is nonspecific and does not provide a definitive diagnosis. Treatment of *Candida* bronchopneumonia or hematogenous disseminated candidiasis is initiated with amphotericin B with or without

5-FC. Among patients unable to tolerate amphotericin B, fluconazole may be considered for treatment of infection due to *C. albicans.*

Candida **Epiglottis and Laryngeal Candidiasis**

Candida epiglottis and laryngeal candidiasis may emerge as life-threatening causes of airway obstruction in neutropenic children, very low birth weight infants, and patients with chronic mucocutaneous candidiasis.[2, 5-9] *Candida* epiglottis manifests initially as refractory odynophagia in the hypopharyngeal and epiglottic regions. The patient may point directly to these areas as the most intense locations of pain. Laryngeal stridor may develop in more advanced cases. Diagnosis is corroborated by an otolaryngologist using appropriate methods for laryngoscopy-guided visualization and swabbing of the epiglottis. The swab material is cultured, smeared, strained, and examined microscopically. Treatment consists of intravenous amphotericin B and airway protection.

ASPERGILLOSIS

Aspergillosis is composed of a spectrum of pathologic processes due to *Aspergillus* spp. which includes hypersensitivity conditions of the respiratory tract, saprophytic involvement of lung cavities, invasive pulmonary disease, and disseminated infection (Table 3). Such a classification carries important therapeutic implications, as

---

TABLE 3.
Classification of Aspergillosis of the Respiratory Tract

Allergic
   Extrinsic allergic alveolitis
   Extrinsic asthma
   Allergic bronchopulmonary aspergillosis
   Allergic *Aspergillus* sinusitis
Saprophytic
   Pulmonary aspergilloma
Invasive
   Bronchopneumonia
   Necrotizing tracheobronchitis
   Invasive sinusitis
   Chronic necrotizing aspergillosis
   Local extension to intrathoracic structures
   Disseminated aspergillosis

TABLE 4.

Summary of Approaches to Treatment of Fungal Infections of the Respiratory Tract in Children

Allergic aspergillosis	
Extrinsic allergic alveolitis	Removal patients from exposure to antigen
Extrinsic asthma	Bronchodilators
Allergic bronchopulmonary aspergillosis (ABPA)	Corticosteroids Itraconazole (ABPA)
Saprophytic aspergillosis	Observation
Pulmonary aspergilloma	Itraconazole
	Amphotericin B
	Surgical resection (usually indicated for intractable hemoptysis and pain)
Invasive aspergillosis	
Bronchopneumonia	Amphotericin B (1.0–1,5 mg/kg/daily)
Necrotizing tracheobronchitis	Itraconazole (8–10 mg/kg/daily) Combination antifungal therapy (?)
Invasive sinusitis	Lipid formulation of amphotericin B
Chronic necrotizing aspergillosis	Reversal of immunosuppression (see Table 6) Surgery:
Local extension to intrathoracic structures	1. Hemoptysis from a single cavitary lesion 2. Progression of a cavitary lesion despite antifungal therapy
Disseminated aspergillosis	3. Infiltration into pericardium, great vessels, bone, or thoracic soft tissue while receiving antifungal therapy 4. Progressive sinusitis
Zygomycosis	Amphotericin B (1.0–1.5 mg/kg/daily)
Rhinocerebral	Lipid formulation of amphotericin B
Pulmonary	Surgical debridement of rhinocerebral infection to viable tissue
	Surgery for pulmonary infection (see invasive aspergillosis)
	Reversal of immunosuppression
	Correction of metabolic acidosis
	Removal of desferrioxamine

Pseudallescheria boydii
  Pulmonary infection
	Miconazole (20−40 mg/kg/daily) or
	  itraconazole (8−10
	  mg/kg/daily)
	Antifungal azole plus amphotericin B
	Surgery for pulmonary infection (see
	  invasive
	  aspergillosis)
	Reversal of immunosuppression

Fusarium infection	Amphotericin B (1.0−1.5 mg/kg/daily)
	  plus flucytosine (5-FC; 50−
	  100 mg/kg/daily)
	Investigational triazole
	Lipid formulation of amphotericin B
	Reversal of immunosuppression

Bipolaris sinusitis	Itraconazole (8−10 mg/kg/daily) or
	  amphotericin B (0.5−1.0
	  mg/kg/daily)
	Surgical resection
	Reversal of immunosuppression

Pulmonary histoplasmosis	Observation in selected normal hosts Itraconazole (4−10 mg/kg/daily) Ketoconazole (4−8 mg/kg/daily) Amphotericin B (0.5−1.0 mg/kg/daily) Reversal of immunosuppression
Pulmonary coccidioidomycosis	Observation in selected normal hosts Itraconazole (4−10 mg/kg/daily) Ketoconazole (4−8 mg/kg/daily) Amphotericin B (0.5−1.0 mg/kg/daily) Reversal of immunosuppression
Pulmonary blastomycosis	Itraconazole (4−10 mg/kg/daily) Ketoconazole (4−8 mg/kg/daily) Amphotericin B (0.5−1.0 mg/kg/daily)

Pulmonary
  paracoccidioidomycosis
	Itraconazole (4−10 mg/kg/daily)
	Ketoconazole (4−8 mg/kg/daily)
	Amphotericin B (0.5−1.0 mg/kg/daily)
	Trimethoprim-sulfamethoxazole (8−10 mg
	  trimethoprim/kg/daily)

(continued)

TABLE 4 (continued).
Summary of Approaches to Treatment of Fungal Infections of the Respiratory Tract in Children

Penicilliosis	Itraconazole (4–10 mg/kg/daily) Amphotericin B (0.5–1.0 mg/kg/daily)
Pulmonary sporotrichosis	Amphotericin B (0.5–1.0 mg/kg/daily)

Pulmonary candidiasis	Amphotericin B (0.5–1.5 mg/kg/daily)
	  with or without 5-FC or
	  fluconazole
	Fluconazole (8–10 mg/kg/daily)
	Lipid formulation of amphotericin B
	Reversal of immunosuppression

Trichosporon infection	Amphotericin B (1.0–1.5 mg/kg/daily)
	  with 5-FC (50–100
	  mg/kg/daily) *and* fluconazole
	  (8–10 mg/kg/daily)
	Reversal of immunosuppression

outlined in Table 4. The allergic conditions induced by *Aspergillus* are further classified as involving the alveoli (extrinsic allergic alveolitis), the airways (extrinsic asthma and allergic bronchopulmonary aspergillosis [ABPA]), or the paranasal sinuses (allergic *Aspergillus* sinusitis). Saprophytic processes include aspergilloma and otomycosis.

The most common species causing aspergillosis are *Aspergillus fumigatus, Aspergillus flavus*, and *Aspergillus niger. Aspergillus* spp. invade human tissue as angular dichotomously branching septate hyphae, which range from 3 to 6 μm in diameter. *Aspergillus* spp. are distinguished by distinctive structures in culture or the saprophytic state: hyphae, conidiophores, vesicles, phialides, metulae, and conidia. Conidiophores, vesicles, and phialides also may be found in saprophytic states, such as lung cavities, ectatic bronchi, and otomycosis.

ALLERGIC BRONCHOPULMONARY ASPERGILLOSIS

The process of ABPA involves an allergic response to *Aspergillus* hyphae without direct tissue invasion by the organism.[117] Bronchospasm in this process is thought to be mediated by IgE (type I reaction) immediate hypersensitivity; the bronchial and peribronchial inflammation in ABPA appears to be induced by immune complex formation (type III reaction).

Allergic bronchopulmonary aspergillosis often appears in a patient with asthma and evanescent, unexplained pulmonary infiltrates. Patients with ABPA may describe expectoration of brown eosinophil-laden mucous plugs containing *Aspergillus* spp. The diagnostic criteria for ABPA include the presence of bronchospasm and bronchial obstruction, fleeting pulmonary infiltrates, central bronchiectasis, peripheral blood eosinophilia, type I (immediate) cutaneous hypersensitivity to *Aspergillus* antigens, elevated total serum IgE concentrations, and elevated anti-*Aspergillus* IgE and IgG concentrations. The diagnosis of ABPA should be considered in any patient with recurrent episodes of asthma and unexplained pulmonary infiltrates. Children with cystic fibrosis may demonstrate a constellation of clinical manifestations similar to that of ABPA.[119]

The current treatment of choice of for exacerbations of ABPA is prednisone, such as 1.0 mg/kg, followed by 0.5 mg/kg/daily for approximately 2 weeks. Early aggressive therapy may attenuate progression to an irreversible fibrotic phase. Some patients may require chronic suppressive therapy. Recent studies indicate that itraconazole may be a valuable adjunct to management of ABPA by apparently reducing the total antigen burden of patients. Allergic bronchopulmonary aspergillosis has a variable prognosis; some patients may sustain numerous recurrent episodes without sequelae, whereas others may develop corticosteroid-dependent asthma and severe chronic obstructive airway disease.

SAPROPHYTIC ASPERGILLOSIS: ASPERGILLOMA AND OTOMYCOSIS

Saprophytic involvement of the respiratory tract develops in the setting of preexisting cavities or ectatic bronchi.[119] Children with cystic fibrosis and bronchiectasis may also have saprophytic involvement of the airways due to *Aspergillus*. Otomycosis is another saprophytic manifestation of *Aspergillus*, where the organism grows on cerumen and desquamated debris with no invasion of cartilage. Otomycosis in profoundly immunocompromised patients may progress relentlessly into the mastoid air cells and CNS.

Saprophytic aspergillosis of the respiratory tract involves the development of a mass of hyphae amid a proteinaceous matrix to form a fungus ball known as an aspergilloma. *Aspergillus niger*, which is often the causative agent in this process, may elaborate large quantities of oxalic acid into the fungus ball and surrounding cavity.[120, 121] Local hemorrhage may ensue into the cavity either as the result of erosion of the fungus ball into the wall of the cavity or because of underlying cavitary disease, such as sarcoidosis.

Aspergilloma of the respiratory tract is often a clinically occult process until the patient complains of hemoptysis. Aspergillomas also may be found during routine follow-up of patients with cavitary tuberculosis or sarcoidosis. The radiographic appearance of a rounded density within a cavity and partially surrounded by a radiolucent crescent halo (Monod's sign) is characteristic of an aspergilloma. However, filamentous fungi other than *Aspergillus,* such as *Pseudallescheria boydii* and Zygomycetes, may also cause intracavitary fungus balls and simulate an aspergilloma.

Aspergillomas often remain quiescent, and as many as 10% may resolve spontaneously. Because aspergillomas often develop in patients with concomitant chronic lung disease, the prognosis for asymptomatic individuals is often determined by their primary pulmonary process, as well as underlying secondary medical problems. The extent of chronic lung disease is an important factor in considering therapeutic options for patients with aspergilloma.

Treatment of aspergilloma is individualized according to the severity of symptoms and the underlying chronic lung disease. Current therapeutic approaches include conservative management (e.g., pulmonary toilet), antifungal chemotherapy, and surgical resection. Many patients are best managed by treatment of the underlying pulmonary process. Patients with locally invasive aspergilloma (chronic necrotizing aspergillosis) may respond to amphotericin B or itraconazole. The latter agent is more practical and better tolerated in an outpatient setting.[122] Intracavitary amphotericin B is another alternative if systemic therapy fails to control the process. Severe underlying chronic lung disease limits surgical resection of aspergillomas in most patients. Recurrent or life-threatening hemoptysis despite antifungal chemotherapy is a relative indication for surgical intervention.

INVASIVE ASPERGILLOSIS

Invasive aspergillosis typically develops in immunocompromised patients. The most common predisposing factors to the development of invasive aspergillosis in children are granulocytopenia, corticosteroid therapy, and quantitative immunodeficiencies, such as chronic granulomatous disease (CGD).[123–136] Patients receiving high doses of corticosteroid therapy include those with lymphoma, brain tumors, autoimmune diseases, organ transplants, and bone marrow transplants (particularly with graft-vs.-host disease). Endogenous hypercortisolemia, such as that due to Cushing's syndrome, also predisposes to development of invasive aspergillosis. Persistent and profound granulocytopenia, which is a major risk factor for invasive aspergillosis, typically is encountered in patients receiving intensive cytotoxic chemotherapy for leukemia, lymphoma, and bone marrow transplantation.

Chronic granulomatous disease is composed of an uncommon heterogeneous group of defects that share an impairment of the respiratory burst and consequent ineffective superoxide production in neutrophils, monocytes, and macrophages. It is strongly associated with a predilection for invasive aspergillosis.[137–140] Although *A. fumigatus* is the most common cause of invasive aspergillosis in children with CGD, *Aspergillus nidulans* occurs with an unusually high frequency in patients with CGD compared with other groups of immunocompromised hosts. Invasive aspergillosis may be the presenting manifestation of CGD.[141] More recently, children with the acquired immunodeficiency syndrome (AIDS) have been recognized with invasive aspergillosis. Some of these HIV-infected patients did not have concomitant corticosteroid therapy or granulocytopenia, suggesting an intrinsic impairment in fungicidal activity.

Low birth weight infants are at particularly high risk for invasive aspergillosis.[142] Schwartz et al.[143] described eight patients with disseminated neonatal aspergillosis. Cultures during life were virtually always negative for *Aspergillus* spp., and the diagnosis was established only after death. The lungs appeared to have been a frequent portal of entry. Rowen et al.[142] reported that among five newborns, moist macerated skin in two patients and an infiltrated percutaneous catheter site in another patient served as points of entry for *Aspergillus*. Early recognition of these cutaneous portals of entry and prompt initiation of amphotericin B may improve outcome. The gastrointestinal tract in the setting of necrotizing enterocolitis may be yet another portal of entry in neonates with invasive aspergillosis.[142, 144]

Immunosuppressed patients may acquire *Aspergillus* in a community or hospital setting.[145] Numerous outbreaks and clusters of nosocomial aspergillosis have been reported in immunosuppressed patients. The most commonly implicated sources for these episodes of nosocomial aspergillosis are contaminated air-conditioning units, hospital construction, and renovation.[146]

Pathogenesis and Pathology

Invasive pulmonary aspergillosis is best understood from the perspective of impaired pulmonary host defenses. The diameter and hydrophobic properties of the conidia allow them to be carried on air currents and gain access to the alveolar air spaces. Pulmonary alveolar macrophages, which are the first line of host defense against inhaled conidia, prevent germination of conidia into hyphae.[147] Should any conidia escape this surveillance system and germinate to form hyphae, neutrophils are capable of damaging hyphae, particularly through oxidative microbicidal pathways.[148]

Invasive pulmonary aspergillosis in the setting of impaired pulmonary host defenses, particularly in neutropenic and corticosteroid-treated hosts, develops through a sequence of (1) inhalation of conidia into distal subsegmental airways and alveolar spaces, (2) germination of inhaled conidia, (3) endobronchial and intraalveolar proliferation of hyphae, (4) invasion into pulmonary blood vessels and lung parenchyma, and (5) thrombosis and ischemic necrosis.[147, 149] The propensity of *Aspergillus* hyphae to invade blood vessels also can lead to extensive hemorrhagic infarction and hemoptysis in thrombocytopenic patients. Blood vessel invasion also increases the risk of hematogenous dissemination. This property of angioinvasiveness is observed with several pathogenic filamentous fungi, particularly *Aspergillus* spp., Zygomycetes, *P. boydii*, and *Fusarium* spp. The patterns of infection observed with such angioinvasive filamentous are summarized in Table 5.

Clinical Manifestations

Invasive aspergillosis usually occurs as a pneumonic process or as sinusitis. Pulmonary aspergillosis in immunocompromised cancer patients has several manifestations, including pneumonia, hemoptysis, and invasion of contiguous intrathoracic structures. A common manifestation of invasive pulmonary aspergillosis is persistent or recurrent fever in a persistently granulocytopenic patient or corticosteroid-treated patient with pulmonary infiltrates. Development of pulmonary infiltrates may be initially absent due to the weak inflammatory response. Pleuritic pain, nonproductive cough, hemoptysis, pleural rub, and occasional adventitious breath sounds are present in the course of invasive pulmonary aspergillosis, reflecting the propensity of *Aspergillus* for invasion of blood vessels.

Hemoptysis is an important manifestation of invasive pulmonary aspergillosis, particularly in granulocytopenic patients. Fungal pneumonia was found in a retrospective study to be the most

TABLE 5.
Patterns of Invasive Pulmonary Infection Caused by
Angioinvasive Filamentous Fungi: *Aspergillus* spp.,
Zygomycetes, *Pseudallescheria boydii, Fusarium* spp.
in Children

- Bronchopneumonia
- Segmental or lobar consolidation
- Cavity formation
- Pleural effusion
- Pulmonary vascular invasion, thrombosis, and infarction
- Dissemination to extrapulmonary tissues
- Invasion of chest wall, diaphragm, pericardium, and myocardium
- Involvement of trachea to cause airway obstruction
- Acute Pancoast's sndrome
- Hemoptysis
- Fistulas
    Bronchoarterial
    Bronchopleural
    Bronchocutaneous
- Chronic necrotizing infection*
- Necrotizing tracheobronchitis*

*Best described with *Aspergillus* spp.

common cause of fatal hemoptysis in patients with hematological malignancies.[116] Two patterns of pulmonary hemorrhage and hemoptysis may develop in granulocytopenic patients. The first is that of hemorrhagic infarction due to vascular invasion during granulocytopenia. A persistently febrile granulocytopenic patient with hematologic malignancy, pulmonary infiltrate, and hemoptysis has a high probability of having invasive aspergillosis. The second pattern is the formation of mycotic aneurysms during recovery from granulocytopenia. Neutrophils invade the walls of infected blood vessels during recovery from granulocytopenia, resulting in destruction of the elastic media in the pulmonary and bronchial blood vessels. As a result, mycotic aneurysms form and rupture to cause potentially fatal hemoptysis.

Invasive pulmonary aspergillosis is not constrained by anatomic barriers to the parenchyma of the lung. *Aspergillus* spp. may invade through the visceral pleura to the pleural space, intercostal muscles, ribs, parietal pericardium, or great vessels. Once within the pericardial space, hyphal elements may cause a pericardial effusion and may continue to extend into the epicardium and myocardium, causing a myocardial infarction. The pericardial effusion may accumulate rapidly, leading to pericardial tamponade.[150] Invasion of the ribs and intercostal nerves may cause severe pain.

The radiographic manifestations of invasive pulmonary aspergillosis include bronchopneumonia, lobar consolidation, segmental pneumonia, cavitary nodules, and multiple nodular lesions resembling septic emboli. The chest radiograph in neutrophenic patients may evolve rapidly with pulmonary infiltrates, causing complete opacification of entire lobes. Computed tomography scans of the chest usually demonstrate more extensive lesions than those seen on chest radiographs. Early lesions visible on CT scan often appear as peripheral or subpleural nodules contiguous with the pulmonary vasculature. These lesions on CT scan are highly suggestive of invasive pulmonary aspergillosis.[151] Cavitary lesions may be observed on chest radiograph; however, cavitary lesions appear to be a later stage of development representing necrosis within the lesion. Computed tomography scans may reveal crescentic cavitation in lesions where none is apparent on chest radiograph. Early recognition of these lesions should prompt initiation of antifungal therapy appropriate for pulmonary aspergillosis.[151, 152]

Aspergillosis of the paranasal sinuses occurs in children who are neutropenic or are receiving corticosteroids.[144] Early in the course of this infection, immunosuppressed patients may have a paucity of symptoms, complaining only of nasal or sinus congestion with no conspicuous discharge. These symptoms should not be dismissed as viral rhinitis. Nasal speculum examination at this time may reveal sentinel eschars along the mucosa of the nasal turbinates. Oral examination may disclose erythema along half of the palatal mucosa ipsilateral to the infected sinus. Tenderness over the maxillary sinuses is not common early in the course of infection. Progression of the infection may involve the orbit, resulting in proptosis, chemosis, and cutaneous necrosis. Direct extension from the orbit to cause frontal lobe infection and cavernous sinus thrombosis may rapidly ensue. Radiographs and CT scan of the sinuses demonstrate air-fluid levels or complete opacification. Bony destruction, retroorbital infiltration, and central nervous system infection also may be evident. A new generation of CT scanning technology known as high-resolution ultrafast (HRU) CT may complete a chest scan within a fraction of the usual time. This approach may be especially appropriate for children where rapid scanning may reduce the need for sedation and diminish the anxiety of the procedure. Barloon et al.[152] showed that rapid scans by HRU CT facilitated early recognition of pulmonary infections in febrile immunocompromised patients whose chest radiographs were equivocal or negative.

The skin may also be the portal of entry, as reported in cases of intraoperative acquisition and in those with contaminated arm boards. Contaminated IV arm boards have been reported as sources of nosocomial outbreaks of invasive aspergillosis in children.[123, 127] These lesions typically develop as erythematous to violaceous indurated plaques that evolve into necrotic ulcers, particularly at the sites of insertion of the peripheral IV cannula or point of contact with the tape and arm board.[127] Nosocomial palmar aspergillosis was reported in five neutropenic children, whose hands were in contact with the contaminated arm board.[123] Early recognition and treatment of these lesions are important in preventing further local invasion or hematogenous dissemination to distant sites.

Disseminated aspergillosis in granulocytopenic and corticosteroid-treated patients is usually an ominous complication of pulmonary infection. The CNS is the most common target organ of hematogenous disseminated aspergillosis. Manifestations of CNS aspergillosis include focal seizures, hemiparesis, and cranial nerve palsies.[133] In a multivariate discriminant analysis of autopsy-proven fungal infections of the CNS, the presence of pulmonary infiltrates and focal neurologic deficits in an immunocompromised patient were significantly more predictive of CNS aspergillosis than for CNS candidiasis or cryptococcosis.[104] Computed tomography scans with contrast enhancement initially may reveal no focal lesions but in a later stage may demonstrate focal ring-enhancing or hemorrhagic lesions. Biopsy of these lesions reveals the same pattern of vascular invasion and infarction seen in lung biopsy specimens. Magnetic resonance imaging techniques may further facilitate early detection of CNS aspergillosis. Disseminated aspergillosis may also involve the eye, skin, liver, gastrointestinal tract, kidneys, bone, and thyroid. *Aspergillus* cutaneous lesions of hematogenous origin in granulocytopenic patients tend to appear on the extremities and may initially appear as purpuric nodules.

Diagnosis and Differential Diagnosis

Invasive pulmonary aspergillosis in immunocompromised patients often develops in those already receiving broad-spectrum antibacterial therapy. The appearance of new focal pulmonary infiltrates developing in the setting of granulocytopenia suggests a differential diagnosis, which includes resistant bacteria (e.g., *Pseudomonas aeruginosa and Xanthomonas maltophilia*), early cytomegalovirus infection, and invasive mycoses, including *Aspergillus* spp. (especially *A. fumigatus and a. flavus*), *T. beigelii, Fusarium* spp. *P. boydii,* and the Zygomycetes (e.g., *Rhizopus* spp., *Cunninghamella bertholettiae*). Among patients receiving corticosteroid therapy as part of their immunosuppressive regimen or those with HIV infection, *Mycobacterium tuberculosis,* atypical mycobacteria, *Nocardia asteroides, Pneumocystis carinii, Cryptococcus neoformans, Histoplasma capsulatum,* and *Coccidioides immitis* are included within the differential diagnosis of pulmonary infiltrates due to *Aspergillus* spp. Because these organisms carry different therapeutic and prognostic implications, distinguishing among the various causes of respiratory mycoses is important (see Table 4).

Biopsy and culture of tissue are the most definitive means by which to establish a diagnosis of invasive aspergillosis. However, because many patients at risk for invasive aspergillosis also have unsupportable thrombocytopenia or other conditions that preclude invasive diagnostic procedures, alternative approaches to establish a presumptive diagnosis are often initially pursued. Isolation of *Aspergillus* spp. from respiratory secretions in febrile granulocytopenic patients with pulmonary infiltrates is strongly associated with invasive pulmonary aspergillosis. A prospective study found that isolation of *Aspergillus* spp. from respiratory secretions of high-risk immunosuppressed patients was highly predictive of invasive pulmonary aspergillosis; invasive aspergillosis was not found in nonimmunosuppressed patients or in nongranulocytopenic patients with solid tumors.[135] Multivariate analysis demonstrated that granulocytopenia was the most significant predictor of invasive aspergillosis in patients with respiratory tract cultures growing *Aspergillus* spp. Conversely, there is a low predictive value for invasive aspergillosis when *Aspergillus* spp. were recovered from respiratory secretions of nongranulocytopenic patients with chronic lung disease. Thus, isolation of *Aspergillus* spp. from respiratory tract cultures of febrile granulocytopenic patients with pulmonary infiltrates should be considered a priori evidence of invasive pulmonary aspergillosis.

Aspergillus sinusitis may develop before or concomitantly with invasive pulmonary aspergillosis. A biopsy of mucosal eschars may be performed, and culture of these "sentinel eschar" lesions may reveal invasive aspergillosis and prompt initiation of appropriate therapy. Similarly, if nasal septal lesions are not observed, a sinus aspirate may preclude the need for bronchoscopy if fungus is demonstrated in the aspirate. Although *Aspergillus* is the most common cause of fungal sinusitis in immunocompromised patients, other fungi, including *Zygomycetes*, *Fusarium*, *P. boydii*, *Curvularia*, and *Alternaria*, may be isolated. Biopsy of suspicious cutaneous lesions may also establish the diagnosis of disseminated aspergillosis.

Bronchoalveolar lavage has been studied by several investigators and found to yield variable results with sensitivities ranging from less than 25% to as much as 75% compared with tissue-proven infection.[153–155] The presence of *Aspergillus* spp. in BAL fluid in a febrile granulocytopenic patients with new pulmonary infiltrates is indicative of invasive aspergillosis; however, the absence of hyphal elements or positive culture does not exclude the diagnosis. The BAL fluid should be divided between cytopathology and clinical microbiology. Fluid should be spun and the sediment or cell block examined by calcofluor white in microbiology and methenamine silver in cytology.

Should the foregoing methods not yield a microbiologic diagnosis of new infiltrates in the recurrently febrile granulocytopenic or otherwise immunosuppressed patient, open lung biopsy (OLB) should be performed. For patients with a localized infiltrate, however, OLB will require a major thoracotomy using either a lateral or mediastinal approach. It is imperative that the surgeon obtain biopsy specimens of both the periphery and central areas of abnormal lung tissue, because the distribution of *Aspergillus* hyphae may vary. These hyphae usually are well seen in tissue and appear basophilic (blue-purple) with hematoxylin-eosin, pink-red with periodic acid–Schiff, and brown-black with methenamine silver stains. *Aspergillus* hyphae, however, often are seen only faintly with Gram's stain. The appearance of such hyphae is characteristic of but not unique to the genus *Aspergillus*. When interpreting the histopathologic appearance of angular, dichotomously branching septate hyphae in an open lung biopsy specimen, one should consider that this is most often caused by *Aspergillus* spp. but may also be caused by *Fusarium* spp., *P. boydii* and dematiaceous hyphomycetes. *Pseudallescherichia boydii* may be resistant to amphotericin B and require azole antifungal compounds.

The differential diagnosis of pneumonia in immunocompromised children is extensive and includes *P. carinii*, cytomegalovirus, *Aspergillus* spp., emerging opportunistic filamentous fungi, *C. neoformans*, dimorphic yeasts, and mycobacteria.[23] Less commonly, *Nocardia* spp., *Legionella pneumophilia*, respiratory syncytial virus, varicella zoster virus, and multiple resistant gram-negative bacillary infections may be etiologic agents. These different infections clearly require specific antimicrobial agents often administered at high dosages. If bronchoalveolar lavage is nondiagnostic, OLB is required to establish a definitive diagnosis.

Detection of invasive pulmonary aspergillosis by immunodiagnostic methods remains investigational. Circulating galactomannan and similar heat-stable carbohydrate antigens have been found by several investigators during invasive aspergillosis in animal models and in patients.[156–159] Analysis of serial samples improves the diagnostic yield of this antigen. Detection of galactomannan and similar carbohydrate antigens in serum and urine offers promise of a sensitive and simple means of enhancing the diagnosis of invasive aspergillosis. Laboratory detection of *Aspergillus* by molecular techniques, such as polymerase chain reaction (PCR), may further advance early diagnosis of invasive aspergillosis. For example, initial studies in four patients with invasive aspergillosis demonstrated the utility of identifying *A. fumigatus* and *A. flavus* by PCR from BAL in 4 patients with proven or probable aspergillosis, whereas 6 (13%) of 46 BAL specimens from control patients had a positive PCR signal.[160] The sensitivity, specificity, and potential for therapeutic monitoring by PCR methods are unknown.

Prognosis and Treatment

Invasive pulmonary aspergillosis and disseminated aspergillosis, by comparison, may progress to overwhelming pneumonia and death within several days to a few weeks unless the underlying immunosuppression is reversed and antifungal therapy is initiated early.[161–163] Amphotericin B is the treatment of choice in profoundly compromised patients. Invasive pulmonary aspergillosis often develops in granulocytopenic patients who are already receiving empirical amphotericin B, 0.5 mg/kg/daily. In such cases, amphotericin B is administered at 1.0 to 1.5 mg/kg/daily. Such dosages require close medical management to avert azotemia. Administration of 3 to 5 mEq of saline solution/kg every 24 hours (saline loading), with close attention to total body weight, electrolyte levels, and cardiopulmonary function, may attenuate azotemia. Other strategies, including pentoxifylline and low-dose dopamine (1–2 μg/kg/per minute) may also control azotemia. Prevention of amphotericin B–induced azotemia becomes more difficult by these measures in patients receiving other nephrotoxic agents (cyclosporine or aminoglycosides), as well as in those with underlying renal disease due to diabetes or hypertension. Amphotericin B in profoundly immunocompromised patients does not cure invasive pulmonary or disseminated aspergillosis but only stabilizes the infection. Instead, survival and resolution of infection are predicated on reversal of immunosuppression. Recovery from granulocytopenia, reduction of corticosteroid therapy, and amelioration of other potential immunosuppressive factors are critical factors for the successful treatment of invasive aspergillosis in immunocompromised hosts. Unless immunosuppression is reversed or substantially ameliorated, the prognosis of opportunistic invasive aspergillosis is dismal.

Combining amphotericin B with rifampin or 5-FC is controversial. Although early laboratory animal studies suggested that rifampin may enhance the antifungal activity of low-dose amphotericin B, recent studies demonstrated that rifampin does not augment the antifungal activity of high-dose amphotericin B (1.0–1.5 mg/kg/daily) in experimental disseminated aspergillosis.[164] Some strains of *Aspergillus* spp. are susceptible to 5-FC. However, no compelling laboratory animal data support or refute the role of 5-FC for aspergillosis. Yet, when pulmonary aspergillosis progresses despite maximum tolerated daily dosages of amphotericin B, use of 5-FC seems prudent. The combination of high-dose amphotericin B plus 5-FC was utilized as initial therapy in the treatment of invasive pulmonary aspergillosis by Burch et al.[162] and Karp et al.[163] If 5-FC is used, careful attention to serum levels is required to avoid myelotoxicity, as discussed later on.[165]

Itraconazole offers new options for treatment of invasive aspergillosis.[131, 166–172] In initial studies this antifungal triazole has been found to have some efficacy in patients with invasive aspergillosis. Although itraconazole is clearly less toxic than amphotericin B, its comparative efficacy is uncertain. Moreover, the bioavailability of itraconazole may be impaired in patients with chemotherapy-induced mucosal disruption and those receiving antacid therapy, including H_2-receptor-blocking agents. Moreover, itraconazole currently is available only as an oral agent, thus further limiting its use in critically ill patients. For neutropenic patients with invasive aspergillosis, high-dose amphotericin B (1.0–1.5 mg/kg/daily) remains the drug of choice.[162] Invasive pulmonary aspergillosis in neutropenic patients may rapidly evolve with ensuing hemorrhagic infarction, hemoptysis, respiratory failure, and disseminated infection. Antifungal therapy in this critical setting must be delivered reliably and in high doses. The unpredictable bioavailability of itraconazole in the profoundly neutropenic host precludes its use as a single agent. Although there is considerable interest in combination therapy with amphotericin B and itraconazole, further studies are warranted to establish an understanding of this approach.

Bone marrow transplant recipients who develop invasive aspergillosis in the postengraftment period also may be candidates for itraconazole therapy if the infection is initially stabilized and reduced by amphotericin B. Serum concentrations should be monitored in all patients receiving itraconazole for serious invasive fungal infections to assure adequate bioavailability. The concerns of the bioavailability of itraconazole were illustrated in a recently reported double-blind, placebo-controlled study of the efficacy of itraconazole in the prevention of fungal infections among neutropenic patients with hematologic malignancies and intensive chemotherapy,[179] as well as in nonrandomized trials.[173] This study was unable to demonstrate a significant effect of itraconazole, underscoring the issue of tissue levels and antifungal activity. A parenteral formulation of itraconazole, which is currently being developed, would be an important therapeutic advance for treatment of such high-risk patients.

Itraconazole also has been reported to be effective in treatment of mycotic keratitis, an infection that afflicts patients of all ages.[174] Previously only topically applied pimaricin was effective for mycotic keratitis. Rajasekaran et al.[174] reported 110 cases of keratomycosis, most of which were caused by *Aspergillus,* dematiaceous fungi, and *Fusarium.* The overall response rate to itraconazole of these patients was 69%. Keratitis due to *Aspergillus* and dematiaceous fungi responded better than did that due to *Fusarium.*

The pharmacokinetics of itraconazole in children are not well understood. Nevertheless, several cases of successful treatment with itraconazole of pulmonary and CNS aspergillosis have been reported.[168, 169] Itraconazole also may be useful in non-neutropenic patients, such as those with chronic granulomatous disease, where management of chronic aspergillosis with an oral agent is especially important.[132] The new oral suspension of itraconazole may ensure improved bioavailability during ambulatory therapy.

Surgical intervention can be an important therapeutic adjunct to antifungal chemotherapy of invasive aspergillosis.[175] Surgical resection of invasive pulmonary aspergillosis may be employed in several specific conditions: (1) hemoptysis from a single cavitary lesion; (2) progression of a cavitary lesion despite antifungal therapy; (3) infiltration into bone or thoracic soft tissue while receiving antifungal therapy; (4) progression of infection in a critical target organ, such as the CNS or pericardium. Decisions for each patient must be individualized. Other indications for surgery in the management of invasive aspergillosis include progressive sinusitis, single refractory symptomatic brain lesion, pericardial infection, endocarditis osteomyelitis, and endophthalmitis. Such indications are not absolute and require thoughtful assessment and experienced clinical judgment for each patient.

Illustrating the need for individual assessment, not all bony involvement may necessarily require extensive surgical debridement. For example, Flynn et al.[125] reported the successful treatment of a child with *Aspergillus* osteomyelitis of the greater trochanter and adjacent soft tissue of the thigh with 2 months of amphotericin B therapy after a diagnostic biopsy. More extensive surgical excision was withheld because of the weight-bearing location of the infection.

Control of environmental transmission of conidia can be an important adjunct in managing an outbreak of nosocomial aspergillosis.[146] Floor to ceiling barriers for prevention of transmission of *Aspergillus* conidia to high-risk populations should be established in hospital areas of construction or renovation. Air-conditioning systems should be microbiologically monitored especially during periods of repair or malfunction. High-efficacy particulate air (HEPA) filters should be used, when possible, in hospital areas where patients with protracted granulocytopenia (e.g., allogeneic bone marrow transplant recipients) are housed.

Currently no antifungal chemotherapeutic regimens have been shown in a large randomized controlled trial to prevent invasive aspergillosis in granulocytopenic patients. Limited open-label studies have suggested that itraconazole may be useful for this purpose; however, further studies are warranted. Intranasal amphotericin B is not sufficient to prevent invasive pulmonary aspergillosis. Fluconazole in the currently used dosages is not effective in the prevention of invasive aspergillosis.

Most children with leukemia, lymphoma, and various solid tumors undergo several cycles of intensive chemotherapy. The challenge in managing such children with invasive fungal infections is to treat the underlying neoplastic disease while continuing to treat the concomitant mycosis during neutropenia.[176] If pulmonary aspergillosis develops in such a patient who will require subsequent cytotoxic chemotherapy, the risk of recurrence of pulmonary aspergillosis is approximately 50%.[163] Thus, one approach to the prevention of recurrent aspergillosis in such patients is to administer amphotericin B (1.0–1.5 mg/kg/daily) at the earliest onset of fever and granulocytopenia. Treatment of the underlying neoplastic process is essential for survival. Cytotoxic chemotherapy may be continued in cancer patients with history of invasive aspergillosis, provided that the fungal infection is controlled. Itraconazole may also be an appropriate alternative for this purpose but requires further study.

The advent of the human recombinant cytokines has led to new potential immunomodulatory modalities for prevention of invasive aspergillosis. Interferon-γ is one such recently approved recombinant cytokine. Approved on the basis of a large, randomized, prospective, placebo-controlled trial, IFN-γ was found to significantly reduce the frequency of serious primary infections.[177] Although this trial demonstrated a trend toward reduction of invasive aspergillosis in patients receiving IFN-γ, the antifungal properties of this recombinant cytokine require further investigation. Among patients with CGD who were receiving IFN-γ, three times per week, nonoxidative mechanisms of microbicidal activity were enhanced in association with increased damage to hyphae of *A. fumigatus.*[178] Granulocyte colony-stimulating factor (G-CSF) and granulocyte-macrophage colony-stimulating factor (GM-CSF) shorten the duration of neutropenia and may contribute to decreasing the risk of invasive aspergillosis. Transfusion of large quantities of granulocytes from G-CSF-treated donors may also provide additional effector cells until patients recover from neutropenia.

ZYGOMYCOSIS

Zygomycosis is an uncommon but frequently fatal group of infections caused by members of the class Zygomycetes. These infections manifest most commonly as rhinocerebral, pulmonary, and disseminated infections.[179, 180] Less frequent patterns of manifestation include cutaneous, abdominal-pelvic, and gastric zygomycosis. The most common organism causing invasive zygomycosis is *Rhizopus oryzae.* Most of the Zygomycetes causing respiratory tract infections in immunocompromised or debilitated hosts have a high propensity for thrombotic invasion of blood vessels, a rapidly evolving clinical course, high mortality, and a relative resistance to antifungal therapy.

Zygomycosis in children may develop in settings similar to those of adults such as in neutropenia, corticosteroid therapy, solid organ transplantation, bone marrow transplantation, burns, and deferoxamine therapy for management of iron and aluminum overload states. Zygomycosis in children occurs in other distinct settings as well: juvenile onset (type 1) diabetes mellitus, particularly with uncontrolled diabetic ketoacidosis; congenital metabolic aciduria[181]; and very low birth weight.[182]

Among the primary risk factors in 41 reported cases of rhinocerebral zygomycosis in children (ages 2 months–18 years) reviewed by Kline,[180] 20 (49%) had diabetes mellitus, 7 (17%) had gastroenteritis, and 6 (15%) had leukemia. Rhinocerebral zygomycosis usually begins as an infection of the paranasal sinuses (especially maxillary and ethmoid sinus), which progresses to invade the orbit, retroorbital region, cavernous sinus, and brain. Thromboses of tissue causes ischemic necrosis. A black eschar on the palatine or nasal mucosa and drainage of a black discharge from the eye are characteristic clinical manifestations of infarction due to this rapidly progressive angioinvasive pathogen. However, black, necrotic lesions on the palate or nasal mucous membranes may also be caused by other fungi, including *Aspergillus* spp., *Fusarium* spp., and *P. boydii*. Newborn infants are another group of hosts who are vulnerable to invasive zygomycosis. Grim et al.[182] recently reviewed the uncommon but well-characterized problem of disseminated zygomycosis in newborn infants.

Symptoms of rhinocerebral zygomycosis may include unilateral headache, ocular irritation, chemosis, lacrimation, periorbital swelling, blurred vision, periorbital numbness, nasal congestion, and epistaxis. The complaint of diplopia or new onset of blurred vision from a diabetic patient, a patient receiving deferoxamine, or a pharmacologically immunosuppressed patient should prompt a careful evaluation for early signs of rhinocerebral zygomycosis. Rhinocerebral zygomycosis may progress rapidly, resulting in death within a few days, or may be a slowly progressive but relentless process. Rarely the disease may regress and remain quiescent when the diabetes is controlled, only to be reactivated by another episode of metabolic acidosis. Radiographic evaluation is needed to assess the anatomic extent of suspected rhinocerebral zygomycosis. Plain sinus films are helpful but CT scans and MRI better define the extent of infection and guide surgical resection of infected tissue.

The mainstay of treatment of rhinocerebral and pulmonary zygomycosis consists of surgery and amphotericin B (1.0–1.5 mg/kg/daily). Amphotericin B is also used as the preferred drug for treatment of disseminated zygomycoses. Critical to the successful outcome of zygomycoses is reversal of the immunologic or metabolic defects that precipitated the infection. These strategies include reversal of granulocytopenia, discontinuation of corticosteroids, and correction of metabolic acidosis.

FUSARIOSIS

Fusarium spp., once considered to cause only infections of the skin, nail, and cornea, have been recognized during the past decade to cause disseminated infection, particularly in granulocytopenic patients undergoing intensive antileukemic chemotherapy or bone marrow transplantation.[183–185] *Fusarium solani, Fusarium oxysporum, Fusarium moniliforme,* and *Fusarium chlamydosporum* all have been reported to cause disseminated infection in immunosuppressed patients. The lung, sinuses, and skin are the primary portals of entry.[186] The periungual regions of the toes notably may be a particularly important site of initial invasion. *Fusarium* infections produce a pattern similar to that of invasive aspergillosis. *Fusarium* infections in granulocytopenic patients are characterized by pulmonary infiltrates, cutaneous lesions, positive blood cultures, and sinusitis. Biopsy of the cutaneous lesions often reveals fine, dichotomously branching, acutely angular, septate hyphae. Unlike *Aspergillus* spp., *Fusarium* spp. are detectable by advanced blood culture detection systems, such as lysis centrifugation. This emerging fungal pathogen often responds only to high doses of amphotericin B (1.0–1.5 mg/kg) and depends on rapid recovery from neutropenia for successful outcome. For example, Merz et al.[187] reported that five out of six patients with disseminated fusariosis survived when treated with high-dose amphotericin B (1.0–1.5 mg/kg/daily) and 5-FC. Cases of invasive *Fusarium* infection may be completely refractory to amphotericin B, therefore requiring investigational antifungal compounds.[188]

PHAEOHYPHOMYCOSIS

Phaeohyphomycosis is defined as deep tissue infection due to a pigmented hyphal fungus.[189, 190] *Bipolaris* spp., *Cladosporium bantianum* or *Xylohypha bantiana, Dactylaria* spp., *P. boydii,* and *Wangiella dermatitidis* are the common agents of phaeohyphomycosis. *Pseudallescheria boydii* and *X. bantiana (C. bantianum)* are among the more lethal causes of phaeohyphomycosis. *Xylohypha bantiana* has a high propensity for CNS infection, which is often fatal.[191] Patients with CNS infections due to *X. bantiana* may have no apparent immunosuppression yet still sustain a high morbidity and mortality.

Pseudallescheria boydii, another agent of phaeohyphomycosis, causes pneumonia disseminated infections in immunocompromised hosts and mycetoma in immunocompetent patients. Deeply invasive infections due to *P. boydii* carry a high mortality. For example, among 31 patients with deeply invasive *Pseudallescheria* infection of the CNS, lungs, and heart, 19 patients (61%) died of infection.[184, 192–197] As the most common cause of eumycotic mycetoma in North America, *P. boydii* may be highly refractory to antifungal therapy. Mycetoma refractory to antifungal chemotherapy unfortunately may require repeated debridement or amputation. Pneumonia and CNS infection due to *P. boydii* are clinically indistinguishable from that due to *Aspergillus* spp.

Diagnostic procedures and approaches, including thoracic CT scan, BAL, and lung biopsy, are also similar to those for invasive pulmonary aspergillosis. The organism in tissue and direct smears resembles *Aspergillus* spp. as angular, septate, dichotomously branching hyphae. However, terminal annelloconidia may be observed histologically in some infected tissues. The definitive microbiologic diagnosis is established by culture, in which the organism may grow as the synanamorph *Scedosporium apiospermum* or as the teleomorph *P. boydii* with cleistothecia.

Infections due to *P. boydii* are frequently refractory to antifungal chemotherapy, including amphotericin B. Poor outcome with *P. boydii* infections may be due to impaired host response or intrinsic microbiologic resistance to antifungal compounds.[196] Antifungal azoles are often cited as the agents of choice for infections due to *P. boydii*. Indeed, a recent case report describes the successful treatment of *S. apiospermum* septic arthritis with itraconazole in a previously healthy 6-year-old boy.[197] Yet, immunocompromised patients often fail to respond to single-agent azole therapy. New therapeutic approaches are clearly needed for treatment of infections due to this organism. A recent study found that although 7 (32%) of 22 clinical isolates of *P. boydii* were resistant in vitro to concentrations of amphotericin B ($\geq$ 2.0 μg/mL), 8 (36%) consistently had MICs of 0.5 μg/mL or less. This strain-dependent response to amphotericin B suggests a potentially wider utility of amphotericin B, perhaps in combination with antifungal azoles, against *P. boydii* infections than has been previously recognized. The study found enhanced in vitro antifungal activity when amphotericin B was combined with miconazole, itraconazole, or fluconazole.[198] Immunomodulatory interventions with recombinant cytokines as an adjunct to antifungal therapy also offer another novel approach to management of infections due to *P. boydii* and other pathogenic dematiaceous molds.

Among the many emerging pathogens of phaeohyphomycosis are *Scedosporium inflatum* and *Bipolaris* spp. *Scedosporium inflatum*, a newly recognized pathogen closely related to *P. boydii*, may cause pneumonia and disseminated infection with cutaneous lesions in immunocompromised patients.[199] Infections due to this organism have been highly resistant to antifungal therapy.

Bipolaris spp. are the most common causes of phaeomycotic sinusitis. *Bipolaris* sinusitis may be particularly refractory to amphotericin B. Recent findings, however, indicate that itraconazole is particularly active against *Bipolaris* sinusitis, including those cases refractory to amphotericin B.[200] This encouraging report from Sharkey et al.[200] also indicates that itraconazole was beneficial in treatment of refractory phaeohyphomycosis due to other dematiaceous molds, suggesting a primary role for this triazole in the initial management of these infections.

INFECTIONS DUE TO DIMORPHIC FUNGI

Histoplasma capsulatum var. *capsulatum*, *Blastomyces dermatitidis*, *C. immitis*, *Paracoccidioides brasiliensis*, and *Penicillium marneffei* are endemic dimorphic fungi that may infect children. *Sporothrix schenckii*, although manifesting the typical thermal dimorphism of the endemic dimorphic organisms, does not appear to follow a geographically defined endemic pattern of distribution. These fungi also have been termed primary, or systemic, fungal pathogens. In the inanimate environment at temperatures less than 35° C, they produce a mycelial form with hyaline, branching, septate hyphae. The hyphae of *H. capsulatum*, *B. dermatitidis*, *P. brasiliensis*, and *P. marneffei* will convert to budding yeast cells in tissue or on enriched media at 37° C in the laboratory. *Coccidioides immitis* produces spherules in tissue.[201] The majority of infections with any of these fungi are initiated by inhalation of conidia in nature. The pulmonary infection may be asymptomatic and resolve spontaneously, but reactivation may occur subsequently. Any one of these fungi may disseminate from the lungs to other organs. The rate of infection is high in the specific geographic areas of endemicity, but the preponderance of these endemic infections result in a self-limiting illness. Possibly due to differences in environmental exposure, clinical infections due to dimorphic fungi are relatively uncommon in children compared with that of adults.

In most cases, the only evidence of infection is the development of an immune response, which is manifested by the acquisition of a positive delayed-type skin test reaction and the production of specific antibodies, development of precipitins and complement-fixing antibodies, as well as conversion to positive results of skin tests. The small percentage of these episodes that advance to progressive pulmonary infection or clinically overt disseminated infection are often associated with predisposing risk factors, particularly underlying defects in cell-mediated immunity, such as those encountered in HIV-infected hosts or patients receiving corticosteroids.

HISTOPLASMOSIS

Most cases of asymptomatic infections due to the *H. capsulatum* var. *capsulatum* have a clinically asymptomatic fungemia. Asymptomatic and otherwise healthy individuals in endemic areas may have splenic and pulmonary calcifications on chest and abdominal radiographs. Resembling the pathogenesis of tuberculosis, this "cryptic dissemination" to multiple organs permits subsequent reactivation at pulmonary and extrapulmonary sites if the host becomes immunocompromised. Histoplasmosis may reactivate years later in extrapulmonary tissues, particularly the CNS, adrenal glands, mucocutaneous surfaces, and other sites.[202] This pattern of histoplasmosis, which often occurs in elderly and immunocompromised patients, must be differentiated from other mycoses, tuberculosis, or neoplastic disease. The syndrome of disseminated histoplasmosis typically develops in older immunocompromised patients with cellular immunodeficiencies, including HIV-infected patients. However, disseminated histoplasmosis of infancy may develop in otherwise apparently healthy infants younger than 2 years old.

Disseminated histoplasmosis of infancy is a primary infection due to *H. capsulatum*, which progresses from a primary pulmonary focus to widespread dissemination.[203] The immunologic immaturity of infants likely predisposes to this primary progressive infection. Untreated, the infection is often fatal. Disseminated histoplasmosis of infancy has been extensively reviewed by Leggiadro et al.[203] Among 19 patients with this syndrome, fever, hepatosplenomegaly, cough, and "flulike" symptoms were the most common symptoms and signs on admission. Fever, hepatosplenomegaly, and pancytopenia of disseminated histoplasmosis of infancy may lead to an initial diagnosis of leukemia or aplastic anemia. In addition to these findings, Steele and Kleiman[204] report that disseminated histoplasmosis of infancy also may manifest as failure to thrive and hypercalcemia. The wide variation of clinical manifestations of disseminated histoplasmosis may delay a definitive diagnosis unless the clinician deliberately searches for this infection. Untreated, disseminated histoplasmosis of infancy is uniformly fatal. By comparison, timely administration of IV amphotericin B

(0.5–1.0 mg/kg/daily), the initial treatment of choice, is highly effective.

Although *H. capsulatum* is well described as an infectious agent in children, particularly in infants, only limited data exist regarding its role in HIV-infected children.[205, 206] One infant, who had a 2-week history of fever, was found to have disseminated histoplasmosis as the AIDS-defining illness.[206] A distinctive syndrome of severe disseminated histoplasmosis can consist of cutaneous lesions, pulmonary infiltrates, and thrombocytopenia, which may progress to septic shock in HIV-infected patients. *Histoplasma capsulatum* is recoverable from bone marrow and blood cultures in HIV-infected patients with disseminated histoplasmosis.

Culture and examination of a bone marrow aspirate and biopsy are among the most rapid and reliable methods to establish the diagnosis of disseminated histoplasmosis. Direct examination by Giemsa or Wright's stains of touch preps, smears, paraffin-embedded clot sections, or decalcified biopsy specimen reveals small 2- to 4-μm diameter yeastlike cells within the cytoplasm of macrophages. Blood cultures, using the lysis centrifugation blood culture system, also may recover the organism. Biopsy of lesions of the skin, lung, liver, and lymph nodes may demonstrate noncaseating and caseating granulomas with intracytoplasmically located blastoconidia within macrophages. The chest radiograph in histoplasmosis in HIV-infected hosts may demonstrate a variety of patterns, including reticulonodular, miliary, and lobar infiltrates. Organisms may be identified on bronchoalveolar lavage or lung biopsy. Differentiating nonbudding yeast cells of *H. capsulatum* from the cysts of *P. carinii* may be difficult. Use of calcofluor white and monoclonal antibodies may facilitate this differential diagnosis. However, recent studies have identified a carbohydrate *H. capsulatum* antigen in urine as a valuable marker in diagnosis and therapeutic monitoring of disseminated histoplasmosis.[207]

The treatment of choice for severe disseminated histoplasmosis is amphotericin B. Itraconazole has been recently approved by the Food and Drug Administration in adults for treatment of stable disseminated histoplasmosis and is a reasonable alternative to amphotericin B in patients with fever and fungemia but no clinically overt CNS infection or hemodynamic deterioration. Although short courses of amphotericin B have been advocated for disseminated histoplasmosis of infancy, an indefinite course of antifungal therapy will likely be necessary for treatment of disseminated histoplasmosis complicating HIV infection. Such a course may follow the pattern of an "induction" regimen with amphotericin B, as in treatment of cryptococcal meningitis, followed by a "maintenance" course of itraconazole or amphotericin B. Recent advances in antigen detection systems for *H. capsulatum* offer the potential for noninvasive monitoring of antifungal therapy.[207]

COCCIDIOIDOMYCOSIS

The incidence of pulmonary coccidioidomycosis has increased strikingly in endemic areas in the United States.[208] Clinical manifestations of coccidioidomycosis have been classified in three general groups: initial pulmonary infection, which is usually self-limiting; pulmonary complications; and extrapulmonary disease. Primary infections in normal hosts usually resolve spontaneously without antifungal therapy. The presence of erythema nodosum in an immunocompetent patient with pulmonary coccidioidomycosis signifies a favorable host response and good prognosis. However, primary pulmonary infection, particularly in immunocompromised patients, may evolve into one of several complications: pulmonary nodules, thin-walled cavities, progressive pneumonia, pyopneumothorax, and bronchopleural fistula. Certain patient populations with defective cellular immunity, such as those with HIV infection and those receiving corticosteroids, are more susceptible to progressive pneumonia, complicated pneumonia, and dissemination.

Disseminated coccidioidomycosis in early infancy may ensue, possibly due to the immunologic immaturity of adequate cell-mediated host defenses.[209] MacDonald et al.[210] analyzed a series of immunocompromised children with coccidioidomycosis and found that all children with extrapulmonary involvement died, whereas those with disease limited to the lungs survived the infection. Dissemination to extrapulmonary sites may result in cutaneous and soft tissue infection, osteomyelitis, arthritis, and meningitis. Cerebrospinal fluid, other body fluids, and biopsy specimens of tissues infected by *C. immitis* may be submitted to the clinical microbiology laboratory for microscopic examination and culture. More detailed discussion of the laboratory diagnosis of coccidioidomycosis may be found elsewhere.[201]

Because of the risks to laboratory personnel when they are working with the mold form of *C. immitis*, direct examinations of sputum, exudates, and tissues are highly recommended. Mature spherules are thick walled, usually 20 to 60 μm in diameter, and easily recognized on wet mounts using potassium hydroxide or calcofluor white. Endospores (2−4 μm) then can be observed in intact or recently disrupted spherules.

Immunocompetent patients with self-limiting pulmonary coccidioidomycosis have been managed with observation only. However, patients with any form of immunosuppression or debilitation prudently warrant antifungal therapy. The advent of ketoconazole, itraconazole, and fluconazole has permitted a wider range of patients to be treated for coccidioidomycosis without the toxicity of amphotericin B. Immunocompetent children with limited coccidioidomycosis may be treated with an initial course of amphotericin B, followed by an antifungal azole.[211] However, amphotericin B is warranted for treatment of progressive pulmonary or disseminated coccidiodomycosis in HIV-infected patients and in other immunocompromised patients. Antifungal azoles also have a role in long-term management of coccidioidal meningitis in children.[212]

In treating coccidioidal meningitis refractory to amphotericin B in nine children, Shehab et al.[213] described the use of orally administered ketoconazole and intraventricularly administered miconazole. Although this study reported no relapse or recrudescence of coccidioidal meningitis during a follow-up of 32 to 90 months, the main cause of morbidity was the ventriculoperitoneal shunt for increased intracranial pressure. The recent successful experience in treatment of coccidioidal meningitis with fluconazole in adults[214] suggests that this approach may be an appropriate alternative before inserting an Ommaya reservoir for intraventricular administration of amphotericin B or miconazole. The experience with immunocompromised patients, including those in early infancy, reveals that apparently successfully treated cases of coccidioidomycosis have a high potential for relapsed infection.[209] Continued clinical and serologic monitoring is important in the management of these infections in high-risk children.

BLASTOMYCOSIS

Blastomyces dermatitidis causes self-limited respiratory tract infection, which manifests as a localized chronic pulmonary or cutaneous lesion in immunocompetent patients. Dissemination to one or more organs, including the genitourinary tract, bone, or CNS, may ensue.[215, 216] Blastomycosis, which is relatively infrequent in children, was described in two groups of children in a well-characterized outbreak at an environmental camp in northern Wisconsin.[217] Of 89 elementary school–age children and 10 adults, 48 (51%) had blastomycosis. Among those 48, 26 (54%) were symptomatic. The median incubation period was 45 days (range 21–106 days). *Blastomyces dermatitidis* was recovered from soil at the site of the outbreak. Despite such outbreaks, Steele and Abernathy[215] reported that among pediatric patients with blastomycosis, the incidence in Arkansas was stable over 10 years and that therapy with single-agent amphotericin B was successful, provided that the infection was diagnosed early and antifungal therapy initiated promptly. Although most reported cases of blastomycosis occur in children, occasional reports of infants and intrauterine transmission underscore the vulnerability of this younger population to blastomycosis.[218, 219] Although response to amphotericin B has been favorable, pulmonary blastomycosis may be fatal in some children.[218]

Concomitant cutaneous lesions may be ulcerative or verrucous and resemble a variety of chronic infections or skin cancer. Biopsy specimens demonstrate pseudoepitheliomatous hyperplasia, acanthosis, and intraepidermal and dermal abscesses containing blastoconidia of *B. dermatitidis*. Osteomyelitis develops in up to one third of patients with blastomycosis. The genitourinary tract, especially the prostate and epididymis, is another target of blastomycosis. Meningitis due to blastomycosis is uncommon, often manifesting as a basilar process, and is difficult to diagnose by culture of lumbar CSF; recovery of *B. dermatitidis* may be improved with culture of ventricular or cisternal fluid.

Sputum samples, bronchial lavage fluid, or lung biopsy specimens should be submitted for microscopy, culture, and cytology. Sputum cytology may reveal unsuspected yeast cells of *B. dermatitidis*. Lung biopsy may reveal a pyogranulomatous reaction with marked fibrosis. Unless special stains for fungi are used on such tissue, conventional hematoxylin-eosin stains may not detect the presence of organisms. Direct calcofluor white or KOH mounts of sputum, exudates, and tissues can demonstrate the yeast cells of *B. dermatitidis*, which are large, spherical, and thick walled and measure approximately 8 to 15 μm in diameter. The yeast cells bud singly and have a wide base of attachment between the bud and parent yeast cell. The bud of *B. dermatitidis* often attains the same size as the parent yeast before becoming detached. Infected tissues stained with Gomori methenamine silver will reveal these characteristic yeast forms.

Treatment of pulmonary blastomycosis in adults has been advanced greatly by the use of ketoconazole and itraconazole.[220] The experience of treating blastomycosis in children with antifungal azoles is more limited compared with that of adults. Itraconazole, which is approved for treatment of blastomycosis in adults, has less reported toxicity and possibly greater antifungal activity against blastomycosis than does ketoconazole.[221] Thus, itraconazole is the preferred drug for mild to moderate blastomycosis, and amphotericin B is the drug of choice for severe respiratory blastomycosis.

PENICILLIOSIS

Increasingly recognized as a cause of disseminated infection in HIV-infected patients from Southeast Asia, *P. marneffei* has emerged as in important endemic pathogen.[222, 223] The infection has a striking resemblance to disseminated histoplasmosis in HIV-infected patients. Among 92 recently reported children and adults from Chiang Mai Province in Northern Thailand, the most common presenting symptoms and signs were fever (92%), anemia (77%), weight loss (76%), and skin lesions (71%). Of patients with skin lesions, 87% had generalized papules with central umbilication. Fever, hepatosplenomegaly, and umbilicated papular lesions were the most common manifestations of penicilliosis in five HIV-infected children.[223] The diagnosis of *P. marneffei* is readily established by direct smear and culture of umbilicated centrally necrotic lesions, bone marrow aspirate, or peripheral lymph nodes. Such diagnostic measures are preferred before a more invasive procedure, such as BAL, is pursued. Itraconazole and amphotericin B have been found to be effective as single agents in the treatment of disseminated *P. marneffei* infection. Itraconazole at a dose of 200 mg twice daily for 2 months, followed by a dose of 100 mg once daily for 1 month, has been found to be effective for the treatment and maintenance of remission in adult patients with disseminated penicilliosis.[224] Limited data in children suggest that an initial course of amphotericin B, followed by maintenance fluconazole or itraconazole, is effective in management of penicilliosis.

SPOROTRICHOSIS

Sporotrichosis may be diagnostically elusive by resembling atypical mycobacterial infection (particularly *Mycobacterium marinum*), nocardiosis, and leishmaniasis. Injury from wood and contact exposure to sphagnum moss are common sources of organism acquisition. Cutaneous sporotrichosis appears as multiple erythematous maculonodular lesions or as a single solitary lesion usually located on an extremity. Although usually painless and subcutaneous, these lesions also may be painful and ulcerative. The diagnosis is established by clinical suspicion and culture of tissue from a biopsy specimen. Direct histologic examination should be performed but typically has a low yield. Although saturated solution of potassium iodide has been the preferred treatment of cutaneous sporotrichosis, recent studies in adults demonstrate encouraging results with the use of itraconazole (100 mg/day). Restrepo et al.[225] found that lesions disappeared and cultures became negative after 90 to 180 days of therapy with no major side effects in 17 cases. Posttherapy evaluations conducted over an average of 115 days found no relapses. Amphotericin B is used for treatment of disseminated sporotrichosis.

CRYPTOCOCCOSIS

There are few studies of pulmonary or CNS cryptococcosis in children.[226, 227] The patterns of pulmonary cryptococcosis develop in extent and severity according to the level of immune impairment and underlying diseases.[228–230] Pulmonary cryptococcosis usually causes a saprophytic process or limited pulmonary infection in patients with chronic pulmonary disease, whereas it is a more aggressive infection leading to disseminated cryptococcal disease in immunocompromised patients, such as organ transplant recipients and HIV-infected patients.[231]

Pulmonary and CNS cryptococcosis appears to be less frequent among HIV-infected children compared with that of adults. For example, extrapulmonary cryptococcosis occurred in only 0.6% of children compared with 6.8% of the total population and in 5.2% to 11.5% of subpopulations of adult AIDS patients.[4] To better understand cryptococcal infection in children with HIV infection, Leggiadro et al.[227] surveyed investigators from 38 institutions concerning their experience with extrapulmonary cryptococcosis. Investigators from 33 (87%) of the institutions responded, resulting in data on 13 patients from 11 centers. This survey demonstrated that approximately 1% of HIV-infected children were found to have extrapulmonary cryptococcosis. The reasons for the reduced frequency may be related to a lower risk of exposure to sources of *C. neoformans* at a younger age. Meningitis was the most common manifestation of extrapulmonary cryptococcosis, occurring in 8 (62%) of the 13 patients. Extrapulmonary cryptococcosis was the AIDS indicator disease in 9 (69%) of the 13 patients. The median age was 8 years, with a range of 2 to 17 years. The spectrum of infection of cryptococcosis in these patients ranged from a rapidly fatal fungemia to chronic meningitis to an indolent fever of unknown origin.

Fever, headache, and altered mental status in cryptococcal meningoencephalitis are usually indolent, often evolving over the course of weeks to months. Unlike some CNS mycoses, such as aspergillosis, cryptococcal meningoencephalitis seldom manifests with focal neurologic deficits.[104] Cryptococcal meningoencephalitis in HIV-infected patients often has few clinically overt signs early in the course of infection but may manifest in some patients with meningismus, photophobia, and seizures.[226, 227, 230] Cryptococcomas, a less common manifestation of CNS cryptococcosis, are evident on CT scan as multiple or solitary nodular lesions. Cryptococcomas may cause focal neurologic deficits and cerebral edema.

Cryptococcosis may develop in the setting of sarcoma treated with intensive cytotoxic chemotherapy, where cell-mediated immunity is impaired by factors other than corticosteroid therapy. Moreover, pulmonary cryptococcosis in these patients simulates metastatic sarcoma. Because there were no radiographic features that can reliably distinguish between pulmonary cryptococcosis and metastatic sarcoma, an open biopsy is required to ascertain the distinction between metastatic sarcoma and pulmonary cryptococcosis. Empirical antineoplastic therapy for the new development of pulmonary nodules should be undertaken after biopsy of these lesions. Such an approach establishes a pathologic diagnosis of new pulmonary metastases and excludes a diagnosis of a concomitant infectious process.

Pulmonary cryptococcosis in HIV-infected children is usually associated with disseminated infection. Extrapulmonary infection, including meningoencephalitis and cutaneous lesions in HIV-infected patients, should be sought in attempting to establish a diagnosis. Cutaneous lesions may resemble molluscum contagiosum.

Cultures of blood and CSF, biopsy of cutaneous lesions, and bronchoalveolar lavage are most likely to yield a diagnosis of cryptococcosis. Cryptococcal antigen titers measured by latex agglutination or by enzyme immunoassay in CSF and serum of HIV-infected patients are typically elevated to levels often exceeding 1:1,000. The CSF cell count and glucose and protein levels in patients with HIV infection may be virtually normal due apparently to the paucity of an inflammatory response. Detection of organisms in biopsy specimens can be enhanced by use of mucicarmine or Alcian blue stains of the capsular acid mucopolysaccharide (glucuronoxylomannan). Because isolated lesions of *C. neoformans* osteomyelitis may manifest in apparently immunocompetent children,[231] diagnosis may be confirmed by bone biopsy and culture, as well as serum cryptococcal antigen titer. A lumbar puncture also is warranted to detect clinically occult CNS infection. Amphotericin B with 5-FC may be initially administered on an inpatient basis and changed to outpatient administration. Chronic lifelong antifungal therapy is not necessary in immunocompetent children.

Treatment of cryptococcosis in non-HIV-infected patients may be accomplished with a defined course of amphotericin B with 5-FC for 2 to 6 weeks, depending on the severity of infection and level of immunosuppression, followed by fluconazole for a total of 4 to 6 weeks, assuming that no extrapulmonary disease is present. If immunosuppression persists or HIV infection persists, an initial 2- to 4-week course of amphotericin B with or without 5-FC, followed by maintenance therapy with fluconazole, is recommended.[232] There is a high propensity for relapse of cryptococcal meningitis in HIV-infected and chronically immunosuppressed patients if maintenance therapy is not continued.[223] Among non-HIV-infected children with severe cryptococcal disease, serum or CSF cryptococcal antigen titer of 1:8 or more at the end of initial induction therapy or within 4 weeks of follow-up is also an important predictive factor of relapse,[234] thus warranting continued fluconazole suppression.

DISSEMINATED *TRICHOSPORON* INFECTIONS

Invasive *Trichosporon* infections are uncommon but frequently fatal infections in granulocytopenic patients or those receiving corticosteroids.[235, 236] Children with this infection have been reported to have neutropenia, corticosteroids, low birth weight, or the hemophagocytic syndrome as predisposing factors.[237–242] No apparent predisposing illness in a previously healthy neonate also has been reported.[243] Clinical manifestations of disseminated trichosporonosis are characterized by refractory fungemia, funguria, renal dysfunction, cutaneous lesions, chorioretinitis, and pneumonia. The pulmonary infiltrates of *Trichosporon* pneumonia consist of either bronchopneumonia after aspiration from an oropharyngeal source or multiple nodular pulmonary infiltrates from hematogenous dissemination. Biopsy specimens of cutaneous lesions generally reveal typical arthroconidia, blastoconidia, pseudohyphae, true hyphae, and vascular invasion. The serum cryptococcal latex agglutination test result may be positive due to shared antigens and resultant cross-reactivity between *T. beigelii* and *C. neoformans*.

Despite the administration of amphotericin B, fungemia may persist. Recent in vitro and in vivo studies indicate safety achievable serum concentrations of amphotericin B were fungistatic but not fungicidal.[244, 245] The combination of amphotericin B plus 5-FC may be synergistic or additive in vitro. Newer antifungal triazoles, such as fluconazole, have been found to be active in vivo and clinically against this organism.[245, 246] Thus, a rational strategy for treatment of disseminated *Trichosporon* infection is (1) amphotericin

B (1.0–1.5 mg/kg/daily), (2) initiation of 5-FC (50–100 mg/kg/daily), (3) high-dose fluconazole (8–10 mg/kg/daily) and (4) reversal of immunosuppression. Recent studies demonstrate GM-CSF, IFN-γ, and macrophage colony-stimulating factor (M-CSF) each augment antifungal activity of peripheral blood mononuclear cells against *T. beigelii*.[247] Antifungal therapy under these circumstances requires continuation until resolution of all clinical manifestations of infection. Recurrent infection may nevertheless occur during a subsequent period of cytotoxic chemotherapy among patients with neoplastic diseases.

INFECTIONS DUE TO *MALASSEZIA FURFUR*

Malassezia furfur is a lipophilic commensal yeast that rapidly colonizes the skin of newborn infants. Over the course of time, *M. furfur* becomes the common cause of tinea versicolor, resulting in hyperpigmented macules on the shoulders, neck, and upper half of the chest.[248] Typical skin scraping reveals the clusters of blastoconidia and hyphae in the classical "spaghetti and meatballs" pattern. Treatment of this infection is accomplished with selenium sulfide (Selsun) shampoo or topical antifungal agents. Alternatively, a short course of oral antifungal azoles, such as ketoconazole, fluconazole, or itraconazole, for 2 weeks may result in substantial resolution of the infection. There is, however, a high propensity for recurrence.

Although *M. furfur* causes tinea versicolor as a cosmetic inconvenience, it may also cause catheter-related fungemia and a life-threatening syndrome in newborn infants.[249–253] Characterized by fungemia, respiratory distress, and thrombocytopenia in infants receiving lipid-supplemented total parenteral nutrition, this fungemic syndrome due to *M. furfur* may be fatal unless lipid supplements are discontinued and the vascular catheter is removed. Our strategy in immunocompromised patients also includes the administration of an antifungal azole for specific antifungal chemotherapy. Fluconazole is the logical choice in newborn infants given its parenteral route of administration. More stable patients may be able to receive ketoconazole, fluconazole, or itraconazole by mouth. Persistent fungemia may ensue in patients with central venous catheter–related fungemia due to *M. furfur* fungemia.[252] Consistent with these findings are scanning electron microscopic data that demonstrate a biofilm of *M. furfur* along the intraluminal surface of the catheter, suggesting that the biofilm may prevent adequate penetration of antifungal agents into the organism. The clinical microbiology should be apprised of the clinical suspicion of *M. furfur* fungemia. Subcultures of blood cultures may then be supplemented with olive oil to promote more rapid and reliable recovery of *M. furfur*.

DERMATOPHYTOSES

Dermatophytosis are caused by *Microsporum* spp., *Trichophyton* spp., and *Epidermophyton floccosum*. Among the dermatophyte infections commonly encountered in children are tinea capitis, tinea corporis, and tinea facialis. Unless the child is immunocompromised, onychomycosis is unusual. The most common agent of tinea capitis in the United States is *Trichophyton tonsurans*. The lesions of dermatophytosis may be highly pleomorphic and mimic contact dermatitis, psoriasis, pityriasis rosea, and cutaneous drug reactions. Management of dermatophytoses has been discussed extensively elsewhere.[248, 253, 255] Nevertheless, several recent advances in management of dermatophytoses warrant discussion.

Tinea capitis is a frequently encountered mycologic problem in pediatric clinics. As summarized by Ginsburg,[254] griseofulvin (15 mg/kg) administered once daily with a glass of whole milk and biweekly selenium sulfide shampoos are the treatments of choice for tinea capitis and kerion. Gan et al.[255] compared the therapeutic efficacy of griseofulvin (15 mg/kg/daily) with ketoconazole (5 mg/kg/daily) in a randomized trial for treatment of tinea capitis in 63 children. The percentages of patients with positive cultures on therapy at 4-, 6-, 8-, and 10-week intervals and the mean time to a sterile culture were significantly greater ($P \le 0.01$) in ketoconazole- (8 weeks) than in griseofulvin-treated (4 weeks) patients. The time for complete scalp clearing also was significantly longer in patients who received ketoconazole (median 108 days) compared with those who were treated with griseofulvin (median 60 days) ($P = 0.01$). In addressing the problem of tinea capitis in children, Ginsburg et al.[256] conducted a randomized controlled trial of intralesional corticosteroid and griseofulvin compared with griseofulvin alone. This study found that there were no significant differences between the two treatment groups in the time to negative culture, time of onset of new hair growth, complete regrowth of hair, and time to scalp clearing. Thus, intralesional injection of corticosteroids is an unnecessary adjunct to therapy for children with kerion. For control of the carrier state, any one of a number of topical compounds is acceptable, including selenium sulfide–containing shampoos, antifungal shampoos, povidone-iodine, or even regular shampoos.[257]

Current studies with novel dosing strategies of itraconazole and fluconazole for treatment of tinea capitis in children appear promising for improving the efficacy and decreasing the duration of therapy of tinea capitis. For example, Elewski et al.[258] reported that three children who did not respond to or could not tolerate griseofulvin therapy achieved a clinical and mycologic cure after a 30-day course of itraconazole 100 mg daily. Recognition of tinea corporis and tinea capitis in hospitalized and ambulatory patients may prevent transmission to other patients, as well as to hospital staff. Undiagnosed tinea capitis can serve as a source of nosocomial tinea corporis among hospital personnel.[259]

Topically or orally administered terbinafine is a new strategy for treatment of dermatophytoses.[260, 261] For example, a 1-week course of 1% terbinafine cream was more effective mycologically and clinically in the treatment of tinea pedis than a 4-week course of 1% clotrimazole cream.[261] A preliminary study of tinea capitis in children found that a 6-week course of oral terbinafine was effective and well tolerated.[262] Thus, the management of tinea capitis is evolving as new therapeutic modalities, such as antifungal triazoles and terbinafine, become available.

PROPERTIES OF ANTIFUNGAL COMPOUNDS

AMPHOTERICIN B

Amphotericin B is the cornerstone of therapy in most critically ill patients with deeply invasive fungal infections. Amphotericin B is amphoteric, forming soluble salts in both basic and acidic environments. It is virtually insoluble in water. The IV infusion is commercially formulated as a desoxycholate micellar suspension consisting of 50 mg of amphotericin and 41 mg of desoxycholate. The principal mechanism of action of amphotericin B, as well as other polyenes, is binding to ergosterol, the principal sterol present in the cell membrane of sensitive fungi.[263] This binding alters the membrane permeability, causing leakage of sodium, potassium, and hydrogen ions, eventually leading to cell death. Amphotericin B also binds to a lesser extent to other sterols, such as cholesterol, which accounts for much of the toxicity associated with its usage. Oxidation-dependent amphotericin B–induced stimulation of macrophages is another proposed mechanism of the chemotherapeutic effect of this polyene.[264]

The pharmacokinetic profile of amphotericin B is somewhat different in children than in adults.[265–268] For example, Starke et al.[268] reported a smaller (<4 L/kg) volume of distribution and a larger (>0.026 L/hour/kg) clearance than that usually found in adults. The peak serum concentrations were significantly lower (approximately half) than those obtained in adults receiving equivalent doses. Benson and Nahata,[265] reported a strong inverse correlation between patient age and total clearance of amphotericin B, suggesting that higher dosages may be better tolerated in patients younger than age 9 years.

The pharmacokinetics of antifungal compounds frequently differ from those in adults. The clearance of amphotericin B is more rapid in infants. Among infants younger than 3 months and among older children (>9 years), amphotericin B clearance is decreased. The rapid clearance of amphotericin B in older infants and younger children, however, may result from more rapid urinary and biliary excretion, drug decomposition, or increased drug metabolism. The delayed clearance in infants is likely related to the renal immaturity found in these patients. When amphotericin B plasma pharmacokinetics were studied in a neonatal population, a marked interindividual variability was found in amphotericin B compared with a more uniform level of variation in the older pediatric population.

Toxicity of amphotericin B may be classified as acute or chronic. Acute or infusion-related toxicity is characterized by fever, chills, rigor, nausea, vomiting, and headache. Fever, chills, and rigors may be mediated by tumor necrosis factor and interleukin-1 (IL-1), cytokines that are released from human peripheral monocytes in response to the drug.[269] These acute reactions may possibly be blunted by corticosteroids, acetaminophen, aspirin, other nonsteroidal anti-inflammatory drugs, or meperidine.[270] To avoid pharmacologic immunosuppression, corticosteroids should be used only in low dosages, such as 0.5 to 1.0 mg of hydrocortisone/kg. Meperidine in low doses (0.2–0.5 mg/kg) interdicts development of rigors; paracetamol may decrease fever but appears to have little effect on rigors. Aspirin should be avoided in thrombocytopenic patients. Thrombophlebitis is a common local side effect associated with amphotericin B infusion. Slow infusion of the drug, rotation of the infusion site, addition of a small dose of heparin to the infusion, application of hot packs, use of in-line filters, and avoidance of amphotericin B concentrations in excess of 0.1 mg/mL may ameliorate thrombophlebitis in patients without central lines.[271] Infusion of amphotericin B through a central venous line avoids these complications.

Nephrotoxicity is the most significant chronic adverse effect of amphotericin B. Nephrotoxicity may be classified as glomerular or tubular.[272] The clinical and laboratory manifestations of glomerular toxicity include a decrease in glomerular filtration rate and renal blood flow, whereas tubular toxicity manifests with urinary casts, hypokalemia, hypomagnesemia, renal tubular acidosis, and nephrocalcinosis.[273]

Amphotericin B can cause changes in tubular cell permeability to ions both in vivo and in vitro. Thus, one possible explanation for amphotericin B–induced azotemia may be tubuloglomerular feedback, a mechanism whereby increased delivery and reabsorption of chloride ions in the distal tubule initiates a decrease in the glomerular filtrate rate of the nephron.[274, 275] Tubuloglomerular feedback is amplified by sodium deprivation and suppressed by previous sodium loading. Other mechanisms for amphotericin B nephrotoxicity include renal arteriolar spasm, calcium deposition during periods of ischemia, and direct tubular or renal cellular toxicity. More recent studies implicate roles for prostaglandin and tumor necrosis factor-α in mediating amphotericin B–induced azotemia.[276] The actual mechanism is likely a combination of these events. Azotemia is usually reversible, and renal function usually returns to normal levels after cessation of therapy. However, return to pretreatment levels may take several months in some cases.

Administration of sodium in the form of normal saline solution initially at 2 to 3 mEq/L/per 24 hours to 4 to 6 mEq/L is often effective in preventing or attenuating the development of azotemia. However, sodium loading requires close monitoring of patients to avoid hypernatremia, hyperchloremia, metabolic acidosis, and pulmonary edema. Furthermore, sodium loading will not ameliorate, and may indeed aggravate, hypokalemia.

Tubular toxicity is most commonly evident as hypokalemia and hypomagnesemia. Hypokalemia, which occurs in the majority of patients receiving amphotericin B, may require the parenteral administration of 5 to 15 mmol of supplemental potassium/hour. Amphotericin B–induced hypokalemia appears to be a result of increased renal tubular cell membrane permeability to potassium due to direct toxic effects, or it may be caused by enhanced excretion via activation of sodium/potassium exchange. Cautious use of amiloride, the potassium-sparing diuretic, may attenuate the severity of hypokalemia. Magnesium wasting may also occur in association with amphotericin B therapy.[277] Such hypomagnesemia may be more profound in patients with cancer who develop a divalent cation–losing nephropathy associated with the antineoplastic drug cisplatin. Amphotericin B should be infused under careful monitoring in newborns, patients with hyperkalemia, and those with renal impairment, all of which have been associated with amphotericin B–induced cardiac arrhythmias.[278]

Anemia is another common side effect of amphotericin B therapy. It is characterized as a normochromic and normocytic process that is probably mediated by suppression of erythrocyte and erythropoietin synthesis.[279] The anemia may be exacerbated by deterioration of renal function due to a decrease in red blood cell production. Maximal decreases in hemoglobin levels usually reach a nadir of between 18% and 35% below baseline, with levels usually returning to normal within several months of discontinuing therapy.

Among the important drug interactions with amphotericin B is the renal toxicity caused by aminoglycosides and cyclosporine during administration of amphotericin B. Acute pulmonary reactions (hypoxemia, acute dyspnea, and radiographic evidence of pulmonary infiltrates) have been associated with simultaneous transfusion of granulocytes and infusion of amphotericin B.[280] Although some investigators have disputed the causality of amphotericin B to such reactions,[281] a rational approach is to separate the infusions of amphotericin B and granulocytes by the longest time possible.

Although experience is limited, amphotericin B is the preferred antifungal drug for treatment of life-threatening fungal infections in pregnant women. Intrauterine transmission of blastomycosis and coccidioidomycosis from maternal infection has been documented.[218] However, amphotericin B has had an important impact on successfully reducing morbidity and mortality in mother and fetus, particularly in coccidioidomycosis.[282, 283] Amphotericin B has been used in all stages of pregnancy without apparent teratogenesis. At the same time, amphotericin B also has been used successfully in the treatment of maternal infection with delivery of healthy infants without evidence of infection. Dean et al.[284] recently reviewed the use of amphotericin B during pregnancy. They found persistent amphotericin B concentrations in placental tissue, cord serum, and infant serum at delivery 4 weeks after discontinuation of amphotericin B. Persistent levels of amphotericin B may have contributed to the sustained hypokalemia in the mother and the increased creatinine level in the infant.

The dosage of amphotericin B varies according to the specific fungus involved, patterns of infections, and the immune status of the patient as previously discussed. Empirical amphotericin B (0.5–0.75 mg/kg/daily) is the most widely used form of this drug in many oncology centers.

Invasive fungal infections in granulocytopenic patients are difficult to detect and carry a high mortality. Thus, empirical antifungal therapeutic strategies have evolved using amphotericin B. In a randomized prospective clinical trial, persistently febrile granulocytopenic patients had significantly fewer invasive fungal infections when they received empirical amphotericin B therapy.[285] These findings were confirmed in a larger trial that demonstrated decreased attributable mortality and fewer infections due to fungi.[286] This approach provides early therapy for occult fungal infections and systemic prophylaxis for patients at high risk of invasive mycoses, particularly invasive candidiasis in the broader context of protocols for managing infectious complications in febrile neutropenic hosts.[287, 289]

LIPID FORMULATIONS OF AMPHOTERICIN B

The recent introduction of lipid formulations has been an important therapeutic advance in improving the therapeutic index of amphotericin B. Because toxicity is the major dose-limiting factor of amphotericin B, lipid formulations of amphotericin B have been developed to reduce toxicity and permit larger doses to be administered.[290] Initial studies investigated several lipid formulations of amphotericin B prepared in individual laboratories. Although classically considered as "liposomal" formulations of amphotericin B, the investigational and clinically approved formulations of amphotericin B have a wider diversity of lipid structure. Liposomes, defined as phospholipid bilayers of one or more closed concentric structures, as well as other lipid formulations, have been used as vehicles for amphotericin B with encouraging results. The lipid formulation may provide a selective diffusion gradient toward the fungal cell membrane and away from mammalian cell membrane. The lipid composition and molar ratio of lipid and liposomal size all play a role in toxicity.[291] For example, when amphotericin B was incorporated into liposomes composed of dimyristoylphosphatidylcholine and dimyristoylphosphatidylglycerol, toxicity was selective for fungal cells but not for red blood cells.[292] Early clinical studies revealed remarkably little toxicity with administration of higher doses of this multilamellar vesicle formulation of amphotericin B.[293] The engineering of lipid formulations of amphotericin B have required extensive investigation of the impact of different lipids and their proportions on safety and toxicity. Indeed, some formulations may augment the toxicity of amphotericin B.

Several carefully engineered lipid formulations of polyenes are being investigated in North America: a small unilamellar vesicle formulation (AmBisome), amphotericin B lipid complex (ABLC), amphotericin B colloidal dispersion (ABCD; Amphocil), and liposomal nystatin (LN). AmBisome was the first lipid formulation of amphotericin B approved for use in Western Europe. Approvals for clinical use are anticipated in Western Europe for ABLC and ABCD. These polyene lipid formulations are currently being investigated in clinical trials in North America.

Although little is known about the pharmcokinetics of these formulations in children, some general observations may be made. Each lipid formulation of amphotericin B confers distinct pharmacokinetic properties. As a general principle, however, AmBisome, ABLC, ABCD, and LN distribute to organs rich in reticuloendothelial cells, leading to higher levels in liver, spleen, and lung and lower levels in kidneys compared with desoxycholate amphotericin B. Infusion of AmBisome results in strikingly higher area-under-the-curve (AUC) values and peak (maximum) concentrations (C_{max}) than is achieved with conventional amphotericin B or other lipid formulations of amphotericin B. Conversely, the apparent volume of distribution for the compounds ABCD and ABLC after single-dose infusion are substantially greater than that of AmBisome. Given their distinctive properties, the pharmacology of each of the polyene lipid formulations needs to be closely examined as part of their overall evaluation.

Francis et al.[157] recently found that persistently neutropenic rabbits with invasive pulmonary aspergillosis, when treated with 5 mg of AmBisome/kg/daily had no significant increase in serum creatinine levels above baseline compared with rabbits receiving 1 mg of amphotericin B/kg/daily, which caused a significant increase of serum creatinine levels above baseline. Similar findings were found with ABCD in treatment of experimental disseminated aspergillosis in immunocompromised rabbits[159] and experimental invasive pulmonary aspergillosis in persistently neutropenic rabbits.[294] Experimental mycoses also were successfully treated at higher doses of ABLC with less toxicity than was achieved with amphotericin B.[295] Some data suggest that amphotericin B incorporated into liposomes has enhanced and prolonged activity compared with equivalent concentrations of desoxycholate amphotericin B.[296]

Although associated with less nephrotoxicity, lipid formulations may confer their own patterns of toxicity. For example, the multilamellar lipid formulation of amphotericin B composed of DMPG and DMPC induced reversible hypoxemia, pulmonary hypertension, and depression of cardiac output during infusion.[297]

All of the lipid formulations of amphotericin B have been associated with elevated serum transaminase levels at greater frequency than that associated with conventional amphotericin B.

Lopez-Berestein et al.[298] developed extensive experience with a multilamellar liposomal formulation of ABLC in treatment of deep mycoses patients with refractory infection or azotemia. More recently, amphotericin B lipid complex in 228 cases treated under a compassionate release protocol was found to be active in treatment of immunocompromised patients with refractory mycoses or those with intolerance to conventional amphotericin B.[299] This study found little dose-limiting nephrotoxicity of ABLC. Ringden et al.[300] reported successful therapeutic use of AmBisome with minimal nephrotoxicity in neutropenic patients and those undergoing bone marrow transplantation. Tollemar et al.[301] investigated the safety and activity of low-dose AmBisome for prophylaxis in a randomized trial in bone marrow transplant recipients. We consider that the most appropriate use, however, because the lipid formulations of amphotericin B is for treatment of proven or suspected infections (empirical therapy) in profoundly immunocompromised patients. Further basic investigation of AmBisome and other lipid polyene formulations are leading to newer understandings of the mechanisms of antifungal activity of these compounds.[302]

Larger comparative trials are currently underway to investigate AmBisome in proven, invasive, fungal infections, empirical antifungal therapy, cryptococcal meningitis, and histoplasmosis. ABLC and ABCD are currently undergoing investigation in large clinical trials for treatment of aspergillosis and empirical antifungal therapy. These studies, which will include children, will provide an important foundation for understanding the utility of lipid formulations of amphotericin B.

FLUCYTOSINE

The mechanisms of action, pharmacokinetics, safety, antifungal properties, and clinical utility of 5-FC have been recently reviewed.[165] Flucytosine, a fluorine analog of cytosine, was first synthesized in the 1950s as a potential antineoplastic agent. Although not effective against tumors, it was found to have in vitro and in vivo antifungal activity. Flucytosine is most frequently used as an adjunct to amphotericin B therapy. This combination was originally proposed because of the observation that amphotericin B potentiated the uptake of 5-FC by increasing fungal cell membrane permeability. Two mechanisms of action have been reported for

5-FC. These are the disruption of protein synthesis by inhibition of DNA synthesis and by alteration of the amino acid pool by inhibition of RNA synthesis. These occur via a two-step process. Initially flucytosine is taken up into susceptible cells by cytosine permease. Flucytosine is converted intracellularly by cytosine deaminase to 5-fluorouracil, which replaces uracil in the pyrimidine pool and thus disrupts protein synthesis. In addition, 5-fluorouracil may then be converted through several steps to 5-fluorodeoxyuridylic acid monophosphate, a competitive inhibitor of thymidylate synthetase. 5-Fluorouracil cannot be directly used as an antifungal agent because it is not taken up by fungal cells, and it is highly toxic to mammalian cells.

Many fungi are resistant or develop resistance to 5-FC. Resistant fungi may have a deficiency in one of the enzymes necessary for conversion to the active molecule, may have decreased permeability to the drug, or may synthesize constituents that compete with 5-FC and its metabolites. Flucytosine treatment is not thought to induce resistance but selects for resistant strains of *Candida* spp. in a given population, particularly when the compound is used alone. Consequently, when 5-FC is used in treatment of candidiasis, aspergillosis, cryptococcosis, or other opportunistic mycosis, it is used only in combination with amphotericin B.

As a low molecular weight, water-soluble compound, absorption of orally administered 5-FC from the gastrointestinal tract is rapid and nearly complete, providing excellent bioavailability. There is negligible protein binding in serum, and the drug has excellent penetration with a volume of distribution that approximates that of total body water. Administration of 150 mg/kg/daily results in peak serum concentrations of 50 to 80 mg/L within 1 to 2 hours in adults with normal renal function. Cerebrospinal fluid concentrations are approximately 74% of corresponding serum concentrations, accounting for its usefulness in CNS mycoses.[303] However, the compound accumulates in patients with impaired renal function, resulting in potentially toxic serum levels unless the dosage is reduced. The plasma half-life 5-FC in adults with normal renal function is 3 to 5 hours. Dosage adjustments are required in patients with renal insufficiency and those using dialysis. As approximately 90% of a given dose is excreted unchanged in the urine by glomerular filtration, dosage adjustment of 5-FC is directly related to creatinine clearance.

Gastrointestinal side effects, such as diarrhea, nausea, and vomiting, are the most common symptomatic side effects associated with 5-FC therapy, occurring in approximately 6% of patients. Abnormally elevated hepatic transaminase levels also have been reported in approximately 5% of patients receiving the drug. Dose-dependent bone marrow suppression is the most serious toxicity associated with 5-FC administration. Conversion of 5-FC to 5-fluorouracil by gastrointestinal flora may account for the majority of these toxicities. These adverse effects may be controlled by close monitoring of the serum concentrations and adjustment of the dose to maintain peak serum concentrations between 40 and 60 mg/L. Because 5-FC is used in combination with amphotericin B, the conventional dosage of 150 mg/kg/daily is not recommended in most patients. Instead, we use 100 mg/kg/daily as a starting dose in patients with normal renal function. As the glomerular filtration rate decreases because of amphotericin B, 5-FC dosage is reduced to less than 100 mg/kg/daily in three to four divided doses. We have found that these properties are applicable in adults and children.

Synergistic or additive effects have been demonstrated in vivo and in vitro with amphotericin B against *C. albicans* and *C. neoformans*. these findings are consistent with the clinical observations that the combination of 5-FC and amphotericin B in a prospective, randomized trial cleared CSF more rapidly than amphotericin B alone in cryptococcal meningitis in non-HIV-infected patients. This combination has also been shown to be effective against large cryptococcal intracerebral masses (cryptococcomas), eliminating the need for surgical intervention. Larsen et al.[304] recently demonstrated that the combination of amphotericin B plus 5-FC was more effective than fluconazole for primary treatment of cryptococcal meningitis. The combination of 5-FC with amphotericin B is therefore recommended for the treatment of meningeal candidiasis or cryptococcosis, *Candida* endophthalmitis, *Candida* thrombophlebitis of the great veins, renal candidiasis, and hepatosplenic (chronic disseminated) candidiasis.

ANTIFUNGAL AZOLES

The antifungal azoles are synthetic compounds composed of imidazoles (clotrimazole, miconazole, and ketoconazole) and triazoles (itraconazole and fluconazole). The antifungal azoles demonstrate less toxicity than amphotericin B, have flexibility for oral administration, and have comparable efficacy under many circumstances. The antifungal azole agents function principally by inhibition of the fungal cytochrome P_{450} enzyme lanosterol 14-α-demethylase, which is involved in the synthesis of ergosterol.[305]

Antifungal Imidazoles: Clotrimazole, Miconazole, and Ketoconazole

Clotrimazole and miconazole, which belong to the class of imidazoles, were the first two antifungal azoles approved for treatment of human mycoses. Clotrimazole and miconazole are relatively insoluble in aqueous solution and are poorly absorbed from the alimentary tract. Consequently, clotrimazole is now used only as a topical agent. The insolubility of miconazole was overcome by dissolving it in a polyethoxylated castor oil, which is believed to be responsible for causing the majority of the toxic effects of the drug, including pruritis, headache, phlebitis, and hepatitis. Rapid IV infusion of miconazole has been reported to cause cardiac arrest.[306] Parenteral usage is currently limited to treatment of invasive infections due to *P. boydii.*

Introduced in 1979 as the first successful orally absorbable antifungal azole, ketoconazole has a broad spectrum of antifungal activity, relatively long serum half-life, increased water solubility, and lack of significant autoinduction of hepatic degradative enzymes. Because ketoconazole is insoluble at neutral pH but is readily solubilized at pH less than 2, it is dependent on an acidic intragastric milieu for systemic absorption. Ketoconazole is highly bound to plasma proteins and penetrates poorly into CSF, urine, and saliva.[307] The absorption of orally administrated ketoconazole varies greatly from patient to patient.[308] A high-carbohydrate meal ingested with ketoconazole may decrease total drug absorption, whereas a high-lipid meal may increase it.[309] Bioavailability of the drug is reduced in patients with gastric achlorhydria.[310] Bioavailability can be improved by concomitant administration of an acidifying agent, such as acidulin, orange juice, or a carbonated beverage. Ketoconazole is extensively metabolized by the liver, primarily by scission of the imidazole and piperazine rings, and then excreted into the bile as an inactive compound. Less than 1% of active drug is excreted in the urine. No modification of the dosage is required in patients with renal insufficiency, and clearance is not significantly altered by chronic ambulatory peritoneal dialysis.

Plasma levels of ketoconazole are decreased by antacids or histamine H_2-receptor-blocking agents (i.e., cimetidine) due to elevated gastric pH, which impairs absorption of ketoconazole.[311] This erratic bioavailability compromises the role of ketoconazole in neutropenic patients, particularly those with chemotherapy- or radiation-induced mucosal disruption. Consequently, ketoconazole has a very limited role in neutropenic patients and is not recommended for prophylaxis or empirical antifungal therapy.[312]

Ginsburg et al.[313] investigated the pharmacokinetics of ketoconazole administered as either a commercially prepared suspension or as a crushed tablet in applesauce in 12 children. The mean peak plasma concentration of ketoconazole and the area under the plasma time-concentration curve were approximately twofold greater with the suspension than with the crushed tablets. Unfortunately, the oral suspension of ketoconazole is not available in the United States at this time.

Nausea and vomiting are the most frequent dose-limiting side effects of ketoconazole in approximately 10% of adults receiving 400 mg/day but increasing to more than 50% in those receiving more than 800 mg/day.[220, 314] Also directly related to dosage of ketoconazole is the occurrence of endocrinopathies, which arise from the cross-reactive inhibition of mammalian cytochrome P_{450} enzymes. Among these endocrinopathies are antiandrogen effects of gynecomastia, oligospermia, and decreased libido in males due to inhibition of testosterone synthesis.[315] Less frequently observed is a transient dose-dependent decrease in the corticotropin (ACTH)–cortisol response due to inhibition of cytochrome P_{450}–dependent enzymes involved in adrenal corticosteroid synthesis.[316] The impact of these endocrinologic effects due to chronic administration of ketoconazole on child development have not been thoroughly examined.

By comparison, ketoconazole-related hepatotoxicity does not appear to be dose dependent and ranges from transient asymptomatic hepatic transaminase elevations to fulminant hepatitis. Approximately 2% to 8% of patients receiving the drug experience some abnormal elevation of serum transaminase levels.[317] Most cases spontaneously resolve or stabilize during continuation of therapy or reverse once administration is discontinued. Approximately 1 in 10,000 patients receiving ketoconazole develop progressive hepatitis, which has occasionally been fatal.

Important drug interactions between ketoconazole and other agents should be assessed before therapy is initiated in patients receiving other medications. Ketoconazole prolongs the serum half-life of cyclosporine, presumably by inhibition of cytochrome P_{450} enzymes, which may lead to cyclosporine-induced nephrotoxicity. Consequently, serum cyclosporine levels are closely monitored, and dosages of cyclosporine are adjusted in patients receiving ketoconazole. Ketoconazole's inhibition of the metabolism of antihistamines, such as terfenadine and astemizole, may lead to widening QT intervals and ventricular arrhythmias, including torsades de pointes. The serum concentrations of ketoconazole are decreased with concomitant administration of drugs that induce hepatic microsomal enzymes, such as rifampin.[318] Caution should also be used in the coadministration of ketoconazole with sodium warfarin (Coumadin) and oral hypoglycemic agents, because the concentrations of these drugs may increase to cause increased prothrombin time and hypoglycemia, respectively.

As previously reviewed in detail, ketoconazole is active against selected nonmeningeal fungal infections, mucosal candidiasis, including chronic mucocutaneous candidiasis, blastomycosis, chronic cavitary, and disseminated histoplasmosis, and paracoccidioidomycosis. Because ketoconazole penetrates CSF poorly, it is not recommended for any fungal infection of the CNS, particularly cryptococcosis. Because the endemic mycoses seldom complicate the course of neutropenia, ketoconazole is rarely used for this indication in patients with neoplastic diseases. Moreover, itraconazole appears to be safer and at least as effective in the treatment of these infections. In treatment of mucosal candidiasis in neutropenic patients, fluconazole is more consistently bioavailable than is ketoconazole and the current formulations of itraconazole.

ANTIFUNGAL TRIAZOLES

Substitution of the triazole ring for the imidazole ring confers many structure-function advantages, including (1) greater polarity (improving solubility and reduce protein binding for some compounds, (2) reduced nucleophilicity of the triazole ring (improving resistance to metabolic degradation), (3) increased specificity for fungal enzyme systems, (4) broader antifungal spectrum, and (5) increased potency.[319, 320] Itraconazole and fluconazole are the only antifungal triazoles licensed worldwide.

Itraconazole

Compared with ketoconazole, itraconazole has a broader spectrum of antifungal activity, less toxicity, a longer plasma half-life, and the capacity to penetrate into brain tissue. The spectrum of itraconazole includes *Candida* spp., *C. neoformans*, *Trichosporon* spp., *Aspergillus* spp., dematiaceous molds, and the thermally dimorphic fungi, including *H. capsulatum*, *B. dermatitidis*, *C. immitis*, *P. braziliensis*, and *S. schenckii*. Despite this extended spectrum and greater safety profile, itraconazole still retains the properties of bioavailability that are similar to those of ketoconazole. Itraconazole is soluble only at low pH, as in the normal gastric milieu. There is wide intersubject variation in the plasma concentration curves of itraconazole in healthy volunteers.[321] Oral bioavailability is compromised and becomes more erratic in patients receiving intensive cytotoxic chemotherapy, causing disruption of gastrointestinal mucosal epithelium.[322] Absorption of itraconazole may be markedly diminished in patients receiving antacid therapy, such as oral antacids or H_2-receptor-blocking agents.

There is a paucity of data describing the pharmacokinetic properties of itraconazole in children. Mean peak serum concentrations of 0.02 mg/L are attained in adults when a single 100-mg dose is administered during fasting, whereas peak concentrations of 0.18 mg/L are attained when the drug is administered after feeding, suggesting enhanced absorption with feeding. Bioavailability may be further enhanced by administration of itraconazole with acidulin or a carbonated beverage. Initial findings indicate that the bioavailability and interpatient variation in absorption of itraconazole is improved by incorporation of the molecule into cyclodextrin. Studies are currently underway to investigate the safety and plasma pharmacokinetics of this novel formulation of itraconazole. These properties should expand the utility of itraconazole to a wider range of patients undergoing intensive cytotoxic chemotherapy.

Itraconazole follows nonlinear plasma pharmacokinetics. Dosage increase between 100, 200, and 400 mg/day produce nonlinear increases in the area under the plasma concentration-time curve, suggesting the possibility of saturable metabolic processes.[319] The drug has a serum half-life of 15 to 20 hours after a single dose and 30 to 35 hours after multiple dosing.[321] Further reflection of its nonlinear pharmacokinetic properties, twice daily dosing of itraconazole leads to improved total area under the curve (AUC) compared with that of once daily itraconazole. Whether AUC or peak plasma concentrations, however, correlate with antifungal response is not known.

Attainment of adequate plasma concentrations is critical for optimal antifungal effect of itraconazole. For example, a recent study demonstrated in immunocompromised animals that when itraconazole was absorbed to achieve peak plasma concentrations (measured by bioassay) of more than 5 μg/mL, antifungal activity in vivo approximated that of amphotericin B.[324] Levels less than 5 μg/mL were associated with significantly less antifungal activity. Translation of these pharmacodynamic findings to clinical conditions are suggested in a study of itraconazole in patients with prolonged neutropenia, where there was a direct relationship between plasma concentrations of drug and antifungal activity.[174]

Because itraconazole is highly protein bound (>99%), with only 0.2% available as free drug,[325] concentrations in body fluids equivalent to body water, such as saliva and CSF, are negligible. However, tissue concentrations are two to five times higher than those in plasma, and they persist for longer, explaining the efficacy of the drug despite low plasma concentrations.[326] Itraconazole is extensively metabolized by the liver to hydroxyitraconazole, which also possesses intrinsic antifungal activity. Less than 1% of the active drug and approximately 35% of the inactive metabolites are excreted in the urine. Because the primary route of excretion is the biliary tract, no adjustment of dosage is necessary in patients with renal impairment.

Several interactions between itraconazole and other drugs bear note. Cyclosporine levels in whole blood may become elevated with the concomitant administration of itraconazole.[324, 327, 328] Cyclosporine levels should be monitored closely when these drugs are coadministered. Itraconazole plasma concentrations are diminished by concurrent administration of rifampin, phenytoin, and phenobarbital. Caution is warranted in its coadministration with antihistamines, sodium warfarin, and oral hypoglycemic agents, because competitive inhibition of metabolism may lead to elevated levels of these compounds.

Itraconazole is well tolerated with long-term use. Most of the adverse reactions reported are transient and include gastrointestinal disturbances, dizziness, headache, and, rarely, leukopenia. Compared with ketoconazole, itraconazole has a lower incidence of hepatic toxicity, no apparent dose-dependent nausea and vomiting, and no adverse effect on testicular steroidogenesis.[166] A syndrome of hypertension and hypokalemia has been observed in some patients receiving high doses of the itraconazole, particularly at levels greater than 10 mg/kg/daily.

Fluconazole

Fluconazole is a water-soluble m-difluorophenyl bistriazole compound that has been shown to be effective against infections due to *Candida* spp., *C. neoformans*, and other fungi in patients with neoplastic diseases, HIV infection, and other immunocompromised states. In the initial development of fluconazole, there was a disparity between its relatively low activity in vitro and its high in vivo activity. Subsequent studies have further clarified the standardized in vitro susceptibility to fluconazole. These methods and those employing new biochemically defined media (RPMI-1640 and HR media) more accurately reflect the MICs that would be anticipated from in vivo and clinical data.[330–332]

Compared with itraconazole and ketoconazole, which are relatively large lipophilic molecules with erratic bioavailability, fluconazole is a relatively small water-soluble molecule with rapid absorption and high bioavailability.[272, 319, 333, 334] Also unlike ketoconazole and itraconazole, fluconazole is only weakly bound to serum proteins (12%), and thus most fluconazole circulates as free drug. Itraconazole follows nonlinear plasma kinetics and is extensively metabolized, whereas fluconazole exhibits linear plasma kinetics and is only slightly metabolized. In the setting of renal impairment, itraconazole and ketoconazole require no dosage adjustment, whereas the dosage of fluconazole is adjusted to reflect glomerular filtration. A 50% reduction of dosage is recommended in those with a creatinine clearance of 21 to 50 mL/min and a 75% reduction of dose with a creatinine clearance less than 21 mL/min. The pharmacokinetics of fluconazole are independent of both the route of administration and formulation such that the concentration-time curves of orally and parenterally administered fluconazole are very similar. Unlike ketoconazole or itraconazole, oral absorption of fluconazole does not depend on a low intragastric pH, feeding, fasting, or gastrointestinal disease.[335]

Although extensive pharmacokinetic studies of fluconazole were initially performed in adults, little was known until recently about fluconazole's properties in children. Consequently, Lee et al.[336] investigated the safety, tolerance, and pharmacokinetic properties of fluconazole in neutropenic children with neoplastic diseases. This study found that the plasma half-life of fluconazole in children was substantially reduced in comparison to that of adults; for example, a mean plasma half-life of 17 hours was found in children vs. 27 and 37 hours previously reported in adults. The linear dose proportionality to peak plasma concentrations were similar to those of adults. In light of the more rapid clearance of fluconazole in children, we suggest that life-threatening fungal infection be treated with fluconazole at 6 mg/kg twice daily, assuming normal renal function. This shorter half-life in high-risk children underscores that antifungal therapeutic trials, which are conducted in adults, cannot be implicity extrapolated to children. Instead, separate therapeutic trials are required to accurately ascertain responsiveness in children at a given dosage.

Recent studies of the pharmacokinetics of fluconazole in premature neonates reveal that its properties are distinctive from those of older children and adults.[337, 338] The volume of distribution of fluconazole is greatest in neonates (1.8−2.2 L/kg) compared with that of adults (approximately 0.7 L/kg). Fluconazole in these very low birth weight infants was eliminated slowly with a mean elimination half-life of 89 hours at birth, 67 hours 1 week later, and 55 hours approximately 2 weeks after birth. The authors recommended that fluconazole in very low birth weight infants be administered at 6 mg/kg every 3 days in the first week, followed by 6 mg/kg every 1 to 2 days thereafter. Similar findings were previously reported by Krzeska et al.[339] in 14 infants (9 days–4.4 months). The volume of distribution was large (1.2 L/kg), with a range from 0.76 to 2.6 L/kg. The mean terminal half-life of elimination, however, was smaller in this older population of infants (22 ± h).

Fluconazole penetrates well into CSF.[108, 340–342] This distribution property results in CSF/serum concentration ratios of between 0.5 and 0.9, increasing to between 0.8 and 0.9 in the setting of meningeal disease. Such CSF penetration may contribute substantially to the important role of fluconazole in the management of cryptococcal meningitis as previously discussed.

Fluconazole has been well tolerated with very few dose-limiting side effects in different pediatric populations.[343–345] Nausea, other gastrointestinal symptoms, and elevated hepatic transaminase levels occur infrequently and are usually reversible. The incidence of reversible, asymptomatic hepatic transaminase elevations attributable to fluconazole may be as high as 12% in children receiving intensive cytotoxic chemotherapy for neoplastic diseases.[336] Exfoliative skin reactions (Stevens-Johnson syndrome) have been reported in patients with AIDS, although the exact role of fluconazole in these reactions is unclear. Fluconazole does not appear to affect the synthesis of steroid hormones.

The drug interactions of fluconazole in principle are potentially similar to those of other azoles.[346] For example, fluconazole has been reported to precipitate phenytoin toxicity due to inhibition of metabolism, thus warranting monitoring of phenytoin concentrations during coadministration of fluconazole. Concentrations of cyclosporine may be increased and the effects of sodium warfarin may be potentiated.[346] Nevertheless, the number of drug interactions reported with fluconazole appear to be substantially fewer than those that have been reported with ketoconazole. Narang et al.[347] recently reported that HIV-infected patients receiving rifabutin and fluconazole had fewer mycobacterial infections than those receiving rifabutin alone, suggesting that fluconazole's inhibition of the metabolism of rifabutin leading to higher plasma levels and improved antimycobacterial efficacy. At the same time, the potential for added hepatotoxicity must also be monitored when the combination of rifabutin and fluconazole is used.

Among neutropenic patients, fluconazole has achieved an important role for the prevention of invasive candidiasis. The experimental basis for administering fluconazole to prevent disseminated candidiasis is reviewed in detail elsewhere.[348] The potential use of fluconazole for prevention and treatment of disseminated candidiasis in granulocytopenic patients was studied by investigating the in vivo activity and pharmacokinetics of this agent in persistently granulocytopenic rabbit models of experimental disseminated candidiasis. This model reflected critical variables that influenced outcome in granulocytopenic patients: depth and duration of granulocytopenia, indwelling central Silastic venous catheter, broad-spectrum antibiotics, different patterns of disseminated candidiasis (acute, subacute, and chronic), sites of infection, and timing of initiation of antifungal agents. Pharmacokinetic studies in rabbits demonstrated a long plasma half-life and large volume of distribution, corresponding to high levels of tissue penetration in multiple organ sites.

Fluconazole in these experiments was administered for systemic prophylaxis, early treatment and delayed treatment. Fluconazole was more effective when used for systemic prophylaxis or early treatment of disseminated candidiasis in comparison to delayed treatment. Moreover, fluconazole was as effective as amphotericin B plus 5-FC in prevention and early treatment of disseminated candidiasis but was significantly less effective than amphotericin B plus 5-FC in delayed treatment of chronic disseminated candidiasis. Dose-response studies demonstrated that the antifungal effect of fluconazole was dose dependent and time dependent, suggesting that more protracted courses of fluconazole would be required for treatment of chronic disseminated candidiasis.

These experimental findings with fluconazole were predictive of the results obtained in a randomized, double-blind, multicenter trial of fluconazole for prevention of deeply invasive candidiasis in adult bone marrow transplant recipients.[349] Fluconazole, 400 mg/daily given orally or intravenously, was initiated on day 1 of marrow-ablative chemotherapy. Among 356 evaluable bone marrow transplant recipients, invasive candidiasis developed in 28 (15.7%) of 178 patients who received placebo and 5 (2.8%) of 179 who received fluconazole ($P < 0.001$). Fluconazole in this study also delayed the initiation of amphotericin B from day 17 to day 21 ($P < 0.004$). Infections due to *C. krusei* were noted in both arms and were not significantly different. Fluconazole was associated with minimal adverse effects in this setting. Another randomized, placebo-controlled trial reported by Slavin et al.[350] from the Fred Hutchinson Cancer Center studied fluconazole at 400 mg/daily given orally or intravenously in bone marrow transplant recipients. Fluconazole in this study was administered throughout the period of granulocytopenia and 100 days after recovery from granulocytopenia. Among the 301 transplant recipients enrolled, most of whom were adult allogeneic recipients, 261 evaluable cases were analyzed. The number of fungal infections was significantly reduced (6 of 131 of fluconazole-treated patients vs. 16 of 130 in placebo-treated patients [$P = 0.01$]), as was the use of empirical amphotericin B in the fluconazole-treated group; mortality also significantly declined.

In adults with acute leukemia, fluconazole failed to prevent deep invasive mycoses.[351] Among 257 evaluable patients, invasive mycoses developed in 10 (7.5%) of 133 placebo-treated patients vs. 5 (4%) of 124 fluconazole-treated patients ($P = 0.3$). The lack of statistical significance in this large clinical trial may result from a low frequency of proven invasive mycosis and an early usage of empirical amphotericin B. Candidemia and tissue-proven invasive candidiasis were diagnosed infrequently in this population, possibly due to an early and aggressive use of empirical amphotericin B. These findings also suggest that the risk for invasive candidiasis in this population of adults with acute leukemia was less than that of patients undergoing allogeneic bone marrow transplantation in the randomized fluconazole studies. Both multicenter fluconazole studies also reported a striking paucity of invasive aspergillosis in treated and placebo groups. This effect may have resulted from stringent criteria for demonstrating invasive pulmonary aspergillosis. For example, patients with CT scans consistent with invasive pulmonary aspergillosis and treated as such were not considered to have possible or probable infection. Moreover, patients who had completed the study but who were later found at autopsy to have invasive pulmonary aspergillosis were not considered as having this infection during study.

Although the findings for prevention of invasive candidiasis by fluconazole in bone marrow transplant recipients are encouraging, antifungal activity has several limitations. For example, fluconazole at the current dosages of 200 to 400 mg/daily has little or no activity against *C. krusei*, *T. glabrata*, *Aspergillus* spp., Zygomycetes, and some hyalohyphomycetes, such as *Fusarium* spp. Moreover, there is a dearth of data investigating fluconazole in febrile neutropenic children.[352–354] Early studies appear encouraging. However, the results of larger clinical trials in children are currently being analyzed and should provide more definitive conclusions.

INVESTIGATIONAL ANTIFUNGAL COMPOUNDS
INVESTIGATIONAL ANTIFUNGAL TRIAZOLE AGENTS

DO-870, formerly known as ICI 195739, is an orally active bistriazole with broad-spectrum antifungal activity.[355] Subsequent in vitro and in vivo studies have demonstrated activity of this agent against pathogens relevant to neutropenic cancer patients, including *C. tropicalis* and *A. fumigatus.* Clinical trials are currently being planned for this promising compound. Other promising antifungal triazoles include compounds in early trials in western Europe. However, little preclinical or clinical data have been reported for these agents at this early stage. The development of earlier potent antifungal triazoles, SCH 39304 and saperconazole, was discontinued because of the development of hepatic and adrenal tumors, respectively.

ECHINOCANDINS

The echinocandins are cell wall–active cyclic lipopeptide fungicidal antifungal compounds that inhibit 1,3-β-glucan synthetase in vitro and in vivo.[354] The inhibition is specific with little or no effect on chitin, mannan, DNA, RNA, or protein synthesis.[331] Cilofungin, which was the first echinocandin compound used in patients, is a semisynthetic lipopeptide derived from echinocandin B by the enzymatic removal of its linoleoyl side chain and chemical replacement with a 4-N-octyloxybenzoyl group.[356, 357] Cilofungin administered by high-dose continuous or intermittent infusion results in nonlinear saturation plasma pharmacokinetics, which are associated with sustained, high plasma concentrations and significantly enhanced antifungal activity against experimental disseminated candidiasis.[358] However, given their mechanism of action, echinocandins also have in vivo activity against *P. carinii.*[359] High doses of cilofungin were also active against aspergillosis in vivo.[360] Unfortunately, cilofungin was withdrawn from clinical trials because the carrier for the drug, polyethylene glycol, caused metabolic acidosis in impaired renal function. However, highly potent extended-spectrum echinocandins are currently being developed that may permit the use of safer vehicles.[361]

TERBINAFINE AND OTHER ALLYLAMINES

Terbinafine is the first derivative that is commercially available in both oral and topical formulations. Allylamines are a class of agents derived from heterocyclic spironaphthalenones, which function by inhibiting squalene epoxidase, a key enzyme in sterol biosynthesis.[362, 363] Although their spectrum of antifungal activity includes

Aspergillus spp., *Candida* spp., and *S. schenkii*,[364] they are used only for topical or systemic dermatophyte infections. The pharmacokinetics and tissue distribution of terbinafine favor distribution to the skin and its appendages. Because the allylamines do not inhibit cytochrome P_{450}, they do not alter mammalian steroidal hormone levels as observed with the azole derivatives.[259] Terbinafine (SF 86327), considered the most active of the allylamine derivatives currently produced, is used worldwide as an oral agent for the treatment of onychomycosis and other dermatophyte infections. Only the topical form is available in the United States. The lipophilic terbinafine molecule accumulates in the epidermis and subcutaneous fat tissue and binds to most fractions of plasma proteins (including albumin and high-, low-, and very low-density lipoproteins); it also is rapidly metabolized, all of which impair distribution into visceral tissue.[365] Current studies of both oral and topical formulations indicate that this compound is an important advance in management of dermatophytoses.

PRADIMICINS AND BENANOMICINS

The pradimicins and benanomicins are sterol-like molecules with amino acid–containing side chains that form calcium-linked complexes with mannose-containing components of the fungal cell membrane.[366] They are fungicidal against a wide variety of fungi, including isolates resistant to other antifungal agents. Pradimicin A is not toxic to cultured mammalian cells at concentrations 100 times higher than the antifungal MICs (0.8–12.5 mg/L).[367] The benanomicins also appear to have low toxicity. Of additional interest is the ability of pradimicin A to inhibit influenza virus replication and its possible anti-HIV effects at the stage of viral adsorption and cell-to-cell infection. These compounds are currently being studied in laboratory animals, and plans for future clinical trials are being developed.

RECOMBINANT HUMAN CYTOKINES AND IMMUNE RECONSTITUTION

Reversal of immunosuppression is a critical factor in improving survival and decreasing morbidity in patients with invasive fungal infections. Table 6 delineates several of the strategies that can be used to ameliorate immunosuppression in the therapy of invasive mycoses. Recombination hematopoietic cytokines are an important advance in the management of neutropenic patients receiving cytotoxic chemotherapy. Few studies have investigated recombinant cytokines in prospective randomized trials in neutropenic chil-

TABLE 6.
Reversal of Immunosuppression: Immunologic Adjuncts
to Prevention and Treatment of Invasive Fungal Infections
in Children

- Recombinant cytokines
  Granulocyte colony-stimulating factor
  Granulocyte-macrophage colony-stimulating factor
  Interferon-γ
  Macrophage colony-stimulating factor
- Stem cell reconstitution
- Immune reconstitution
- Granulocyte transfusions
- Adoptive immunotherapy
- Discontinuation of corticosteroids

dren. Moreover, no clinical trials demonstrate an effect of recombinant hematopoietic cytokines on reducing the frequency of invasive mycoses. Administration of the recombinant hematopoietic human cytokines, such as G-CSF, granulocyte-GM-CSF, and M-CSF may decrease duration of neutropenia (G-CSF, GM-CSF), increase microbicidal function of neutrophils, monocytes, and macrophages (G-CSF, GM-CSF, M-CSF), and possibly improve mucosal integrity (G-CSF, GM-CSF) after cytotoxic chemotherapy under experimental and clinical conditions.[332, 368] Shortening the duration of neutropenia by use of recombinant human cytokines may permit more intensive cytotoxic chemotherapy. The impact of these cytokines on invasive fungal infections cannot be readily determined from the clinical trials performed thus far due to the relatively small numbers of patients studied. Clearly, decreasing the duration of granulocytopenia should decrease the frequency of invasive fungal infections. For example, autologous bone marrow transplantation with intensive cytotoxic chemotherapy is being conducted in some centers as an outpatient procedure as the result of recombinant human cytokines and administration of peripheral blood stem cells.

Nevertheless, some patients with profound, persistent granulocytopenia such as those with acute nonlymphocytic leukemia or those undergoing allogeneic bone marrow transplantation may have only a modest shortening of their duration of granulocytopenia, thereby still carrying a high risk for invasive fungal infections.

Patients also undergoing repeated cycles of intensive cytotoxic therapy may become colonized with *Candida* spp. during the course of repeated cycles, resulting in the potential for invasive candidiasis despite an abbreviated course of granulocytopenia. Nevertheless, cytokines such as G-CSF and GM-CSF appear to have ameliorated one of the important risk factors for invasive fungal infections.

Whether cytokines are effective in treatment of proven fungal infections in cancer patients is not known. Recent studies with GM-CSF suggest that this recombinant cytokine may be active as adjunctive therapy in the management of invasive fungal infections in patients with cancer.[369] A phase I clinical trial of recombinant human M-CSF in patients with invasive fungal infections demonstrated that M-CSF was well tolerated but did produce a transient dose-related thrombocytopenia.[370] The study design did not permit evaluation of the potential antifungal properties of M-CSF vs. optimal antifungal therapy alone. A randomized placebo-controlled clinical trial is being planned to delineate the potential role of M-CSF in prevention of invasive fungal infections in neutropenic hosts.

The American Society for Clinical Oncology recently recommended for children and adults that G-CSF or GM-CSF be used in those situations of febrile neutropenia when the expected incidence is 40% or more or after documented febrile neutropenia in a prior chemotherapy cycle to avoid infectious complications and maintain dose intensity in subsequent treatment cycles when chemotherapy dose reduction is not appropriate and after high-dose chemotherapy with autologous progenitor-cell transplantation.[371] We would further recommend the administration of recombinant G-CSF or GM-CSF to persistently neutropenic patients who have a proven invasive fungal infection and who are not receiving a recombinant colony-stimulating factor. The rationale for this approach is based on the observations that accelerated recovery from neutropenia improves the prognosis of neutropenic patients with invasive aspergillosis.

Recombinant hematopoietic cytokines also augment functional activity of immunosuppressed non-neutropenic hosts against fungi. However, the in vivo significance of these observations remains to be determined. For example, G-CSF reverses the neutrophil dysfunction against *Aspergillus* hyphae in HIV-infected children.[372] Granulocyte colony-stimulating factor also reverses the corticosteroid-induced immunosuppression of neutrophils against *Aspergillus* hyphae.[373] Further investigation of these therapeutic modalities to ameliorate non-neutropenic immunosuppression in children are warranted.

Newer recombinant cytokines such as IL-1, IL-3, IL-6, stem cell factor, and hematopoietic dipentapeptides may result in improved recovery from marrow aplasia, lead to increased microbicidal function, and reduce the risk of invasive mycoses. Transfusion of elutriated monocytes or of neutrophils from donors treated with G-CSF may be important therapeutic or preventive adjuncts, which merit further study. Such immune reconstitution with transfused effector cells would also provide a larger cell population for activation by cytokines in neutropenic patients.

FUTURE DIRECTIONS

Based on the current trends and patterns of invasive fungal infections, one can anticipate an increasingly important role for these infections in causing excess morbidity and mortality in children, particularly in immunocompromised hosts. If one wishes to understand the future trends of these host-pathogen interactions, discussion of new pediatric hosts, new fungal pathogens, and new antifungal interventions is a useful approach. The evolution of new pediatric hosts will likely continue to develop. Indeed, within the past 20 years, there has been a chronologic expansion of vulnerable populations to include inherited immunodeficiencies, profound neutropenia, graft-vs.-host disease in allogeneic bone marrow transplantation, organ transplantation, surgical trauma, severe burns, very low birth weight infancy, and more recently, HIV infection.[374, 375] One can only anticipate further expansion of these susceptible patient populations, as well as the probable development of new immunocompromised pediatric populations in the coming years.

Invasive fungal infections may emerge in immunocompromised hosts with new patterns of infection, as recently exemplified in HIV-infected children. For example, disseminated histoplasmosis, CNS cryptococcosis, and mucosal candidiasis in HIV-infected patients may manifest with unusually extensive heavy tissue burden, leading to extensive deep tissue and mucocutaneous manifestations.[376–380] The persistence of immunosuppression in HIV-infected children also leads to a high propensity for recurrent infection. As success is achieved in managing HIV-infected children and increased survival is obtained,[381] these children will be placed at increased risk of exposure to a wider range of endemic and nosocomial fungal pathogens.

The emergence of new immunocompromised hosts will also lead to new paradigms of host-pathogen interaction. The recent emergence of invasive aspergillosis in HIV-infected patients reinforced old concepts about this infection and illustrated new dimensions of host susceptibility.[372, 382–386] Other pediatric populations, such as low birth weight infants and neutropenic hosts, will likely continue to present formidable challenges to the management of invasive mycoses, particularly disseminated candidiasis and invasive aspergillosis, respectively.[387–391]

As previously mentioned, there has been a striking increase in the frequency of new and emerging fungal pathogens in immunocompromised hosts.[184, 186, 189, 237, 392] These pathogens are often resistant to conventional antifungal agents and may be difficult to diagnose early in the course of their infection. Such organisms will represent continuing impediments not only of antifungal therapy but of early detection of diagnosis.

Bedside evaluation is fundamental to assessing immunocompromised patients at risk for invasive fungal infections; particular attention is paid to characteristic clinical patterns of infection.[23, 176, 394] Difficulty in early diagnosis coupled with severe immunodeficiency can lead to high mortality and morbidity, as illustrated in deeply invasive candidiasis in HIV-infected children.[58] The development of new blood culture systems, such as the lysis centrifugation and the Bact/Alert methods, have substantially improved the yield and early detection of fungemia compared with older broth techniques.[394–397] Continued technologic advances in blood detection systems should enable earlier recognition of fungemia. However, fungemia may still be a late manifestation of deeply invasive fungal infection, particularly in profoundly immunocompromised hosts.[28] Simple bedside or histologic approaches may permit an early diagnosis[398, 399] but are limited in utility to a small subpopulation of immunocompromised patients.

Newer approaches to nonculture methods of diagnosis of invasive fungal infections may provide important advances in early detection and therapeutic monitoring. For example, detection of biochemically defined antigens, such as *Candida* enolase, mannans, protease, and heat-shock proteins have identified patients with invasive candidiasis early in the course of deep tissue infection and in the absence of fungemia.[400–404] Rapid analytic detection of fungal metabolites or cell wall components are not influenced by host response and may provide a potential means of early detection, as well as therapeutic monitoring.[405, 406] Particularly promising in the early detection of invasive fungal infections is the application of

PCR methodology to the detection of pathogenic fungi in blood and respiratory secretions.[407-409] Further work in characterizing PCR-based systems is required for optimizing sensitivity, specificity, and utility in clinical microbiology laboratories.

Concurrent with the development of new diagnostic systems is the expansion of antifungal drug research aimed at novel targets specific for fungi.[410] During the past decade, considerable advances have been achieved in development and understanding of antifungal triazoles.[411, 412] These agents are being used increasingly with success in management of severe fungal infections in children. Newer more potent and pharmacologically versatile compounds are undergoing early clinical trials. New lipid formulations of amphotericin B have seldom been used in children,[413-415] but experience is continuing to be accrued with these important compounds. Cell wall–active agents may enter clinical studies, pending further laboratory animal studies and resolution of problems of formulations. Although many of these agents may have important therapeutic benefit, antifungal prophylaxis is another strategy for early interdiction of organisms.[416] Although this approach may be feasible in some neutropenic hosts, the emergence of antifungal drug resistance raises ominous questions concerning this approach in HIV-infected and other chronically immunosuppressed patients.

Augmentation of host defense and treatment of the underlying neoplastic disease and resolution of the principal immune impairment is paramount to successful treatment of invasive mycoses in immunocompromised children.[417] The advent of recombinant cytokines offers hope for the prevention and treatment of invasive fungal infections[418]; however, thoughtfully designed and carefully executed clinical trials in children are needed to assess the clinical antimicrobial impact of the agents, particularly against invasive fungal infections.

In summary, given the expanding population of immunocompromised children and HIV-infected children, there is an increasing recognition of the need for early studies of investigational antifungal compounds in children. The urgency of implementation of these compounds in children warrants the simultaneous investigation of new compounds in children, as well as in adults. Such a model has been well demonstrated for antiretroviral drugs in children. Among the new antifungal compounds, such as antifungal triazoles, lipid formulations of amphotericin B, echinocandins, allylamines, and other promising classes of compounds, rationally designed studies will hopefully lead to improved treatment for life-threatening infections. Moreover, the development of recombinant cytokines and the potential application for immune reconstitution with granulocyte transfusions and elutriated monocyte transfusions offer hope that these agents may provide important adjunctive immunotherapy to antifungal chemotherapy.

ACKNOWLEDGMENTS

We thank Patricia Andrews for her excellent secretarial assistance in preparation of this manuscript.

REFERENCES

 1. Leggott P, Robertson P, Greenspan D, et al: Oral manifestations of primary and acquired immunodeficiency diseases in children. *Pediatr Dent* 9:98–104, 1987.
 2. Leggott PJ: Oral manifestations of HIV infection in children. *Oral Surg Oral Med Oral Pathol* 73:187–192, 1992.
 3. Buckley RH: Immunodeficiency diseases. *JAMA* 268:2797–2806, 1992.
 4. Selik R, Starcher E, Curran J: Opportunistic diseases reported in AIDS patients: frequencies, associations, and trends. *AIDS* 1:175–182, 1987.
 5. Walsh TJ, Gray W: *Candida* epiglottitis in immunocompromised patients. *Chest* 91:482–485, 1987.
 6. Balsam D, Sorrano D, Barax C: *Candida* epiglottis presenting as stridor in a child with HIV infection. *Pediatr Radiol* 22:235–236, 1992.
 7. Hass A, Hyatt AC, Kattan M, et al: Hoarseness in immunocompromised children: Association with invasive fungal infection. *J Pediatr* 111:731–733, 1987.
 8. Tashjian LS, Peacock JE Jr: Laryngeal candidiasis. *Arch Otolaryngol* 10:806–809, 1984.
 9. Jacods RF, Yasuda K, Smith AL, et al: Laryngeal candidiasis presenting as inspiratory stridor. *Pediatrics* 69:234–236, 1982.
10. Hay RJ, Clayton YM: Fluconazole in the management of patients with chronic mucocutaneous candidosis [letter]. *Br J Dermatol* 119:683–684, 1988.
11. Hernandez-Sampelayo T: Fluconazole versus ketoconazole in the treatment of oropharyngeal candidiasis in HIV-infected children. *Eur J Clin Microbiol Infect Dis* 13:340–344, 1994.
12. Burke WA: Use of itraconazole in a patient with chronic mucocutaneous candidiasis. *J Am Acad Dermatol* 21:1309–1310, 1989.
13. DePadova-Elder SM, Ditre CM, Kantor GR, et al: Candidiasis endocrinopathy syndrome. Treatment with itraconazole. *Arch Dermatol* 130:19–22, 1994.
14. Kobayashi RH, Rosenblatt HM, Carney JM, et al: *Candida* esophagitis and laryngitis in chronic mucocutaneous candidiasis. *Pediatrics* 66:380–384, 1980.
15. Walsh T, Peter J, Damron S, et al: Emergence of resistance to flucona-

zole in HIV-infected children [abstract]. Paper presented at the Annual Meeting of the Infectious Diseases Society of America, 1994.

16. Kodsi BE, Wickremesinghe PC, Kozinn PJ, et al: *Candida* esophagitis: A prospective study of 27 cases. *Gastroenterology* 71:715–719, 1976.

17. Walsh T, Belitsos N, Hamilton S: Bacterial esophagitis in immunocompromised patients. *Arch Intern Med* 146:1345–1348, 1986.

18. Hoppe JE, Klingebiel T, Niethammer D: Selection of *Candida glabrata* in pediatric bone marrow transplant recipients receiving fluconazole. *Pediatr Hematol Oncol* 11:207–210, 1994.

19. Wingard JR, Merz WG, Rinaldi MG, et al: Increase in *Candida krusei* infection among patients with bone marrow transplantation and neutropenia treated prophylactically with fluconazole. *N Engl J Med* 325:1274–1277, 1991.

20. Alter SJ, Farley J: Development of *Hansenula anomala* infection in a child receiving fluconazole therapy. *Pediatr Infect Dis J* 13:158–159, 1994.

21. DuBois D, van Burik JA, Davis C, et al: Emergence of non-*Candida albicans* fungemia in bone marrow transplant patients receiving flkuconazole prophylaxis. In *Abstract of the 34th ICAAC*. Washington DC, American Society for Microbiology, Abstract no J-6, p 9.

22. Haron E, Vartivarian S, Anaissie E, et al: Primary *Candida* pneumonia. Experience at a large cancer center and review of the literature. *Medicine (Baltimore)* 72:137–142, 1993.

23. Hughes WT: Pneumonia in the immunocompromised child. *Semin Respir Infect* 2:177–183, 1987.

24. Loke HL, Szymonowicz W, Yu VYH: Systemic candidiasis and pneumonia in preterm infants. *Aust Paediatr J* 24:138–142, 1988.

25. Mamlok RJ, Richardson CJ, Mamlok V, et al: A case of intrauterine pulmonary candidiasis. *Pediatr Infect Dis* 4:692–693, 1985.

26. Wey SB, Mori M, Pfaller MA, et al: Risk factors for hospital-acquired candidemia. A matched case-control study. *Arch Intern Med* 149:2349–2353, 1989.

27. Walsh TW, Lyman CA, Pizzo PA: Laboratory diagnosis of invasive fungal infections in patients with neoplastic diseases. *Bailliéres Clin Infect Dis Int Pract Res* (in press).

28. Berenguer J, Buck M, Witebsky F, et al: Lysis-centrifugation blood cultures in the detection of tissue-proven invasive candidiasis: Disseminated versus single organ infection. *Diagn Microbiol Infect Dis* 17:103–1109, 1993.

29. Faix RG: *Candida parapsilosis* meningitis in premature infants. *Pediatr Infect Dis* 2:462–464, 1983.

30. Brooks R: Prospective study of *Candida* endophthalmitis in hospitalized patients with candidemia. *Arch Intern Med* 149:2226–2228, 1989.

31. Dato V, Dajani A: Candidemia in children with central venous catheters: Role of catheter removal and amphotericin B therapy. *Pediatr Infect Dis J* 9:309–314, 1990.

32. Eppes SC, Troutman JL, Gutman LT: Outcome of treatment of candidemia in children whose central catheters were removed or retained. *Pediatr Infect Dis J* 8:99–104, 1989.

33. Weems JJ, Chamberland ME, Ward J, et al: *Candida Parapsilosis* fungemia associated with parenteral nutrition and contaminated blood pressure transducers. *J Clin Microbiol* 25:1029–1032, 1987.

34. Walsh T, Hutchins GM: Postoperative *Candida* infections of the heart in children: Clinicopathologic study of a continuing problem of diagnosis and therapy. *J Pedatri Surg* 15:325–331, 1980.

35. Finkelstein R, Reinhertz G, Hashman N, et al: Outbreak of *Candida tropicalis* fungemia in a neonatal intensive care unit. *Infect Control Hosp Epidemiol* 14:587–590, 1993.

36. Shian W, Chi C, Wang C, et al: Candidemia in the neonatal intensive care unit. *Acta Paediatr Sin* 34:349–355, 1993.

37. Weese-Mayer D, Fondriest DW, Brouillette R, et al: Risks factors associated with candidemia in the neonatal intensive care unit: A case control study. *Pediatr Infect Dis* 6:190–197, 1987.

38. Wiley JM, Smith N, Lenethal B, et al: Invasive fungal disease in pediatric leukemia patients with fever and neutropenia during induction chemotherapy. A multivariate analysis of risk factors. *J Clin Oncol* 8:280–286, 1990.

39. Hughes WT: Systemic candidiasis: A study of 109 fatal cases. *Pediatr Infect Dis J* 1:11–18, 1982.

40. Flynn PM, Marina NM, Rivera GK, et al: *Candida tropicalis* infections in children with leukemia. *Leuk Lymphoma* 10:369–376, 1993.

41. Lecciones JA, Lee JW, Navarro E, et al: Vascular catheter–associated fungemia in cancer patients: analysis of 155 episodes. *Rev Infect Dis* 14:875–883, 1992.

42. Faix R: Invasive neonatal candidiasis: Comparison of *albicans* and *parapsilosis* infection. *Pediatr Infect Dis J* 11:88–93, 1992.

43. Bodey GP, Luna M: Skin lesions associated with disseminated candidiasis. *JAMA* 229:1466–1468, 1974.

44. Jarowski CI, Fialk MA, Murray HW, et al: Fever, rash and muscle tenderness. A distinctive clinical presentation of disseminated candidiasis. *Arch Intern Med* 138:544–546, 1978.

45. Dick JD, Rosenguard BR, Merz WG, et al: Fatal disseminated candidiasis due to amphotericin B–resistant *Candida guilliermondii*. *Ann Intern Med* 102:67–68, 1985.

46. Faix R: Systemic *Candida* infections in infants in intensive care nurseries: High incidence of central nervous system involvement. *J Pediatr* 105:616–622, 1984.

47. Johnson DE, Thompson TR, Green TP, et al: Systemic candidiasis in very low-birth-weight infants (<1500 grams). *Pediatrics* 73:138–143, 1984.

48. Maaksymiuk AW, Thongprasert S, Hopfer R, et al: Systemic candidiasis in cancer patients. *Am J Med* 77(suppl):20–27, 1984.

49. Tashjian LS, Abramson JS, Peacock JE Jr: Focal hepatic candidiasis: A distinct clinical variant of candidiasis in immunocompromised patients. *Rev Infect Dis* 6:689–703, 1984.
50. Miller JH, Greenfield LD, Wald BR: Candidiasis of the liver and spleen in childhood. *Radiology* 142:375–380, 1982.
51. Thaler M, Pastakia B, Shawker TH, et al: Hepatic candidiasis in cancer patients: The evolving picture of the syndrome. *Ann Intern Med* 108:88–100, 1988.
52. Rex JH, Bennett JE, Sugar AM, et al: A randomized trial comparing fluconazole with amphotericin B for the treatment of candidemia in patients without neutropenia. *N Engl J Med* 331:1325–1330, 1994.
53. Faix R, Feick H, Frommelt P, et al: Successful medical treatment of *Candida parapsilosis* endocarditis in a premature infant. *Am J Perinatol* 7:272–275, 1990.
54. El-Mohandes AE, Johnson-Robbins L, Keiser JF, et al: Incidence of *Candida parapsilosis* colonization in an intensive care nursery population and its association with invasive fungal disease. *Pediatr Infect Dis J* 13D:520–524, 1994.
55. Walsh TJ, Merz W: Pathologic features in the human alimentary tract associated with invasiveness of *Candida tropicalis*. *Am J Clin Pathol* 85:498–502, 1986.
56. Malfroot A, Verboven M, Levy J, et al: Suppurative thrombophlebitis with sepsis due to *Candida albicans*: An unusual complication of intravenous therapy in cystic fibrosis. *Pediatr Infect Dis* 5:376–377, 1986.
57. Walsh TJ, Bustamente C, Vlahov D, et al: *Candida* suppurative peripheral thrombophlebitis: Prevention, recognition and management. *Infect Control* 7:16–22, 1986.
58. Leibovitz E, Rigaud M, Chandwani S, et al: Disseminated fungal infections in children infected with human immunodeficiency virus. *Pediatr Infect Dis J* 10:888–894, 1991.
59. Walsh TJ, Gonzalez C, Roilides E, et al: Fungemia in HIV-infected children: New epidemiologic patterns, emerging pathogens, and improved antifungal outcome. *Clin Infect Dis* (in press).
60. Ashkenazi S, Pickering LK, Robinson LH: Diagnosis and management of septic thrombosis of the inferior vena cava caused by *Candida tropicalis*. *Pediatr Infect Dis J* 9:446–447, 1990.
61. Christenson JC, Guruswamy A, Mukwaya G, et al: *Candida lusitaniae:* An emerging human pathogen. *Pediatr Infect Dis J* 6:755–757, 1987.
62. Merz WG: *Candida lusitaniae:* Frequency of recovery, colonization, infection, and amphotericin B resistance. *J Clin Microbiol* 20:1194–1195, 1984.
63. Yinnon AM, Woodin KA, Powell KR: *Candida lusitaniae* infection in the newborn: Case report and review of the literature. *Pediatr Infect Dis J* 11:878–880, 1992.
64. Yagupsky P, Dagan R, Chipman M et al: Pseudooutbreak of *Candida*

guilliermondii fungemia in a neonatal intensive care unit. *Pediatr Infect Dis J* 10:928–932, 1991.

65. Dick JD, Rosenguard BR, Merz WG, et al: Fatal disseminated candidiasis due to amphotericin B resistant *Candida guilliermondii*. *Ann Intern Med* 102:67–68, 1985.

66. Tam JY, Blume KG, Prober CG: Prophylactic fluconazole and *Candida krusei* infections [letter]. *N Engl J Med* 326:891, 1992.

67. Glick C, Graves G, Feldman S: *Torulopsis glabrata* in the neonate: An emerging fungal pathogen. *South Med J* 86:969–970, 1993.

68. Quirke P, Hwang WS, Validen CC: Congenital *Torulopsis glabrata* infection. *Am J Clin Pathol* 73:137–140, 1980.

69. Walter EB, Gingras JL, McKinney RE: Systemic *Torulopsis glabrata* infection in a neonate. *South Med J* 86:837–838, 1990.

70. Walsh TJ, Salkin I, Dixon DM, et al: *Candida lipolytica*. Clinical, microbiological, and animal studies. *J Clin Microbiol* 27:927–931, 1989.

71. Butler K, Baker C: *Candida*: An increasingly important pathogen in the nursery. *Pediatr Clin North Am* 35:543–563, 1988.

72. Kauffman CA, Bradley SF, Ross SC, et al: Hepatosplenic candidiasis: Successful treatment with fluconazole. *Am J Med* 91:137–141, 1991.

73. Anaissie E, Bodey GP, Kantarjian H, et al: Fluconazole therapy for chronic disseminated candidiasis in patients with leukemia and prior amphotericin B therapy. *Am J Med* 91:142–150, 1991.

74. Walsh TJ, Whitcomb P, Ravankar S, et al: Successful treatment of hepatosplenic candidiasis during repeated episodes of neutropenia. In *Program and Abstracts of the 33rd Intersci Conf Antimicrob Agents Chemother*. Washington DC, American Society for Microbiology, abstract no 809, 1993.

75. Schwartz DA, Reef S: *Candida albicans* placentitis and funisitis: Early diagnosis of congenital candidemia by histopathologic examination of umbilical cord vessels. *Pediatr Infect Dis J* 9:661–665, 1990.

76. Baley JE, Kliegeman RJ, Fanaroff A: Disseminated fungal infections in very low-birth-weight infants: Clinical manifestations and epidemiology. *Pediatrics* 73:144–152, 1984.

77. Baley JE, Kliegman RM, Fanaroff AA: Disseminated fungal infections in very low-weight infants: Therapeutic toxicity. *Pediatrics* 73:153–157, 1984.

78. Johnson DE, Bass JL, Thompson TR, et al: *Candida septicemia* and right atrial mass secondary to umbilical vein catheterization. *Am J Dis Child* 135:275–277, 1981.

79. Johnson DE, Conroy MM, Thompson TR, et al: *Candida* peritonitis in the newborn infant. *Pediatrics* 97:298–300, 1980.

80. Johnson DE, Thompson TR, Ferrieri P: Congenital candidiasis. *Am J Dis Child* 135:273–275, 1981.

81. Smith H, Congdon P: Neonatal systemic candidiasis. *Arch Dis Child* 60:365–369, 1985.

82. Conway SP, Dear PRF, Smith I: Immunoglobulin profile of the preterm baby. *Arch Dis Child* 60:208–212, 1985.
83. Xanthou M, Valassi-Adam E, Kintzonidou E, et al: Phagocytosis and killing ability of *Candida albicans* by blood leukocytes of healthy term and preterm babies. *Arch Dis Child* 50:72–75, 1975.
84. Ho NK: Systemic candidiasis in premature infants. *Aust Pediatr J* 20:127–130, 1984.
85. Karlowicz MG: Risk factors associated with fungal peritonitis in very low birth weight neonates with severe necrotizing enterocolitis: A case-control study. *Pediatr Infect Dis J* 12:574–577, 1993.
86. Kaplan M, Eidelman A, Dollberg L, et al: Necrotizing bowel disease with *Candida* peritonitis following severe neonatal hypothermia. *Acta Pediatr Scand* 79:876–879, 1990.
87. Glick C, Graves G, Feldman S: Neonatal fungemia and amphotericin B. *South Med J* 86:1368–1371, 1993.
88. Butler KM, Rench MA, Baker CJ: Amphotericin B as a single agent in the treatment of systemic candidiasis in neonates. *Pediatr Infect Dis J* 9:51–56, 1990.
89. Bhandari V, Narang A: Oral itraconazole therapy for disseminated candidiasis in low birth weight infants [letter]. *J Pediatr* 120:330, 1992.
90. Viscoli C, Castagnola E, Corsini M, et al: Fluconazole therapy in an underweight infant. *Eur J Microbiol Infect Dis* 8:925–926, 1993.
91. Saxen H, Hoppu K, Pohjavuori M: Pharmacokinetics of fluconazole in very low birth weight infants during the first two weeks of life. *Clin Pharmacol Ther* 54:269–277, 1993.
92. Deleted in proofs.
93. Epelbaum S, Laurent C, Morin G, et al: Failure of fluconazole treatment in *Candida* meningitis [letter]. *J Pediatr* 123:168–169, 1993.
94. Fasano C, O'Keeffe J, Gibbs D: Fluconazole treatment of neonates and infants with severe fungal infections not treatable with conventional agents. *Eur J Clin Microbiol Infect Dis* 13:351–354, 1994.
95. Lackner H, Schwinger W, Urban C, et al: Liposomal amphotericin B (AmBisome) for treatment of disseminated fungal infections in two infants of very low weight. *Pediatrics* 89:1259–1261, 1992.
96. Betremieux P, Chevrier S, Quindos G, et al: Use of DNA fingerprinting and biotyping methods to study a *Candida albicans* outbreak in a neonatal intensive care unit. *Pediatr Infect Dis J* 13:899–905, 1994.
97. Eisenberg ES, Leviton I, Soeiro R: Fungal peritonitis in patients receiving peritoneal dialysis: Experience with 11 patients and review of the literature. *Rev Infect Dis* 8:309–321, 1986.
98. McClung MR: Peritonitis in children receiving continuous ambulatory peritoneal dialysis. *Pediatr Infect Dis J* 2:328–332, 1983.
99. Oh SH, Conley SB, Rose GM, et al: Fungal peritonitis in children undergoing peritoneal dialysis. *Pediatr Infect Dis* 4:62–66, 1985.
100. Tapson JS, Mansy H, Freeman R, et al: The high morbidity of CAPD fungal peritonitis—description of 10 cases and review of treatment strategies. *Q J Med New S* 61:1047–1053, 1986.

101. Johnson RJ, Blair AD, Ahmad S: Ketoconazole kinetics in chronic peritoneal dialysis. *Clin Pharmacol Ther* 37:325–329, 1985.
102. Reuman PD, Neiberger R, Kondor DA: Intraperritoneal and intravenous fluconazole pharmacokinetics in a pediatric patient with end state renal disease. *Pediatr Infect Dis J* 11:132–133, 1992.
103. Buchs S: *Candida* meningitis: A growing threat to premature and full-term infants. *Pediatr Infect Dis* 4:122–291, 1985.
104. Walsh TJ, Hier DB, Caplan LR: Fungal infections of the central nervous system: Analysis of risk factors and clinical manifestations. *Neurology* 35:1654–1657, 1985.
105. Leggiadro RJ, Collins T: Postneurosurgical *Candida lusitaniae* meningitis. *Pediatr Infect Dis J* 7:368–369, 1988.
106. Chiou C, Wong T, Lin H, et al: Fungal infection of ventriculoperitoneal shunts in children. *Clin Infect Dis* 19:1049–1053, 1994.
107. Sanchez P, Cooper B: *Candida lusitaniae:* Sepsis and meningitis in a neonate. *Pediatr Infect Dis J* 6:758–759, 1987.
108. Byers M, Chapman S, Feldman S, et al: Fluconazole pharmacokinetics in the cerebrospinal fluid of a child with *Candida tropicalis* meningitis. *Pediatr Infect Dis* 11:895–896, 1992.
109. Walsh TJ, Lee JW, Seibel N, et al: Failure of fluconazole treatment in *Candida* meningitis. *J Pediatr* 123:168–169, 1993.
110. Oleinik E, Della-Latta P, Rinaldi M, et al: *Candida lusitaniae* osteomyelitis in a premature infant. *Am J Perinatol* 10:313–315, 1993.
111. Poplack DG, Jacobs SA: *Candida* arthritis treated with amphotericin B. *J Pediatr* 87:989–900, 1975.
112. Johnston P, Lee J, Demanski M, et al: Late recurrent *Candida* endocarditis. *Chest* 99:1531–1533, 1991.
113. Sanchez PJ, Siegel JD, Fishbein J: *Candida* endocarditis: Successful medical management in three preterm infants and review of the literature. *Pediatr Infect Dis J* 10:239–243, 1991.
114. Edwards JE Jr: *Candida* endophthalmitis. In Bodey GP, Fainstein V (eds): *Candidiasis.* New York, Raven Press, 1985, 211–225.
115. Annable WL, Kachmer ML, De Santis D: Long term follow-up of *Candida* endophthalmitis in th premature infants. *J Pediatr Ophthalmol Strabismus* 27:103–106, 1990.
116. Panos R, Barr L, Walsh TJ, et al: Factors associated with fatal hemoptysis in cancer patients. *Chest* 94:1008–1013, 1988.
117. Ricketti AJ, Greenberger PA, Mintzer RA, et al: Allergic bronchopulmonary aspergillosis. *Arch Intern Med* 143:1553, 1983.
118. Laufer P, Fink JN, Bruns WT, et al: Allergic bronchopulmonary aspergillosis in cystic fibrosis. *J Allerg Clin Immunol* 73:44, 1984.
119. Glimp RA, Bayer AS: Pulmonary aspergilloma: Diagnostic and therapeutic considerations. *Arch Intern Med* 143:303, 1983.
120. Nime FA, Hutchins GM: Oxalosis caused by *Aspergillus* infection. *Johns Hopkins Med J* 113:183–194, 1973.
121. Walsh T, Hutchins GM: Metabolite in diagnosis of pulmonary as-

pergillosis and oxalic acid factor. *Am Rev Resp in Dis* 121:190–191, 1980.

122. Dupon B: Itraconazole/aspergilloma.
123. Barson WJ, Ruymann FB: Palmar aspergillosis in immunocompromised children. *Pediatr Infect Dis* 5:264–268, 1986.
124. Berkow RL, Weisman SJ, Provisor AJ, et al: Invasive aspergillosis of paranasal tissues in children with malignancies. *J Pediatr* 103:49–53, 1983.
125. Flynn PM, Magill HL, Jenkins JJ, et al: *Aspergillus* osteomyelitis in a child treated for acute lymphoblastic leukemia. *Pediatr Infect Dis J* 9:733–736, 1990.
126. Gerson SL, Talbot GH, Hurwitz S, et al: Prolonged granulocytopenia: The major risk factor for invasive pulmonary aspergillosis in patients with acute leukemia. *Ann Intern Med* 100:345, 1984.
127. Grossman ME, Fithian EC, Behrens C, et al: Primary cutaneous aspergillosis in six leukemic children. *J Am Acad Dermatol* 12:313–318, 1985.
128. Meyer RD, Young LS, Armstrong D, et al: Aspergillosis complicating neoplastic disease. *Am J Med* 54:6, 1973.
129. Walsh TJ: Invasive pulmonary aspergillosis in patients with neoplastic diseases. *Semin Respir Infect* 5:111–122, 1990.
130. Prystowsky SD, Vogelstein B, Ettinger DS, et al: Invasive aspergillosis. *N Engl J Med* 295:655, 1976.
131. Pervez N, Kleinerman J, Kattan M, et al: Pseudomembranous necrotizing bronchial aspergillosis. A variant of invasive aspergillosis in patient with hemophilia and acquired immune deficiency syndrome. *Am J Med* 131:961, 1985.
132. Spencer DA, John P, Ferryman SR, et al: Successful treatment of invasive pulmonary aspergillosis in chronic granulomatous disease with orally administered itraconazole suspension. *Am J Respir Crit Care Med* 149:239–241, 1994.
133. Walsh TJ, Caplan LR, Hier DB: *Aspergillus* infections of the central nervous system: A clinicopathological analysis. *Ann Neurol* 18:574–582, 1985.
134. Buffington J, Reporter R, Lasker BA, et al: Investigation of an epidemic of invasive aspergillosis: Utility of molecular typing with the use of random amplified polymorphic DNA probes. *Pediatr Infect Dis J* 13:386–393, 1994.
135. Meis JF, Donnelly JP, Hoogkamp-Korstanje JA, et al: *Aspergillus fumigatus* pneumonia in neutropenic patients during therapy with fluconazole for infection due to *Candida* species [letter]. *Clin Infect Dis* 16:734–735, 1993.
136. Yu VL, Muder RR, Poorsattar A: Significance of isolation of *Aspergillus* from the respiratory tract in diagnosis of invasive pulmonary aspergillosis. Results of a three-year prospective study. *Am J Med* 81:249, 1986.

137. Lehrerr RI, Ganz T, Selsted ME, et al: Neutrophils and host defense. *Ann Intern Med* 109:127, 1988.

138. Quie PG: Chronic granulomatous disease of childhood: A saga of discovery and understanding. *Pediatr Infect Dis J* 12:395–398, 1993.

139. Gallin JI: Phagocytic cells: Disorders of function. In Gallin JI, Goldstein JM, Snyderman R (eds): *Inflammation: Basic Principles and Clinical Correlates*. New York, Raven Press, 1988, p 493.

140. Baehner RL, Nathan DG: Quantitative nitroblue tetrazolium test in chronic granulomatous disease. *N Engl J Med* 278:971, 1968.

141. Schoumacher RA, Berkow RL: Invasive pulmonary aspergillosis in an infant: An unusual presentation of chronic granulomatous disease. *Pediatr Infect Dis J* 6:215–216, 1987.

142. Rowen JL, Correa AG, Sokol DM, et al: Invasive aspergillosis in neonates: report of five cases and literature review. *Pediatr Infect Dis J* 11:576–582, 1992.

143. Schwartz DA, Jacquette M, Chawla HS: Disseminated neonatal aspergillosis: Report of a fatal case and analysis of risk factors. *Pediatr Infect Dis J* 7:349–353, 1988.

144. Mangurten HH, Fernandez B: Neonatal aspergillosis accompanying fulminant necrotising enterocolitis. *Arch Dis Child* 54:559–562, 1979.

145. Walsh TJ, Pizzo PA: Nosocomial fungal infections. *Ann Rev Microbiol* 42:517–545, 1988.

146. Walsh TJ, Dixon DM: Nosocomial aspergillosis: Environmental microbiology, hospital epidemiology, diagnosis, and treatment. *Eur J Epidemiol* 5:131–142, 1989.

147. Schaffner A, Douglas H, Braude A: Selective protection against conidia by mononuclear and against mycelia by polymorphonuclear phagocytes in resistance to *Aspergillus*. *J Clin Invest* 69:617, 1982.

148. Diamond RD, Krzesicki R, Epstein B, et al: Damage to hyphal forms of fungi by human leukocytes in vitro. *Am J Pathol* 91:313, 1978.

149. Dixon DM, Polak A, Walsh TJ: Fungus dose-dependent primary pulmonary aspergillosis in immunosuppressed mice. *Infect Immun* 57:1452–1456, 1989.

150. Walsh TJ, Bulkley BH: Aspergillus pericarditis: Clinical and pathological features in the immunocompromised patient. *Cancer* 49:48–54, 1982.

151. Kuhlman JE, Fishman EK, Burch PA, et al: Invasive pulmonary aspergillosis in acute leukemia. The contribution of CT to early diagnosis and aggressive management. *Chest* 92:95–99, 1987.

152. Barloon TJ, Galvin JR, Mori M, et al: High-resolution ultrafast chest CT in the clinical management of febrile bone marrow transplant patients with normal or nonspecific roentgenograms. *Chest* 99:928–933, 1991.

153. Kahn FW, Jones JM, England DM: The role of bronchoalveolar lavage in the diagnosis of invasive pulmonary aspergillosis. *Am J Clin Pathol* 86:518, 1986.

154. Albelda SM, Talbot GH, Gerson SL, et al: Role of fiberoptic broncho-
     scopy in the diagnosis of invasive pulmonary aspergillosis in patients
     with acute leukemia. *Am J Med* 76:1027, 1984.
155. Saito H, Anaissie EJ, Morice RC, et al: Bronchoalveolar lavage in the
     diagnosis of pulmonary infiltrates in patients with acute leukemia.
     Chest 94:745−749, 1988.
156. Dupont B, Huber M, Kim SJ, et al: Galactomannan antigenemia and
     antigenuria in aspergillosis: Studies in patients with experimentally
     infected rabbits. *J Infect Dis* 155:1, 1987.
157. Francis P, Lee JW, Hoffman A, et al: Efficacy of unilamellar liposomal
     amphotericin B in treatment of pulmonary aspergillosis in persistently
     granulocytopenic rabbits: The potential role of bronchoalveolar lavage
     D-mannitol and galactomannan as markers of infection. *J Infect Dis*
     169:356−368, 1994.
158. Andriole VT, Miniter P, George D, et al: Animal models: Usefulness
     for studies of fungal pathogenesis and drug efficacy in aspergillosis.
     Clin Infect Dis 14(suppl):S134−S138, 1992.
159. Patterson TF, Miniter P, Dijkstra J, et al: Treatment of experimental
     invasive aspergillosis with novel amphotericin B/cholesterol-sulfate
     complexes. *J Infect Dis* 159:717−724, 1989.
160. Tang CM, Holden DW, Aufauvre-Brown A, et al: The detection of *As-
     pergillus* spp. by the polymerase chain reaction and its elevation in
     bronchoalveolar lavage fluid. *Am Rev Respir Dis* 148:1313−1317,
     1993.
161. Aisner J, Schimpff SC, Wiernik PH: Treatment of invasive aspergillo-
     sis: Relationship of early diagnosis and treatment to response. *Ann
     Intern Med* 86:539, 1977.
162. Burch PA, Karp JE, Merz WG, et al: Favorable outcome of invasive
     aspergillosis in patients with acute leukemia. *J Clin Oncol* 5:1985−
     1993, 1987.
163. Karp JE, Burch PA, Merz WG: An approach to intensive antileukemia
     therapy in patients with previous invasive aspergillosis. *Am J Med*
     85:203−206, 1988.
164. George D, Kordick D, Miniter P, et al: Combination therapy in experi-
     mental invasive aspergillosis. *J Infect Dis* 168:692−698, 1993.
165. Francis P, Walsh TJ: The evolving role in flucytosine in immunocom-
     promised patients: New insights into safety, pharmacokinetics, and
     antifungal therapy. *Rev Infect Dis* 15:1003−1018, 1992.
166. Cauwenbergh G, DeDoncker P, Stoops K, et al: Itraconazole in the
     treatment of human mycoses: Review of three years of clinical expe-
     rience. *Rev Infect Dis* 9(suppl 1):S146−S152, 1987.
167. Denning DW, Lee JY, Hostetler JS, et al: NIAID mycoses study group
     multicenter trial of oral itraconazole therapy for invasive aspergillo-
     sis. *Am J Med* 97:135−144, 1994.
168. Moore L, Ellis DH, Suppiah R, et al: Complete eradication of *Aspergil-
     lus fumigatus* from the lung in an immunocompromised patient by
     oral itraconazole. *J Paediatr Child Health* 29:141−143, 1993.

169. Neijens HJ, Frenkel J, de Muinck Keizer-Schrama SM, et al: Invasive *Aspergillus* infection in chronic granulomatous disease: Treatment with itraconazole. *J Pediatr* 115:1016–1019, 1989.

170. Odds FC: Itraconazole—a new oral antifungal agent with a very broad spectrum of activity in superficial and systemic mycoses. *J Dermatol Sci* 5:65–72, 1993.

171. Viviani MA, Tortorano AM, Pagano A, et al: European experience with itraconazole in systemic mycoses. *J Am Acad Dermatol* 23:587–593, 1990.

172. Vreugdenhil G, Van Dijke BJ, Donnelly JP, et al: Efficacy of itraconazole in the prevention of fungal infections among neutropenic patients with hematological malignancies and intensive chemotherapy. A double blind, placebo controlled study. *Leuk Lymphoma* 11:353–358, 1993.

173. Boogaerts MA, Verhoef GE, Zachee P, et al: Antifungal prophylaxis with itraconazole in prolonged neutropenia: Correlation with plasma levels. *Mycoses* 32(suppl 1):103–108, 1989.

174. Rajasekaran J, Thomas PA, Kalavathy CM, et al: Itraconazole therapy for fungal keratitis. *Indian J Ophthalmol* 35:157–160, 1987.

175. Denning DW, Stevens DA: Antifungal and surgical treatment of invasive aspergillosis: Review of 2,121 cases. *Rev Infect Dis* 12:1147–1201, 1990.

176. Pizzo PA, Walsh TJ: Fungal infections in the pediatric cancer patient. *Semin Oncol* 17(suppl):6–9, 1990.

177. Gallin JI, Malech HL, Melnick DA, et al: A controlled trial of interferon gamma to prevent infection in chronic granulomatous disease. The International Chronic Granulomatous Diseases Study Group. *N Engl J Med* 324:509–516, 1991.

178. Rex JH, Bennett JE, Gallin JI, et al: In vivo interferon gamma therapy augments the in vivo ability of chronic granulomatous disease neutrophils to damage *Aspergillus* hyphae. *J Infect Dis* 163:849–852, 1991.

179. Walsh TJ, Rinaldi MG, Pizzo PA: Zygomycosis of the respiratory tract. In Sarosi G, Davies S: *Fungal Diseases of the Lung*, ed 2. New York, Raven Press, 1993, pp 149–170.

180. Kline MW: Mucormycosis in children: Review of the literature and report of cases. *Pediatr Infect Dis* 4:672–676, 1985.

181. Lewis LL, Hawkings HK, Edwards MS: Disseminated mucormycosis in an infant with methylmalonicaciduria. *Pediatr Infect Dis J* 9:851–854, 1990.

182. Grim PF, Demello D, Keenan WJ: Disseminated zygomycosis in a newborn. *Pediatr Infect Dis* 3:61–63, 1984.

183. Chaulk CP, Smith PW, Feagler JR, et al: Fungemia due to *Fusarium solani* in an immunocompromised child. *Pediatr Infect Dis* 5:363–366, 1986.

184. Anaissie E, Bodey GP, Kantarjian H, et al: New spectrum of fungal infections in patients with cancer. *Rev Infect Dis* 11:369–378, 1989.

185. Anaissie E, Kantarjian H, Ro J, et al: The emerging role of *Fusarium* infections in patients with cancer. *Medicine (Baltimore)* 67:77–83, 1988.
186. Martino P, Gastaldi R, Raccah R, et al: Clinical patterns of *Fusarium* infections in immunocompromised patients. *J Infect* 28(suppl 1):7–15, 1994.
187. Merz W, Karp J, Hoagland M, et al: Diagnosis and successful treatment of fusariosis in the compromised host. *J Infect Dis* 158:1046–1055, 1988.
188. Anaissie EJ, Kontoyiannis DP, Vartivarian S, et al: Effectiveness of an oral triazole for opportunistic mold infections in patients with cancer: experience with SCH 39304. *Clin Infect Dis* 17:1022–1031, 1993.
189. Matsumoto T, Ajello L, Matsuda T, et al: Recent developments in phaeohyphomycosis and hyalohyphomycosis. *J Med Vet Mycol* (in press).
190. Berry AJ, Kerkering TM, Giordano AM, et al: Phaeohyphomycotic sinusitis. *Pediatr Infect Dis* 3:150–152, 1984.
191. Dixon DM, Walsh TJ, Merz WG, et al: Human central nervous system infections due to *Xylohypha bantiana (Cladosporium trichoides)*. *Rev Infect Dis* 11:515–525, 1989.
192. Berenguer J, Diaz-Mediavilla J, Urra D, et al: Central nervous system infection caused by *Pseudallescheria boydii*. Case report and review. *Rev Infect Dis* 11:890–896, 1990.
193. Galgiani JN, Stevens DA, Graybill JR, et al: *Pseudallescheria boydii* infections treated with ketoconazole. Clinical evaluations of seven patients and *in vitro* susceptibility results. *Chest* 86:219–224, 1984.
194. Hachimi-Drissi S, Willemsen M, Desprechins B, et al: *Pseudallescheria boydii* and brain abscesses. *Pediatr Infect Dis J* 9:737–741, 1990.
195. Welty FK, McLeod GX, Ezratty C, et al: *Pseudallescheria boydii* endocarditis of the pulmonic valve in a liver transplant recipient. *Clin Infect Dis* 15:858–860, 1992.
196. Travis LB, Roberts GD, Wilson WR: Clinical significance of *Pseudallescheria boydii*: A review of 10 years' experience. *Mayo Clin Proc* 60:531–537, 1985.
197. Piper JP, Golden J, Brown D, et al: Successful treatment of *Scedosporium apiospermum* suppurative arthritis with itraconazole. *Pediatr Infect Dis J* 9:674–675, 1990.
198. Walsh TJ, Peter J, McGough DA, et al: Activity of amphotericin B and antifungal azoles alone and in combination against *Pseudallescheria boydii*. *Antimicrob Agents Chemother* (in press).
199. Wood GM, McCormack JG, Muir DB, et al: Clinical features of human infection with *Scedosporium inflatum*. *Clin Infect Dis* 14:1027–1033, 1992.
200. Sharkey K, Graybill JR, Rinaldi MG, et al: Itraconazole treatment of phaeohyphomycosis. *J Am Acad Dermatol* 23:577–586, 1990.
201. Walsh TJ, Mitchell T, Larone DH: *Histoplasma, Blastomyces, Coccid-*

ioides, and other dimorphic fungi causing systemic mycoses. In *Manual of Clinical Microbiology,* ed 6. Washington, DC, American Society for Microbiology, Chapter 62 (in press).

202. Wheat LJ: Systemic fungal infections: Diagnosis and treatment: I. Histoplasmosis. *Infect Dis Clin North Am* 2:841–859, 1988.

203. Leggiadro RJ, Barrett FF, Hughes WT: Disseminated histoplasmosis of infancy. *Pediatr Infect Dis J* 7:799–805, 1988.

204. Steele CJ, Kleiman MB: Disseminated histoplasmosis, hypercalcemia and failure to thrive. *Pediatr Infect Dis J* 13:421–422, 1994.

205. Schutze GE, Tucker NC, Jacobs RF: Histoplasmosis and perinatal human immunodeficiency virus [letter]. *Pediatr Infect Dis J* 11:501–502, 1992.

206. Byers M, Feldman S, Edwards J: Disseminated histoplasmosis as the acquired immunodeficiency syndrome-defining illness in an infant. *Pediatr Infect Dis J* 11:127–128, 1992.

207. Fojtasek MF, Kleiman MB, Connolly-Stringfield P, et al: The *Histoplasma capsulatum* antigen assay in disseminated histoplasmosis in children. *Pediatr Infect Dis J* 13:801–805, 1994.

208. Einstein HE, Johnson RH: Coccidioidomycosis: New aspects of epidemiology and therapy. *Clin Infect Dis* 16:349–356, 1993.

209. Golden SE, Morgan CM, Bartley DL, et al: Disseminated coccidioidomycosis with chorioretinitis in early infancy. *Pediatr Infect Dis* 5:272–274, 1986.

210. MacDonald N, Steinhoff MC, Powell KR: Review of coccidioidomycosis in immunocompromised children. *Am J Dis Child* 135:553–556, 1981.

211. O'Brien JJ, Gilsdorf JR: Primary cutaneous coccidioidomycosis in children. *Pediatr Infect Dis* 5:485–486, 1986.

212. Harrison H, Galgiani J, Reynolds A, et al: Amphotericin B and imidazole therapy of coccidioidal meningitis in children. *Pediatr Infect Dis* 2:216–221, 1983.

213. Shehab ZM, Britton H, Dunn JH: Imidazole therapy of coccidioidal meningitis in children. *Pediatr Infect Dis J* 7:440–444, 1988.

214. Galgiani JN, Catanzaro A, Cloud GA, et al: Fluconazole therapy for coccidioidal meningitis. The NIAID-Mycoses Study Group. *Ann Intern Med* 119:28–35, 1993.

215. Hughes WT, Franco S, Oh MHK: Systemic blastomycosis in childhood. *Clin Pediatr* 8:597–601, 1969.

216. Steele RW, Abernathy RS: Systemic blastomycosis in children. *Pediatr Infect Dis* 2:304–307, 1983.

217. Klein BS, Vergeront JM, Weeks RJ, et al: Isolation of *Blastomyces dermatitidis* in soil associated with a large outbreak of blastomycosis in Wisconsin. *N Engl J Med* 314:529–534, 1986.

218. Chesney JC, Gourley GR, Peters ME, et al: Pulmonary blastomycosis in children. *Am J Dis Child* 133:1134–1139, 1979.

219. Watts EA, Gard PD, Tuthill SW: First reported case of intrauterine transmission of blastomycosis. *Pediatr Infect Dis* 2:308–310, 1983.

220. Dismukes WE, Stamm AM, Graybill JR, et al: Treatment of systemic mycoses with ketoconazole: Emphasis on toxicity and clinical responsiveness. *Ann Intern Med* 98:13–20, 1983.

221. Bradsher RW: Blastomycosis: Fungal infections of the lung update: 1989. *Semin Respir Infect* 5:105–110, 1990.

222. Sirisanthana V, Sirisanthana T: *Penicillium marneffei* infection in children infected with human immunodeficiency virus. *Pediatr Infect Dis J* 12:1021–1025, 1993.

223. Supparatpinyo K, Khamwan C, Baosoung V, et al: Disseminated *Penicillium marneffei* infection in southeast Asia. *Lancet* 344:110–113, 1994.

224. Supparatpinyo K, Chiewchanvit S, Hirunsri P, et al: An efficacy study of itraconazole in the treatment of *Penicillium marneffei* infection. *J Med Assoc Thai* 75:688–691, 1992.

225. Restrepo A: Treatment of sporotrichosis with itraconazole.

226. Leggiadro R, Barrett F, Hughes W: Extrapulmonary cryptococcosis in immunocompromised infants and children. *Pediatr Infect Dis J* 11:43–47, 1992.

227. Leggiadro R, Kline M, Hughes W: Extrapulmonary cryptococcosis in children with acquired immunodeficiency syndrome. *Pediatr Infect Dis J* 10:658–662, 1991.

228. Cohen I: Isolated pulmonary cryptococcosis in a young adolescent. *Pediatr Infect Dis* 4:416–418, 1985.

229. Allende M, Horowitz M, Pass HI, et al: Pulmonary cryptococcosis presenting as metastases in children with sarcoma. *Pediatr Infect Dis J* 12:240–243, 1993.

230. Pippard M, Dalgleish A, Gibson P, et al: Acquired immunodeficiency with disseminated cryptococcosis. *Arch Dis Child* 61:289–302, 1986.

231. Baldwin S, Stagno S, Odrezin GT, et al: Isolated *Cryptococcus neoformans* osteomyelitis in an immunocompetent child. *Pediatr Infect Dis J* 7:289–292, 1988.

232. Powderly WG, Saag MS, Cloud GA, et al: A controlled trial of fluconazole or amphotericin B to prevent relapse of cryptococcal meningitis in patients with the acquired immunodeficiency syndrome. *N Engl J Med* 326:793–798, 1992.

233. Zuger A, Louie E, Holzman R, et al: Cryptococcal disease in patients with the acquired immunodeficiency syndrome. Diagnostic features and outcome of treatment. *Ann Intern Med* 104:234–240, 1986.

234. Moncino MD, Gutman LT: Severe systemic cryptococcal disease in a child: Review of prognostic indicators predicting treatment failure and an approach to maintenance therapy with oral fluconazole. *Pediatr Infect Dis J* 9:363–368, 1990.

235. Walsh TJ, Newman KR, Moody M, et al: Trichosporonosis in patients with neoplastic disease. *Medicine (Baltimore)* 65:268–279, 1986.

236. Hoy J, Hsu KC, Rolston K, et al: *Trichosporon beigelii* infection: A review. *Rev Infect Dis* 8:959–967, 1986.

237. Walsh TJ, Melcher GP, Rinaldi MG, et al: *Trichosporon beigelii,* an emerging pathogen resistant to amphotericin B. *J Clin Microbiol* 28:1616–1622, 1990.
238. Apaliski SJ, Moore MD, Reiner BJ, et al: Disseminated *Trichosporon beigelii* in an immunocompromised child. *Pediatr Infect Dis* 3:451–454, 1984.
239. Evans HL, Kletzel M, Lawson RD, et al: Systemic mycosis due to *Trichosporon cutaneum:* A report of two additional cases. *Cancer* 45:367, 1980.
240. Rivera R, Cangir A: *Trichosporon* sepsis and leukeima. *Cancer* 36:1106, 1975.
241. del Palacio A, Perez-Revilla A, Albanil R, et al: Disseminated neonatal trichosporonosis associated with hemophagocytic syndrome. *Pediatr Infect Dis J* 9:520–522, 1990.
242. Fisher DJ, Christy C, Spafford P, et al: Neonatal *Trichosporon beigelii* infection: Report of a cluster of cases in a neonatal intensive care unit. *Pediatr Infect Dis J* 12:149–155, 1993.
243. Henwick S, Henrickson S, Storgion SA, et al: Disseminated neonatal *Trichosporon beigelii. Pediatr Infect Dis J* 11:50–52, 1992.
244. Walsh TJ, Melcher G, Rinaldi M, et al: *Trichosporon beigelii:* An emerging pathogen resistant to amphotericin B. *J Clin Microbiol* 28:1616–1622, 1990.
245. Walsh TJ, Lee JW, Melcher GP, et al: Experimental disseminated trichosporonosis in persistently granulocytopenic rabbits: Implications for pathogenesis, diagnosis, and treatment of an emerging opportunistic infection. *J Infect Dis* 166:121–133, 1992.
246. Anaissie E, Gokaslan A, Hachem R, et al: Azole therapy for trichosporonosis: Clinical evaluation of eight patients, experimental therapy for murine infection, and review. *Clin Infect Dis* 15:781–787, 1992.
247. Lyman CA, Garrett KF, Pizzo PA, et al: Response of human polymorphonuclear leukocytes and monocytes to *Trichosporon beigelii.* Host defense against an emerging pathogen. *J Infect Dis* 170:1557–1565, 1994.
248. Ginsburg CM: Superficial fungal and mycobacterial infections of the skin. *Pediatr Infect Dis* 4(suppl 3):S19–S22, 1985.
249. Dankner WM, Spector SA, Fierer J, et al: *Malassezia* fungemia in neonates and adults: Complication of hyperalimentation. *Rev Infect Dis* 9:743–753, 1987.
250. Long JG, Keyserling HL: Catheter-related infection in infants due to an unusual lipophilic yeast: *Malassezia furfur. Pediatrics* 76:896–900, 1985.
251. Marcon MJ, Powell DA: Epidemiology, diagnosis and management of *Malassezia furfur* systemic infection. *Diagn Microbiol Infect Dis* 7:161–175, 1987.
252. Powell DA, Marcon MJ: Failure to eradicate *Malassezia furfur* broviac catheter infection with antifungal therapy. *Pediatr Infect Dis J* 6:579–580, 1987.

253. Redline RW, Redline SS, Boxerbaum B, et al: Systemic *Malassezia furfur* infections in patients receiving Intralipid therapy. *Hum Pathol* 16:815–822, 1985.
254. Ginsburg CM: Tinea capitis. *Pediatr Infect Dis J* 10:48–49, 1991.
255. Gan VN, Petruska M, Ginsburg CM: Epidemiology and treatment of tinea capitis: Ketoconazole vs. griseofulvin. *Pediatr Infect Dis J* 6:46–49, 1987.
256. Ginsburg CM, Gan VN, Petruska M: Randomized controlled trial of intralesional corticosteroid and griseofulvin vs. griseofulvin alone for treatment of kerion. *Pediatr Infect Dis J* 6:1084–1087, 1987.
257. Neil G, Hanslo D, Buccimazza S, et al: Control of the carrier state of scalp dermatophytes. *Pediatr Infect Dis J* 9:57–58, 1990.
258. Elewski BE: Tinea capitis: Itraconazole in *Trichophyton tonsurans* infection. *J Am Acad Dermatol* 31:65–67, 1994.
259. Arnow PM, Houchins SG, Pugliese G: An outbreak of tinea corporis in hospital personnel caused by a patient with *Trichophyton tonsurans* infection. *Pediatr Infect Dis J* 10:355–359, 1991.
260. Villars VV, Jones TC: Special features of the clinical use of oral terbinafine in the treatment of fungal diseases. *Br J Dermatol* 126(suppl 39):61–69, 1992.
261. Evans EG, Dodman B, Williamson DM, et al: Comparison of terbinafine and clotrimazole in treating tinea pedis. *BMJ* 307:645–647, 1993.
262. Haroon TS, Hussain I, Mahmood A, et al: An open clinical pilot study of the efficacy and safety of oral terbinafine in dry noninflammatory tinea capitis. *Br J Dermatol* 126(suppl 39):47–50, 1992.
263. Kerridge D: Mode of action of clinically important antifungal drugs. *Adv Microbiol Physiol* 27:1–72, 1986.
264. Sokol-Anderson ML, Brajtburg J, Medoff G: Amphotericin B–induced oxidative damage and killing of *Candida albicans. J Infect Dis* 154:76–83, 1986.
265. Benson JM, Nahata MC: Pharmacokinetics of amphotericin B in children. *Antimicrob Agents Chemother* 33:1989–1993, 1989.
266. Baley JE, Meyers C, Kliegman RM, et al: Pharmacokinetics, outcome, treatment and toxic effects of amphotericin B and flucytosine in neonates. *J Pediatr* 116:791–797, 1990.
267. Koren G, Lau A, Klein J, et al: Pharmacokinetics and adverse effects of amphotericin B in infants and children. *J Pediatr* 113:559–563, 1988.
268. Starke JR, Mason O, Kramer WG, et al: Pharmacokinetics of amphotericin B in infants and children. *J Infect Dis* 155:766–774, 1987.
269. Gelfand JA, Kimball K, Burke JF, et l: Amphotericin B treatment of human mononuclear cells in vitro results in secretion of tumor necrosis factor and interleukin-1. *Clin Res* 36:456A, 1988.
270. Burks LC, Aisner J, Fortner CL, et al: Meperidine for the treatment of shaking chills and fever. *Arch Intern Med* 140:483–484, 1980.
271. Graybill JR: New antifungal agents. *Eur J Clin Microbiol Infect Dis* 8:402–412, 1989.

272. Walsh TJ, Pizzo PA: Treatment of systemic fungal infections: Recent progress and current problems. *Eur J Clin Microbiol* 7:460–475, 1988.
273. Sabra R, Branch RA: Amphotericin B nephrotoxicity. *Drug Safety* 5:94–108, 1990.
274. Heidemann HT, Gerkens JF, Spickard WA, et al: Amphotericin B nephrotoxicity in humans decreased by salt repletion. *Am J Med* 75:476–481, 1983.
275. Branch RA: Prevention of amphotericin B-induced renal impairment: A review on the use of sodium supplementation. *Arch Intern Med* 148:2389–2394, 1988.
276. Wasan KM, Vadiei K, Lopez-Berestein G, et al: Pentoxifylline in amphotericin B toxicity rat model. *Antimicrob Agents Chemother* 34:241–244, 1990.
277. Barton CH, Pahl M, Vaziri ND, et al: Renal magnesium wasting associated with amphotericin B therapy. *Am J Med* 77:471–474, 1984.
278. Googe JH, Walterspiel JN: Arrhythmia caused by amphotericin B in a neonate. *Pediatr Infect Dis J* 7:73, 1988.
279. MacGregor RR, Bennett JE, Erslev AJ: Erythropoietin concentration in amphotericin B-induced anemia. *Antimicrob Agents Chemother* 14:270–273, 1978.
280. Wright DG, Robichaud KJ, Pizzo PA, et al: Lethal pulmonary reactions associated with the combined use of amphotericin B and leukocyte transfusions. *N Engl J Med* 304:1185–1189, 1981.
281. Dana BW, Durie BGM, White RF, et al: Concomitant administration of granulocyte transfusions and amphotericin B in neutropenic patients: Absence of significant pulmonary toxicity. *Blood* 57:90–94, 1981.
282. Cohen I: Absence of congenital infection and teratogenesis in three children born to mothers with blastomycosis and treated with amphotericin B during pregnancy. *Pediatr Infect Dis* 6:76–77, 1987.
283. Peterson CM, Schuppert K, Kelly PC, et al: Coccidioidomycosis and pregnancy. *Obstet Gynecol Surv* 48:149–156, 1993.
284. Dean JL, Wolf JE, Ranzini AC, et al: Use of amphotericin B during pregnancy: Case report and review. *Clin Infect Dis* 18:364–368, 1994.
285. Pizzo PA, Robichaud KJ, Gill FA, et al: Empiric antibiotic and antifungal therapy for cancer patients with prolonged fever and granulocytopenia. *Am J Med* 72:101, 1982.
286. EORTC International Antimicrobial Therapy Cooperative Group: Empiric antifungal therapy in febrile granulocytopenic patients. *Am J Med* 86:668–672, 1989.
287. Hughes WT, Pizzo PA, Wade JC, et al: Evaluation of new anti-infective drugs for the treatment of febrile episodes in neutropenic patients. *Clin Infect Dis* 16:341, 1993.
288. Pizzo PA: After empiric therapy or what to do until the granulocyte count comes back. *Rev Infect Dis* 9:214–219, 1987.
289. Pizzo PA, Rubin M, Freifeld A, et al: The child with cancer and in-

fection: II. Approach to nonbacterial infections. *J Pediatr* 119:845–857, 1991.

290. de Marie S, Janknegt R, Bakker-Woudenberg IA: Clinical use of liposomal and lipid-complexed amphotericin B. *J Antimicrob Chemother* 33:907–916, 1994.

291. Szoka FC Jr, Milholland D, Barza M: Effect of lipid composition and liposome size on toxicity and in vitro fungicidal activity of liposome-intercalated amphotericin B. *Antimicrob Agents Chemother* 31:421–429, 1987.

292. Mehta T, Lopez-Berestein G, Hopfer R, et al: Liposomal amphotericin B is toxic to fungal cells but not to mammalian cells. *Biochem Biophys Acta* 770:230–234, 1984.

293. Lopez-Berestein G, Fainstein V, Hopfer R, et al: Liposomal amphotericin B for the treatment of systemic fungal infections in patients with cancer: A preliminary study. *J Infect Dis* 151:704–710, 1985.

294. Allende MC, Lee JW, Francis P, et al: Dose-dependent antifungal activity and nephrotoxicity of amphotericin B colloidal dispersion (ABCD) in experimental pulmonary aspergillosis. *Antimicrob Agents Chemother* 38:518–522, 1994.

295. Clark JM, Whitney RR, Olsen SJ, et al: Amphotericin B lipid complex therapy of experimental fungal infections in mice. *Antimicrob Agents Chemother* 35:615–621, 1991.

296. Meunier F: New methods for delivery of antifungal agents. *Rev Infect Dis* 11(suppl 7):S1605–S1612, 1989.

297. Levine SJ, Walsh TJ, Martinez A, et al: Hypoxemia, pulmonary hypertension, and depression of cardiac output as sequelae of liposomal amphotericin B infusion. *Ann Intern Med* 114:664–666, 1991.

298. Lopez-Berestein G: Liposomal amphotericin B in the treatment of fungal infections. *Ann Intern Med* 105:130–131, 1986.

299. Walsh TJ, Hiemenz JW, Seibel N, et al: Amphotericin B lipid complex in the treatment of 228 cases of invasive mycosis. In *Abstracts of the 34th Intersci Conf Antimicrob Agents Chemother.* Washington, DC, American Society for Microbiology, abstract no M69, p 247, 1994.

300. Ringden O, Meunier F, Tollemar J, et al: Efficacy of amphotericin B encapsulated in liposomes (AmBisome) in the treatment of invasive fungal infections in immunocompromised patients. *J Antimicrob Chemother* 28(suppl B):63–72, 1991.

301. Tollemar J, Ringden O, Andersson S, et al: Prophylactic use of liposomal amphotericin B (AmBisome) against fungal infections: A randomized trial in bone marrow transplant recipients. *Transplant Proc* 25:1495–1497, 1993.

302. Alder-Moore JP, Proffitt RT: Development, characterization, efficacy and mode of action of AmBisome, a unilamellar liposomal formulation of amphotericin B. *J Liposomal Res* 3:429–450, 1993.

303. Utz JP, Garriques IL, Sande MA, et al: Therapy of cryptococcosis with a combination of flucytosine and amphotericin B. *J Infect Dis* 132:368–373, 1975.

304. Larsen RA, Leal MAE, Chan LS: Fluconazole compared with amphotericin B plus flucytosine for cryptococcal meningitis in AIDS. *Ann Intern Med* 113:183–187, 1990.

305. van der Bossche H: Biochemical targets for antifungal azole derivatives: Hypothesis on the mode of action. In McGinnis M (ed): *Current Topics in Medical Mycology.* New York, Springer-Verlag, 1985, pp 313–351.

306. Fainstein V, Bodey GP: Cardiorespiratory toxicity due to miconazole. *Ann Intern Med* 93:432–433, 1980.

307. Daneshmend TK, Warnock DW: Clinical pharmacokinetics of ketoconazole. *Clin Pharmacokinet* 14:13–34, 1988.

308. Shadomy S, Espinel-Ingroff A, Tartaglione TA, et al: Treatment of systemic mycosis with ketoconazole: Studies of ketoconazole serum levels. *Mykosen* 29:195–209, 1986.

309. Lelawongs P, Barone JA, Colaizzi JL, et al: Effect of food and gastric acidity on absorption of orally administered ketoconazole. *Clin Pharm* 7:228–235, 1988.

310. Lake-Bakaar G, Tom W, Lake-Bakaar D, et al: Gastropathy and ketoconazole malabsorption in the acquired immunodeficiency syndrome. *Ann Intern Med* 109:471–473, 1988.

311. Daneshmend TK, Warnock DW, Ene MD, et al: Influence of food on the pharmacokinetics of ketoconazole. *Antimicrob Agents Chemother* 25:1–3, 1984.

312. Walsh TJ, Rubin M, Hathorn J, et al: Amphotericin B versus high-dose ketoconazole empirical antifungal therapy among febrile granulocytopenic cancer patients: A prospective randomized study. *Arch Intern Med* 151:765–770, 1991.

313. Ginsburg CM, McCracken GH Jr, Olsen K: Pharmacology of ketoconazole suspension in infants and children. *Antimicrob Agents Chemother* 23:787–789, 1983.

314. Sugar AM, Alsip S, Galgiani JN, et al: Pharmacology and toxicity of high-dose ketoconazole. *Antimicrob Agents Chemother* 31:1874–1878, 1987.

315. Pont A, Graybill JR, Craven PC, et al: High-dose ketoconazole and adrenal and testicular function in man. *Arch Intern Med* 144:2150, 1984.

316. Loose DS, Kan PB, Hirst MA, et al: Ketoconazole blocks adrenal steroidogenesis by inhibiting cytochrome P450-dependent enzymes. *J Clin Invest* 71:495–499, 1983.

317. Lewis JH, Zimmerman HJ, Benson GD, et al: Hepatic injury associated with ketoconazole therapy: Analysis of 33 cases. *Gastroenterology* 86:503–513, 1984.

318. Engelhard D, Stutman HR, Marks MI: Interaction of ketoconazole with rifampin and isoniazid. *N Engl J Med* 311:1681–1683, 1984.

319. Grant SM, Clissold SP: Fluconazole: A review of its pharmacodynamic and pharmacokinetic properties, and therapeutic potential in superficial and systemic mycoses. *Drugs* 39:877–916, 1990.

320. Richardson K, Cooper K, Marriott MS, et al: Discovery of fluconazole, a novel antifungal agent. *Rev Infect Dis* 12(suppl 3):S267–S271, 1990.

321. Hardin TC, Graybill JR, Fetchick R, et al: Pharmacokinetics of itraconazole following oral administration to normal volunteers. *Antimicrob Agents Chemother* 32:1310–1313, 1988.

322. Tricot G, Joosten E, Boogaerts MA, et al: Ketoconazole vs. itraconazole for antifungal prophylaxis in patients with severe granulocytopenia: Preliminary results of two nonrandomized studies. *Rev Infect Dis* 9(suppl 1):94–99, 1987.

323. Deleted in proofs.

324. Berenguer J, Ali N, Allende MC, et al: Itraconazole in experimental pulmonary aspergillosis: comparison with amphotericin B, interaction with cyclosporin A, and correlation between therapeutic response and itraconazole plasma concentrations. *Antimicrob Agents Chemother* 38:1303–1308, 1994.

325. Heykants J, Michiels M, Meuldermans W, et al: The pharmacokinetics of itraconazole in animals and man: An overview. In Fromtling RA (ed): *Recent Trends in the Discovery, Development and Evaluation of Antifungal Agents.* Barcelona, JR Prous Science Publishers, 1987, pp 223–249.

326. Denning DW, Tucker RM, Hanson LH, et al: Itraconazole therapy for cryptococcal meningitis and cryptococcosis. *Arch Intern Med* 149:2301–2308, 1989.

327. Novakova I, Donnelly P, DeWitte T, et al: Itraconazole and cyclosporin nephrotoxicity. *Lancet* 2:920–921, 1987.

328. Trenk D, Brett W, Jahnchen E, et al: Time course of cyclosporine/itraconazole interaction. *Lancet* 2:1335–1336, 1987.

329. Deleted in proofs.

330. National Committee for Clinical Laboratory Standards: Reference method for broth dilution antifungal susceptibility testing of yeasts. Proposed Standard. NCCLS document M27-P. NCCLS, Villanova, Pa.

331. Pfaller M, Riley J, Koerner T: Effects of cilofungin LY121019 on carbohydrate and sterol composition of *Candida albicans. Eur J Clin Microbiol Infect Dis* 8:1067–1070, 1989.

332. Rex JH, Pfaller MA, Rinaldi MG, et al: Antifungal susceptibility testing. *Clin Microbiol Rev* 6:367–381, 1993.

333. Walsh TJ, Foulds G, Pizzo PA: Pharmacokinetics and tissue penetration of fluconazole in rabbits. *Antimicrob Agents Chemother* 33:467–469, 1989.

334. Brammer KW, Farrow PR, Faulkner JK: Pharmacokinetics and tissue penetration of fluconazole in humans. *Rev Infect Dis* 12(suppl 3):S318–S326, 1990.

335. Drew RH, Perfect JR, Gallis HE: Use of fluconazole in a patient with documented malabsorption of ketoconazole. *Clin Pharm* 7:622–623, 1988.

336. Lee JW, Seibel NI, Amantea MA, et al: Safety, tolerance, and pharma-

cokinetics of fluconazole in children with neoplastic diseases. *J Pediatr* 120:987–993, 1992.

337. Brammer KW, Coates PE: The pharmacokinetics of fluconazole in children. *Eur J Clin Microbiol Infect Dis* 13:325–329, 1994.

338. Lazo de la Vega S, Volkow P, Yeates RA, et al: Administration of the antimycotic agents fluconazole and itraconazole to leukaemia patients: A comparative pharmacokinetic study. *Drugs Exp Clin Res* 20:69–75, 1994.

339. Krzeska I, Yeates RA, Pfaff G: Single dose intravenous pharmacokinetics of fluconazole in infants. *Drugs Exp Clin Res* 19:267–271, 1993.

340. Perfect JR, Durack DT: Penetration of imidazoles and triazoles into cerebrospinal fluid in rabbits. *J Antimicrob Chemother* 16:81–86, 1985.

341. Arndt CAS, Walsh TJ, McCully CL, et al: Fluconazole penetration into cerebrospinal fluid: Implications for treating fungal infections of the central nervous system. *J Infect Dis* 157:178–180, 1988.

342. Foulds G, Brennan DR, Wajszczuk C, et al: Fluconazole penetration into cerebrospinal fluid in humans. *J Clin Pharmacol* 28:363–366, 1988.

343. Viscoli C, Castagnola E, Fioredda F, et al: Fluconazole in the treatment of candidiasis in immunocompromised children. *Antimicrob Agents Chemother* 35:365–367, 1991.

344. Marchisio P, Princiipi N: Treatment of oropharyngeal candidiasis in HIV-infected children with oral fluconazole. *Eur J Clin Microbiol Infect Dis* 13:338–340, 1994.

345. Bode S, Pedersen-Bjergaard L, Hjelt K: *Candida albicans* septicemia in a premature infant successfully treated with oral fluconazole. *Scand J Infect Dis* 24:673–675, 1992.

346. Lazar JD, Wilner KD: Drug interactions with fluconazole. *Rev Infect Dis* 12(suppl 3):S327–S333, 1990.

347. Narang PK, Trapnell CB, Schoenfelder JR, et al: Fluconazole and enhanced effect of rifabutin prophylaxis [letter]. *N Engl J Med* 330:1316–1317, 1994.

348. Walsh TJ, Lee J, Aoki S, et al: Experimental basis for usage of fluconazole for preventive or early treatment of disseminated candidiasis in granulocytopenic hosts. *Rev Infect Dis* 12:S307–S317, 1990.

349. Goodman JL, Winston DJ, Greenfield RA, et al: A controlled trial of fluconazole to prevent fungal infections in patients undergoing bone marrow transplantation. *N Engl J Med* 326:845–851, 1992.

350. Slavin MA, Osborne B, Adams R, et al: Efficacy and safety of fluconazole prophylaxis for fungal infections after marrow transplantation—A prospective, randomized, double-blind study. *J Infect Dis* 171:1545–1552, 1995.

351. Winston DJ, Chandrasekar PH, Lazarus HM, et al: Fluconazole prophylaxis of fungal infections in patients with acute leukemia. Results of a randomized placebo-controlled, double-blind, multicenter trial. *Ann Intern Med* 118:495–503, 1993.

352. Ninane J: A multicentre study of fluconazole versus oral polyenes in the prevention of fungal infection in children with hematological or oncological malignancies. *Eur J Clin Microbiol Infect Dis* 13:330–337, 1994.

353. Cap J, Mojzesova A, Kayserova E, et al: Fluconazole in children: First experience with prophylaxis in chemotherapy-induced neutropenia in pediatric patients with cancer. *Chemotherapy* 39:438–442, 1993.

354. Cesaro S, Rossetti F, Perilongo G, et al: Fluconazole prophylaxis and *Candida* fungemia in neutropenic children with malignancies. *Haematologica* 78:249–251, 1993.

355. Ryley JF, McGregor S, Wilson RG: Activity of ICI 195,739—a novel, orally active bistriazole—in rodent models of fungal and protozoal infections. *Ann N Y Acad Sci* 544:310–328, 1988.

356. Gordee RS, Zeckner DJ, Howard LC, et al: Anti-*Candida* activity and toxicology of LY121019, a novel semisynthetic polypeptide antifungal antibiotic. *Ann N Y Acad Sci* 544:294–309, 1988.

357. Sawistowska-Schroder ET, Kerridge D, Perry H: Echinocandin inhibition of 1,3-β-D-glucan synthase from *Candida albicans*. *Fed Eur Biochem Soc Lett* 173:134–138, 1984.

358. Walsh TJ, Lee JW, Kelly P, et al: The antifungal effects of the nonlinear pharmacokinetics of cilofungin, a 1,3-β-glucan synthase inhibitor, during contnuous vs. intermittent infusion of cilofungin in treatment of experimental disseminated candidiasis. *Antimicrob Agents Chemother* 35:1321–1328, 1991.

359. Schmatz DM, Romancheck MA, Pittarelli LA, et al: Treatment of *Pneumocystis carinii* pneumonia with 1,3-beta-glucan synthesis inhibitors. *Proc Natl Acad Med* 87:5950–5954, 1990.

360. Denning DW, Stevens DA: Efficacy of cilofungin alone and in combination with amphotericin B in a murine model of disseminated aspergillosis. *Antimicrob Agents Chemother* 35:1329–1333, 1991.

361. Balkovec JM, Black RM, Hammond ML, et al: Echinocandin analogues: Synthesis and *in vivo* efficacy of L-693,989 and other water soluble echinocandins in *Candida* and *Pneumocystis* rodent models. In *31st Interscience Conference on Antimicrobial Agents and Chemotherapy*, Washington, DC, American Society for Microbiology, abstract no 204, 1991.

362. Petranyi G, Ryer NS, Stutz A: Allylamine derivatives: New class of synthetic antifungal agents inhibiting fungal squalene epoxidase. *Science* 224:1239–1241, 1984.

363. Balfour JA, Faulds D: Terbinafine. A review of its pharmacodynamic and pharmacokinetic properties, and therapeutic potential in superficial mycoses. *Drugs* 43:259–284, 1992.

364. Shadomy S, Espinel-Ingroff A, Gebhart RJ: In vitro studies with SF 86-327, a new orally active allylamine derivative. *Sabouraudia* 23:125–132, 1985.

365. Jones TC, Villars VV: Terbinafine. In Ryley JF (ed): *Chemotherapy of*

Fungal Diseases. New York, Springer-Verlag New York, 1990, pp 483–503.

366. Oki T, Konishi M, Tomatsu K, et al: Pradimicin, a novel class of potent antifungal antibiotics. *J Antibiotics (Tokyo)* 41:1701–1704, 1988.

367. Oki T, Saitoh K, Tomatsu K, et al: Novel antifungal antibiotic BMY-28567. *Ann N Y Acad Sci* 544:184–187, 1988.

368. Walsh TJ, van Cutsem J, Polak A, et al: Pathogenesis, immunomodulation, and antifungal therapy of experimental invasive candidiasis, histoplasmosis, and aspergillosis: Recent advances and concepts. *J Med Vet Mycol* 30(suppl 1):225–240, 1992.

369. Bodey GP, Anaissie E, Gutterman J, et al: Role of granulocyte-macrophage colony stimulating factor as adjuvant therapy for fungal infection in patients with cancer. *Clin Infect Dis* 17:705–707, 1993.

370. Neumanaitis J, Meyers JD, Buckner CD, et al: Phase I trial of recombinant human macrophage colony-stimulating factor in patients with invasive fungal infections. *Blood* 4:907–913, 1991.

371. American Society of Clinical Oncology: Recommendations for the use of hematopoietic colony-stimulating factors: Evidence-based, clinical practice guidelines. *J Clin Oncol* 12:2471–2508, 1994.

372. Roilides E, Holmes A, Blake C, et al: Impairment of neutrophil fungicidal activity against *Aspergillus fumigatus* in HIV-infected children. *J Infect Dis* 167:905–911, 1993.

373. Roilides E, Uhlig K, Venzon D, et al: Prevention of corticosteroid-induced suppression of human polymorphonuclear leukocyte-induced damage of *Aspergillus fumigatus* hyphae by granulocyte colony-stimulating factor and gamma interferon. *Infect Immun* 61:4870–4877, 1993.

374. Buckley RH: Immunodeficiency diseases. *JAMA* 268:2797–2806, 1992.

375. Albano EA, Pizzo PA: The evolving population of immunocompromised children. *Pediatr Infect Dis J* 7:S79–S86, 1988.

376. Byers M, Feldman S, Edwards J: Disseminated histoplasmosis as the acquired immunodeficiency syndrome-defining illness in an infant. *Pediatr Infect Dis J* 11:127–128, 1992.

377. Hazelhurst J, Vismer H: Histoplasmosis presenting with unusual skin lesions in acquired immunodeficiency syndrome. *West J Med* 113:345–348, 1985.

378. Diamond RD: The growing problem of mycoses in patients infected with the human immunodeficiency virus. *Rev Infect Dis* 13:480–486, 1991.

379. Dismukes W: Cryptococcal meningitis in patients with AIDS. *J Infect Dis* 157:624–628, 1988.

380. Jimenez-Acosta F, Casado M, Borbujo J, et al: Cutaneous cryptococcosis mimicking molluscum contagiosum in a haemophiliac with AIDS. *Clin Exp Dermatol* 12:446–450, 1987.

381. Wilfert CM, Wilson C, Luzuriaga K, et al: Pathogenesis of pediatric

human immunodeficiency virus type 1 infection. *J Infect Dis* 170:286–292, 1994.

382. Denning DW, Follansbee SE, Scolaro M, et al: Pulmonary aspergillosis in the acquired immunodeficiency syndrome. *N Engl J Med* 324:654–662, 1991.

383. Minamoto GY, Barlam TF, Vander Els NJ: Invasive aspergillosis in patients with AIDS. *Clin Infect Dis* 14:66–74, 1992.

384. Purcell KJ, Telzak EE, Armstrong D: *Aspergillus* species colonization and invasive disease in patients with AIDS. *Clin Infect Dis* 14:141–148, 1992.

385. Schaffner A: Pulmonary aspergillosis in AIDS [letter]. *N Engl J Med* 325:355, 1991.

386. Stevens DA, Denning DW: Pulmonary aspergillosis in AIDS [letter]. *N Engl J Med* 325:356–357, 1991.

387. Annable WL, Kachmer ML, De Santis D: Long term follow-up of *Candida* endophthalmitis in the premature infants. *J Pediatr Ophthalmol Strabismus* 27:103–106, 1990.

388. Arisoy ES, Correa A, Seilheimer DK, et al: *Candida rugosa* central venous catheter infection in a child. *Pediatr Infect Dis J* 12:961–963, 1993.

389. Baley JE, Annable WL, Kliegman RM: *Candida* endophthalmitis in the premature infant. *J Pediatr* 98:458–461, 1981.

390. Mazor M, Chaim W, Shinwell ES, et al: Asymptomatic amniotic fluid invasion with *Candida albicans* in preterm premature rupture of membranes. Implications for obstetric and neonatal management. *Acta Obstet Gynecol Scand* 72:52–54, 1993.

391. Sadiq HF, Devaskar S, Keenan WK, et al: Broviac catheterization in low birth weight infants: Incidence and treatment of associated complications. *Crit Care Med* 15:47–50, 1987.

392. Silliman CC, Lawellin DW, Lohr JA, et al: *Paecilomyces lilacinus* infection in a child with chronic granulomatous disease. *J Infect* 24:191–195, 1992.

393. Commers J, Robichaud KJ, Pizzo PA, et al: New pulmonary infiltrates in granulocytopenic patients being treated with antibiotics. *Pediatr Infect Dis* 3:423–428, 1984.

394. Guerra-Romero L, Edson RS, Cockerill FR III, et al: Comparison of Du-Pont Isolator and Roche Septi-chek for detection of fungemia. *J Clin Microbiol* 25:1623–1625, 1987.

395. Kiehn TE, Wong B, Edwards FF, et al: Comparative recovery of bacteria and yeasts from lysis-centrifugation and a conventional blood-culture system. *J Clin Microbiol* 18:300–304, 1983.

396. Bille J, Edson R, Roberts G: Clinical evaluation of the lysis centrifugation blood culture system for the detection of fungemia and comparison with a conventional biphasic broth blood culture system. *J Clin Microbiol* 19:126–128, 1984.

397. Wilson ML, Weinstein MP, Reimer LG, et al: Controlled comparison

of the BacT/Alert and BACTEC 660/730 nonradiometric blood culture systems. *J Clin Microbiol* 30:323–329, 1992.

398. Cattermole HEJ, Rivers RPA: Nenonatal *Candida* septicaemia: Diagnosis on buffy smear. *Arch Dis Child* 62:302–304, 1987.

399. Walsh TJ, Catchatourian R, Cohen H: Disseminated histoplasmosis complicating bone marrow transplantation. *Am J Clin Pathol* 79:509–511, 1983.

400. Matthews RC, Burnie JP, Tabaqchali S: Immunoblot analysis of the serological response in systemic candidosis. *Lancet* 2:1415–1418, 1984.

401. Schreiber JR, Maynard E, Lew MA: *Candida* antigen detection in two premature neonates with disseminated candidiasis. *Pediatrics* 74:838–841, 1984.

402. Walsh TJ, Hathorn JW, Sobel JD, et al: Detection of circulating *Candida* enolase by immunoassay in patients with cancer and invasive candidiasis. *N Engl J Med* 324:1026–1031, 1991.

403. Reiss E, Morrison CJ: Nonculture methods for diagnosis of disseminated candidiasis. *Clin Microbiol Rev* 6:311–323, 1993.

404. McNeill MM, Gerber AR, McLaughlin DW, et al: Mannan antigenemia during invasive candidiasis caused by *Candida tropicalis*. *Pediatr Infect Dis J* 22:493–496, 1992.

405. Walsh TJ, Merz WG, Lee JW, et al: Diagnosis and therapeutic monitoring of invasive candidiasis by rapid enzymatic detection serum D-arabinitol. *Am J Med* (in press).

406. Obayashi T, Yoshida M, Mori T, et al: Plasma (1 → 3)-beta-D-glucan measurement in diagnosis of invasive deep mycosis and fungal febrile episodes. *Lancet* 345:17–20, 1995.

407. Erlich HA, Gelfand D, Sninsky JJ: Recent advance in the polymerase chain reaction. *Science* 252:1643–1651, 1991.

408. Hopfer RL, Walden P, Setterquist S, et al: Detection and differentiation of fungi in clinical specimens using polymerase chain reaction (PCR) amplification and restriction enzyme analysis. *J Med Vet Mycol* 31:65–75, 1993.

409. Tang CM, Holden DW, Aufauvre-Brown A, et al: The detection of *Aspergillus* spp. by the polymerase chain reaction and its evaluation in bronchoalveolar lavage fluid. *Am Rev Respir Dis* 148:1313–1317, 1993.

410. Georgopapadakou NH, Walsh TJ: Human mycoses: Drugs and targets for emerging pathogens. *Science* 264:371–372, 1994.

411. Koldin MH, Medoff G: Antifungal chemotherapy. *Pediatr Clin North Am* 30:49–61, 1983.

412. Como JA, Dismukes WE: Oral azole drugs as systemic antifungal therapy. *N Engl J Med* 330:263–272, 1994.

413. de Marie S, Janknegt R, Bakker-Woudenberg IA: Clinical use of liposomal and lipid-complexed amphotericin B. *J Antimicrob Chemother* 33:907–916, 1994.

414. Gates C, Pinney RJ: Amphotericin B and its delivery by liposomal and lipid formulations. *J Clin Pharm Ther* 18:147–153, 1993.

415. Mustafa MM, Sandler ES, Bernini JC, et al: Amphotericin B colloidal dispersion therapy for invasive mycosis: Report of successful therapy in two pediatric patients. *Pediatr Infect Dis J* 13:326–328, 1994.
416. Walsh TJ, Lee JW: Prevention of invasive fungal infections in patients with neoplastic diseases. *Clin Infect Dis* 17:S468–S480, 1993.
417. Pizzo PA: Management of fever in patients with cancer and treatment-induced neutropenia. *N Engl J Med* 328:1323–1332, 1993.
418. Lau AS: Cytokines in the pathogenesis and treatment of infectious diseases. *Adv Pediatr Infect Dis* 9:211–236, 1994.

Nematode Infections in Children*

Niranjan Kanesa-thasan, M.D., M.T.M.H.
Division of Communicable Diseases and Immunology, Walter Reed
Army Institute of Research, Washington, D.C.

Michael J. Bangs, M.S.P.H.
Division of Tropical Public Health, Department of Preventive Medicine
and Biometrics, Uniformed Services University of the Health Sciences,
Bethesda, Maryland

John H. Cross, Ph.D.
Professor, Department of Preventive Medicine and Biometrics,
Uniformed Services University of the Health Sciences, Bethesda,
Maryland

N ematodes, or roundworms, are the most common helminth parasites of humans. Infections with nematodes are most prevalent in the tropics, where human infections with multiple nematode species (nematodiases) are common. However, nematodes are ubiquitous and pose a hazard to humans throughout the world. This review will delineate the range of nematode infections likely to be encountered in children within the United States but is not intended to be comprehensive. Capsular summaries of individual infections will be provided with reference to more detailed works. The review is arranged by mode of transmission of parasite to humans (soil transmitted, insect-borne, and foodborne infections); this progression also reflects the increasing complexity of nematode life cycles as parasites evolve to infect hosts other than humans. This review will focus particularly on the intestinal nematode parasites of humans, because exciting insights have been gained in recent years into the epidemiology and immunology of these infections. It is hoped that the review will furnish a framework for understanding and appreciating these varied and often intricate infections.

---

*The opinions contained herein are those of the authors and are not to be construed as official or as reflecting the views of the U.S. Department of Defense.

Advances in Pediatric Infectious Diseases®, vol. 11
© 1996, Mosby–Year Book, Inc.

NEMATODE INFECTIONS

The nematodes comprise a diverse class of the phylum Aschelminthes.[1] Most nematodes are free living, but some are major parasites of humans. The life cycle of nematodes is often complex, requiring intermediate hosts for particular larval stages. However, the typical life cycle includes oviposition by gravid females, maturation of eggs with subsequent release of larvae, and development of larvae through a typical series of five stages, resulting in creation of fecund adult male and female worms. These worms mate to create fertile embryos, which are encapsulated and released within distinctive eggs. The exception to this life cycle is *Strongyloides stercoralis*, where the females are parthenogenic (i.e., do not require a male worm to produce fertile eggs).

Nematodes are true round worms that are attenuated at both ends. They have a characteristic cuticle that encompasses the worm in a relatively impervious but elastic and semipermeable shield. These cuticles are shed through a series of four molts by larvae. This has implications for the immune response to the nematode parasite, because each larval stage may have quite distinct expression of specific antigens.[2] In addition, larvae and adult worms shed secretory-excretory molecules through cuticular pores, which often provoke host immunologic responses.[3]

Parasitic nematodes have adapted part of all of their life cycle inside a host animal or plant (endoparasitism). In contrast to free-living nematodes, parasitic nematodes have varying requirements for support and shelter from the external environment.[4] Filarial nematodes are so highly adapted to human hosts that no life cycle stage is free living. Other parasitic nematodes, such as hookworms as *Ascaris* spp., retain a free-living portion of their life cycle as either eggs or larvae.

Nematode infections are parasitic infections of the human host. Infection occurs either through ingestion of mature eggs or larvae or through penetration of skin by nematode larvae or insect vectors. The symbiotic relationship between nematode and humans usually results in varying degrees of harm to the human host. Humans may be either the definitive host (sole or primary animal where adult stages of the parasite develop and reproduce), intermediate host (animal where only larval stages develop), or accidental host (parasite fails to develop) for parasitic nematodes. Usually the infective stage for mammals is the third larval stage. There is often an arrest in development of larvae after their entry into human hosts.[5] In addition, there is no replication of adult nematodes within the human host except for *S. stercoralis* and *Capillaria philippinensis*. In these cases, autoinfection may result in completion of the life cycle within the intestine, resulting in amplification of adult worm number.

The variety of nematode parasites is truly astounding; they are a common cause of intestinal infection but can also penetrate tissues and inflict significant damage. Intestinal infections are often subclinical, and disease is usually apparent only in heavily infected individuals. Overt clinical disease for intestinal parasites ranges from nonspecific abdominal symptoms to malabsorption (strongyliasis, capillariasis), iron deficiency anemia (hookworm), and acute conditions of the abdomen (ascariasis and trichuriasis). Mortality is usually attributable to complications of high parasitic infestations; although this rate is low, the total burden of deaths from parasitic nematodes is high because of their widespread prevalence. Invasive infections of nematodes often result in tissue inflammatory responses such as granulomas (visceral larva migrans, anisakiasis, and angiostrongyliasis) and dermatologic manifestations (cutaneous larva migrans, larva currens, and edema [trichinosis and gnathostomiasis]). Rarely more serious disease occurs because of nematode larval invasion of neurologic (angiostrongyliasis and gnathostomiasis), subcutaneous (dracunculosis) and lymphatic tissues (filariases). In many cases, the host immune response is contributory to tissue damage from parasite passage or entrapment.[6]

GLOBAL IMPACT

Nematode infections are very common worldwide. Infections spread wherever there is poor sanitation, poverty, and crowding, unsafe food practices, or unchecked proliferation of insect vectors. Conservatively there are more than 1 to 2 billion nematode infections; it is predicted that more than 1 billion individuals are infected with either *Ascaris lumbricoides*, hookworm (*Ancylostoma duodenale* and *Necator americanus*), or whipworm *Trichuris trichuria*).[7] Many individuals are multiply infected, classically with all three of these worms.[8] The global worm burden is stunning; the total mass of eggs laid daily would exceed several thousand tons![9] Most infections occur in childhood, because nematodes are particularly efficient in infecting pediatric populations. Enhanced transmission among children is attributed to increased exposure to soil nematodes, lack of acquired resistance, and other ill-defined contributory factors such as malnutrition or presence of maternal-blocking antibodies.[10]

It is now realized that the global health impact of nematode infections may extend far beyond the consequences of severe infection.[11] Moderate and mixed nematode infections have been shown to adversely affect physical growth, development,[12] and nutritional status[13, 14] of children. Previous studies were correlational and had difficulty in controlling adequately for socioeconomic, nutritional, and other potential confounding factors. New intervention studies have been used to demonstrate the increment in growth and nutritional status after vermicidal treatment. Preliminary investigations using this methodology have indicated a possible small deleterious effect of intercurrent helminthic infection on mental processing and school performance.[15] Infection with one intestinal worm can also predispose to infections with other helminth species, such as other nematodes or possibly even trematodes.[16, 17] Helminth infections may even predispose to superinfection and transmission of bacterial disease.[18] It is apparent that there is yet more to be learned about the ecology and impact of nematode infections, especially their impact on an immunologically and nutritionally vulnerable population of preschool-age children.

NEMATODE INFECTIONS IN THE UNITED STATES

In the United States, pediatricians are most likely to see nematode infections in imported cases (i.e., those acquired outside the country from areas endemic for nematode parasitic infections).[19] There is still limited autochthonous transmission of nematode parasites, particularly geohelminths (parasites transmitted by soil) such as hookworm in regions of Appalachia or the Southeast, but these indigenous cases are uncommon. Most recent reports of nematode infection occur within certain subpopulations, namely immigrants (e.g., refugees,[20] foreign-born adoptees[21]), travellers returning from endemic regions,[22] or possibly institutionalized individuals.[23] Contrasting general features between nematode infections globally and in the United States are listed in Table 1.

In the near future, it is likely that there will be more nematode infections coming to the attention of the infectious disease specialist because of increased travel and increased entry of immigrant populations, movements of parasite nematodes within human and other hosts,[24] and perhaps newer attentiveness and diagnostic interest for specific nematodes or nematode groups (e.g., foodborne nematodes). Thus, there is reason for reconsidering this diverse class of agents. This review will provide an overview of nematode infections in children. It is organized into three parts: soil-

TABLE 1.

General Features of Nematode Infections in Humans

	Global	**United States**
Prevalence of infection	Generally high	Low
Intensity of infection	Overdispersed (many with light to moderate infections; few individuals with heavy infections)	Light
Multiple infections	Common (nematodiases)	Unlikely
Affected populations	Predominantly children (5–10 yr old)	Special populations (immigrants; travellers)
Symptomatic disease	Clinically apparent disease in heavily infected individuals	None or hypersensitivity reactions
Mortality	Low, attributable to high parasitic infestations; total burden of deaths high	Rare (predominantly immunocompromised individuals)
Morbidity	Probably high (see text)	None
Treatment requirement	Not absolute; generally selective	Generally yes
Public health significance	High	Low
Particular diseases of importance	Intestinal helminthiases, filariases	*Enterobius* and *Strongyloides* infections; foodborne infections

transmitted nematode infections, vector-borne nematode infections, and foodborne nematode infections. Chemotherapy of these infections will be discussed but is not a focus for this review, because the principal antiparasitic drugs are well reviewed elsewhere,[25, 26] and regimens are updated periodically.[27, 28]

SOIL-TRANSMITTED NEMATODES

The soil-transmitted nematodes are disbursed in temperate and tropical regions. Because they are transmitted through contact of humans with soil, they must rely on environmental and social ecology to continue their survival (geohelminths). Environmental factors influencing transmission include humidity, type of soil, temperature, and rainfall present in a biome; these nematodes flourish under conditions of moist warm climate, with loamy shaded soil. Because many of these worms have a direct cycle with humans as definitive or sole host, transmission also relies on the prevalence and intensity of infection in the community. As is well known, the soil-transmitted nematodes thrive among impoverished populations living under crowded and unsanitary conditions.[29] Manifest contamination of the environment with nematode eggs promotes transmission, because most nematodes rely on high rates of egg excretion to maintain their ecologic niches.

Most soil-transmitted nematodes cause intestinal infections. They are acquired by ingestion of eggs or larvae from fecally contaminated material (*A. lumbricoides, T. trichuria,* and *Enterobius vermicularis*) or by penetration of skin by free-living larvae (*S. stercoralis* and hookworm). With the exception of S. *stercoralis,* intestinal nematodes do not multiply in the human host. *Ascaris lumbricoides,* hookworm, and S. *stercoralis* adult worms reside within the small intestine. Other nematodes live in the cecum (*E. vermicularis,* a pinworm) and the large intestine (*T. trichuria*). Some parasites remain entirely in the intestine; others pass through tissues for part of their life cycle. The consequences of severe infestation with these parasites are well appreciated and attributed to mechanical or physiologic disruption of the human host. In rare cases, dissemination of parasites occurs, usually in immunocompromised hosts (e.g., S. *stercoralis* superinfection).

EPIDEMIOLOGY

Recent efforts have attempted to establish a quantitative framework for investigation of host interactions with nematode parasites.[30] These have been facilitated by the accessibility of worms and eggs for quantitation of worm burden and by their direct life cycles with a single animal host (humans).[31] These studies have shown that intestinal parasites are distributed unevenly (overdispersed) throughout a community. Worm numbers per person tend to be highly aggregated, so that few individuals retain heavy parasite burdens, whereas the majority harbor only few parasites (best approximated by the negative binomial probability distribution). The prevalence of nematode infection fails to reveal as much as the density of infection such that the mere presence of worms is less significant than the actual individual worm burden.[32] The significance of this observation is most evident in populations with high intensity of infection, generally school-age and teenage children.[33] Those individuals with peak intensity of infection are at most risk for adverse consequences of infection, such as morbidity and mortality. Intriguing observations show that individuals may be predisposed to light or heavy parasitic infections, that individual levels of infection remain remarkably stable over time, and that individuals will reacquire infection at the same level of intensity even after chemotherapeutic removal of worm burden.[34] Intensity of infection may be governed by a combination of ecologic, genetic,[35] and immunologic influences. These factors are apparent at individual and familial level.[36]

IMMUNOLOGY

The immune responses to nematodes depend in large part on the location and stage of the parasite. Generally the most immunogenic phase is during larval invasion of tissues. Sterile immunity is rarely achieved against intestinal or tissue invasive worms; although a few members of each population retain zero worm burden, these are the exception rather than the rule. More commonly, individuals manifest premunition, the ability of the body to protect against concomitant or massive infection once an adult worm has established residence. The function of immune responses against nematodes might be best interpreted as efforts primarily to control against pathologic consequences on infection rather than rid the body of every worm.[37] A form of acquired immunity exists in populations with endemic transmission of nematodes; the intensity of infection decreases sharply after the second decade of life, returning slightly at older ages.

The mechanisms of protection against nematodes have been subject to intense investigation. Features seen in characteristic responses of mammalian hosts to intestinal and tissue nematodes include local and systemic eosinophilia and local and systemic IgE production[38]; in intestinal nematode infection, a mucosal mastocytosis is also seen.[39] These aspects suggested an allergic or immediate type of hypersensitivity pattern to controlling nematode infections. Work done with mouse models of nematode infection showed that these responses required the presence of T cells (gut-associated lymphoid tissue [GALT]), and there appears to be selective proliferation of particular CD4$^+$ T cells (Th$_2$ subset) in many intestinal nematode infections. Subsequent study showed that particular T cell–derived lymphokines (interleukin-4 [IL-4], interleukin-5 [IL-5], and interleukin-3 [IL-3]) were the dominant

TABLE 2.
Parasitologic Features of Soil-Transmitted Nematodes

Primary Parasite Spp.	Primary Host	Modes of Transmission	Location of Larvae	Location of Adults	Egg Production/ Worm (Daily)	Life Span
Ascaris lumbricoides	Humans	Fecal-oral and fertilized eggs in soil	Larvae pass through lungs and expectorated to gut	Small intestine	200,000	<1 yr
Ancylostoma duodenale and *Necator americanus*	Humans	Larvae penetrate skin; occasional oral (*A doudenale*), transmammary (*A. doudenale*), and transplacental (?) (*A. doudenale*)	Free-living larvae enter skin and pass through pulmonary circulation	Small intestine (duodenum and jejunum)	20,000 (*A. duodenale*) 10,000 (*N. americanus*)	6–7 yr

Strongyloides stercoralis (*Strongyloides fulleborni*, parasite of primates)	Humans	Larvae penetrate skin; autoinfection; occasional oral; transmammary (S.f)	Larvae enter skin and pass through lungs	Small intestine, lungs and gut (hyperinfection), disseminated	13,000	Up to 35 yr
Trichuris trichuria	Humans	Eggs ingested	Mature to larvae by passage through gut	Cecum and upper colon	10,000	6–7 yr
Enterobius vermicularis	Humans	Eggs ingested; autoinoculation; retroinfection	Large intestine and perineal skin (?)	Cecum	1,000	30–45 days
Toxocara canis (dog roundworm) and *Toxocana cati* (cat roundworm)	Dogs/cats	Eggs ingested	Larvae develop and migrate to viscera	Fail to mature to adults	—	—
Ancylostoma braziliense (dog and cat hookworm)	Dogs/cats	Skin penetration	Larvae move through skin	Fail to mature to adults	—	—

mediators of local and systemic responses.[40] Similar responses have been detected in human nematode infections.[41] Depletion of these Th_2 cytokines did not result in decreased immunity[42]; thus, whether these responses are truly host protective is still a matter for debate.[43] In contrast, in certain mouse models, engendering a counter-Th_1 response resulted in protection.

Other areas regarding immunity to nematodes are under investigation. What causes these responses seems to be worm-derived products[44]; the appearance of these antigens may be key to generating a protective vs. a diverted host response. Effector mechanisms to kill nematode parasites include oxygen and nitric oxide radicals and complement. The parasites have in most cases evolved means to evade these destructive responses.[45] The puzzle of immunity to nematodes may be part of the "discontinuous variations in resistance"; some individuals are able to develop effective responses against (intestinal) nematodes, whereas others seem incapable of doing so.[37]

Description of specific diseases caused by soil-transmitted helminths follows, and Table 2 summarizes parasitologic features of these nematodes. Transmission of parasitic nematodes through soil may proceed either by ingestion of ova (ascariasis, trichuriasis, enterobiasis, and visceral larval migrans) or after skin penetration by larvae (hookworm, strongyloidiasis, and cutaneous larva migrans).

ASCARIASIS

Ascaris lumbricoides is one of the largest and most common parasites of humans.[46] The worms are smooth, round, and pinkish white. Adult worms reside in the small bowel and may grow 15 to 35 cm. Adult female worms may produce up to 200,000 embryonated and unembryonated eggs daily. Ingestion of embryonated eggs from soil (through contamination of fingers or geophagy) or contaminated foods (through use of night soil for fertilizer) results in release of second-stage larvae within the gut. These infective larvae penetrate the intestinal wall and enter the venous circulation to the lungs, where they break into the alveolar spaces. A local hypersensitivity reaction (Splendore-Hoeppli's phenomenon) may occur at sites of larval entry into lung tissue. Third-stage larvae then ascend to the trachea, where they are expectorated and swallowed, resulting in introduction of fourth-stage larvae into the gut. During their passage through the gut, these larvae develop into mature adults, which preferentially establish residence in the jejunum and ileum. Adult worms retain their location by actively swimming against peristaltic action of the gut. This motion sometimes results in migration of adults into pancreatic and biliary tracts.[47]

Ascariasis is most common in children of preschool or early school age.[48] The most common clinical manifestations are non-specific abdominal colic and sometimes abdominal distention. High intensities of infection may result in obstruction of the small bowel by tangled masses of adult worms; this complication occurs in approximately 1 in 1,000 infected individuals and may represent 30% to 50% of children who have acute obstruction in endemic areas.[49, 50] Clinical manifestations during larval migration in the lungs are generally minimal in endemic areas[51]; however, Loeffler's pneumonitis, with eosinophilia, wheezing, and pulmonary infiltrates, may occur in areas with seasonal transmission of *Ascaris*.[52] The nutritional impact of ascariasis has been controversial,[53] but it appears that the infection may result in subtle malnutrition[54] and may interfere with absorption of specific nutrients, such as vitamin A.[55]

The diagnosis is made by quantitative examination of the stools for distinctive golden-coated ovoid embryonated or unembryonated eggs; concentration techniques are rarely needed for examination. Adult worms may sometimes be passed per rectum or coughed up through the nose or mouth. Eosinophilia may be evident during pulmonary migration of third stage; in uncomplicated intestinal infections, eosinophils do not exceed 10% of total white blood cell count. Treatment is with mebendazole for uncomplicated intestinal ascariasis. Pyrantel pamoate may be used for heavy infestations.

TRICHURIASIS (WHIPWORM)

Trichuris trichuria is also transmitted by ingestion of eggs contaminating the soil or foods.[56] The eggs are extremely resistant to the external environment and mature after 3 weeks. After ingestion, larvae mature to adult forms during their passage through the gut. On arrival at the large intestine, adult worms are whip shaped with a narrow anterior end buried in intestinal mucosa and a coiled thicker posterior segment exposed to the lumen. Adult size ranges from 30 to 50 mm. *Trichuris* worms cause minute blood losses (0.005 mL/worm/daily) from trauma and proteolysis at their sites of attachment to mucosa. Inflammation secondary to these worms may be significant and even systemic.[57] Adult females shed approximately 13,000 eggs/worm/daily. The entire life cycle in humans is contained within the intestinal environment. It is reasoned that *Trichuris* must be a very efficient parasite because worm fecundity is relatively low.

Trichuriasis (whipworm) affects especially children 5 to 10 years old. Light infections are generally asymptomatic, whereas moderate infections may cause epigastric or lower abdominal pain, chronic diarrhea, or nausea and vomiting.[58] In hyperendemic areas severe infections may develop into a dysentery-like syndrome with tenesmus, right-sided abdominal pain, bloody diarrhea, and wasting. Severe inflammation of the colon and rectum with heavy infections can result in significant losses of water and electrolytes. A large worm burden may build up in the rectal vault; persistent straining, coupled with decreased muscle tone, may result in rectal prolapse. Stunted growth and severe anemia are well recognized in severe cases of trichuriasis, often complicated by multiple parasitic infections.[59] More recently, subtle deficits in school performance have been associated with moderate infections.[60]

The diagnosis of trichuriasis is established by finding characteristic barrel-shaped, twin-plugged eggs in stool. Direct examination of stool may be unreliable in light infections, and concentration techniques may be required. Diagnosis can be confirmed by visualization of adult worms at proctoscopy. Moderate peripheral eosinophilia (5%–15% of total white blood cell differential) may be seen after infection. Mebendazole and pyrantel pamoate are the drugs of choice for treatment of trichuriasis.

ENTEROBIASIS (PINWORM AND THREADWORM)

Enterobius vermicularis may be the most prevalent nematode parasite in the United States and Europe.[61] Humans are the only host, and transmission is maintained through fecal-oral spread and uncommonly by inhalation or ingestion of eggs from fomites. In temperate climes, transmission is facilitated by decreased washing, increased clothing and contact, and prolonged survival of eggs. The short-lived female worm resides in the cecum but wanders out into the perineal area to oviposit eggs. Rarely adult worms may migrate to other sites such as the vulva, peritoneum, and appendix. Pinworm eggs mature very quickly, so there is further potential for wide transmission of the parasite.[62] In addition, retroinfection may result from larvae that hatch from eggs and return to the cecum.

The classical clinical manifestation of enterobiasis is nocturnal pruritus ani due to hypersensitivity to worm antigens. A local tingling of perineal skin may also be reported. Aberrant migration of the adult females into the vulva occasionally results in vulvovaginitis and may predispose to urinary tract infections.

Cellophane tape applied to the perineum on awakening in the morning is used to detect eggs deposited on skin. Eggs are not usually seen on stool examination because of the low level of excretion; occasionally adult worms can be seen but are quite small (10 by 0.5 mm). Blood eosinophilia (6%–12% white blood cell differential) may be associated with infection. Mebendazole or pyrantel pamoate are curative after a single dose, but a second course of therapy is generally required because of reinfection with the parasite.

TOXOCARIASIS (VISCERAL LARVAL MIGRANS)

Toxocara canis (dog roundworm) and *Toxocara cati* (cat roundworm) larvae are the causative agents of visceral larval migrans.[63] Infections are found worldwide in both temperate and tropical climates.[64] Dogs and cats are carriers of adult worms, often after being infected with larvae in utero; the roundworms complete life cycles in the intestines of their hosts with the passage of ova. Infections in humans are acquired by ingestion of eggs shed by household pets or found outside the home (e.g., sandboxes), release and limited development of larvae within the intestine after ingestion of eggs and larva penetration of the bowel wall, and access portal blood to the liver and lungs. They form granulomas within these viscera and induce prominent peripheral eosinophilia and IgE responses. Due to their small size, larvae may escape into the peripheral circulation to lodge in small vessels of other tissues (e.g., retina and brain).

Clinical manifestations include tender hepatomegaly, hepatitis, or wheezing caused by larval migration.[65] The extent of symptoms reflects the amount of ingested embryonated eggs and the intensity of host immune response to the larvae. Manifestation may also be occult, with constitutional symptoms of fever, night sweats, and anorexia. Symptoms may persist for months to years without resolution because the inciting larvae often remain alive but encapsulated within host granulomas. Retinitis may develop as a result of subretinal trapped larvae.

Diagnosis is usually made by serologic determination of *Toxocara* titers because cross-reactive antigens within the *Ascaris* group of nematodes makes indirect methods (immunofluorescent antibody and indirect hemagglutination antibody) unreliable. Demonstration of the parasites in tissue is definitive. Diethylcarbamazine is the drug of choice to resolve the infection.

HOOKWORM

Hookworm results from infection by *A. duodenale* or *N. americanus* nematodes.[66] *Ancylostoma duodenale*, previously referred to as Old World hookworm, is found throughout the Mediterranean to India and some parts of Far East Asia. *Necator americanus*, the

New World hookworm, is widely distributed throughout North and South America, Africa, and Asia. Hookworm was present throughout the southeastern United States, but a successful eradication campaign and improved standards of living have greatly reduced transmission. Most cases are imported or occur within susceptible groups.

Larvae hatch from eggs deposited on ground by infected humans. After maturation, larvae penetrate exposed skin or are ingested through drinking water. After entry into the venous circulation, infective larvae are carried to the lungs, penetrate alveoli, and enter the tracheal airspace to be coughed and swallowed. Other modes of transmission, such as oral or transmammary passage of larvae, may account for some *Ancylostoma* infections.[67] The larvae then mature into adults, which attach to the jejunal mucosa. Buccal structures pierce the mucosa and anchor the worm, which sucks minute quantities of blood from intestinal capillaries. Adults move every 4 to 8 hours, resulting in multiple minute ulcerations to intestinal mucosa. Fertile female adult worms produce 9,000 to 30,000 eggs daily.

Humans are the primary host; endemicity of hookworm in an area is sustained by infections acquired by children and adolescents.[68] The major clinical manifestations of infection in children are iron deficiency anemia and hypoalbuminemia resulting from chronic worm burden and poor host diet. Growth retardation is seen in children with heavy infections in the second decade of life; whether this reflects malabsorption of proteins or malnutrition associated with hookworm infection is controversial.[69] Minor clinical manifestations include pruritus, erythema, and vesicular rash (ground itch) resulting from larval invasion of skin and occasional gastrointestinal and respiratory complaints. Symptoms may be more directly related to intensity of parasitic infection rather than host immune responses.[70]

The diagnosis is made from finding characteristic ovoid eggs in feces; concentration techniques may be required for light infections. Rhabditiform larvae may hatch from embryonated eggs and should be differentiated from *Strongyloides* larvae (large buccal cavity, small genital primordium). Treatment is with mebendazole and supplemental iron salts.

STRONGYLOIDIASIS

Strongyloides stercoralis has a variety of disease manifestations from asymptomatic infection to disseminated fatal hyperinfections.[71] The worms are widely distributed throughout the world;

the southeastern United States was once endemic for *S. stercoralis*, and indigenous infections are still occasionally seen.[72] Cases are also found among immigrants and other exposed populations, but severe infections are increasingly recognized among malnourished or immunosuppressed individuals.[73]

Larvae in stool develop into free-living adults or infective filariform larvae in the soil. The infective larvae penetrate skin to enter circulation, then pass to the lungs and finally to the upper small intestine, where they develop into adults. Adult worms produce eggs from which first-stage or rhabditiform larvae may hatch during transit through the bowel. In addition, *Stronglyoides* infections can result in autoinfection when rhabditiform larvae develop to infective larvae while still within the bowel. Because the infective larvae proceed through the lungs to reinfect the small intestine, the parasite is able to maintain infections for prolonged periods (over decades). This continuing cycle has the potential to increase dramatically when host immune status fails to control worm burden or invasion, resulting in hyperinfection (expansion of worms in lungs and intestine) and dissemination (penetration of viscera, e.g., liver and brain), respectively.

Humans are the primary host. In endemic areas, children often have asymptomatic strongyloidiasis.[74] Gastrointestinal symptoms (epigastric pain, vomiting, and diarrhea) may be prominent in some individuals. A chronic malabsorption-like syndrome with weight loss and protein-losing enteropathy may develop in severe infections. Repeated exposure of skin to infective larvae results in typical skin lesions (larva currens): large, erythematous urticarial lesions with rapidly moving edges. A Loeffler-like pulmonary syndrome with eosinophilia may occur on passage of larvae through the lungs, but it is generally milder than that seen in ascariasis and hookworm infections. In patients with severe malnutrition or immunosuppression, disseminated strongliodosis can manifest as acute abdominal distress, paralytic ileus, asthma, or spruelike disease.[75] Only a few cases support a linkage between strongyliodiasis and retroviral infections.[71] Moderate peripheral eosinophilia (mean 18% white blood cell differential) is a frequent accompaniment to infection.[76]

The diagnosis of strongyliodiasis must be considered in any patient from an endemic region who is to be treated with immunosuppressive agents (e.g., chemotherapy and transplant drugs). Definitive diagnosis requires demonstration of characteristic rhabditiform larvae (short buccal cavity and large genital primordium), because eggs hatch within the intestine. Diagnosis of uncomplicated infection can be difficult because repeated stool examinations often fail to demonstrate larvae, even after concentration. Yield may be further improved using duodenal fluid recovered by the string test. Serologic diagnostic assays offer increased sensitivity of detecting disease but have some cross-reactions with concurrent parasitic infections.[77] In *Strongyloides* hyperinfection, larvae may be readily recovered from sputum and other body fluids, as well as stool. Treatment of strongyloidiasis with thiabendazole is successful but has frequent side effects.[78] Albendazole or ivermectin have been used for treatment of disseminated strongliodiasis.

Strongyloides fulleborni is a parasite of primates that has been reported to cause human infections in Papua New Guinea and Africa.[79] In these areas, there is a high incidence of infections among nursing infants resulting in hyperinfection, malabsorption, and often fatal disease.[80] The parasite has been demonstrated in breast milk, supporting the possibility of transmammary transmission.[81]

CUTANEOUS LARVA MIGRANS (CREEPING ERUPTION)

Animal hookworm larvae, especially *Ancylostoma braziliense*, are responsible for this dermatologic disease, which is increasingly recognized.[82] Infective larvae penetrate skin but are unable to pass through to the circulation and the lungs. Infection commonly manifests as a dermatitis, typically on the extremities; the larvae move within the skin, resulting in migrating erythemas with pruritus. Treatment with topical thiabendazole is successful in controlling the rash and pruritus.[83] Accidental ingestion of larvae may induce eosinophilic enteritis in humans.

VECTOR-TRANSMITTED NEMATODES

There are relatively few nematode infections with an obligatory arthropod or crustacean intermediate host or vector. The most common vector-borne pathogens are filarid worms, which can be conveniently grouped into blood or tissue parasites, depending on location. Occasionally infections with dracunculid worms may be transmitted by ingestion of intermediate copepod hosts.

FILARIAL INFECTIONS

Human filariasis is not endemic in North America, with the exception of extraordinarily rare zoonotic infections.[84] In the United States, diagnosis of filarial infections in individuals immigrating or returning from endemic countries appears to be uncommon; this may reflect very low prevalence or underdiagnosis of infected individuals. In addition, onset of clinical disease may occur many years after one leaves an endemic area because filarial worms are relatively long lived.

Filarial worms are long, threadlike parasites that reside in tissues or body cavities. Fertilized females extrude mature microfilariae; these highly motile forms circulate in the peripheral blood or move within the cutaneous tissues. Some filarial species maintain distinct periodic shifts in the density of microfilariae detected in the peripheral blood, where maximal densities occur at times synchronous with peak feeding cycles of primary arthropod vectors. Such circadian fluctuations are important for diagnosis. Filariases are nonfatal but often chronic infections that may lead to disfiguring and debilitating sequelae. Pediatric reports of clinical filarial diseases are uncommon. In most cases, treatment is effective but frequently requires follow-up and retreatment. No vaccines are available for any human filarid parasite.

Filarid worms cause lymphatic (bancroftian and brugian filariasis) and cutaneous or subcutaneous disease (onchocerciasis, loiasis, and mansonellosis).[85] Lymphatic disease caused by *Wuchereria bancrofti*, *Brugia malayi*, and *Brugia timori* account for more than 90 million human cases throughout the tropics, far more than other filarid parasites combined. Descriptions of specific filarial diseases follow, and parasitologic features are summarized in Table 3. Zoonotic filariases and dracunculosis are discussed separately.

Bancroftian filariasis

Wuchereria bancrofti is the most common filarial parasite in humans; there are an estimated 82 million infected individuals and more than 900 million people at risk of infection.[86] Bancroftian filariasis is worldwide in distribution but occurs predominately in urban coastal areas in tropical and subtropical regions.[87]

Wuchereria bancrofti is exclusively a human parasite with no known animal reservoir. In endemic areas, exposure begins early in childhood and continues throughout life; rates of microfilaremia in children can be significant in areas of high transmission. One survey found more than 15% of all children less than age 9 years with microfilaremia before control programs began in Tahiti.[88] A wide variety of culicine and anopheline mosquito vectors can transmit infection; infective larvae are deposited on skin and crawl into the bite wound. The time required for adults to develop, mate, and release microfilariae detectable in the circulation (biological incubation period or prepatent period) is 9 to 12 months or longer, and infections can persist for 6 to 8 years.

There is a wide spectrum of responses to infection, which de-

TABLE 3.

Parasitologic Features of Human Filarial Parasites

Primary Parasite Spp.	Geographic Distribution	Primary Host	Transmission Vector	Location of Microfilaria	Location of Adult Worms	Periodicity	Life Span (yr)
Wuchereria bancrofti	Cosmopolitan and tropics/ subtropics	Humans	Mosquitoes	Blood	Lymphatics	Nocturnal and subperiodic	6–8
Brugia malayi and *Brugia timori*	Asia	Humans	Mosquitoes	Blood	Lymphatics	Nocturnal and subperiodic	6–8
Onchocerca volvulus	Africa, South and Central America	Humans	*Simulium* (black fly)	Skin	Subcutaneous tissues	None	≤15
Loa loa	West and Central Africa	Humans	*Chrysops* (deer fly)	Blood	Subcutaneous tissues	Diurnal	≤17
Mansonella streptocerca	West Africa	Humans	*Culicoides* (midge)	Skin	Subcutaneous tissues	None	?
Mansonella perstans	Africa, South and Central America	Humans	*Culicoides* (midge)	Blood	Mesenteries and retroperitoneal tissues	None	?
Mansonella ozzardi	South and Central America	Humans	*Culicoides* and *Simulium*	Blood	Mesenteries and body cavities	None	?

pend in part on cumulative exposure (intensity × length of exposure) to the parasite. Some innate immunity to filarial infection may exist, but most immunity is partial and increases with age and exposure; acquired immunity probably regulates chronic worm burdens and protects from superinfection. Development of partial immunity coincides with the presence of adult worm antigens, elevated antifilarial IgE, IgM and IgG antibody levels, and skin test positivity to filarial antigens.[89] Asymptomatic exposed individuals in endemic areas are protected against infective larvae by antibody-mediated immunity.

In endemic areas, many infections occur without evident disease; individuals commonly remain asymptomatic despite detectable microfilaremia. Pathologic conditions result from continual lymphatic irritation and are strongly associated with variable host immunologic responsiveness between early and chronic infections.[90] Generally lymphatic disease can be divided into inflammatory manifestations (characterized by adenolymphangitis, lymphedema, lymphatic ulceration, orchitis, chyluria, and hydrocele) and obstructive manifestations associated with tissue fibroses and skin thickening. Cases with inflammatory and obstructive lymphatic disease generally represent a small percentage of the infected community.

Acute inflammatory responses are not uncommon in naíve individuals on exposure to filarial parasites. Filarial fevers are caused by immediate hypersensitivity reactions to microfilariae and developing adult worms. Mechanisms involving primarily IgE and eosinophils are responsible for absence of circulating microfilariae despite infection (occult or cryptic filariasis).[91] Recurrent bouts of filarial fever can occur for many years after one leaves an endemic area. In endemic areas, prominent suppressor immune mechanisms involving the IgG4 subclass and cytokines diminish immunologic responsiveness and greatly reduce pathology.

Chronic lymphatic pathologic conditions and obstruction (elephantiasis) generally manifest in young adults after chronic infection and repeated exposure to filarial parasites. Upper and lower limbs and genitalia can be affected with massive proliferation of lymphatic tissues. Clinical signs of elephantiasis are usually more common in males than females. Microfilariae are usually reduced or absent from peripheral blood. Lymphatic abnormalities are associated with delayed-type hypersensitivity responses to filarial antigens; specific IgE, IgG2, and IgG4 antifilarial antibodies and eosinophilia are also present.[92] Inadequate immunity against infective larvae permits continual invasion of new worms and promotes pathologic conditions.

Tropical pulmonary eosinophilia is an asthmalike disorder found in endemic populations, generally among young men.[93] It is also an occult filariasis associated with marked immunologic hyperresponsiveness to microfilariael antigens. Massive accumulation of activated eosinophils in the lung (Loeffler's syndrome) result in a chronic obstructive or restrictive pulmonary syndrome. Diagnosis is often complicated by the enhanced antibody responses that result in clearance of microfilaremia.

A complete travel history is important for diagnosis of any filarial disease, because location and length of stay provide important information on potential risk for infection. Demonstration of microfilariae in the peripheral blood, urine (chyluria), or hydrocele fluid provides definitive diagnosis of bancroftian filariasis. Wet mounts, stained thick smears, and concentration techniques may be used for cases where low microfilariael densities are suspected[94]; common methods include filtration of whole blood (1–2 mL) through a 3-μm Millipore filter or examining cellular sediment after mixing blood and 2% formaldehyde (Formalin) solution in 1:10 dilution.[95] It is best to sample blood at suspected peak parasite densities, usually during evening to midnight hours; individuals with known exposure to infection in the South Pacific should ideally be examined in late afternoon.

Patients with suspected filarial fever and associated symptoms (low-grade fever, eosinophilia, chest symptoms, or lymphedema) often need diagnostic assays to determine infection status because it is often hard to detect circulating microfilariae. Research in this area has been difficult because of the lack of a good animal model. The microfilarial antigen skin test and assays based on serum IgE levels have had low predictive or prognostic value. Assays to detect circulating filarial antigens hold promise for accurately detecting all microfilaremic, as well as a proportion of amicrofilaremic, infections. Recently a highly specific and sensitive monoclonal antibody–based enzyme-linked immunosorbent assay has been developed and is commercially available.[96] In addition, IgG4 antifilarial antibodies indicate the presence of active infection with greater specificity and may aid diagnosis.[97] Diagnostic DNA probes and polymerase chain reaction technology offer promise for the future.

In pediatric age groups, the drug of choice for lymphatic filariasis is diethylcarbamazine citrate (DEC), which kills blood-stage microfilariae. It has a short half-life and very low toxicity in humans. However, antihistamines or corticosteroids may be required to abrogate allergic reactions to antigens released by dying microfilariae. Persons with lymphatic disease are prone to developing local reactions with treatment (lymphadenitis, transient lymphedema, and abscess formation).[98] Complete cures can be difficult to obtain without repeated courses, because adult worms may not be effectively killed by the drug. Ivermectin, a newly developed macrocyclic lactone antibiotic, can also reduce microfilaremia, but like DEC, it may require retreatment at 6-month intervals.[99] Ivermectin does not appear to be effective in treatment of tropical pulmonary eosinophilia syndrome. Chronic inflammation and elephantiasis (a rare event in childhood) may require surgical intervention or compression bandage therapy. Hydrocele can be aspirated or surgically repaired.

Malayan and Timorian Filariasis

Brugia malayi and *B. timori* are related parasites with similar disease manifestations. Infections are limited to rural areas of Asia, with *B. malayi* being most common in Southeast Asia and *B. timori* restricted to southeastern Indonesia.[87] An estimated 9 million infections are caused by the 2 parasites. Their life cycles resemble that of *W. bancrofti*, but varying microfilarial periodicities are found with *B. malayi* infection.

Malayan and timorian filariasis manifest with inflammation of the lymphatics and recurrent acute symptoms.[100] Acute episodes may occur with greater frequency and severity than in bancroftian filariasis. Elephantiasis usually affects areas below the knees and elbows. Inguinal lymphatic abscesses and scarring are common, whereas hydrocele and chyluria are very uncommon manifestations of disease.

Diagnosis is based on detection of characteristic microfilariae in peripheral blood with symptomatic manifestation in endemic areas. Monoclonal antibody–based assays and DNA probes have been developed but are not routinely used. Treatment is with DEC. High rates of adverse side effects have been reported in asymptomatic individuals and in persons from hyperendemic areas.[101] Ivermectin and DEC have shown similar rates of efficacy in treatment.

Onchocerciasis (River Blindness)

Onchocerca volvulus occurs in West and Central Africa, Yemen, and Central and South America; about 18 million people are infected, and an estimated 78 million remain at risk for infection. The worm is transmitted from person to person by the bites of female black flies (*Simulium* spp.) that breed in fast-flowing streams. The multinational Onchocerciasis Control Program greatly reduced incidence of the disease in West Africa over the past 20 years, yet disease control remains a formidable problem.[102]

Infection begins at an early age in endemic areas; children as young as 6 months have had detectable infections.[103] Infective larvae may require 12 months to develop into adult worms; fertile female parasites normally live up to 15 years and discharge millions of microfilariae. Microfilariae can persist in the skin, eyes, and other tissues for up to 24 months. No known animal reservoirs exist.

Adult worms in subcutaneous tissues are surrounded by characteristic fibrous nodules, particularly notable about the head and shoulders (the Americas) or pelvic girdle and lower extremities (Africa). Skin nodules can be easily detected, particularly over bony prominences, yet nodules will occur in deeper tissues with no observable signs in some cases. Nodules occur at lower frequency in children compared with adults. An immunologically mediated onchocercal dermatitis may accompany severe infections, causing intense rash and itching, changes in skin pigmentation (leopard skin), and swelling, thickening and atrophy of the skin (hanging groin). In chronic infections, large numbers of microfilariae in the eyes eventually die and calcify, causing ocular lesions and impaired sight or blindness.

Pathologic conditions are related to microfilarial density and the balance of host inflammatory and suppressor responses.[104] Infection progresses through life and can result in both skin (inflammation and fibrosis) and corneal (sclerosing keratitis and blindness) involvement. Fibrous encapsulation of adult worms is also a host-derived reaction but is not considered immunopathologic.

Onchocerciasis is more likely to be diagnosed in a nonendemic area than lymphatic filariasis because of skin nodule formation. Demonstration of microfilariae in skin snips or the isolation of adult worms from excised nodules is definitive. Microfilariae are not found in the blood. The Mazzotti reaction, based on an immediate hypersensitivity response to dying microfilariae after giving DEC treatment, gives further evidence of active disease.[105] Serologic tests are of value in light infections or where nodules reside in deep tissue. Ultrasonography has proved useful for detection of deep tissue nodules.

All palpable nodules should be surgically removed. Although DEC effectively kills microfilariae, it can produce undesirable side effects, particularly inducing Mazzotti's reactions in the eyes or skin. Ivermectin is a safe and effective microfilaricidal drug, providing longer lasting control with fewer side effects. It is effective in a single oral dose, and given annually, it prevents accumulation of microfilariae and decreases risk of blindness.[106] Neither drug is effective for prophylaxis or kills adult worms. The prognosis after chemotherapy is good if lesions do not endanger the eyes. Patients should be examined for microfiladermia on a semiannual or annual basis.

Loaisis

Loa loa, the African eye worm, is confined to West and Central Africa, where an estimated 13 million individuals are infected. The worm is transmitted by several species of day-biting deer flies (*Chrysops* spp.). The prepatent period is about 6 months but may be considerably longer. Adult worms may live 17 years or more.

Adult worms migrating in subcutaneous tissues can provoke a temporary inflammation ("Calabar swellings") in any part of the body. Whites are particularly susceptible to allergic reactions to adult worm antigens, which include peripheral eosinophilia, fever, and urticarial swellings of skin and mucous membranes.[107] Commonly microfilaremia is less often found in children than in adults, although adult worms are present. *Loa loa* may rarely invade the central nervous system (CNS), causing encephalitis or spinal cord damage.

Loiasis is often diagnosed clinically because of the conspicuous transient swellings associated with fever and prominent eosinophilia. During acute phases of infection, microfilariae are frequently not detectable in peripheral blood; then immunodiagnosis using an immunofluoresce antibody test is the preferred choice for detection of disease. Surgical removal of adult worms provides the best prognosis for treating disease. Migrating worms can sometimes be removed when they traverse the cornea beneath the conjunctiva or are located across the bridge of the nose. Special caution in the use of chemotherapy to eradicate infection is warranted because of reported severe Mazzotti-like allergic reactions, including encephalopathy, that can occur in heavy infections as a result of rapid killing of the microfilariae.[108] Antihistamines or corticosteroids may be required to decrease allergic reactions. Suramin and DEC are effective against both microfilariae and adult parasites. Ivermectin and albendazole have also been found to reduce microfilariae.[109] Apheresis has been reported effective in reducing microfilaremia in heavily infected patients.[93] For weekly prophylaxis against loiasis in endemic areas, DEC has been recommended.[110]

Mansonellosis

Three species of *Mansonella* are responsible for human infection.[111] The epidemiology and health impact of these nematodes are poorly understood. Prevalence of infection with *Mansonella perstans* and *Mansonella ozzardi* can reach more than 90% in some endemic populations.

Mansonella streptocerca occurs only in West Africa. The number of infected people is unknown. Adult worms live in subcutaneous tissue, usually less than 1 mm below the skin surface. Microfilariae are nonperiodic and found in the skin during day and night. The vectors for this infection are *Culicoides* spp. (biting midges). The disease varies from asymptomatic microfiladermia to dermatitis (pruritus, hypopigmented macules, and lichenification). These conditions should be distinguished from leprosy and granuloma multiforme. Diagnosis involves examination of blood smears, as well as skin snips in saline solution as described for onchocerciasis, and microfilariae must be differentiated from *Onchocerca* spp. Treatment with DEC is effective against both microfilariae and adults.

Mansonella perstans occurs in Africa, South America, and the Caribbean. Adults reside in the body cavity and deep connective tissue. Microfilariae are found in the blood and show no marked periodicity. The vectors include biting midges. This parasite produces little overt disease but may result in eosinophilia, angioderma, arthralgia, and itching. Diagnosis is made by recovery of microfilariae from blood. Variable treatment success has been reported with DEC. Mebendazole chemotherapy is preferred but is considered investigational for this condition in the United States.[27]

Mansonella ozzardi is found in Central and South America and the Caribbean. The adult worms are located in the body cavity, whereas nonperiodic microfilariae are found in the blood. Arthropod vectors include both *Culicoides* spp. and *Simulium* spp. Although considered nonpathogenic, infection has been associated with pruritus, articular pain, eosinophilia, and lymphadenopathy. Diagnosis is based on recovery of microfilariae from the blood. Although DEC has no effect, ivermectin might be effective against both microfilariae and adult worms.[112]

Zoonotic Filariases

Several species of *Dirofilaria* animal parasites have been reported to cause human pulmonary and cutaneous disease.[84] Humans constitute dead-end hosts because microfilariae are not produced in these zoonotic infections.

Dirofilaria immitis, dog heartworm, has been responsible for more than 50 documented cases of human pulmonary disease in the United States. Transmission is mosquito borne. This infection has not been reported in children, and only 15% of documented cases have been less than age 40 years. The worm, often found in an occluded branch of the pulmonary artery, can lead to local coagulation, necrosis, and fibrosis. Common symptoms are chest pain, cough, and hemoptysis. Eosinophilia is infrequent. A characteristic fibrotic nodule ("coin lesion") is sometimes present in the lung on radiograph. Treatment consists of surgical removal of the nematode.

Cutaneous disease may rarely be caused by *Dirofilaria* spp., which are common parasites of raccoons, bears, dogs, and cats. Typically the conjunctivae and subcutaneous tissues are involved. In most cases, the female worms are infertile, and infection is abortive. Diagnosis is made by finding worms in surgically removed lesions.

Dracunculosis (Guinea Worm)

Dracunculus medinensis is the largest known nematode parasite (60–100 cm) in humans. It represents a serious health and economic risk in arid and semiarid parts of Africa and south Asia, infecting as many as 2 million people, with another 100 million at risk. The goal of eradicating dracunculosis by 1995 was declared by the World Health Assembly, and important achievements have been made in endemic countries.[113]

Individuals are infected by drinking water containing infective larvae developing within the bodies of tiny crustacean intermediate hosts (*Cyclops* spp. [water fleas]). Within 12 months of ingestion, fertile adult female worms migrate to subcutaneous tissues and produce skin blisters on a distal part of the body (usually the foot or lower leg). The female worms evacuate motile larvae into the water during immersion of the limb. These larvae then infect the copepod intermediate hosts essential for their survival.

Inflammatory reactions to the adult female often cause painful swelling and debilitating joint pain. Fever, nausea, vomiting, diarrhea, dyspnea, urticaria, and eosinophilia may accompany or precede formation of skin blisters. Although infection is not fatal, serious secondary infections and tetanus are not uncommon. All age groups appear to be susceptible to infection, and multiple and repeated infections can occur because there is no acquired infection. Diagnosis is by microscopic identification of larvae or recognition of the adult female worm and blister formation. No drugs eradicate worms from infected individuals. Benzimidazole drugs (metronidazole, niridazole, and thiabendazole) appear to decrease inflammation, relieve pain and itching, and facilitate parasite removal. However, the drugs do not appear to have an adverse effect on the worms. The worm is difficult to remove surgically without promoting sepsis. Administration of tetanus toxoid is recommended for patients with open lesions.

TABLE 4.
Parasitologic Features of Foodborne Nematodes

Principal Parasite Spp.	Primary Host	Intermediate Host	Modes of Transmission	Location of Larvae	Time to Clinical Manifestation in Humans
Trichinella spiralis	Humans	Pigs; also polar bears, seals	Ingestion of contaminated meats containing encysted larvae	Larvae pass through intestine and migrate to muscle (daughter cells)	May be silent (found at autopsy)
Anisakis simplex	Cetacea (whales, dolphins)	Saltwater fish	Larvae penetrate intestinal mucosa and occasionally perforate viscus	Stomach and small intestine, particularly duodenum	Hr–days after ingestion

Angiostrongylus cantonensis	Rats	Snails and freshwater fish	Larvae penetrate skin and occasionally enter CNS* tissues	CNS* and eyes	Few days–wk
Angiostrongylus costaricensis	Rats	Veroncilid slugs	Abdominal tissue granulomas	Mesentric arteries	Days–wk
Capillaria philippinensis	Birds	Freshwater fish	Small intestine and autoinfection	Small intestine	Several wk
Gnathostoma spinigerum	Dogs/cats	Copepods, fish, etc.	Ingestion of infected intermediate host	Variable	Wk

*CNS = central nervous system.

FOODBORNE NEMATODES

Foodborne nematodes are less known, rarely reported, and often more pathogenic nematode infections that are associated with eating habits.[114] Humans are usually not the natural host for these worms but are accidental or paratenic hosts.[115] Changes in diet and unique eating habits contribute to the increased incidence of these parasitoses.[116] Recognition of symptoms and the development of new diagnostic techniques are also important in the increasing incidence of these diseases. Table 4 summarizes parasitologic features of some of these parasitoses.

TRICHINOSIS

Five species of *Trichinella* are now recognized: *Trichinella spiralis, Trichinella nativa, Trichinella nelsoni, Trichinella pseudospiralis,*and *Trichinella britovi.* However, *T. spiralis* is the species responsible for most human illness and has the widest geographic distribution, including temperate regions.[117] Adult worms are small (females 2–4 mm by 60–100 μm and males 1.0–1.5 mm).

Trichinosis is acquired by ingestion of animal muscle containing encysted larvae. Larvae are liberated from cysts in the small intestine and enter the gut columnar epithelium. The larvae become adults within 24 hours, and mating occurs within a further 12 to 24 hours. Five days after infection, fertile female worms produce living larvae that enter the intestinal vasculature and are disseminated throughout the body. On reaching striated muscle, the larvae penetrate individual muscle cells, which transform into nurse cells. In a few weeks, the larvae become infective, and the nurse cell becomes a thick-walled capsule. Larval production ceases after several weeks after the adult worms are expelled by immune reactions associated with T cells, IgG antibodies, and peripheral eosinophilia.

In most individuals, infections are asymptomatic, but severity of infection rises with ingestion of a large number of larvae. Adult worms embedded in the intestinal mucosa may cause abdominal pain, nausea, weight loss, anorexia, diarrhea, and fever. Migrating larvae produce symptoms of muscle and joint pain, along with emaciation, dyspnea, and periorbital edema. Neurologic and myocardial complications may occur in severe infections.

Diagnosis is based on symptoms, a history of eating potentially infected meat, and demonstration of the parasite (usually by muscle biopsy). Serologic tests are of little value early in the course of infection. Antigen detection systems are available, and the use of molecular technology will eventually be applicable in detecting parasite genetic material.[118] Treatment with thiabendazole, mebendazole, or pyrantel pamoate is effective. Corticosteroids may be necessary for individuals with severe symptoms.

Pork and improperly cooked pork products are the major sources of infection. Wild animal meat from bears, boars, walruses, or wolves has also been involved in scattered epidemics. Thorough cooking of all meats prevents infection.

ANISAKIASIS

Anisakiasis is the accidental human infection with the larval stage of marine anisakine nematodes; adult anisakids do not infect humans.[119] Adult worms are found in marine mammals such as whales, porpoises, dolphins, and seals, whereas the larval stages are found in various species of fish and squid. Adult female worms pass eggs in the feces; after a period of development on the ocean floor, developed larvae hatch from the eggs and are eaten by small crustaceans. The larvae become infective, and when the crustaceans are eaten by fish, they migrate to the peritoneal cavity and musculature of fish. When the fish is eaten by the definitive host, the worms probably migrate through the host's body and eventually develop into adults in the intestine. Humans become infected after eating the intermediate fish or squid hosts raw. The larvae may then penetrate intestinal mucosa and provoke an intense inflammatory reaction.

Two species most often associated with human illness are *Anisakis simplex* and *Pseudoterranova decipiens*.[120] The former is associated with invasive disease, and the latter is usually noninvasive. The larva of *A. simplex* is tapered at both ends and measures 20 to 35 mm long and 0.3 to 0.06 mm wide. *Pseudoterranova decipiens* is larger, 25 to 50 mm long and 0.3 to 1.22 mm wide. Anisakine larvae, especially those of *P. decepiens*, enter the pharyngeal area and cause "tickle throat." *Anisakis simplex* larvae usually involve the gastric mucosa and initially elicit a foreign body reaction with the infiltration of neutrophils, scant eosinophils, and giant cells. Protease secretions by the parasite may cause tunnels or burrows in the gastric mucosa. An abscess develops in a few days after massive infiltration of phagocytic cells, lymphocytes, histiocytes, and plasma cells, with eventual necrosis and hemorrhage. The worms eventually die as a result of the inflammatory reaction. Larvae may also enter the peritoneal cavity and other organs.

Symptoms may occur within a few hours or a few days after an infectious meal. Symptoms associated with *A. simplex* may resemble peptic ulcer disease. Abdominal pain, nausea, vomiting, fever, and possibly diarrhea are early symptoms, which may persist for a few weeks. Blood may be found in the stools and gastric aspirates. The diagnosis of anisakiasis is usually misdiagnosed as an acute condition of the abdomen, ulcer, or other gastrointestinal conditions. A confirmed diagnosis is made by recovery of the parasite in vomitus or feces or after removal by endoscopy or surgery. Tissue sections obtained by gastric biopsy may also reveal the parasite. Serologic tests may provide a presumptive diagnosis. Removal by surgery or fiberoptic endoscopy is recommended, and prognosis is good after treatment. Chemotherapy with mebendazole and albendazole has not been completely tested.

ANGIOSTRONGYLIASIS

There are approximately 20 species of *Angiostrongylus;* but only *Angiostrongylus cantonensis* and *Angiostrongylus costaricensis* are foodborne and accidental parasites of humans.[121]

Angiostrongylus cantonensis lives in the pulmonary arteries of rats; female adult worms lay eggs, and first-stage larvae hatch and enter the alveoli. The larvae then migrate up the pulmonary tree, are swallowed, and are passed in the feces. Second-stage larvae then enter terrestrial or aquatic snails and develop into third-stage, or infective, larvae. When the mollusks are eaten by rats, these larvae are released, enter the intestinal tissues, and are carried by the circulation to the brain. They develop into young adult worms in the CNS and after 3 weeks migrate to the pulmonary arteries to complete their life cycle. When humans eat infected mollusks, infective larvae can enter the CNS and cause eosinophilic meningitis or eosinophilic meningoencephalitis.[122]

Angiostrongyliasis cantonensis is reported from many parts of Asia, Pacific Islands, Australia, India, parts of Africa, and a few of the Caribbean Islands.[24] A young boy has recently been reported with the disease in New Orleans.[123] Many species of mollusks can serve as intermediate hosts, but *Achatina fulica, Pila* spp., and the garden snails *Bradybaena similasis* are the most important. There are also known paratenic hosts, such as land crabs, frogs, and toads.

Most angiostrongyliasis patients in Taiwan are children, whereas most in Thailand are adults.[124, 125] Furthermore, it is believed that more parasites are acquired by eating the giant African snail *(A. fulica)* in Taiwan, a snail often found harboring hundreds, if not thousands, of larvae. *Pila* spp. of snails are the common source of infection in Thailand, and they usually have light infections with third-stage larvae. Therefore, symptoms are considered related to the number of larvae ingested.

Symptoms may develop soon after eating raw mollusks. Penetration of intestinal mucosa by the released larvae may cause nausea, vomiting, abdominal pain, and diarrhea. A skin rash with itching has also been reported from some areas in Thailand. Mild fever, malaise, cough, sneezing, and rhinorrhea then develop. Central nervous system manifestations (headache, fever, stiff neck, and paresthesias of the trunk and extremities) may occur soon afterward, and cranial nerve palsies have also been observed. Coma is common in Taiwanese children but is not often seen in Thai patients. In cases of meningitis there is an eosinophilic pleocytosis, and worms may be recovered from spinal fluid, especially in children.[126] Worms have been recovered from the eye chamber, and in these cases there are usually no symptoms of meningitis. The disease may persist for several weeks, and then symptoms eventually resolve. Deaths have been reported but are rare.

A confirmed diagnosis requires the recovery of worms from cerebrospinal fluid or the eye. A presumptive diagnosis may be based on symptoms and history of ingestion of or association with snails from endemic areas. Serologic tests only support a presumptive diagnosis; antibody or antigen detection tests of sera and cerebrospinal fluid using monoclonal antibodies are of value.[127] Radiographic scans (computed tomography and magnetic resonance imaging) are reportedly of value.[128]

Specific antihelminthic treatment is not recommended by some physicians because dead worms may contribute to the pathologic condition. Mebendazole and albendazole are reported to be effective in treating children in Taiwan. Supportive treatment and sometimes surgery are necessary when worms are present in the eyes. Infections are easily prevented by simply cooking the intermediate and paratenic hosts thoroughly before eating them.

Angiostrongylus costaricensis lives in the mesenteric arteries of rodents in Costa Rica and other American countries.[129] The natural intermediate host is a slug, *Vaginulus plebeius*, which allows development of third-stage larvae after the host ingests rodent feces containing first-stage larvae. Humans are accidental hosts after ingestion of slugs concealed in produce or vegetables contaminated with infectious mucous secretions. The parasite enters the mesenteric arteries and causes formation of a large eosinophilic granuloma near the cecum (abdominal angiostrongyliasis).[130] The clinical manifestation may resemble appendicitis, and many cases are discovered on surgical exploration. Surgical resection is often required, and chemotherapy with thiabendazole or mebendazole has been used as adjunctive treatment. A case has recently been reported in the United States.[131]

CAPILLARIASIS

Although a number of species of *Capillaria* are reported from animals, only three species have been reported to cause infection in humans: *Capillaria aerophila* (a parasite of the respiratory tract of canines and felines; rare in humans), *Capillaria hepatica*, and *Capillaria philippinensis*. *Capillaria hepatica* is found in the liver of rats and other rodents worldwide, but fewer than 30 infections, mostly in children, are reported in the literature.[132] In contrast, *C. philippinensis* was first reported from humans and is responsible for severe disease.[133] The parasite is found in the small intestine and causes a life-threatening gastroenteritis. More than 2,000 infections have been reported from Asia, particularly the Philippines and Thailand, with sporadic cases elsewhere. Infection is most common in middle-aged men; only a few children have been reported with the disease. Infections are associated with the dietary habit of eating uncooked freshwater or brackish water fish. Fish-eating birds are thought to be the natural hosts.

Capillaria philippinensis is one of the smallest worms found in humans (males are 1.3–3.9 mm; females are 2.5–5.3 mm). Eggs passed in the feces of infected humans and embryonate in 5 to 10 days. When eggs are swallowed by small freshwater fish, they hatch in the intestine, and the released larvae become infective in a few weeks. When the fish are eaten uncooked by humans, the larvae released from the digested fish become adults in 2 weeks. Some fertile female worms will produce eggs, and others produce larvae that develop into adults in the small intestines. This autoinfection leads to hyperinfection with thousands of parasites. The rapidly increasing worm population is responsible for increasing disease and death if untreated.

Few symptoms are experienced early in the infection with *C. philippinensis*. As the worm burden increases, patients experience abdominal pain, borborygmi, and diarrhea with increasing intensity. Patients may have 5 to 10 voluminous watery stools daily, with malaise, vomiting, and weight loss. Over months, the patients develop muscle wasting, weakness, hypotension, edema, and anasarca. Electrolyte imbalances develop with hypokalemia and hypocalcemia; hypoproteinemia may result from protein-losing enteropathy and malabsorption. Death will result if specific treatment is not given.

Specific diagnosis is made by finding typical striated bipolar eggs (40 by 20 μm) or larvae and adult worms in the feces. Thiabendazole, mebendazole, and albendazole are effective curative chemotherapy. The recommended regimen includes an antidiarrheal, electrolyte replacement, and treatment with mebendazole or albendazole.

GNATHOSTOMIASIS

Gnathostomes are nematode parasites usually found in tumorlike masses in the stomach of carnivorous mammals.[134] The larval stages are responsible for disease in humans, which follows cutaneous or subcutaneous larval migration. The parasite may also cause serious illness by invading the eye or CNS. The disease is reported from children, as well as adults, with most infections being reported from Thailand and Japan.

Gnathostoma spinigerum is the most common species reported in humans. Males measure 11 to 25 mm and females 25 to 54 mm. The worm live in tumors in the stomach, with the posterior end extending into the stomach lumen. Eggs produced by fertile females pass into the feces, reach water, and embryonate in 7 to 10 days. First-stage larvae hatch from the eggs and are eaten by freshwater copepods (*Cyclops* spp.), where second-stage larvae develop. After a second intermediate host (fish, birds, amphibians, reptiles, and mammals) eats the copepod, the larvae enter the tissue of the animal and become infective third-stage larvae. When the definitive host eats an infected second intermediate host, the larvae emerge from the digested tissue, penetrate the stomach wall, migrate to the liver and other organs, the peritoneal cavity, and finally penetrate the stomach wall to form tumors.

Humans acquire the parasite by eating a second intermediate host, such as the snakeheaded fish.[135] Infections occur in males and females of all age groups. Larvae migrate throughout tissue and eventually enter subcutaneous tissue. Tracks made by the migrating worm cause inflammatory lesions, necrosis, and hemorrhage. Swelling may also develop, along with pain and edema. These reactions are transient and migratory; they disappear only to reappear several days later at a different location. The parasite may cause direct damage to the eye, and encephalitis, myelitis, radiculitis, and subarachnoid hemorrhage may evolve if the CNS is invaded.[136]

Consideration in differential diagnosis must be given to syndromes caused by other nematode- or cestode-migrating larvae. The diagnosis is made by finding characteristic worms in surgical specimens, urine, sputum, or vaginal discharge. A presumptive diagnosis is made in endemic areas by history, symptoms, or serologic findings. There is no specific anthelminthic therapy, but preliminary findings suggest that albendazole given daily over several weeks may cause the worms to migrate out of subcutaneous tissues.[137]

CONCLUSION

A wide variety of human diseases are associated with the diverse group of nematode parasites. The cost of these billions of infections in human morbidity alone is staggering. Although treatment is still relatively uncomplicated, new issues of control of these infections will pose the future global challenge. For clinicians in the United States, the primary issue will be recognition of these infections as they arrive or resurface among children, the target population for so many of these parasites.

A framework for formulating pathogenesis of nematode infections in humans arises from understanding their modes of transmission and from an appreciation of their general life cycles. Nematodes that have evolved a direct life cycle with humans as the primary host, such as intestinal nematodes, are most successful at maintaining their ecologic niche. As one moves from the soil-transmitted parasites to foodborne parasites, there is increasing complexity of interaction, and humans become an incidental host. There is often a consequent increase in pathologic conditions, because parasites have less chance to develop evasion strategies to circumvent the immune system.

No single review will encompass the nematode parasites. Perhaps this one will spark further interest in the often neglected nematode infections and restore some well-deserved importance to the very clever nematode parasites.

REFERENCES

1. Parasites, parasitism and host relations. In Markell EK, Voge M, John D (eds): *Medical Parasitology*, ed 7. Philadelphia, WB Saunders, 1992.
2. Ogilvie BM, Selkirk ME, Maisels RM: The molecular revolution and nematode parasitology: yesterday, today, and tomorrow. *J Parasitol* 76:607–618, 1990.
3. Selkirk ME, Maisels RM: Nematode antigens. In Englund PT, Sher A (eds): *The Biology of Parasitism.*
4. The intestinal nematodes. In Markell EK, Voge M, John D (eds): *Medical Parasitology*, ed 7. Philadelphia, WB Saunders, 1992.
5. Schad GS, Chwodhury AB, Dean CG, et al: Arrested development in human hookworm infections: An adaptation to a seasonally unfavorable external environment. *Science* 180:502–504, 1973.
6. Beaver PC: Wandering nematodes as a cause of disability and disease. *Am J Trop Med Hyg* 6:433–437, 1957.

7. Savioli L, Bundy D, Tomkins A: Intestinal parasitic infections—a soluble public health problem. *Trans R Soc Trop Med Hyg* 86:353, 1992.

8. Cook GC: The clinical significance of gastrointestinal helminths—a review. *Trans R Soc Trop Med Hyg* 80:675, 1986.

9. Stoll NR: This wormy world. *J Parasitol* 33:1–18, 1947.

10. Schweitzer N, Anderson RM: Immunology, helminths, and equations. In Ash C, Gallagher RB (eds): *Immunoparasitology Today*. Cambridge, Elsevier, 1991, pp A76–A81.

11. Bundy DAP: The global burden of intestinal nematode disease. *Trans R Soc Trop Med Hyg* 88:259–261, 1994.

12. Stephenson LS, Latham MC, Kinoti SN, et al: Improvements in physical fitness of Kenyan schoolboys infected with hookworm, *Trichuris trichuria* and *Ascaria lumbricoides* following a single dose of albendazole. *Trans R Soc Trop Med Hyg* 84:277–282, 1990.

13. Crompton DWT: Nutritional aspects of infection. *Trans R Soc Trop Med Hyg* 80:697–705, 1986.

14. Stephenson LS: *Impact of Helminth Infections on Human Nutrition*. London, Taylor & Francis, 1987.

15. Nokes C, Bundy DAP: Does helminth infection affect mental processing and educational achievement? *Parasitol Today* 10:14–18, 1994.

16. Haswell-Elkins MR, Elkins DB, Anderson RM: Evidence for predisposition of humans to infection with *Ascaris*, hookworm, *Enterobius*, and *Trichuris* in a South Indian fishing community. *Parasitology* 95:323–337, 1987.

17. Chamone M, Marques CA, Atuncar GS, et al: Are there interactions between schistosomes and intestinal nematodes? *Trans R Soc Trop Med Hyg* 84:557–558, 1990.

18. Woodruff AW: Helminths as vehicles and synergists of microbial infections. *Trans R Soc Trop Med Hyg* 62:446–452, 1968.

19. Kappus KK, Juranek DD, Roberts JM: Results of testing for intestinal parasites by state diagnostic laboratories. *MMWR* 40:25–45, 1991.

20. Hoffman SJ, Barrett-Connor E, Norcross W, et al: Intestinal parasites in Indochinese immigrants. *Am J Trop Med Hyg* 30:340, 1981.

21. Jannista JA, Chapman D: Medical problems of foreign-born adopted children. *Am J Dis Child* 141:298–302, 1987.

22. Chattopadhyay B, Fricker E, Gelia CB: Incidence of parasitic infestations in minority group travellers to and new immigrants arriving from the Third World countries. *Public Health* 102:245–250, 1988.

23. Yoeli M, Most H, Hammond J, et al: Parasitic infections in a closed community. Results of a 10-year survey in Willowbrook State School. *Trans R Soc Trop Med Hyg* 66:764, 1972.

24. Kliks MM, Palumbo NE: Eosinophilic meningitis beyond the Pacific Basin: the global dispersal of a peridomestic zoonosis caused by *Angiostrongylus cantonensis*, the nematode lungworm of rats. *Soc Sci Med* 34:199–212, 1992.

25. Cook GC: Anthelminthic agents: Some recent developments and their clinical application. *Postgrad Med J* 67:16–22, 1991.
26. Marr JJ: Antiprotozoal and anthelminthic chemotherapy. In Hoeprich PD, Jordan MC, Ronald AR (eds): *Infectious Diseases: A Treatise of Infectious Processes*, ed 5. Philadelphia, JB Lippincott, 1994, pp 296–297.
27. Drugs for parasitic infections. *Med Lett* 35:111–122, 1993.
28. Committee on Infectious Diseases, American Academy of Pediatrics: *Report of the Committee on Infectious Diseases*, ed 23. 1991, p 575.
29. Jernigan J, Guerrant RL, Pearson RD: Parasitic infections of the small intestine. *Gut* 35:289–293, 1994.
30. Crofton HD: A model of host-parasite relationships. *Parasitology* 63:343–364, 1971.
31. Anderson RM: The population dynamics and epidemiology of intestinal nematode infections. *Trans R Soc Trop Med Hyg* 80:686, 1986.
32. Anderson RM, May RM: Helminth infections of humans: Mathematical models, population dynamics and control. *Adv Parasitol* 24:1–101, 1985.
33. Anderson RM, May RM: Herd immunity to helminth infection: Implications for disease control. *Nature* 315:493–496, 1985.
34. Elkins DB, Haswell-Elkins M, Anderson RM: The epidemiology and control of intestinal helminths in the Pulicat Lake region of Southern India. I. Study design and pre- and post-treatment observations on *Ascaris lumbricoides* infection. *Trans R Soc Trop Med Hyg* 80:774–792, 1986.
35. Wakelin D: Genetic and other constraints on resistance to infection with gastrointestinal nematodes. *Trans R Soc Trop Med Hyg* 80:742–747, 1986.
36. Chan L, Bundy DAP, Kan SP: Aggregation and predisposition to *Ascaris lumbricoides* and *Trichuris trichuria* at the familial level. *Trans R Soc Trop Med Hyg* 88:46–48, 1994.
37. Befus D: Immunity in intestinal helminth infections: Present concepts, future directions. *Trans R Soc Trop Med Hyg* 80:735–741, 1986.
38. Finkelmann FD, Pearce EJ, Urban JF Jr, et al: Regulation and biological function of helminth-induce cytokine responses. *Parasitol Today* 7:A62, 1991.
39. Urban JF Jr, Gamble HR, Katona IM: Intestinal immune responses of mammals to nematode parasites. *Am Zool* 29:469–478, 1989.
40. Finkelmann FD, Pearce EJ, Urban JF Jr, et al: Regulation and biological function of helminth-induce cytokine responses. *Parasitol Today* 7:A62–A66, 1991.
41. Mahanty S, King CL, Kumaraswami V, et al: IL-4- and IL-5-secreting lymphocyte populations are preferentially stimulated by parasite-derived antigens in human tissue invasive nematode infections. *J Immunol* 151:704–711, 1993.
42. Urban JF Jr, Madden KB, Svetic A, et al: The importance of Th2 cyto-

kines in protective immunity to nematodes. *Immunol Rev* 127:206–220, 1992.

43. Pritchard DI: Immunity to helminths: Is too much IgE parasite—rather than host-protective? *Parasite Immunol* 15:5–9, 1993.
44. Reiner SL, Locksley RM: The worm and the protozoa: stereotyped responses or distinct antigens? *Parasitol Today* 9:258–260, 1993.
45. Behnke JM: Evasion of immunity by nematode parasites causing chronic infections. *Adv Parasitol* 26:1–71, 1987.
46. Pawlowski ZS: Ascariasis. *Clin Gastroenterol* 7:157–178, 1978.
47. Khuroo MS, Zargar SA, Mahajan R: Hepatobiliary and pancreatic ascariasis in India. *Lancet* 335:1503, 1990.
48. Crompton DWT: The prevalence of ascariasis. *Parasitol Today* 4:162–169, 1989.
49. Blumenthal DS, Schultz MG: Incidence of intestinal obstruction in children infected with *Ascaris lumbricoides*. *Am J Trop Med Hyg* 24:801–805, 1975.
50. Louw JH: Abdominal complications of *Ascaris lumbricoides* in children. *Br J Surg* 53:510, 1966.
51. Spillman RK: Pulmonary ascariasis in tropical communities. *Am J Trop Med Hyg* 24:791–800, 1975.
52. Gelpi AP, Mustafa A: *Ascaris* pneumonia. *Am J Med* 44:377, 1968.
53. Schultz MG: Ascariasis: Nutritional implications. *Rev Infect Dis* 4:814–816, 1982.
54. Thein Hlaing, Thane-Toe, Than-Saw, et al: A controlled chemotherapeutic intervention trial on the relationship between *Ascaris lumbricoides* infection and malnutrition in children. *Trans R Soc Trop Med Hyg* 85:523–528, 1991.
55. Mahalanabis D, Simpson TW, Chakraborty ML, et al: Malabsorption of water miscible vitamin A in children with giardiasis and ascariasis. *Am J Clin Nutr* 32:313–318, 1979.
56. Bundy DAP, Cooper ES: Trichuria and trichuriasis in humans. *Adv Parasitol* 28:107–173, 1989.
57. MacDonald TT, Spencer J, Murch SH, et al: Immunoepidemiology of intestinal helminthic infections. 3. Mucosal macrophages and cytokine production in the colon of children with *Trichuris trichuria* dysentery. *Trans R Soc Trop Med Hyg* 88:265–268, 1994.
58. Jung RC, Beaver PC: Clinical observations on *Trichocephalus trichuris* (whipworm) infestation in children. *Pediatrics* 18:548–557, 1951.
59. Gilman RH, Chong YH, Davis C: The adverse consequences of heavy *Trichuris* infections. *Trans R Soc Trop Med Hyg* 77:432, 1983.
60. Cooper E, Bundy DAP: *Trichuris* is not trivial. *Parasitol Today* 4:301–306, 1988.
61. Wolfe MS: *Oxyuris, Trichostrongylus, and Trichuris. Clin Gastroenterol* 7:201–217, 1978.
62. Keystone JS: Enterobiasis. In Goldsmith R, Heyneman D (eds): *Tropical Medicine and Parasitology*. East Norwalk, Conn, Appleton & Lange, 1989, pp 357–361.

63. Marsden PD: Other nematodes. *Clin Gastroenterol* 7:219–229, 1978.
64. Magnaval J-F, Michault A, Calon N, et al: Epidemiology of human toxocariasis in La Reunion. *Trans R Soc Trop Med Hyg* 88:531–533, 1994.
65. Beaver PC: Parasitological reviews. Larva migrans. *Exper Parasitol* 5:587–621, 1956.
66. Banwell JG, Schad GA: Hookworm. *Clin Gastroenterol* 7:128–156, 1978.
67. Hotez PJ: Hookworm disease in children. *Pediatr Infect Dis J* 8:516–520, 1989.
68. Miller TA: Hookworm infection in man. *Adv Parasitol* 17:315–383, 1979.
69. Gilman RH: Hookworm disease: Host-pathogen biology. *Rev Infect Dis* 4:824–829, 1982.
70. Maxwell C, Hussain R, Nutman TB, et al: The clinical and immunologic responses of normal human volunteers to low dose hookworm (*Necator americanus*) infection. *Am J Trop Med Hyg* 37:126–134, 1987.
71. Liu Lx, Weller PF: Strongyloidiasis and other intestinal nematode infections. *Infect Dis Clin North Am* 7:655–682, 1993.
72. Walzer PD, Milder JE, Banwell JG, et al: Epidemiologic features of *Strongyloides stercoralis* infection in an endemic area of the United States. *Am J Trop Med Hyg* 31:313–319, 1982.
73. Carvalho Filho E: Strongyliodiasis. *Clin Gastroenterol* 7:179–200, 1978.
74. Burke JA: Stronglyloidiasis in childhood. *Am J Dis Child* 132:1130–1136, 1978.
75. Smith SB, Schwartzman M, Mencia LF, et al: Fatal disseminated strongyloidiasis presenting as acute abdominal distress in an urban child. *J Pediatr* 91:607–609, 1977.
76. Milder JE, Walzer PD, Kilgore G, et al: Clinical features of *Strongyloides stercoralis* infection in an endemic area of the United States. *Gastroenterology* 80:1481–1488, 1981.
77. Gam A, Neva FA, Krotoski WA: Comparative sensitivity and specificity of ELISA and IHA for serodiagnosis of strongyloidiasis with larval antigens. *Am J Trop Med Hyg* 37:157–161, 1987.
78. Grove DI: Treatment of strongyloidiasis with thiabendazole: An analysis of toxicity and effectiveness. *Trans R Soc Trop Med Hyg* 76:114–118, 1982.
79. Kelly A, Little MD, Voge M: *Strongyloides fulleborni*–like infections in man in Papua New Guinea. *Am J Trop Med Hyg* 25:694–699, 1976.
80. Ashford RW, Vince JD, Gratten MJ, et al: *Strongyloides* infection associated with acute infantile disease in Papua, New Guinea. *Trans R Soc Trop Med Hyg* 72:554, 1978.
81. Brown RC, Girardeau MHF: Transmammary passage of *Strongyloides* sp. larve in the human host. *Am J Trop Med Hyg* 26:215–219, 1977.

82. Elliot DL, Tolle SW, Goldberg L, et al: Pet associated illnesses. *N Engl J Med* 313:985–995, 1985.
83. Cutaneous larva migrans in travelers: Synopsis of histories, symptoms, and treatment of 98 patients. *Clin Infect Dis* 19:1062–1066, 1994.
84. Beaver PC, Jung RC, Cupp EW: *Clinical Parasitology*, ed 3. Philadelphia, Lea & Febiger, 1984.
85. Ottesen EA: Filarial infections. In Maguire JH, Keystone JS (eds): *Infectious Disease Clinics of North America*. Philadelphia, WB Saunders, pp 619–633, 1993.
86. World Health Organization: Lymphatic filariasis: The disease and its control—fifth report of the WHO Expert Committee on Filariasis. *WHO Tech Rep Ser* 86:1–7, 1992.
87. Sasa M: *Human Filariasis*. Baltimore, University Park Press, 1976.
88. Beye HK, Edgar SA, Mille R, et al: Preliminary observations on the prevalence, clinical manifestations and control of filariasis in the Society Islands. *Am J Trop Med Hyg* 1:637–661, 1952.
89. Ottesen EA: Filariasis now. *Am J Trop Med Hyg* 41:9–17, 1989.
90. WHO Expert Committee on Filariasis: Lymphatic filariasis: Diagnosis and pathogenesis. *Bull WHO* 71:135–141, 1993.
91. Beaver PC: Filariasis without microfilaremia. *Am J Trop Med Hyg* 19:181–189, 1970.
92. King CL, Nutman TB: Regulation of the immune response in lymphatic filariasis and onchocerciasis. *Parasitol Today* 7:A54–A57, 1991.
93. Ottesen EA, Nutman TB: Tropical pulmonary eosinophilia. *Annu Rev Med* 43:417–424, 1992.
94. World Health Organization: *Control of Lymphatic Filariasis: A Manual for Health Personnel*. Geneva, World Health Organization, 1987.
95. Ash LR, Orihel TC: *Parasites: a Guide to Laboratory Procedures and Identification*. Chicago, ASCP Press, 1991, pp 83–84, 111–114.
96. More SJ, Copeman DB: A highly specific and sensitive monoclonal antibody-based ELISA for the detection of circulating antigen in bancroftian filariasis. *Trop Med Parasitol* 41:403–406, 1990.
97. Kwan LG, Forsyth KP, Maizels RM: Filarial-specific IgG4 response correlates with active *Wuchereria bancrofti* infection. *J Immunol* 145:4298, 1990.
98. Ottesen EA: Description, mechanisms, and control of post-treatment reactions in human filariasis. *Ciba Found Symp* 127:265–283, 1987.
99. Campbell WC: Ivermectin as an antiparasitic agent for use in humans. *Annu Rev Microbiol* 45:445–474, 1991.
100. World Health Organization: Lymphatic filariasis: Diagnosis and pathogenesis. *Bull WHO* 71:135–141, 1993.
101. Partono F: Diagnosis and treatment of lymphatic filariasis. *Parasitol Today* 1:52–57, 1985.
102. Webbe G: The Onchocerciasis Control Programme. *Trans R Soc Trop Med Hyg* 86:113–114, 1992.

103. Onchocerciasis. In Benenson AS (ed): *Control of Communicable Diseases in Man.* ed 15. Washington, DC, American Public Health Association, 1990, pp 308–311.

104. Ottesen eA: Immune responsiveness and the pathogenesis of human onchocerciasis. *J Infect Dis* 171:659–671, 1995.

105. Taylor AER, Denham DA: Diagnosis of filarial infections. *Trop Dis Bull* 89:R1–R33, 1992.

106. Greene BM, Taylor Hr, Cupp EW, et al: Comparison of ivermectin and diethylcarbamazine in the treatment of onchocerciasis. *N Engl J Med* 313:133, 1985.

107. Nutman TB, Miller KD, Mulligan M, et al: *Loa loa* infection in temporary residents of endemic regions: Recognition of a hyperresponsive syndrome with characteristic clinical manifestations. *J Infect Dis* 154:10–17, 1986.

108. Carme B, Boulesteix J, Boutyes H, et al: Five cases of encephalitis during treatment of loiasis with diethylcarbamazine. *Am J Trop Med Hyg* 44:684–690, 1991.

109. Martin-Prevel Y, Cosnefroy J-Y, Tshipamba P, et al: Tolerance and efficacy of single high-dose ivermectin for the treatment of loiasis. *Am J Trop Med Hyg* 48:186–192, 1993.

110. Nutman TB, Miller KD, Mulligan M, et al: Diethylcarbamazine prophylaxis for human loiasis: Results of a double-blinded study. *N Engl J Med* 319:752–756, 1988.

111. Beaver PC, Jung RC, Cupp EW: *Clinical Parasitology,* ed 3. Philadelphia, Lea & Febiger, 1984, pp 350–399.

112. Nutman TB, Nash TE, Ottesen EA: Ivermectin in the successful treatment of a patient with *Mansonella ozzardi* infection. *J Infect Dis* 154:662–665, 1987.

113. Centers for Disease Control and Prevention: Recommendations of the International Task Force for Disease Eradication. *MMWR* 42(RR-16):7–10, 1993.

114. Nelson GS: Parasitic zoonoses. In Englund P, Sher A (eds): *The Biology of Parasitism.* New York, Alan R Liss, 1988, pp 13–41.

115. Cross JH: Fish and invertebrate-borne helminths. Hui YH, Gorhan JR, Murrell KD, et al (eds): *In Food-borne Disease Handbook.* New York, Marcel Dekker, 1994, pp 279–329.

116. Schantz PM, McAuley J: Current status of food-borne parasitic zoonoses in the United States. *Southeast Asian J Trop Med Public Health* 22(suppl):65–71, 1991.

117. Bailey TM, Schantz PM: Trends in the incidence and transmission patterns of trichinosis in humans in the United States: Comparison of the periods 1975–1981 and 1982–1986. *Rev Infect Dis* 12:5–11, 1990.

118. Zarlenga DS, Barta JR: DNA analysis in the diagnosis of infection and in the speciation of nematode parasites. *Rev Sci Tech* 9:533–554, 1990.

119. Sakanari JA, McKerrow JH: Anisakiasis. *Clin Microbiol Rev* 2:278–284, 1989.

120. Schantz PM: The dangers of eating raw fish. *N Engl J Med* 320:1143–1145, 1989.
121. Bhaibulaya M: Snail-borne parasitic zoonoses: Angiostrongyliasis. *Southeast Asian J Trop Med Public Health* 22(suppl):189–193, 1991.
122. Hsu WY, Chen JY, Chien CT, et al: Eosinophilic meningitis caused by *Angiostrongylus cantonensis. Pediatr Infect Dis J* 9:443–445, 1990.
123. New D, Little MD, Cross J: *Angiostrongylus cantonensis* infection from eating raw snails. *N Engl J Med* 332:1105, 1995.
124. Hwang KP, Chen ER: Clinical studies on angiostrongyliasis cantonensis among children in Taiwan. *Southeast Asian J Trop Med Public Health* 22(suppl):194–199, 1991.
125. Punyagupta S, Juttijudata P, Bunnag T: Eosinophilic meningitis in Thailand: Clinical studies of 484 typical cases probably caused by *Angiostrongylus cantonensis. Am J Trop Med Hyg* 24:921–931, 1975.
126. Koo J, Pien F, Kliks MM: *Angiostrongylus (Parastrongylus) cantonensis* eosinophilic meningitis. *Rev Infect Dis* 10:1155–1162, 1988.
127. Jaroonvesama N, Chareonlarp K, Buranasin P, et al: ELISA testing in cases of clinical angiostrongyliasis in Thailand. *Southeast Asian J Trop Med Public Health* 16:110–112, 1985.
128. Hsu WY, Chen JY, Chien CT, et al: Eosinophilic meningitis caused by *angiostrongylus cantonensis. Pediatr Infect Dis J* 9:443–445, 1990.
129. Morera P: Life history and redescription of *Angiostrongylus costaricensis. Am J Trop Med Hyg* 22:613–621, 1973.
130. Loria-Cortes R, Lobo-Sanahuja JF: Clinical abdominal angiostrongylosis. A study of 116 children with intestinal eosinophilic granuloma caused by *Angiogstrongylus costaricensis. Am J Trop Med Hyg* 29:538–544, 1980.
131. Hulbert TV, Larsen RA, Chandrasoma PT: Abdominal angiostrongyliasis mimicking acute appendicitis and Meckel's diverticulum: report of a case in the United States and review. *Clin Infect Dis* 14:836–840, 1992.
132. Ewing GM, Tilden IL: Capillaria hepatica, a report of the fourth case of true human infestation. *J Pediatr* 48:341–348, 1956.
133. Cross JH: Intestinal capillariasis. *Clin Micrbiol Rev* 5:120–129, 1992.
134. Miyazaki I: On the genus *Gnathostoma* and human gnathostomiasis. *Exp Parasitol* 9:338–370, 1960.
135. Dow C, Chiodini PL, Haines AJ, et al: Human gnathostomiasis. *J Infect* 17:147–149, 1988.
136. Schmutzhard E, Boongird P, Vejajiva A: Eosinophilic meningitis and radiculomyelitis in Thailand caused by CNS invasion on *Gnathostoma spinigerum* and *Angiostrongylus cantonensis. J Neurol Neurosurg Psychiatry* 51:80–87, 1988.
137. Kraivichian P, Kulkumthorn M, Yingyourd P, et al: Albendazole for the treatment of human gnathostomiasis. *Trans R Soc Trop Med Hyg* 86:418–421, 1992.

Hepatitis A and B Vaccines in Children

Jay M. Lieberman, M.D.
Assistant Professor of Pediatrics, UCLA School of Medicine,
Harbor-UCLA Medical Center, UCLA Center for Vaccine Research,
Torrance, California

David P. Greenberg, M.D.
Associate Professor of Pediatrics, UCLA School of Medicine,
Harbor-UCLA Medical Center, Associate Director, UCLA Center for
Vaccine Research, Torrance, California

A lthough hepatitis is an ancient disease (Hippocrates provided one of the earliest descriptions of epidemic jaundice), it is only over the past 30 years that the causative viruses have been characterized. In the 1960s, Krugman et al.[1] described two types of viral hepatitis that were designated MS-1 and MS-2. The virus causing MS-1 or infectious hepatitis was later identified as hepatitis A, and the agent of MS-2 or serum hepatitis was identified as hepatitis B. In 1965, Blumberg et al.[2] discovered an antigen in the serum of an Australian aborigine; the "Australia antigen" was subsequently shown to be hepatitis B surface antigen (HBsAg). Later, the Dane particle, the complete hepatitis B virion, was described.[3] In 1973, hepatitis A virus (HAV) was visualized by immune electron microscopy,[4] and later in the decade the virus was successfully propagated in cell culture.[5] Since then, other viral causes of hepatitis have been identified: the delta agent, a defective virus that causes infection only in the presence of active hepatitis B virus (HBV) infection; hepatitis C virus, the agent responsible for most cases of transfusion-related non-A, non-B hepatitis; and hepatitis E virus, a cause of enterically transmitted non-A, non-B hepatitis.

Even as the alphabet of hepatitis viruses has expanded, great strides have been made in the quest to prevent HAV and HBV. Hepatitis B vaccines, the first that can prevent a cancer and a sexually transmitted disease, are now part of routine childhood immunizations. The first hepatitis A vaccine has recently been licensed in the United States. This review focuses on the use of these two vaccines in infants and children.

Advances in Pediatric Infectious Diseases®, vol. 11
© 1996, Mosby–Year Book, Inc.

HEPATITIS B

Hepatitis B virus is the smallest DNA virus known. It is a 42-nm double-shelled spherical particle whose outer layer contains HBsAg proteins and glycoproteins. The inner protein shell is the viral capsid and contains the core antigen (HBcAg) and the e antigen (HBeAg). HBsAg proteins are produced in excess, are released by infected cells, and circulate as small spherical or filamentous particles.

Humans are the only natural host for HBV, which is transmitted primarily by exposure to blood or serous fluids from infected individuals.[6] The blood of infected individuals contains high concentrations of virus, whereas semen and saliva have much lower concentrations. The major modes of transmission are via transfusion of contaminated blood, by inoculation with contaminated needles, through sexual contact with an infected person, and vertical transmission from an infected mother. Perinatal transmission occurs primarily at delivery, and the risk of transmission is significantly increased in women who are HBeAg positive, which correlates with high levels of circulating virus. Horizontal transmission also occurs, particularly in families with young children who are infectious.[7, 8]

The incubation period averages 100 days, with a range of 45 to 180 days. Symptoms of HBV include nausea, vomiting, anorexia, malaise, low-grade fevers, abdominal pain, and jaundice. Arthralgias and rashes can occur early in the course of the illness. However, most infants and young children have asymptomatic infections, and even among adults, fewer than half are symptomatic.[9] The disease is occasionally fulminant, and in the United States about 300 people die annually from acute HBV infection.

As shown in Figure 1, patients are viremic, and therefore infectious, before the onset of symptoms. The development of antibodies against HbsAg signals resolution of the infection, but some people do not develop antibodies and chronic infection ensues, defined as persistent serum HBsAg positivity over a 6-month period. Persons with chronic HBV infection are at increased risk for developing liver cirrhosis, hepatocellular carcinoma, or both.

EPIDEMIOLOGY

In the United States, approximately 200,000 to 300,000 acute HBV infections occur annually, more than 1 million people are chronically infected, and 4,000 to 5,000 people die each year from HBV-induced cirrhosis or hepatocellular carcinoma. Most infections are acquired in early adulthood (Fig 2). However, the risk of chronic

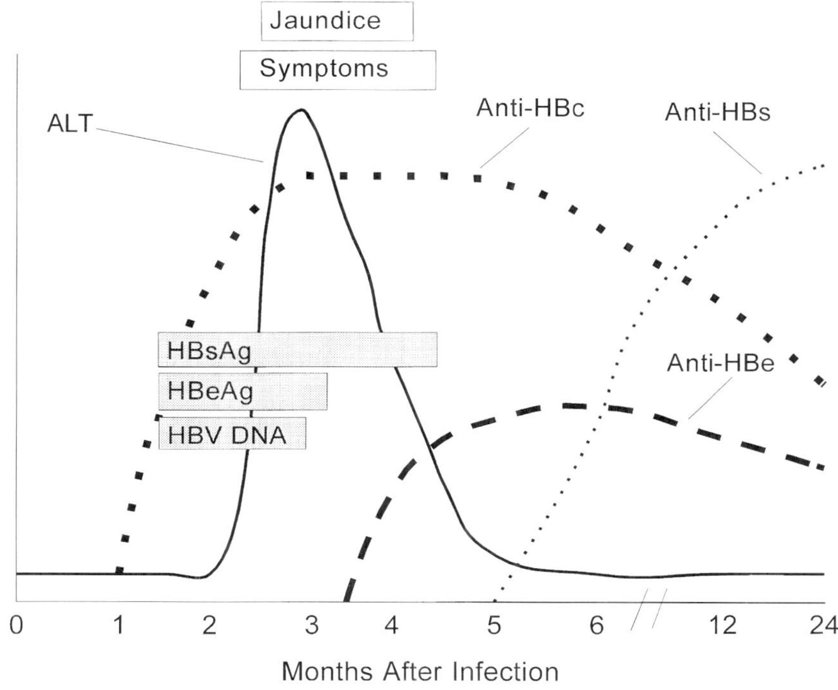

FIGURE 1.

Course of typical acute hepatitis B virus infection with complete recovery. The onset of symptoms is preceded by HBsAg serum positivity. IgM HBcAg-specific antibodies develop early in the course of infection and may be the only marker of infection in the "window"period between the time HBsAg is no longer present in the serum and when HBsAg-specific antibodies appear.

carriage is inversely related to the age at which infection is acquired.[9] Infants who are infected perinatally have a 70% to 90% risk of chronic carriage, whereas the risk is 20% to 50% for children younger than 5 years and only 5% to 10% for older children and adults.[10] Thus, in the United States, although infants and young children account for only about 4% of acute HBV infections, about 25% of chronic carriers acquired their infection early in life.[11]

Worldwide, an estimated 300 million people are chronic carriers of HBV, and 75 to 100 million of them will die from cirrhosis or hepatocellular carcinoma. In certain areas, such as Southeast Asia, China, and Africa, more than 10% of the population is chronically infected, and cirrhosis and hepatocellular carcinoma are leading causes of death. In these areas, a much higher percentage of HBV infections are acquired perinatally, so that 30% to 50% of chronic carriers acquired their infection perinatally.[6]

Risk factors for acute HBV in the United States are shown in Figure 3. About one third of infected persons do not have an identifiable risk factor and therefore fall outside the scope of a targeted immunization strategy.

VACCINES

After the discovery of HBsAg and the development of assays to measure anti-HBs (HBsAg-specific antibodies), several observations suggested the potential utility of HBsAg as a vaccine antigen. During recovery from acute HBV infection, HBsAg is cleared from the serum as anti-HBs appear, and these antibodies protect against reinfection. Subsequently it was shown that serum from an HBsAg-positive patient, heated to inactivate infectious virus, induced anti-HBs in healthy individuals.[12]

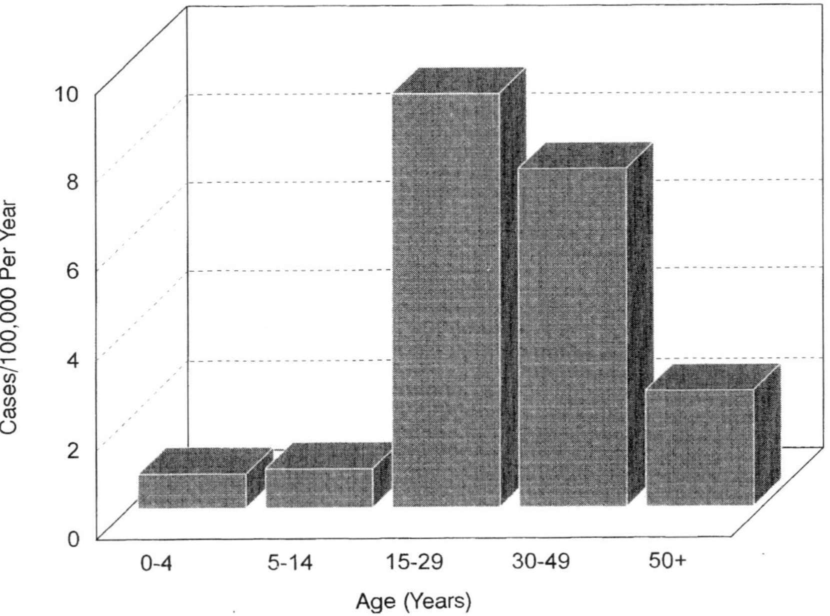

FIGURE 2.

Incidence rates (reported cases per 100,000 population per year) by age for hepatitis B virus, 1993. (Data courtesy of the Viral Hepatitis Surveillance Program, Hepatitis Branch, Centers for Disease Control and Prevention, Atlanta.)

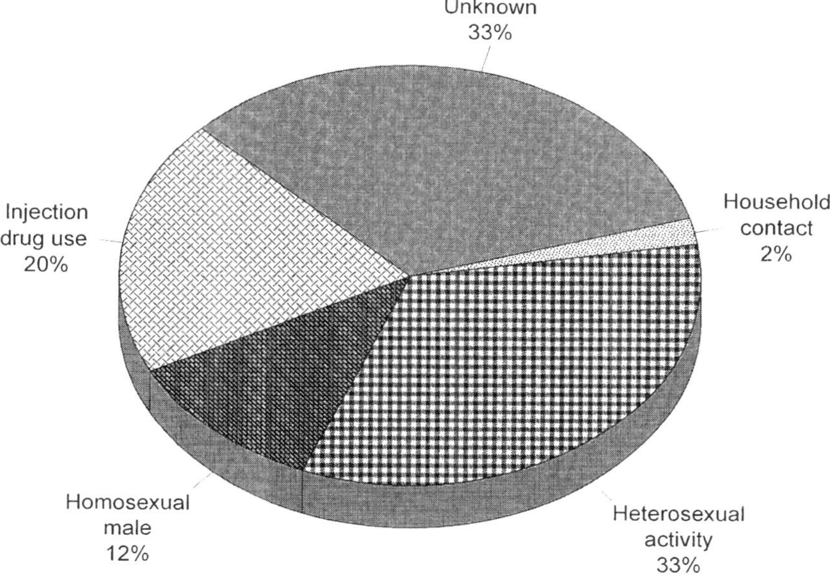

FIGURE 3.

Risk factors for reported cases of hepatitis B virus, 1993. Heterosexual activity includes sexual contact with multiple partners or with persons with acute hepatitis virus or HBsAg carriers. (Data courtesy of the Sentinel Counties Study, Centers for Disease Control and Prevention, Atlanta.)

In the 1970s, the first HBV vaccines were developed from the plasma of asymptomatic HBV carriers.[13, 14] These vaccines contained 22 nm HBsAg particles that were purified by biophysical and biochemical methods and then treated with heat or chemicals to inactivate potential contaminating infectious agents. Testing in chimpanzees and humans demonstrated that these vaccines were safe, immunogenic, and effective in preventing HBV infection. In 1982, the first plasma-derived HBV vaccine (Heptavax B, Merck & Company) was licensed in the United States and was recommended for individuals at high risk of infection.[15] However, the vaccine was costly to produce, the supply of human serum could not be assured, and there were unfounded concerns about the possibility of viral contamination, particularly with human immunodeficiency virus (HIV). These concerns led to very slow public acceptance of the vaccine.

In the mid-1980s, recombinant DNA technology was used to produce HBsAg.[16] The portion of the viral genome (S gene) coding for HBsAg is transferred to an appropriate plasmid that is then inserted into the desired expression vector. The two recombinant vaccines currently licensed in the United States (Recombivax HB, Merck & Company; Engerix-B, SmithKline Beecham [SB]), are produced using common baker's yeast, *Saccharomyces cerevisiae*, although vaccines have also been produced with vectors such as mammalian cell lines (Chinese hamster ovary) and different viruses. After lysing the yeast cells, the HBsAg is purified by biochemical and biophysical techniques.

In the United States, the first yeast-derived recombinant vaccine was licensed in 1986, and the recombinant vaccines have replaced the plasma-derived vaccines. In many parts of the world, however, the plasma-derived vaccines are still used. The two types of vaccine are essentially equivalent in safety, immunogenicity, and protective efficacy. Because both are inactivated subunit vaccines containing only noninfectious HBsAg particles, they cannot cause HBV infection. In both types of vaccine, aluminum hydroxide is used as an adjuvant, and thimerosal is added as a preservative.

SAFETY

Both the plasma-derived and recombinant HBV vaccines are very safe. In adults, adverse reactions occurred at similar rates among individuals given plasma-derived vaccine or placebo.[17, 18] The rates of side effects were also similar in adults given either plasma- or yeast-derived vaccines.[19] The recombinant vaccines have been given to thousands of people in clinical trials and to millions of people around the world. The most frequent side effects are pain and inflammation at the injection site. These and other reactions generally resolve within 48 hours after vaccination and occur less frequently with subsequent doses. There is no correlation between the frequency or severity of adverse reactions and the amount of HBsAg given per dose.

The tolerability of HBV vaccines has been evaluated in more than 10,000 infants and children.[19-22] Reactions occur less frequently in infants and children than in adults. Minor reactions are reported in less than 7% of infants and include mild temperature elevations (usually <38° C), local redness or soreness, and systemic symptoms such as brief periods of poor feeding or irritability. Adverse reactions occur more frequently in older children; 10% to 25% have local tenderness or systemic reactions such as low-grade fever, headache, and malaise. Concurrent administration of other childhood vaccines does not result in an increased rate of adverse reactions.

Severe adverse events have been reported infrequently in adults and rarely in infants and children. A possible association was found between plasma-derived vaccine and Guillain-Barré syndrome (GBS) in adults.[23] Cases of GBS have also been reported after use of the recombinant vaccines,[24, 25] but there is insufficient evidence to determine if there is a causal relationship between HBV vaccines and GBS.[26] Guillain-Barré syndrome has not been observed after vaccination of children.[26, 27] Although severe adverse reactions have been reported anecdotally,[28, 29] these events have not been shown to occur at increased rates in vaccinated persons.

IMMUNOGENICITY

Antibodies against HBsAg are measured by enzyme immunoassay, and an anti-HBs level of 10 mIU/mL or more is generally considered to indicate seroprotection. The antibody level achieved is dependent on the age of the recipient, the dose of vaccine, and the vaccination schedule. The usual schedule consists of three doses, with the first two doses given 1 month apart and a booster dose given 6 months after the first. The third dose can be administered as early as 2 months after the second, but increasing the interval between the second and third doses results in higher antibody levels.[30, 31] A three-dose series leads to protective levels of antibodies in more than 90% of adults and more than 95% of infants and children. Antibody responses are diminished in the elderly, immunocompromised individuals, and patients with chronic diseases.

Children older than 2 years respond very well to HBV immunization, and a lower vaccine dose is needed than in adults. In children 3 months to 10 years old, a three-dose vaccine series results in seroprotection rates of nearly 100%. Both the SB (10-μg dose) and Merck (2.5-μg dose) vaccines result in geometric mean anti-HBs levels greater than 1,000 mIU/mL after the third dose, often with levels in the 3,000 to 8,000 mIU/mL range.[32-36] Infants also respond well to the recombinant vaccines, although higher anti-HBs levels are achieved when immunization is begun after age 2 months.[37] With either recombinant vaccine, 95% to 100% of infants attain seroprotective levels with vaccine given at birth and at 1 and 6 months.[38-40]

Most prelicensure studies of the recombinant HBV vaccines used schedules not easily adapted to current infant immunization practices (i.e., birth, 1, and 6 months or birth, and 1, 2, and 12 months). When the SB vaccine (10 μg) was given (without hepatitis B immune globulin [HBIG]) at birth and at 1, 2, and 12 months to infants born to mothers positive for both HBsAg and HBeAg, 98% of infants attained protective antibody levels after three doses.[41]

Geometric mean titers (GMTs) rose from 2.5 mIU/mL at 1 month to 244 mIU/mL at 4 months but then waned. A booster dose at 12 months resulted in a more than 20-fold increase of the GMT to 3,531 mIU/mL. Similar antibody responses were seen in infants born to mothers positive only for HBsAg and to mothers negative for HBsAg.[19] Comparison of a birth, 1-, and 2-month schedule with a birth, 1-, and 6-month regimen showed that the accelerated schedule resulted in earlier attainment of seroprotection but significantly lower GMTs at 7 months (420 vs. 3,142 mIU/mL, respectively).[42]

When the Merck vaccine was given to infants at doses of 1.25, 2.5, or 5.0 µg at birth and at 1 and 6 months, the two higher dosages induced protective antibody levels in 98% to 100% of infants after the third dose; however, only 81% of the infants given the 1.25-µg dose developed protective levels of antibodies.[43] When infants born to HBsAg-positive mothers were given a 5.0-µg dose at birth (with HBIG), 1, and 6 months, similar high rates of seroprotection were observed.[44, 45] A 2.5-µg dose of the vaccine given at birth, 1, and 6 months to infants born to HBsAg-negative mothers induced protective levels of anti-HBs in 49% of infants after the second dose and in 100% of the infants after the third dose, with a GMT of 314 mIU/mL after the third dose.[46]

Vaccination schedules better suited to routine infant immunization programs in the United States have also been evaluated. In one study, infants were given either SB or Merck vaccine at recommended doses (10 and 2.5 µg, respectively) at 2, 4, and 6 months with other routine childhood immunizations.[47] After the second vaccine dose, the proportion of infants with antibody levels of 10 mIU/mL or more was higher in the SB group than the Merck group (95% and 82%, respectively, $P < 0.01$). After the third dose, more than 99% of infants in both groups were seroprotected. After the second and third doses, anti-HBs levels were significantly higher in infants given the SB vaccine than in those given the Merck vaccine, with GMT values 1 month after the third vaccine dose of 1,832 and 550 mIU/mL, respectively ($P < 0.001$). Despite the differences in antibody levels, nearly all infants given either vaccine are likely to be protected against HBV infection for many years. When administered by another schedule easily incorporated into current practices (at 2, 4, and 12 or 15 months), the Merck vaccine resulted in seroprotective levels of antibodies in more than 98% of recipients.[48]

Nonresponders and Revaccination

Some immunocompetent individuals fail to develop antibodies after the three-dose vaccine series. Although the reasons for the lack of response are not clear, there is some evidence for a genetic component.[49, 50] Repeat administrations of vaccine elicit antibody responses in many previous nonresponders. Up to 40% respond with a single additional dose and 50% to 70% respond to a full three-dose series.[51] Children who did not respond after perinatal immunization responded to a three-dose series when given at 4 years of age in Singapore[52] and when given during the second year of life in Taiwan.[53]

Simultaneous Immunization With Immune Globulins or Other Vaccines

Concurrent administration of HBIG at birth does not interfere with the antibody response to HBV vaccine.[54, 55] In addition, the concurrent administration of other childhood vaccines, including diphtheria-tetanus-pertussis (DTP), oral polio virus, and measles-mumps-rubella, does not interfere with the antibody response to HBV vaccine, nor does hepatitis B vaccine interfere with the response to the other vaccines.[56–61] Vaccine manufacturers are now combining HBV vaccine with DTP and *Haemophilus influenzae* type b–conjugate vaccines to reduce the number of injections children need at each visit. Studies to assess the safety and immunogenicity of these combination vaccines are underway.

Antigenemia

Hepatitis B surface antigenemia can occur transiently after immunization of neonates.[62–64] Antigenemia may last as long as 8 days, and this must be taken into consideration if detection of HBsAg is an important part of a diagnostic evaluation.

EFFICACY

Preexposure Prophylaxis

Several placebo-controlled efficacy trials of the plasma-derived vaccine were conducted in the late 1970s in high-risk populations, including homosexual men[17, 18] and hemodialysis patients.[65] These studies demonstrated that the vaccine was highly effective in preventing HBV infection. For ethical reasons, placebo-controlled efficacy trials were not performed with the recombinant vaccines, although their comparable immunogenicity suggest their efficacy should be similar.

Clinical experience with HBV vaccines in countries that have adopted universal infant immunization suggests a high degree of efficacy. In Taiwan, a mass immunization campaign was begun in 1984, with infants receiving doses of HBV vaccine at birth and at 1, 2, and 12 months. Eight years later, the carrier rate in young children had decreased fivefold.[66] In American Samoa, universal immunization essentially eliminated perinatal transmission and dramatically reduced infection and carrier rates in young children.[67]

Postexposure Prophylaxis

Immunization with recombinant HBV vaccines beginning at birth is highly effective in preventing perinatal transmission of HBV in infants born to chronically infected mothers. Either passive-active immunization with HBIG and HBV vaccine or active immunization alone is 89% to 100% effective in protecting infants born to mothers positive for both HBsAg and HBeAg.[68-71] In most studies, HBIG was given concurrently with the first vaccine dose, but vaccination alone is also highly effective. Thus, in countries where HBV infection is endemic and screening mothers is difficult, immunization at birth is the primary means of preventing perinatal HBV transmission.

ANTIBODY PERSISTENCE AND LONG-TERM PROTECTION

An important concern with universal immunization of infants is the duration of protection. Will persons immunized at birth still be protected when exposed to the virus in adolescence and adulthood? The best data on antibody persistence derives from studies of plasma-derived vaccines. Follow-up studies of Alaska Yupik Eskimos[72, 73] and homosexual men[74] show that the rate of decline of antibody is independent of the original levels but that the persistence of antibody is directly related to the maximal antibody response. Eight years after vaccination of 1,581 Yupik Eskimos, 74% retained anti-HBs levels of 10 mIU/mL or more. Among 773 homosexual men followed for 5 years, 58% of those who initially responded to vaccination had protective levels of anti-HBs. Similar antibody kinetics were found with recombinant vaccine in healthy young adults[30] and children. A study of 122 children ages 1 to 12 years given three doses of Merck vaccine (0.6–5.0 µg/dose) at birth and at 1 and 6 months revealed that 3 months after the third dose, 93% to 100% had anti-HBs levels of 10 mIU/mL or more; the GMTs ranged from 1,088 to 1,699 mIU/mL. Four years later, the GMT declined to 73 to 119 mIU/mL, and the proportion of children with seroprotective levels declined to 70% to 87%.[34]

Although antibody levels wane, the absence of measurable antibodies in a person who initially responded to vaccination does not necessarily indicate susceptibility to infection. The incubation period for HBV is prolonged; thus, a person with immunologic memory should have sufficient time to mount an anamnestic response on exposure to the virus. Among the Yupik Eskimos, only five vaccine responders were infected by HBV (as evidenced by seroconversion to anti-HBc), and none developed detectable HBsAg or clinical hepatitis.[73] Hepatitis B virus infection occurred in 38 homosexual men who initially responded to immunization; 2 men (both HIV infected) were transiently HBsAg positive, and none became carriers.[74] Similarly, long-term protection has been demonstrated in studies involving hundreds of vaccinated infants born to chronically infected mothers in the United States,[70] Taiwan,[75–77] Thailand,[71] China,[78, 79] Senegal,[80] and the Gambia[81] who were followed for up to 9 years. Although antibody levels waned and some children became infected (<4% over all), very few developed clinical disease or became chronic HBV carriers. These studies indicate that infants and children who respond to vaccine, but later lose detectable antibody levels, should continue to be protected from both symptomatic and chronic HBV infection.

Further evidence for the importance of immunologic memory is the response to booster doses of vaccine. Despite the loss of circulating levels of anti-HBs years after immunization, an anamnestic response to a booster dose of vaccine usually occurs. Children given a dose of HBV vaccine 12 years after a primary series consisting of 2 doses 1 month apart in the first year of life showed an anamnestic response 1 week after the booster dose.[82] Four years after 70 infants were immunized with 3 doses of either 1 or 2 μg of plasma-derived vaccine, 21% had antibody levels less than 10 mIU/mL. After a booster dose (2 μg) of recombinant vaccine, the geometric mean antibody level increased 100-fold, and 90% had levels of 1,000 mIU/mL or more.[83] These dramatic and rapid responses to a booster dose suggest that a similar response may occur after exposure to the virus. On the other hand, if waning immunity ultimately is shown to be a problem, a single booster dose in adolescence may be sufficient to provide long-term protection.

RECOMMENDATIONS

After licensure in the United States, HBV vaccine was recommended for adults and children at high risk of HBV infection and for infants born to chronically infected mothers (along with HBIG).[15, 84] For several years after vaccine licensure, the incidence of HBV infection in the United States increased (Fig 4), and it became clear that the existing vaccination programs were not effective in reducing the incidence of HBV infection. Therefore, in 1991, the Committee on Infectious Diseases of the American Academy of Pediatrics and the Advisory Committee on Immunization Practices of the U.S. Public Health Service developed a strategy to eliminate HBV transmission in the United States, with universal immunization of infants as its cornerstone.[85, 86]

The recommendations for routine infant immunization initially met with resistance from many practitioners.[87] Among the reasons was a perception that the prevention of HBV infection was not a public health priority. This was particularly true among pediatricians, who rarely see children with acute symptomatic HBV infections and who do not see the long-term sequelae of chronic infection. Other concerns were the costs, the additional injections required and uncertainty about the duration of protection.

The rationale for universal immunization is clear.[88, 89] Many high-risk individuals are inaccessible to vaccination, and many people who become infected do not have an identifiable risk factor. The only way to reach both of these groups is through universal immunization. Routine immunization of infants is the only practical means to accomplish this because well-established mechanisms to immunize infants are already in place. In addition, the prevention of chronic infection is a major goal of the HBV im-

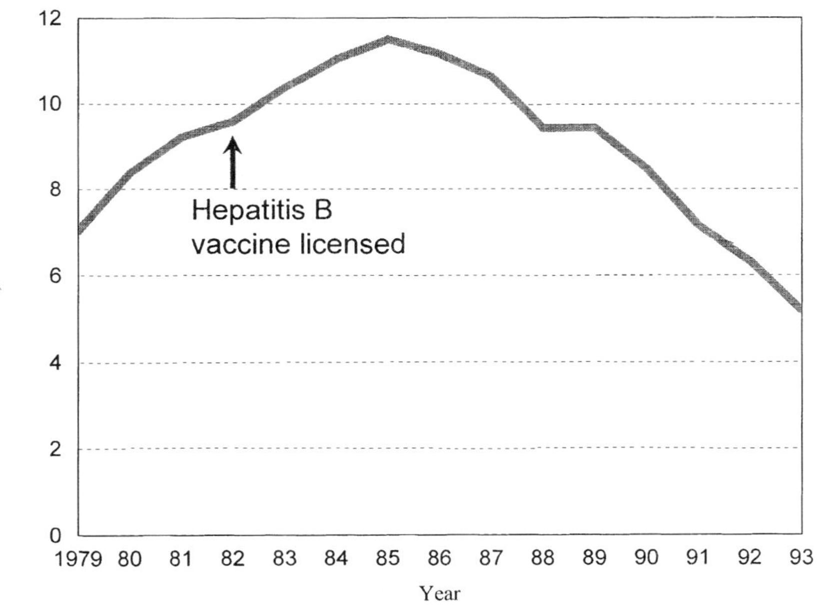

FIGURE 4.

Annual incidence of reported cases of hepatitis B virus, 1979–1993. (Data courtesy of the Viral Hepatitis Surveillance Program, Hepatitis Branch, Centers for Disease Control and Prevention, Atlanta.)

munization program because of the long-term sequelae of chronic HBV infection and because HBsAg-positive persons serve as a source of infection for others. Thus, the high risk of chronic infection when it is acquired early in life makes immunization of infants and young children particularly important.

Although HBV vaccine was also recommended initially only for high-risk adolescents, consensus on the need to immunize all teenagers has been growing. About 75% of HBV infections are acquired between the ages of 15 and 39 years,[90] yet only about 1% of adolescents at risk for infection are immunized. Thus, routine immunization of previously unvaccinated children is now recommended at 11 to 12 years.[91] Routine immunization is also recommended for younger children who are at increased risk for disease because their parents or other household members are of Pacific Islander ethnicity or are first-generation immigrants from countries with high rates of endemic HBV disease.

Schedules and Dosages

For older children and adults, the usual schedule consists of three doses at 0, 1, and 6 months.[85, 86, 91] An alternative schedule, useful when a rapid onset of protection is desired, is approved for the SB vaccine and consists of doses at 0, 1, 2, and 12 months. For infants, substantial flexibility was built into the immunization schedules to facilitate integration of HBV vaccine into current preventive health care practices. For infants born to mothers known to be HBsAg negative, the first vaccine dose can be given any time between birth and 2 months. The second dose can be given between 1 and 4 months, provided that at least 1 month has elapsed since the first dose. The third dose can be given between 6 and 18 months, although effort should be made to complete the series by 6 to 9 months in Pacific Islanders, Alaskan natives, and other children from countries with high rates of endemic HBV. Newborns whose mothers are HBsAg positive should be immunized within 12 hours of birth and should be given HBIG (0.5 mL) concurrently. These infants should be given their second vaccine dose at 1 to 2 months and their third dose at 6 months, and they should be tested for anti-HBs and HBsAg between 9 and 15 months. If maternal HBV status is unknown, the first vaccine dose should be given within 12 hours of birth, and HBIG should be given if serologic results subsequently indicate that the mother is HBsAg positive. For all infants and children, an interruption in the vaccine series does not require restarting the series, regardless of the interval between doses.[92]

Some studies have shown that very low birth weight infants immunized at birth are less likely to develop protective antibody levels than premature infants whose immunizations are begun when they are older and weigh more.[93, 94] Therefore, in premature infants born to mothers who are HBsAg negative, it may be advisable to delay HBV immunization until hospital discharge.[92] However, premature infants born to HBsAg-positive mothers should be given HBIG and HBV vaccine within 12 hours of birth as is recommended for term infants.

The recommended dosages and volumes of the two recombinant vaccines differ based on the age and risk factors of the targeted population (Table 1). Nonetheless, the vaccines may be used interchangeably.

Route of Administration

Hepatitis B vaccine should be administered intramuscularly into the anterior thigh of infants or the deltoid muscle of older children and adults. It should not be given in the buttocks because of suboptimal responses.[95, 96] Intradermal vaccination also is not recommended because of lower response rates and difficulty in properly administering the vaccine.[97, 98]

Serologic Testing

Routine serologic testing of infants and children after immunization is not recommended. Testing should be performed 1 to 2 months after immunization in persons known to respond poorly, such as HIV-infected children, and in those whose future management is dependent on the results, such as hemodialysis patients.

REMAINING ISSUES

The availability of safe, effective HBV vaccines does not mean it is time to close the book on HBV.[99] Vaccines combining HBV vaccine with DTP and *H. influenzae* type b–conjugate vaccines are under investigation. The duration of protection after three vaccine doses given in infancy and the possible need for booster doses at a later age must be assessed. The need for incorporation of additional HBsAg epitopes (pre-S gene products) into the HBV vaccine must be determined.[51] Pre-S regions of HBsAg may improve long-term protection by enhancing immunogenicity of HBsAg, inducing neutralizing antibodies to the virus-binding site, and stimulating cellular immune responses. Questions remain about the need to incorporate other antigens into the vaccines because mutant forms of HBV have been discovered that are not prevented by administration of the current vaccines.[100–102] The implications of this discovery and the scope of the problem are not yet clear.

TABLE 1.

Recommended Dosages of Hepatitis B Recombinant Vaccines*

	Recombivax HB (Merck & Company)		Engerix-B (SmithKline Beecham)	
	Dose (μg)	mL	Dose (μg)	mL
Infants of HBsAg-negative mothers	2.5	0.5†	10	0.5
Infants of HBsAg-positive mothers (HBIG [0.5 mL] should also be given)	5	0.5‡ 1.0†	10	0.5
Children <11 yr	2.5	0.5†	10	0.5
Children and adolescents 11–19 yr	5	0.5‡	10	0.5
Adults ≥20 yr	10	1.0‡	20	1.0
Dialysis patients and other immunosuppressed adults	40	1.0§	40	2.0‖

*See text for dosing schedules.
†Pediatric formulation.
‡Adult formulation.
§Special formulation for dialysis patients.
‖Two 1.0-mL doses given at one site in a 4-dose schedule at 0, 1, 2, and 6–12 mo.

HEPATITIS A

Hepatitis A virus, a member of the picornavirus family, is a small nonenveloped RNA virus measuring about 27 nm in diameter. Although there are several genotypes, only one antigenic serotype exists, and strains from around the world have been found to be highly conserved.[103] Humans are the only natural host, and infection is usually acquired by fecal-oral spread from an infected contact or by ingestion of contaminated food or water. Disease usually occurs sporadically, but fecal contamination of food or water can lead to epidemic disease, such as a 1988 outbreak in Shanghai that resulted in an estimated 300,000 cases.[104] Transmission occurs rarely through transfusion or sexual contact, and nosocomial spread in a neonatal intensive care unit has been reported.[105]

The incubation period is about 4 weeks, with a range of 15 to 50 days. The symptoms of acute HAV infection are clinically indistinguishable from those of acute HBV infection, and the cause must be determined serologically. As with HBV, the likelihood of symptomatic HAV infection is inversely related to the age of the patient. About 90% of infants and young children have subclinical infection, whereas 70% to 80% of adults are symptomatic.[106] The disease usually lasts 2 to 4 weeks, but 10% to 20% of persons have prolonged or relapsing symptoms for up to 6 months. Although the morbidity associated with HAV infection is substantial, the majority of infected individuals recover without sequelae. Mortality is unusual, although the case fatality rate may be as high as 3% in the elderly, and about 100 people die annually in the United States from acute fulminant HAV.

Patients are viremic and fecal shedding begins before the onset of symptoms (Fig 5). High concentrations of virus (10^8 particles/g) are excreted in the stool, and infected persons are most contagious before the clinical syndrome is recognized. In adults, fecal shedding ceases at the time humoral immunity is detected, which generally coincides with the onset of jaundice. Chronic shedding has not been reported, although infected infants can shed HAV for longer periods than do adults.[105]

EPIDEMIOLOGY

Overall, nearly 40% of people in the United States have antibodies against HAV.[107] The infection is highly endemic in certain populations, including Native Americans, Alaskan natives, and certain Hispanic populations. In the United States, the age of acquisition of those with HAV is younger than that of individuals with HBV (Fig 6). The highest rate of reported cases is among children aged 5 to 14 years, and nearly 30% of cases occur in individuals younger than 15 years. In developing countries, the virus is usually acquired in infancy and early childhood because virus transmission is enhanced where there is poor sanitation and crowded living conditions.

Risk factors for HAV infection in the United States are shown in Figure 7. Key considerations in devising an effective vaccination strategy are that almost half of infected persons do not have an identifiable risk factor and that young children (particularly those in diapers) often are a source of infection for adults.[107] About

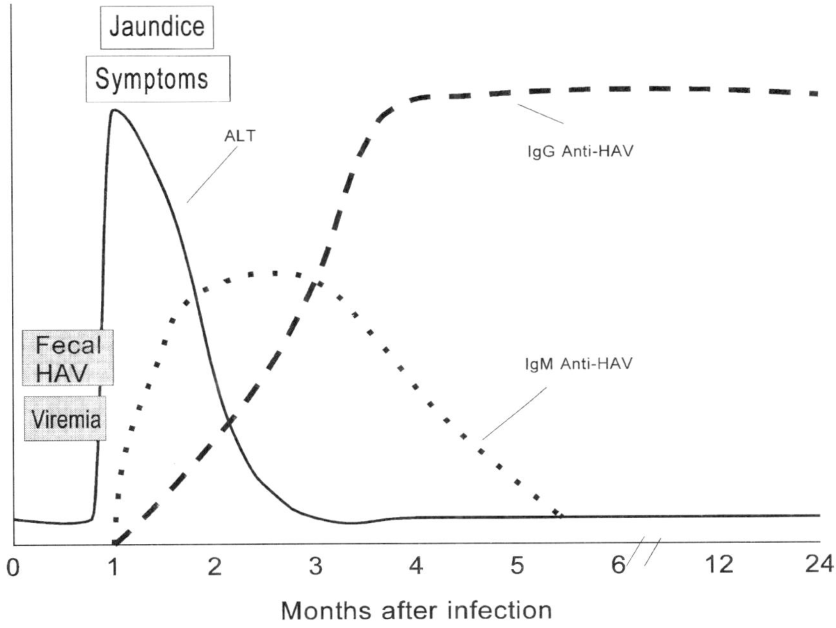

FIGURE 5.

Course of typical acute hepatitis A virus (HAV) infection with complete recovery. Fecal excretion of HAV and viremia precede the onset of symptoms.

15% of cases are day-care related, but because young children are usually asymptomatic, outbreaks in day-care centers often are not recognized until an adult with HAV is identified.[108]

VACCINES

Two vaccines (Havrix, SmithKline Beecham; and VAQTA, Merck & Company) have undergone extensive clinical evaluation. Both are killed whole virus vaccines prepared by serial passage of HAV in cell culture, purification, formaldehyde inactivation, and adsorption to aluminum hydroxide.[109, 110] Because they are killed vaccines they cannot cause hepatitis. The Merck vaccine is a more highly purified product, although the clinical significance of this is unknown.

Havrix was first licensed in 1992 in Switzerland and is now available in more than 30 countries. In February 1995, it was licensed for use in the United States. The adult formulation contains 1,440 enzyme-linked immunosorbent assay (ELISA) units (ELU), whereas the vaccine for children aged 2 to 18 years contains 360 ELU. A product license application for VAQTA has been filed with the U.S. Food and Drug Administration for a 25-unit dose for children older than 2 years and adolescents and for a 50-unit dose in adults older than 18 years. The 25-unit dose is believed to be similar to a 720-ELU-dose of the SB vaccine.

SAFETY

Both vaccines appear to be safe. More than 4.5 million doses of the SB vaccine have been administered worldwide, and in clinical trials the vaccine has been given to more than 50,000 persons, including more than 41,000 children. The vaccine causes fewer adverse reactions in children than in adults. In an efficacy study in Thailand, more than 100,000 doses of vaccine were administered without any serious adverse reactions.[111] Among more than 1,000 children given a 360-ELU dose, greater than 75% had no symptoms after vaccination. About 15% of recipients had soreness at the injection site, and temperatures of 37.5° C or more were reported by fewer than 3% of vaccinees.[112]

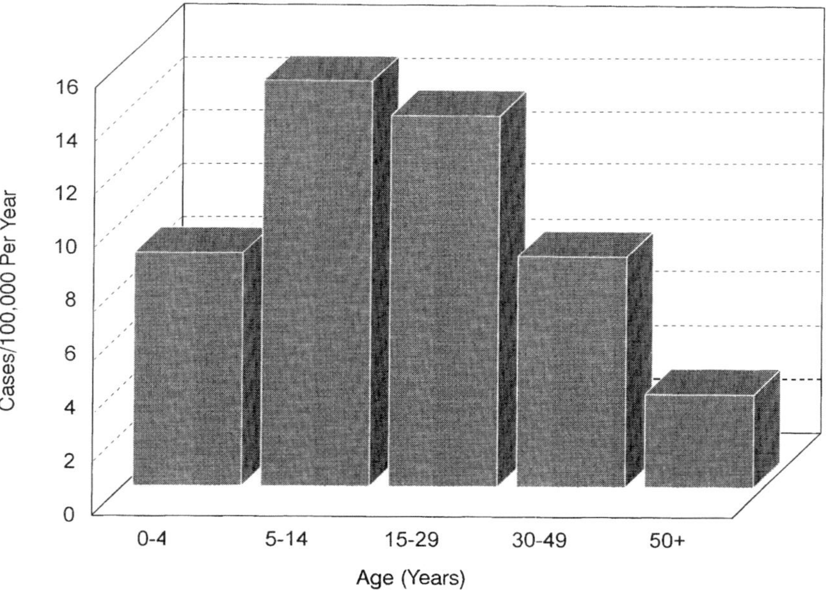

FIGURE 6.

Incidence rates (reported cases per 100,000 population per year) by age for hepatitis A virus, 1993. (Data courtesy of the Viral Hepatitis Surveillance Program, Hepatitis Branch, Centers for Disease Control and Prevention, Atlanta.)

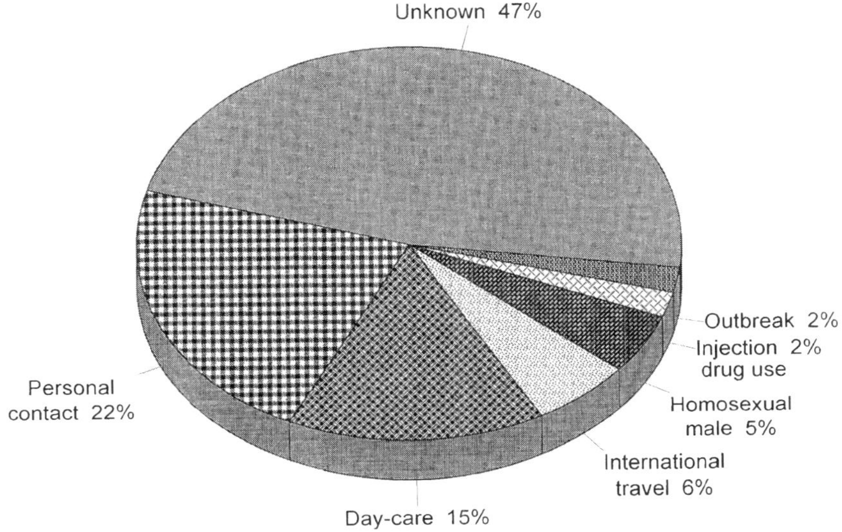

FIGURE 7.

Risk factors for reported cases of hepatitis A virus, 1993. (Data courtesy of the Viral Hepatitis Surveillance Program, Hepatitis Branch, Centers for Disease Control and Prevention, Atlanta.)

In clinical trials, the Merck vaccine has been administered to more than 7,600 persons, including almost 3,000 children. In an efficacy trial in upstate New York, similar rates of local and systemic reactions were seen in the vaccine and placebo groups.[113] In more than 500 children aged 2 to 3 years given a 25-unit dose of vaccine, local reactions were generally mild and occurred in fewer than 13% of vaccine recipients. Systemic complaints were also mild, with fewer than 9% of children having temperatures 37.8° C or higher.[114] Adverse reactions have neither been more severe nor more common after booster doses.

IMMUNOGENICITY

Antibodies to HAV are measured by a commercially available radioimmunoassay (RIA) or by a modified RIA that is more sensitive.[115] Due to the lack of standards for testing and the variability from one assay to another, antibody levels from different studies cannot be directly compared. The antibody level that confers protection is not precisely known, but levels of 10 to 20 mIU/mL or more are generally considered to be protective.

A 720-ELU dose of the SB vaccine leads to seroconversion in more than 95% of healthy adults after one dose and in more than

99% of vaccinees after a second dose.[116, 117] Use of a 1,440 ELU dose results in higher antibody levels,[117, 118] and this dose is now recommended for adults. Children respond better than adults and therefore require a lower dose of vaccine. In children aged 1 to 17 years given the SB vaccine (360 ELU) on a 0-, 1-, and 6-month schedule, the first dose results in seroconversion in more than 95% of recipients. After the second dose, more than 99% of children have responded and the GMT is about 500 mIU/mL. The booster dose induces an anamnestic response, and the GMT increases to about 4,000 mIU/mL.[119, 120] In seronegative infants vaccinated at 2, 4, and 6 months, 97% of children seroconverted after three doses with a GMT of about 300 mIU/mL.[121]

In adults, a single 50-unit dose of the Merck vaccine results in seroconversion in more than 95% of recipients. In children aged 4 to 12 years, a 25-unit dose of vaccine leads to an antibody response in more than 98% of vaccinees.[122, 123] In children between 2 and 3 years old, a single 25-unit dose of vaccine results in seroconversion in more than 97% of vaccinees with a GMT of about 150 mIU/mL. After a booster dose 6 months later, more than 99% of vaccinees are seropositive and the GMT is almost 3,000 mIU/mL.[115] Evaluation of the Merck vaccine in children less than 2 years has recently begun.

Effect of Passive Immunization

In adults, concomitant administration of serum IG suppresses responses to the SB vaccine. In people given IG with the first of their three vaccine doses, geometric mean antibody levels after the third dose were only about half those in people not given IG, although seroconversion rates were comparable.[124, 125] Similarly, limited data in young infants with a 360-ELU dose of the SB vaccine suggest that maternal antibodies may interfere with the antibody response.[121] If transplacental antibodies interfere with the immune response of infants, this could influence recommendations for use of the vaccines because about one third of U.S. women of childbearing age have antibodies against HAV. Possible strategies to overcome the problem include using higher vaccine doses or delaying initiation of the vaccine series.

EFFICACY

The efficacy of the SB vaccine was evaluated in a double-blind controlled trial in Thailand.[111] More than 40,000 children aged 1 to 16 years were randomized to receive either HAV vaccine (360 ELU) or HBV vaccine as a control at 0, 1, and 12 months. Active surveillance, by evaluation of school absences of 2 or more days, revealed 40 cases of HAV, of which 38 occurred among control children, yielding a vaccine efficacy after 2 doses of 94% (95% confidence interval [CI], 79%–99%). Both cases in vaccine recipients were mild and short lived.

The efficacy of the Merck vaccine was evaluated in a double-blind controlled trial in a Hasidic Jewish community in upstate New York that had recurrent outbreaks of HAV.[113] More than 1,000 seronegative children 2 to 16 years old were randomized to receive either a single 25-unit dose of vaccine or placebo. The primary end point was HAV cases occurring 50 days or more (the upper limit of the usual incubation period) after vaccination. No cases occurred in the vaccine group compared with 25 cases in the placebo group ($P < 0.001$) yielding an efficacy of 100% (lower limit of 95% CI 87%). Also of interest is that no cases occurred in vaccine recipients during the interval between 21 and 46 days after immunization compared with 9 cases in placebo recipients.

In each of these clinical trials, a decreased number of cases were observed among unvaccinated community members compared with residents of nearby communities, suggesting possible herd immunity. Similarly, in a demonstration project in Alaska in which more than 5,000 persons received a single dose of SB vaccine, HAV transmission was interrupted in communities where a large proportion of susceptibles were immunized.[126]

RECOMMENDATIONS

Hepatitis A vaccine is currently recommended for individuals at high risk for infection,[127, 128] including travelers to endemic areas, military personnel, male homosexuals, injecting drug users, and patients with chronic liver disease. Routine immunization of children 2 years or older is recommended for high-risk populations such as Native Americans and Pacific Islanders. Vaccination may also be indicated for certain communitywide outbreaks as determined by local public health authorities.

For adults, the SB vaccine (1,440-ELU dose) is recommended as a two-dose regimen, with the second immunization 6 to 12 months after the initial dose. For children and young adults aged 2 to 18 years, three doses (360-ELU dose) are recommended, given at 0, 1, and 6 to 12 months. The vaccine is not yet recommended for children younger than 2 years. When licensed, the Merck vaccine will likely be recommended as a two-dose regimen (0 and 6 months) for children older than 2 years and adolescents (25-unit dose) and also for adults older than 18 years (50-unit dose).

Hepatitis A vaccines can be given at the same time as other vaccines, including HBV. For persons who need immediate protection (e.g., postexposure prophylaxis) and also desire long-term protection, vaccine can be given simultaneously with IG. Vaccine should be administered intramuscularly, although, as with HBV vaccine, it should not be given in the buttocks or administered intradermally.[129]

REMAINING ISSUES

The primary issue regarding HAV vaccine is the best and most cost-effective strategy for its use.[130] Immunizing only high-risk individuals might be cost effective, but because almost half of infected individuals do not have a recognized risk factor, many cases would not be prevented. In addition, young children, who play an important role in disease transmission, are frequently asymptomatic and thus not recognized to be infectious. Therefore, a strategy of universal infant immunization might be the optimal means to reduce the morbidity associated with HAV in the United States and is certainly the only way to eliminate HAV transmission. Routine infant immunization will likely not be recommended until HAV vaccine is combined with other routine childhood immunizations to reduce the number of injections required to vaccinate children. Furthermore, the importance of interference by passive maternal antibody, and thus the optimal dose and schedule for infants, is not yet known.

The duration of protective immunity is unknown and must be determined by long-term follow-up studies. Antibody levels wane over time, but as with HBV, the absence of measurable antibodies may not indicate lack of protection in a person with immune memory.[131] Persons who seroconvert to vaccination mount a brisk anamnestic antibody response to a booster dose. Comparative trials of the two inactivated HAV vaccines need to be performed to determine if there are important differences in safety, immunogenicity, or efficacy. Finally, the possible utility of vaccine in postexposure prophylaxis has not been determined.

SUMMARY

Universal HBV immunization of infants has been recommended since 1991, and now routine immunization of previously unvaccinated 11- to 12-year-old children is also recommended. Recombinant HBV vaccines are safe and highly immunogenic in infants and children using a wide variety of schedules. The vaccines are effective in protecting high-risk newborns against HBV infection when the first dose is given at birth with HBIG. Available data indicate that immunized infants and children are protected from chronic HBV infection for at least 10 years, even if they have lost detectable antibodies. Further research will determine if booster doses are necessary during the second decade of life to provide protection from HBV exposures that occur during adulthood.

The first HAV vaccine has recently been licensed for use in the United States and is recommended for high-risk individuals older than 2 years. Inactivated HAV vaccines appear to be very safe, and one or two doses induce protective levels of antibodies in most recipients. Because of the important role young children play in disease transmission, HAV vaccine will likely be given as part of routine childhood immunizations when combination vaccines are produced.

ACKNOWLEDGMENTS

We gratefully express our appreciation to David S. Krause, M.D., SmithKline Beecham Pharmaceuticals, and David R. Nalin, M.D., Merck & Company, for their critical review of the manuscript and helpful comments.

REFERENCES

1. Krugman S, Giles JP, Hammond J: Infectious hepatitis: Evidence for two distinctive clinical, epidemiological and immunological types of infection. *JAMA* 200:365–373, 1967.
2. Blumberg BS, Alter HJ, Visnich S: A "new" antigen in leukemia sera. *JAMA* 191:541–546, 1965.
3. Dane DS, Cameron CH, Briggs M: Virus-like particles in serum of patients with Australia antigen-associated hepatitis. *Lancet* 1:695–698, 1970.
4. Feinstone SM, Kapikian AZ, Purcell RH: Hepatitis A: Detection by immune electron microscopy of a viruslike antigen associated with acute illness. *Science* 182:1026–1028, 1973.
5. Provost PJ, Hilleman MR: Propagation of human hepatitis A virus in cell culture in vitro. *Proc Soc Exp Biol Med* 160:213–221, 1979.
6. Hadler SC, Margolis HS: Epidemiology of hepatitis B virus infection. In Ellis RW (ed): *Hepatitis B Vaccines in Clinical Practice*. New York, Marcel Dekker, 1993, pp 141–157.
7. Franks AL, Berg CJ, Kane MA, et al: Hepatitis B virus infections among children born in the United States to Southeast Asian refugees. *N Engl J Med* 321:1301–1305, 1989.
8. Hurie MB, Mast EE, David JP: Horizontal transmission of hepatitis B virus infection to United States-born children of Hmong refugees. *Pediatrics* 89:269–273, 1992.

9. McMahon BJ, Alward WLM, Hall DB, et al: Acute hepatitis B infection: Relation of age to the clinical expression of disease and subsequent development of the carrier state. *J Infect Dis* 151:599–603, 1985.
10. Shapiro CN: Epidemiology of hepatitis B. *Pediatr Infect Dis J* 12:433–437, 1993.
11. West DJ, Margolis HS: Prevention of hepatitis B infection in the United States: A pediatric perspective. *Pediatr Infect Dis J* 11:866–874, 1992.
12. Krugman S, Giles JP, Hammond J: Hepatitis virus effect of heat on the infectivity and antigenicity of the MS-1 and MS-2 strain. *J Infect Dis* 122:432–436, 1970.
13. Hilleman MR: Plasma-drived hepatitis B vaccine: A breakthrough in preventive medicine. In Ellis RW (ed): *Hepatitis B Vaccines in Clinical Practice.* New York, Marcel Dekker, 1993, pp 17–39.
14. Krugman S, Stevens CE: Hepatitis B vaccine. In Plotkin SA, Mortimer EA (eds): *Vaccines,* Philadelphia, WB Saunders, 1994, 419–437.
15. Immunization Practices Advisory Committee: Inactivated hepatitis B virus vaccine. *MMWR* 31:317–328, 1982.
16. Sitrin RD, Wampler DE, Ellis RW: Survey of licensed hepatitis B vaccines and their production processes. In Ellis RW (ed): *Hepatitis B Vaccines in Clinical Practice.* New York, Marcel Dekker, 1993, pp 83–101.
17. Szmuness W, Stevens CE, Harley EJ, et al: Hepatitis B vaccine: Demonstration of efficacy in a controlled clinical trial in a high-risk population in the United States. *N Engl J Med* 303:833–841, 1980.
18. Francis DP, Hadler SC, Thompson SE, et al: Prevention of hepatitis B with vaccine: Report from the Centers for Disease Control multi-center efficacy trial among homosexual men. *Ann Intern Med* 97:362–366, 1982.
19. André FE, Path FRC: Summary of safety and efficacy data on a yeast-derived hepatitis B vaccine. *Am J Med* 87:(suppl 3A)14S–20S, 1989.
20. West DJ: Clinical experience with hepatitis B vaccines. *Am J Infect Control* 17:172–180, 1989.
21. Zajac BA, West DJ, McAlerr WJ, et al: Overview of clinical studies with hepatitis B vaccine made by recombinant DNA. *J Infect* 13 (suppl A):39–45, 1986.
22. Greenberg DP: Pediatric experience with recombinant hepatitis B vaccines and relevant safety and immunogenicity studies. *Pediatr Infect Dis J* 12:438–445, 1993.
23. Shaw FE, Graham DJ, Guess HA, et al: Postmarketing surveillance for neurologic adverse events reported after hepatitis B vaccination: Experience of the first three years. *Am J Epidemiol* 127:337–352, 1988.
24. Herroelen L, de Keyser J, Ebinger G: Central-nervous-system demyelination after immunisation with recombinant hepatitis b vaccine. *Lancet* 338:1174–1175, 1991.
25. Tuohy PG: Guillain-Barre syndrome following immunisation with synthetic hepatitis B vaccine. *NZ Med J* 102:114–115, 1989.

26. Institute of Medicine: Hepatitis B vaccines. In Stratton KR, Howe CJ, Johnston RB Jr (eds): *Adverse Events Associated With Childhood Vaccines. Evidence Bearing on Causality*. Washington DC, National Academy Press, 1994, pp 211–235.

27. McMahon BJ, Helminiak C, Wainwright RB, et al: Frequency of adverse reactions to hepatitis B vaccine in 43,618 persons. *Am J Med* 92:254–256, 1992.

28. Goolsby PL: Erythema nodosum after recombinant hepatitis B vaccine. *N Engl J Med* 321:1198–1199, 1989.

29. Fried M, Conene D, Conzelmann M, et al: Uveitis after hepatitis B vaccination. *Lancet* 2:631–632, 1987.

30. Jilg WJ, Schmidt M, Deinhardt F: Vaccination against hepatitis B: Comparison of three different vaccination schedules. *J Infect Dis* 160:766–769, 1989.

31. Hadler SC, Alcala de Monzon M, Lugo DR, et al: Effect of timing of hepatitis B vaccine doses on response to vaccine in Yucpa Indians. *Vaccine* 7:106–110, 1989.

32. Tsega E, Tafesse B, Horton J, et al: Immunogenicity, reactogenicity and comparison of two doses of recombinant DNA yeast-derived hepatitis B vaccine in Ethiopian children. *Trop Geogr Med* 43:220–227, 1991.

33. Moyes C, Milne A: Immunogenicity of a recombinant yeast-derived hepatitis B vaccine (Engerix B) in children. *NZ Med J* 101:162–164, 1988.

34. Goh KT, Tan KL, Kong KH, et al: Comparison of the immune response of four different dosages of a yeast-recombinant hepatitis B vaccine in Singapore children: A four-year follow-up study. *Bull WHO* 70:233–239, 1992.

35. Tan KL, Oon CJ, Goh KT, et al: Immunogenicity and safety of low doses of recombinant yeast-derived hepatitis B vaccine. *Acta Paediatr Scand* 79:593–598, 1990.

36. Zajac BA, West DJ, McAleer WJ, et al: Overview of clinical studies with hepatitis B vaccine made by recombinant DNA. *J Infect 13(suppl A):39–45, 1986.*

37. Yeoh EK, Young B, Chan YY, et al: Determinants of immunogenicity and efficacy of hepatitis B vaccine in infants. In Hollinger FB, Lemon SM, Margolis HS (eds): *Vital Hepatitis and Liver Disease*. Baltimore, Williams & Wilkins, 1991, pp 749–752.

38. Jilg W, Lorbeer B, Schmidt M, et al: Clilnical evaluation of a recombinant hepatitis B vaccine. *Lancet* 2:1174–1175, 1984.

39. Panda SK, Ramesh R, Rao KVS, et al: Comparative evaluation of the immunogenicity of yeast-derived (recombinant) and plasma-derived hepatitis B vaccine in infants. *J Med Virol* 35:297–301, 1991.

40. André FE: Overview of a 5-year clinical experience with a yeast-derived hepatitis B vaccine. *Vaccine* 8:S74–S78, 1990.

41. Poovorawan Y, Sanpavat S, Pongpunlert W, et al: Protective efficacy of a recombinant DNA hepatitis B vaccine in neonates of HBe antigen-positive mothers. *JAMA* 261:3278–3281, 1989.

42. Goldfarb J, Baley J, Medendorp SV, et al: Comparative study of the immunogenicity and safety of two dosing schedules of Engerix-B® hepatitis B vaccine in neonates. *Pediatr Infect Dis J* 13:18–22, 1994.
43. West DJ: Clinical experience with hepatitis B vaccines. *Am J Infect Control* 17:172–180, 1989.
44. Yeoh EK, Chang WK, Ip P, et al: Efficacy and safety of recombinant hepatitis B vaccine in infants born to HBsAg-positive mothers. *J Infect* 13(suppl A):15–18, 1986.
45. Stevens CE, Taylor PE, Tong MJ, et al: Yeast-recombinant hepatitis B vaccine. Efficacy with hepatitis B immune globulin in prevention of perinatal hepatitis B virus transmission. *JAMA* 257:2612–2616, 1987.
46. Seto D, Diwan A, Hesley T, et al: Hepatitis B vaccine alternative vaccination schedules in healthy babies of non-carrier (HBsAg-) mothers [abstract]. *Pediatr Res* 31:179A, 1992.
47. Greenberg DP, Vadheim CM, Marcy SM, et al: Comparative safety and immunogenicity of two recombinant hepatitis B (HBV) vaccines given to infants at 2, 4, and 6 months of age [abstract]. In *Program and Abstracts of 32nd Interscience Conference on Antimicrobial Agents and Chemotherapy*. Anaheim, Calif, 1992, p 264.
48. Keyserling HL, West DJ, Hesley TM, et al: Antibody responses of healthy infants to a recombinant hepatitis B vaccine administered at two, four, and twelve or fifteen months of age. *J Pediatr* 125:67–69, 1994.
49. Craven De, Awdeh ZL, Kunches LM, et al: Nonresponsiveness to hepatitis B vaccine in health care workers: Results of revaccination and genetic typings. *Ann Intern Med* 105:356–360, 1986.
50. Alper CA, Kruskall MS, Marcus-Bagley D, et al: Genetic prediction of nonresponse to hepatitis B vaccine. *N Engl J Med* 321:708–712, 1989.
51. Hadler SC, Margolis HS: Hepatitis B immunization: Vaccine types, efficacy, and indications for immunization. *Curr Clin Topics Infect Dis* 12:282–308, 1992.
52. Tan KL, Goh KT, Oon CJ, et al: Immunogenicity of recombinant yeast-derived hepatitis B vaccine in nonresponders to perinatal immunization. *JAMA* 271:859–861, 1994.
53. Cheng KF, Chang MH, Lee CY, et al: Response to supplemental vaccination with recombinant or plasma hepatitis B vaccine in healthy non-responding children. *Vaccine* 12:899–902, 1994.
54. Wong VCW, Ip HMH, Reesink HW, et al: Prevention of the HBsAg carrier state in newborn infants of mothers who are chronic carriers of HBsAg and HBeAg by administration of hepatitis-B vaccine and hepatitis-B immunoglobulin. Double-blind randomised and placebo-controlled study. *Lancet* 1:921–926, 1984.
55. Xu Z-Y, Liu C-B, Francis DP, et al: Prevention of perinatal acquisition of hepatitis B virus carriage using vaccine: Preliminary report of a randomized, double-blind placebo-controlled and comparative trial. *Pediatrics* 76:713–718, 1985.

56. Huang L-M, Lee C-Y, Hsu C-Y, et al: Effect of monovalent measles and trivalent measles-mumps-rubella vaccines at various ages and concurrent administration with hepatitis B vaccine. *Pediatr Infect Dis J* 9:461–465, 1990.
57. Chiron JP, Coursaget P, Yvonnet B, et al: Simultaneous administration of hepatitis B and diphtheria/tetanus/polio-vaccines. *Lancet* 1:623–624, 1984.
58. Coursaget P, Yvonnet B, Relyveld EH, et al: Simultaneous administration of diphtheria-tetanus-pertussis-polio and hepatitis B vaccines in a simplified immunization program: Immune response to diphtheria toxoid, tetanus toxoid, pertussis, and hepatitis B surface antigen. *Infect Immun* 51:784–787, 1986.
59. Coursaget P, Bringer L, Bourdil C, et al: Simultaneous injection of hepatitis B and measles vaccines. *Trans R Soc Trop Med Hyg* 85:788, 1991.
60. Barone P, Mauro L, Leonardi S, et al: Simultaneous administration of HB recombinant vaccine with diphtheria and tetanus toxoid and oral polio vaccine: A pilot study. *Acta Paediatr Jpn* 33:455–458, 1991.
61. Giammanco G, Li Volti S, Mauro L, et al: Immune response to simultaneous administration of a recombinant DNA hepatitis B vaccine and multiple compulsory vaccines in infancy. *Vaccine* 9:747–750, 1991.
62. Challapalli M, Naidu V, Cunningham DG: Hepatitis B surface antigenemia in a newborn infant after vaccination. *Pediatr Infect Dis J* 12:408–409, 1993.
63. Bernstein SR, Krieger P, Puppula BL, et al: Incidence and duration of hepatitis B surface antigenemia after neonatal hepatitis B immunization. *J Pediatr* 125:621–622, 1994.
64. Weintraub Z, Khamaysi N, Elena H, et al: Transient surface antigenemia in newborn infants vaccinated with Engerix B: Occurrence and duration. *Pediatr Infect Dis J* 13:931–933, 1994.
65. Stevens CE, Alter HJ, Taylor PE, et al: Hepatitis B vaccine in hemodialysis patients: Immunogenicity and efficacy. *N Engl J Med* 311:496–501, 1984.
66. Wong WCW, Tsang KK: A mass hepatitis B vaccination program in Taiwan: Its preparation, results and reasons for uncompleted vaccinations. *Vaccine* 12:229–234, 1994.
67. Mahoney FJ, Woodruff BA, Erben JJ, et al: Effect of hepatitis B vaccination program on the prevalence of hepatitis B virus infection. *J Infect Dis* 167:203–207, 1993.
68. Lee C-Y, Huang L-M, Chang M-H, et al: The protective efficacy of recombinant hepatitis B vaccine in newborn infants of hepatitis B e antigen-positive-hepatitis B surface antigen carrier mothers. *Pediatr Infect Dis J* 10:299–303, 1991.
69. Pongpipat D, Suvatte V, Assateerawatts A: Hepatitis B immunization in high risk neonates born from HBsAg positive mothers: Comparison between plasma derived and recombinant DNA vaccine. *Asian Pac J Allergy Immunol* 7:37–40, 1989.

70. Stevens CE, Toy PT, Taylor PE, et al: Prospects for control of hepatitis B virus infection: Implications of childhood vaccination and long-term protection. *Pediatrics* 90:170–173, 1992.
71. Poovorawan Y, Sanpavat S, Pongpunglert W, et al: Long term efficacy of hepatitis B vaccine in infants born to hepatitis B e antigen-positive mothers. *Pediatr Infect Dis J* 11:816–821, 1992.
72. Wainwright RB, McMahon BJ, Bulkow LR, et al: Duration of immunogenicity and efficacy of hepatitis B vaccine in a Yupik Eskimo population. *JAMA* 261:2362–2366, 1989.
73. Wainwright RB, McMahon BJ, Bulkow LR, et al: Protection provided by hepatitis B vaccine in a Yupik Eskimo population. *Arch Intern Med* 151:1634–1636, 1991.
74. Hadler SC, Francis DP, Maynard JE, et al: Long-term immunogenicity and efficacy of hepatitis B vaccine in homosexual men. *N Engl J Med* 315:209–214, 1986.
75. Lo KJ, Lee SD, Tsai YT, et al: Long-term immunogenicity and efficacy of hepatitis B vaccine in infants born to HBeAg-positive HBsAg-carrier mothers. *Hepatology* 8:1647–1650, 1988.
76. Hwang LY, Lee CY, Beasley RP: Five-year follow-up of HBV vaccination with plasma-derived vaccine in neonates: Evaluation of immunogenicity and efficacy against perinatal transmission. In Hollinger FB, Lemon SM, Margolis HS (eds): *Viral Hepatitis and Liver Disease.* Baltimore, Williams & Wilkins, 1991, pp 759–761.
77. Hsu NHM, Chen DS, Chuang CH, et al: Studies on the efficacy of a mass immunization program against hepatitis B in Taiwan: A three-year follow-up. In Coursaget P, Tong MJ (eds): *Progress in Hepatitis B Immunization.* Paris, John Libby Eurotext, 1990, pp 509–517.
78. Lieming D, Mintai Z, Yinfu W, et al: A 9-year follow-up study of the immunogenicity and long-term efficacy of plasma-derived hepatitis B vaccine in high risk Chinese infants. *Clin Infect Dis* 17:475–479, 1993.
79. Xu Z-Y, Duan S-C, Margolis HS, et al: Long-term efficacy of active postexposure immunization of infants for prevention of hepatitis B virus infection. *J Infect Dis* 171:54–60, 1995.
80. Cousaget P, Yvonnet B, Chotard J, et al: Seven year study of hepatitis B vaccine efficacy in infants from an endemic area (Senegal). *Lancet* 2:1143–1145, 1986.
81. Chotard J, Inskip HM, Hall AJ, et al: The Gambia intervention study: Follow-up of a cohort of children vaccinated against hepatitis B. *J Infect Dis* 166:764–768, 1992.
82. West DJ, Watson B, Lichtman J, et al: Persistence of immunologic memory for twelve years in children given hepatitis B vaccine in infancy. *Pediatr Infect Dis J* 13:745–747, 1994.
83. Moyes CD, Milne A, Waldon J: Very low dose hepatitis B vaccination in the newborn: Anamnestic response to booster at four years. *J Med Virol* 30:216–218, 1990.
84. Immunization Practices Advisory Committee: Postexposure prophylaxis of hepatitis B. *MMWR* 33:285–290, 1984.

85. American Academy of Pediatrics, Committee on Infectious Diseases: Universal hepatitis B immunization. *Pediatrics* 89:795–800, 1992.
86. Centers for Disease Control: Hepatitis B virus: A comprehensive strategy for eliminating transmission in the United States through universal childhood vaccination. Recommendations of the Immunization Practices Advisory Committee (ACIP). *MMWR* 40(RR-13):1–25, 1991.
87. Freed GL, Bordley WC, Clark SJ, et al: Universal hepatitis B immunization of infants: Reactions of pediatricians and family physicians over time. *Pediatrics* 93:747–751, 1994.
88. Alter MJ, Hadler SC, Margolis HS, et al: The changing epidemiology of hepatitis B in the United States. Need for alternative vaccination strategies. *JAMA* 263:1218–1222, 1990.
89. Hall CB, Halsey NA: Control of hepatitis B: To be or not to be. *Pediatrics* 90:274–277, 1992.
90. Margolis HS, Alter MJ, Hadler SC: Hepatitis B: Evolving epidemiology and implications for control. *Semin Liver Dis* 11:84–92, 1991.
91. Centers for Disease Control: Hepatitis B infection: A comprehensive strategy for eliminating transmission in the United States through immunization. Recommendations of the Advisory Committee on Immunization Practices (ACIP). 1995 Update. *MMWR* (in press).
92. Committee on Infectious Diseases: Update on timing of hepatitis B vaccination for premature infants and for children with lapsed immunization. *Pediatrics* 94:403–404, 1994.
93. Lau Y-L, Tam AYC, Ng KW, et al: Responses of preterm infants to hepatitis B vaccine. *J Pediar* 121:962–965, 1992.
94. Chawareewong S, Jirapongsa A, Lokaphadhana K: Immune response to hepatitis B vaccine in premature neonates. *Southeast Asian J Trop Med Public Health* 22:39–40, 1991.
95. Centers for Disease Control: Suboptimal response to hepatitis B vaccine given by injection into the buttock. *MMWR* 34:105, 1985.
96. Shaw FE Jr, Guess HA, Roets JM: The effect of anatomic injection site, age, and smoking on the immune response to hepatitis B vaccination. *Vaccine* 7:425–430, 1989.
97. Centers for Disease Control: Inadequate immune response among public safety workers receiving intradermal vaccination against hepatitis B—United States, 1990–1991. *MMWR* 40:569–572, 1991.
98. Coberly JS, Townsend T, Repke J, et al: Suboptimal response following intradermal hepatitis B vaccine in infants. *Vaccine* 12:984–987, 1994.
99. Hibberd PL, Rubin RH, Dienstag JL: Needs unfulfilled by current hepatitis B vaccines. In Ellis RW (ed): *Hepatitis B Vaccines in Clinical Practice.* New York, Marcel Dekker, 1993, pp 323–336.
100. Carman WF, Zanetti AR, Karayiannis P, et al: Vaccine-induced escape mutant of hepatitis B virus. *Lancet* 2:325–329, 1989.
101. Okamoto H, Yano K, Nozaki Y, et al: Mutations within the S gene of hepatitis B virus transmitted from mothers to babies immunized with

hepatitis B immune globulin and vaccine. *Pediatr Res* 32:264–268, 1992.

102. Fortuin M, Karthigesu V, Allison L, et al: Breakthrough infections and identification of a viral variant in Gambian children immunized with hepatitis B vaccine. *J Infect Dis* 169:1374–1376, 1994.

103. Robertson BH, Khanna B, Nainan OV, et al: Epidemiologic patterns of wild-type hepatitis A virus determined by genetic variation. *J Infect Dis* 163:286–292, 1991.

104. Xu Z-Y, Li Z-H, Wang J-X, et al: Ecology and prevention of a shellfish-associated hepatitis A epidemic in Shanghai, China. *Vaccine* 10(suppl 1):S67–S68, 1992.

105. Rosenblum LS, Villarino ME, Nainan OV, et al: Hepatitis A outbreak in a neonatal intensive care unit: Risk factors for transmission and evidence of prolonged viral excretion among preterm infants. *J Infect Dis* 164:476–482, 1991.

106. Hadler SC: Global impact of hepatitis A virus infection: Changing patterns. In Hollinger FB, Lemon SM, Margolis H (eds): *Viral hepatitis and Liver Disease.* Baltimore, Williams & Wilkins, 1991, pp 14–20.

107. Shapiro CN, Coleman PJ, McQuillan GM, et al: Epidemiology of hepatitis A: Seroepidemiology and risk groups in the USA. *Vaccine* 10(suppl 1):S59–S62, 1992.

108. Hadler SC, McFarland L: Hepatitis in day care centers: Epidemiology and prevention. *Rev Infect Dis* 8:548–557, 1986.

109. Peetermans J: Production, quality control and characterization of an inactivated hepatitis A vaccine. *Vaccine* 10(suppl 1):S99–S101, 1992.

110. Armstrong ME, Giesa PA, Davide JP, et al: Development of the formalin-inactivated hepatitis A vaccine, VAQTA™ from the live attenuated virus strain CR326F. *J Hepatol* 18(suppl 2):S20–S26, 1993.

111. Innis BL, Snitbhan R, Kunasol P, et al: Protection against hepatitis A by an inactivated vaccine. *JAMA* 271:1328–1334, 1994.

112. SmithKline Beecham Pharmaceuticals: Unpublished data, 1995.

113. Werzberger A, Mensch B, Kuter B, et al: A controlled trial of formalin-inactivated hepatitis A vaccine in healthy children. *N Engl J Med* 327:453–457, 1992.

114. Merck & Company: Unpublished data, 1995.

115. Miller WJ, Clark W, Hurni W, et al: Sensitive assays for hepatitis A antibodies. *J Med Virol* 41:201–204, 1993.

116. Andre FE, D'Hondt E, Delem A, et al: Clinical assessment of the safety and efficacy of an inactivated hepatitis A vaccine: Rationale and summary of findings. *Vaccine* 10(suppl 1):S160–S168, 1992.

117. Clemens R, Safary A, Hepburn A, et al: Clinical experience with an inactivated hepatitis A vaccine. *J Infect Dis* 171(suppl 1):S44–S49, 1995.

118. Westblom TU, Gudipati S, DeRousse C, et al: Safety and immunogenicity of an inactivated hepatitis A vaccine: Effect of dose and vaccination schedule. *J Infect Dis* 169:996–1001, 1994.

119. Horng Y-C, Chang M-H, Lee C-Y, et al: Safety and immunogenicity of hepatitis A vaccine in healthy children. *Pediatr Infect Dis J* 12:359–362, 1993.
120. Lee S-D, Lo K-J, Chan C-Y, et al: Immunogenicity of inactivated hepatitis A vaccine in children. *Gastroenterology* 104:1129–1132, 1993.
121. Shapiro C, Letson G, Kuehn D, et al: Immunogenicity and reactogenicity of inactivated hepatitis A vaccine in infants. In *International Symposium on Viral Hepatitis and Liver Disease.* Tokyo, abstract 38, 1993.
122. Block SL, Hedrick JA, Tyler RD, et al: Safety, tolerability and immunogenicity of a formalin-inactivated hepatitis A vaccine (VAQTA) in rural Kentucky children. *Pediatr Infect Dis J* 12:976–980, 1993.
123. Newcomer W, Rivin B, Reid R, et al: Immunogenicity, safety and tolerability of varying doses and regimens of inactivated hepatitis A virus vaccine in Navajo children. *Pediatr Infect Dis J* 13:640–642, 1994.
124. Leentvaar-Kuijpers A, Coutinho RA, Brulein V, et al: Simultaneous passive and active immunization against hepatitis A. *Vaccine* 10(suppl 1):S138–S141, 1992.
125. Green MS, Cohen D, Lerman Y, et al: Depression of the immune response to inactivated hepatitis A vaccine administerred concomitantly with immune globulin. *J Infect Dis* 168:740–743, 1993.
126. McMahon BJ, Beller M, Williams J, et al: A program to control an outbreak of hepatitis A in Alaska using an inactivated hepatitis A vaccine. In *Abstracts of the 34th Interscience Conference on Antimicrobial Agents and Chemotherapy.* Orlando, Fla, abstract H11, 1994, p 103.
127. Centers for Disease Control: Prevention of hepatitis A through active or passive immunization. Recommendations of the Advisory Committee on Immunization Practices (ACIP). *MMWR* (in press).
128. American Academy of Pediatrics, Committee on Infectious Diseases: Recommendations for hepatitis A prophylaxis. *Pediatrics* (in press).
129. Brindle RJ, Morris CA, Berger R, et al: Inadequate response to intradermal hepatitis A vaccine. *Vaccine* 12:483–484, 1994.
130. Margolis HS, Shapiro CN: Who should receive hepatitis A vaccine? Considerations for the development of an immunization strategy. *Vaccine* 10(suppl 1):S85–S87, 1992.
131. Villarejos VM, Serra J, Anderson-Visona K, et al: Hepatitis A infection in households. *Am J Epidemiol* 115:577–586, 1982.

Adenoviral Infections in Children

Nalini Singh-Naz, M.D., M.P.H.
Associate Professor of Pediatrics, George Washington University School of Medicine and Health Sciences, Children's National Medical Center, Washington, D.C.

William Rodriguez, M.D., Ph.D.
Professor of Pediatrics, George Washington University School of Medicine and Health Sciences, Children's National Medical Center, Washington, D.C.

A denoviruses were first isolated in 1953 by two groups of scientists working independently. Rowe et al.[1] during the course of a study of growth of polioviruses in human adenoid tissue noticed a cytopathic change in uninoculated tissue culture and coined the term "adenoid degenerating agent." Hilleman and Werner[2] isolated an agent with a similar cytopathic effect from respiratory secretions demonstrating these agents to be causative for acute respiratory tract disease. Recently two new adenoviruses, candidates 48 and 49 of subgenus D serotype, have been identified, making a total of 49 serotypes of human adenoviruses.[3] A report from the World Health Organization on a survey of respiratory tract infections caused by adenovirus stated that in 1967 to 1976 adenovirus type 3 (Ad3) isolates accounted for 13% of all the strains.[4] These Ad3 strains were most frequently isolated from children.[5–7]

MOLECULAR BIOLOGY

Human adenoviruses belong to the family Mastadenovirus. The human adenoviruses have been divided into six groups. Classification of the currently recognized 49 serotypes is shown in Table 1. The current method for classification is based on DNA base composition of guanine and cytosine and DNA homology, measured by DNA hybridization.[8] The DNA homology grouping is based on oncogenicity, guanine and cytosine content, and molecular characteristics of viral proteins. Members of group A are between 48% and 69% homologous, whereas those of group B to E are more

TABLE 1.

Currently Recognized Adenovirus Serotypes and Diseases

Subgenus	Serotype	DNA Homology	Hemagglutination			Oncogenicity	Selected Diseases
			Guanine and Cytosine (%)	Rat	Rhesus Monkey		
A	12, 18, 31	48–69	48	+/−	−	High	Upper respiratory tract infections, tonsillopharyngitis
B1	3, 7, 16, 21	89–94	51	−	+	Weak	Respiratory tract disease: pneumonia, bronchiolitis, pharyngoconjunctival fever
B2	14, 11, 34, 35						Hemorrhagic cystitis persists in kidney Ad3, Ad4, Ad7, Ad14, and Ad21 cause epidemics

C	1, 2, 5, 6	99–100	58	+	–	Nil	Endemic, upper respiratory tract infection, tonsillopharyngitis persists in lymphoid tissue
D	8–10, 13, 15, 17, 19, 20, 22–30, 32, 33, 36, 37, 38, 39, 42–47, 48, 49	94–99	58	+	+/0	Nil	Keratoconjunctivitis (epidemic)
E	4	—	58	+/–	–	Nil	Conjunctivits, pharyngoconjunctival fever
F	40, 41	62–69	52	+	–	Nil	Gastroenteritis

closely related, approximately 85% homologous.[9] The homology between serotypes is less than 20%. Most adenovirus serotypes also have unique patterns of DNA cleavage if multiple restriction enzymes are used.[10] It is possible to group these related viruses by comparing DNA fragments after digestion with *SmaI*.

Adenoviruses are nonenveloped DNA viruses that measure approximately 60 to 90 nm in diameter.[11] They are composed of 87% protein and 13% DNA. Each virus contains one molecule of linear-stranded DNA, which, together with certain proteins, forms the core of the virus. There is a slight variation in the size of the DNA molecule with each serotype. Adenoviruses are regular icosahedrons, composed of 20 equilateral triangles and 12 vertices, each of which has a fiber projecting from the surface. The length of the fiber varies in different serotypes. The viral capsid is made up of 252 capsomeres, which contain 240 hexons and 12 pentons. The hexons are composed of polypeptide II, VI, VIII, and IX. Each penton and fiber is composed of polypeptide III and polypeptide IV, respectively. Polypeptide V and VII are noncovalently linked to DNA to form the core.

All human adenovirus serotypes share a major cross-reacting family antigen (α) which is carried on the inner surface of the hexon capsomere (group specific) and on the penton (type specific).[12] This antigen elicits antibodies detectable by complement fixation (CF), and enzyme-linked immunosorbent assay (ELISA). Type specific antigens are found on the hexon (ϵ) and fiber (γ) and give rise to neutralizing antibodies. The major type-specific antigen on the fiber is responsible for the hemagglutination patterns seen.

Adenoviruses are absorbed slowly onto the cell surface. Phagocytosis is completed over the next several hours. The virus passes to the cytoplasmic matrix over 1 to 2 hours, and the viral core is then transported to the nucleus. After uncoating and before replication, the viruses cannot be recognized antigenically or microscopically. This phase is known as the eclipse phase. In permissive human cells adenovirus genes are expressed in two phases: early and late phase.[13] Before DNA replication the immediate early genes and early mRNA are transcribed from six separate regions of the genome. The early genes lie in six noncontiguous regions designated as early region 1 (E1), E2A, E2B, E3, E4, and L1. The early genes actually take over the cells' systems to efficiently produce viral mRNA, the viral DNA, and the proteins.[13] During the late phase essentially all cellular resources are directed toward production of the viral macromolecules. Respiratory adenoviruses grow efficiently in tissue culture; however, enteric adenovirus types 40 and 41 are highly fastidious agents that fail to replicate efficiently in many conventional cell lines that support the growth of other human adenoviruses. These enteric adenoviruses grow well in 293 cells, an adenovirus type 5–transformed human embryonic kidney (HEK) cell line. The replication of these enteric viruses is abortive beyond the early stage of the replicative cycle.[14, 15]

A knowledge of the early genes is important to understanding the initiation of adenovirus infection in permissive cells. E1 proteins carry out a number of key regulatory functions; but protein synthesis is not required for the E1A transactivation. E1 gene contains two transcription units: E1A and E2B, which encode the first transcripts to be expressed after infection of permissive human cells. One or more E1A gene products is required to activate most of the remaining viral genes. Both E1A and E1B are nonessential for viral growth in 293 cells. Regions in E1 are required for gene regulation and cell transformation and apparently are used by groups A and E adenoviruses to transform cells in vitro. Only group A viruses are oncogenic in vivo.[16] Cytolysis of group C adenovirus–transformed cells by natural killer (NK) and activated macrophages (AMs) requires E1A.[17, 18] Other interactions of adenovirus and the host await further studies. The capability for oncogenic behavior appears to be species specific. Subgenus A in serotypes A-12, A-18, and A-31 are highly oncogenic, whereas serotype B-1, B-3, B-7, B-11, B-14, B-16, B-21, and B-34 are weakly oncogenic in newborn hamsters (see Table 1). Of note, the guanine-cytosine content of the DNA decreases with increasing oncogenicity. The E1A region of type 4 and 9 are associated with mammary tumors and sarcoma in rats. However, there is no association between adenoviruses and human malignancy.

The E3 region appears to be nonessential for viral replication in tissue culture and in an animal model.[12, 19] The proteins of the E3 region are well conserved among different subgroups of adenovirus. The proteins of this region also contribute to the persistence of infection by masking the infected cells from the immune surveillance mechanism and from the antiviral effect of tumor necrosis factor (TNF).[12]

Replication of the virus begins in the nucleus 6 to 8 hours after infection and reaches its maximum rate at about 20 hours. Late mRNA transcription begins shortly after the onset of DNA replication, resulting in the production of structural proteins. Viral DNA and mRNA are synthesized in the nucleus, whereas viral proteins are made in the cytoplasm. The assembly of virus occurs in the nucleus.

The adenovirus group is particularly suited for gene transfer vectors in the cells because (1) they are widely studied and well characterized, (2) they are easy to grow in vitro and in vivo and (3) large amounts of virus can be produced in infected cells. The genome of adenovirus consists of 36,000 base pairs of double-stranded DNA. Because only a small portion of viral genome appears to be required in *cis*, adenovirus-derived vectors permit the substitution of large DNA fragments once host cell lines have been developed that can provide most of the essential viral functions in *trans*.[12] The size of the DNA insert is limited to 5% of the normal genome length, otherwise the recombinant will not be properly encapsidated. Foreign viral genes can be expressed by endogenous adenoviral regulatory elements, eliminating the need for additional promoters.[20]

Because adenovirus E3 region is nonessential for viral replication in vitro and in vivo, this region can be deleted to accommodate the insertion of large pieces of foreign DNA (up to 7 Kbp). When foreign genes are inserted in place of the deleted E3 sequences, their expression is regulated by the endogenous E3 promoter.[20] Recombinants containing foreign gene insertions in the E1 region have been made with E1 region deletions. These recombinant viruses require cultivation in adenovirus-transformed cell lines that constitutively express E1 proteins. These constructs are capable of expressing large amounts of foreign antigen in cell culture, but are unable to replicate independently in vivo and thus have limited potential as live vaccines.

Experimental adenovirus-vectored vaccines have been developed for several pathogens, including hepatitis B virus, human immunodeficiency virus type 1, and herpes simplex virus.[21-24] Using adenovirus type 5, HBsAg has been expressed in the E1 region, E3 region, and the region between E4 and the right inverted terminal repeat. Evaluation of in vivo expression of HBsAg is difficult because human adenoviruses have a limited host range. Serologic responses have been induced in rabbits, hamsters, and chimpanzees. An Ad5 recombinant-containing envelope glycoprotein in the E3 region has been developed for potential use as a live virus vaccine against acquired immunodeficiency virus (AIDS). Immunization of cotton rats induced a serologic response to the human immunodeficiency virus type 1 envelope protein. An Ad5 recombinant with glycoprotein B of herpes simplex has been developed;

mice immunized with this recombinant are subsequently protected from lethal herpes simplex virus challenge. Helper independent recombinant adenovirus factors have also been developed for the expression of herpes simplex virus thymidine kinase enzyme.[20–24]

PATHOGENESIS

Various cell types and tissues react differently to adenoviruses and have specific degeneration patterns. Respiratory epithelial cells develop large nuclei with basophilic inclusion bodies. Lymphoid cells also may contain viral inclusions. In the eye, an exudative and mononuclear infiltrate forms underneath the epithelium. Despite the demonstration of tropism for specific organs, adenoviruses differ in their capacity to produce disease specific sites. Abnormalities that occur after viral replication in the gastrointestinal tract are specific for both types 40 and 41 and result in acute gastroenteritis, whereas adenovirus 5 replication in the gastrointestinal tract results in few or no abnormalities.[25] Similarly, infections with adenovirus type 8 result in keratoconjunctivitis, whereas types 2 and 5, although capable of causing this condition, produce mild disease. Hemorrhagic cystitis seems to be caused solely by adenovirus 11 and 21. In addition, some adenoviruses are more likely to cause enhanced pathologic conditions such as the severe pneumonia caused by adenovirus type 3.[26]

An understanding of the various genes and the proteins they code for is important to understanding what happens in adenovirus-infected cells. Adenoviral replication in the bronchiolar epithelial cells can be shown in situ by demonstrating early gene expression. Similarly, such gene expression can be demonstrated in macrophages and monocytes in alveoli and hilar lymph nodes. The subject of adenovirus pathogenesis has recently been reviewed.[27] Adenovirus infection leads to expression of late and early genes; however, only early genes are necessary for infection and expression of the disease. In addition, those early genes are characterized by an early and late phase. Early viral genes from group C—Ad2 and Ad5—can be expressed in situ in nasal and bronchiolar epithelial cells, alveolar macrophages, and monocytes in peripheral and hilar lymph nodes of infected lungs.[27]

There are two important proteins in the group C adenoviruses: Ad2 and AD5 in the E3 region during the early phase.[27, 28] The 19-kD glycoprotein reduces expression of the Class I major histocompatibility complex (MHC) antigen on the surface of infected cells, suppressing the response by cytotoxic T cells. Mutation of the 19-kD glycoprotein results in an increase in the late inflammatory response, similar to the wild-type virus. The 14.7-kD protein is associated with a reduction in the polymorphonuclear leukocytes in the initial inflammation. It has been reported that the E3 region is not necessary for adenovirus replication in an animal model.[19] In this study, the cotton rat was subjected to intranasal instillation of virus; the virus caused interstitial pneumonia, characterized by mononuclear cell infiltrates. The demonstration that the pulmonary histopathology and replication of adenovirus type 5 in 1-month-old cotton rats paralleled those observed in natural disease provided a model on which to further study pathogenesis.

In the E1B region, a 55-kD protein is essential for the late inflammatory response. If this gene undergoes mutation, a decreased inflammatory response occurs; however, viral replication is not affected. Therefore, it appears that if only the early genes are present, the virus can still cause pneumonia in the cotton rat model.[27]

The role of TNF and cytokines in the pathogenesis of adenovirus-induced pulmonary disease have also been studied.[27–30] Interleukin-1 (IL-1), IL-6, and TNF-α are elaborated within the first 2 to 3 days of infection, but only TNF-α appears to play a significant role. E3 14.7-kD protein, which is found in all adenoviruses, reduces the elaboration of TNF-α. However, other early viral genes in the pulmonary macrophage induce TNF-α production. The host early-phase inflammatory response is characterized by the production of TNF-α.[29] The delayed phase is associated with a cellular immune response after Class I MHC expansion (CD8[+]).[30] During the first day of infection, the cytokines, TNF-α, IL-1, and IL-6 are found in lung homogenates; of these proteins only IL-6 is found in the blood. Between day 2 and 3, TNF-α and IL-1 levels peak. If antibodies against TNF-α are used, 50% to 75% of the inflammation is prevented. Similarly, when corticosteroids were given early in adenovirus type 5 infection in the cotton rat, the signs of infection ablated and the cytokine production decreased.[27]

Although fibroblasts infected with Group C human adenoviruses are sensitive to cytolysis by TNF-α, E3 14.7-kD protein protects the cells from the TNF-α cytolysis.[31] Cells infected with adenovirus mutants lacking the E3 14.7-kD gene were not lysed by TNF-α. In another study, C3HA fibroblasts were not killed by TNF at any dose tested.[32] However, when they were exposed to adenoviruses that had large deletions in E3, lysis ensued. The investigators concluded that the infection with adenoviruses had rendered the cell sensitive to TNF and that genes within E3 could actually be used by the virus to protect infected cells from lysis by TNF.

Several viruses, including adenoviruses, express gene products that interfere with the antiviral activities of MHC Class I cytotoxic T lymphocytes.[33] Human adenoviruses produce an integral membrane protein of the endoplasmic reticulum, E3-GP-19K, which binds strongly to Class I MHC proteins and is critical for antiviral cytotoxic activity. Human cells infected with adenoviruses that lack this and other E3 proteins remain resistant to TNF killing. However, if there is deficiency in the production of E1B-19K protein, cells are susceptible to TNF lysis.[34] On the other hand, absence of E1B-19K protein and presence of E3 protein results in protection. Thus, E3 proteins appear to function primarily when the virus has been in a long-term asymptomatic relationship with the host.[33]

The ability of the adenoviruses to persist can protect and abet the transforming process. Adenovirus E1A and E1B proteins are required for transformation of primary rodent cells.[35] When expressed in the absence of E1B 19-kD protein, the E1A proteins are acutely cytotoxic and induce wholesale chromosomal DNA fragmentation, cytolysis, and cell death. By suppressing the intrinsic cell death mechanism activated by TNF-β or E1A protein, E1B 19-kD protein enhanced the transforming activity of E1A and enabled the adenovirus to evade TNF-dependent immune surveillance.[35] In another report the absence of E3 14.7-kD, E3 10.4-kD, and E3 14.5-kD proteins was required to protect several of the mouse cell lines against TNF-β lysis. The fact that the E3 10.4-kD protein is coimmuneoprecipitated with the E3 14.5-kD protein suggests that they may exist as a complex. Hence, the three sets of proteins, E3 14.7-kD, E1B 19-kD, and E3 10.4-kD/14.5-kD proteins, are adenoviral encoded, and prevent TNF-α cytolysis of different cell types.[36] In this fashion adenoviral-infected cells can escape this form of immune surveillance.

It is unclear if low-level infection of tonsils and adenoids represents adenoviral persistance or latentcy. Although adenovirus can infect and replicate in some B- and T-cell lymphocytes in vitro, ultimately the infected lymphocytes die. It may be that lymphoid tissue serves as a reservoir for the virus. The proteins from E1A, VA RNA, GP-19K, 14.7K, or other E3 regions function to counteract the host antiviral defenses. Of these, GP-19K is probably one of the most critical in the search for prevention. The E3 19- and 14.7-kD proteins probably help adenovirus types 1, 2, 5, and 6 persist in lymphoid cells.

EPIDEMIOLOGY

Adenovirus infections are species specific and occur worldwide. Adenovirus serotypes 1, 2, 5, and 6 are endemic, whereas serotypes 3, 4, 7, 14, and 21 occur most often in epidemics in most areas of the world. Demonstration of virus-specific antibodies by ELISA is the best laboratory tool for estimating the prevalence of infection within a population. Studies have shown that 40% to 60% of children have antibodies to adenovirus types 1, 2, and 5 but only a few have experienced infection with types 3, 4, or 7. Therefore, adults are more susceptible to infection with these serotypes. Adenoviral infections are common in lower socioeconomic groups. Epidemic adenoviral infections occur in military recruits where the attack rate varies between 40% and 90%.[37] Adenoviruses are an important cause of febrile illness, respiratory tract infections, and gastroenteritis in children. The majority of infections occur between 6 and 12 months of age.[38] Person-to-person spread follows contact with respiratory secretions and by the fecal-oral route. Adenoviruses can be transmitted via contaminated water in swimming pools or with improperly sterilized eye equipment.[39-41]

Epidemics of pharyngoconjunctival fever (PCF) are caused primarily by adenovirus type 8. However, serotypes 19 and 37 also cause epidemic infections.[40, 42] Water has been implicated as the source in many of these outbreaks. Isolation of Ad 4 from patients with PCF and from water taken from the implicated swimming pool support this mode of transmission.[39] In other studies AD8 was recovered from both the Golman tonometer and pneumotonometer after use in infected patients.[40, 41] Adenovirus was recovered after the tips of the tonometer were wiped dry, rinsed, or soaked in water; no virus was recovered when disinfectants such as isopropyl alcohol, hydrogen peroxide, or iodophor were used for 5 minutes.

Although adenoviral infections occur infrequently in immunocompromised individuals such as transplant recipients or patients with AIDS, they are frequently severe and occasionally fatal in this setting.[43, 44] Outbreaks of adenoviral infections have occurred at day-care centers, schools, and children's homes.[45, 46] Pneumonia, permanent lung damage, and death have been reported in young infants with Ad3 infection.[26, 47] Nosocomial adenoviral infections (Ad40 and Ad41) may cause severe pneumonia or gastroenteritis.[48-50]

CLINICAL SIGNIFICANCE

The infection rate of adenovirus disease is approximately 40.8 per 100 person-years for those younger than 1 year and 14.4 for those

10 years or older.[51] Diseases caused by adenoviruses are shown in Table 1. Among them the lower serotypes (except type 4) are often recovered from pediatric patients. Pharyngotonsillitis, upper respiratory tract infections, and gastroenteritis are the most common clinical syndromes. Most manifestations of adenoviral disease are seen in the respiratory tract. Adenovirus causes conjunctivitis, acute otitis, media, and acute sinusitis. Dermatologic manifestations are not common. Prolonged high fever occurs commonly in adenoviral infections. Viremia with lymphocyte-associated virus has been reported with adenovirus type 2 in infants with respiratory tract infections,[52] whereas adenovirus 7 may disseminate to multiple organs.[53] After respiratory tract infection, viruses may be shed in the stool for weeks. Accordingly, isolation of viruses from the stool is no guarantee of an association with enteric diseases. Adenovirus types 40 and 41 have been identified as the second most common cause of gastroenteritis.[46, 54-56] Nosocomial adenovirus enteric disease prolongs hospitalization after gastrointestinal surgery.[57]

In a study of children with viral infections, adenoviruses were the most frequent virus detected (38.5% of 161 viral isolations) from 49 of 62 children.[58] The virus was isolated from the upper respiratory tract in 70% of the patients and from the feces in 44%. Pharyngotonsillitis, bronchopneumonia with wheezy bronchitis, and otitis media were the usual diseases in children with adenovirus recovered from the respiratory tract. The virus was also recovered from several patients with Schönlein-Henoch purpura. The peak incidence of adenoviral infection was approximately 1 year of age; the virus was rarely isolated from children younger than 6 months, presumably because of protection from maternal antibodies.

In a similar study conducted in Finland, 2,500 nasopharyngeal specimens from febrile children without a specific etiologic diagnosis, as well as stools of 1,500 children, were studied for adenovirus.[59] Out of 105 children with presumed adenoviral infection hospitalized at Turku University Hospital, 82 had adenovirus antigen detected in the pharyngeal secretions, 17 had the antigen in feces, and 6 had significant increases in complement-fixing antibody levels. The authors reported a clinical picture characterized by high fever for several days (average 5.4 days); tonsillitis, otitis media, and gastroenteritis were the most common illnesses. In 17% of the patients there was no identifiable focus of infection. Approximately 10% of the children had febrile convulsions with no definable focus. Erythrocyte sedimentation rates were found to be elevated to a mean of 34 mm/hr (range 3–89 mm/hr). In 30% of cases, the sedimentation rate was more than 40 mm/hr. Approximately one third of these patients had no evidence of secondary bacterial complications such as otitis media or pneumonia. The mean white blood cell count was approximately 13,000 cells/mm^3, the counts ranged from 4,100 to 30,700cells/mm^3.[59]

ACUTE OTITIS MEDIA

In a Finnish study of adenoviral infections, approximately one third of the patients had acute otitis media and approximately one fifth had adenovirus tonsillitis.[59] Lim and coworkers[60] developed an animal model of otitis media using adenovirus. They were able to infect chinchillas by intranasal or transbullar inoculation with adenovirus type 1. Clinically the animals developed evidence of infection within 48 hours of inoculation. This infection was consistently maintained for 10 days after inoculation. In other studies in their laboratory, the adenoviral infection acted synergistically with bacterial inoculation, affecting the development and severity of infections of middle ear infections caused by nontypable *Haemophilus influenzae*.

PNEUMONIA

Approximately 20% of childhood pneumonias in children younger than 5 years are caused by adenoviruses.[61] Radiographic findings include patchy or diffuse infiltrates; consolidation and pleural effusion occasionally occur. The diagnosis is based on serologic response or isolation of the virus. The pneumonia syndrome can be accompanied by a sepsislike picture along with respiratory distress. Hepatosplenomegaly, hematologic abnormalities with bleeding, myocarditis, and death have been reported. In children younger than 5 years, the fatality rate for adenovirus pneumonia may be as high as 20%.[51]

Pneumonia in the First Months of Life

Adenovirus pneumonia in neonates can be more severe than that caused by other viruses such as respiratory syncytial virus.[51] Adenovirus types 3, 7, 19, 21, and 30 have been associated primarily with severe systemic manifestations accompanying the pneumonic processes.

In a retrospective study of 40 neonatal pneumonias presumed to be viral, adenoviruses were identified in approximately 10% of patients.[62] Symptoms included decreased feeding, cyanosis, lethargy, retraction, apnea, bradycardia, seizures, and depressed consciousness. The severity of illness ranged from moderate to severe.

There was a fatality rate of approximately 7.5%. Premature infants were ill appearing, had lobar consolidation, and were considered to be at risk for severe disease. Other predisposing risk factors for neonatal adenoviral infection include prolonged ruptured of membranes and maternal fever.[63] These neonatal infections manifest in the first 10 days of life with clinical findings consistent with sepsis (e.g., lethargy, fever or hypothermia, anorexia, apnea, hepatomegaly, and progressive pneumonia). The disease is disseminated and involves multiple organs. The adenoviral isolates are of serotypes 3, 7, 21, and 30.

Pneumonia Outcome

When death occurs, the histopathology of the lungs is characterized by patchy alveolar seropurulent exudates, necrotizing bronchitis, and hyaline membrane formation.[61] Intranuclear inclusions in bronchiolar epithelium and alveolar lining cells can be seen. Survivors may have long-term complications, such as hyperlucent lung syndrome, bronchiectasis, bronchiolitis obliterans, and persistent lobular collapse.

Sequelae are few and, when present, have been associated primarily with chronic pulmonary changes. Persistence or latency of adenovirus in the lungs of patients can be associated with chronic airway obstruction.[64]

Bronchiolitis obliterans can follow adenoviral infection. Recurrent wheezing, chronic cough, and chest infection (asymptomatic in some) can result in obliteration of the lumen of terminal bronchioles with dilation of distal bronchioles, narrow pulmonary arteries, and diminished blood flow to the affected area.[65]

Extrapulmonary manifestations of adenoviral infection have been reported in three children with Ad7 pneumonia.[53] These children had an unexpected onset of coma; biochemical findings were incompatible with Reye's syndrome. These authors reported finding penton antigen in the sera, although they found no extrapulmonary evidence of the whole virus.

OCULAR MANIFESTATIONS

Conjunctivitis

The incubation period is approximately 7 days, and the process may last 1 to 2 weeks. Adenovirus types 3, 4, 7, and 8 are typically implicated.[66–69] Fever may be an accompanying finding. The involvement of the conjunctivae may be unilateral or bilateral. Abnormalities are described as nonspecific and follicular. Children older than 2 years usually have a milder form of the disease than adults; however, younger children may have a severe membranous manifestation.

Keratoconjunctivitis

The disease manifests with lid edema, formation of a membrane over the palpebral conjunctivae, periorbital swelling, foreign body sensation, preauricular adenopathy, and diffuse superficial keratitis with some corneal erosions. These findings are unusual among infants and young children and are more common in those older than 20 years. Sequelae occurring in 50% to 80% of patients include subepithelial corneal infiltrates, which can persist for months to years.[66]

URINARY TRACT

Cystitis is usually a self-limited disease starting with suprapubic pain, fever, and bloody urine. Pathophysiologically, the bladder wall is hemorrhagic around the trigonal area. Types 11 and 21 are associated with this condition.[70, 71]

GASTROENTERITIS

Although other adenovirus serotypes have been recovered from patients with diarrhea, serotypes 40 and 41 have been recognized as an important cause of gastroenteritis in children seeking care in Europe and the United States.[46, 54, 55, 72] Gastroenteritis is nonseasonal and has an incubation period of 7 days. Adenovirus causes a self-limited gastroenteritis usually affecting children younger than 2 years. The children have watery diarrhea for 5 days, associated with vomiting and dehydration. Asymptomatic infections are uncommon.

Other Gastrointestinal Manifestations

Intussusception has been associated with adenoviruses, primarily types 2, 3, and 5. Intranuclear inclusion bodies were found by light microscopy in epithelial cells of one set of infants and children younger than 2 years with ileocecal intussusception. The findings were accompanied by the isolation of the virus, as well as serologic evidence of infection. Respiratory problems were not a common manifestation of this disease.[73–75]

JOINT

Attempts have been made to implicate adenoviruses as a cause of arthritis along with other viruses such as rubella, human parvovirus, mumps, Epstein-Barr virus, and Coxsackie B virus. Adenoviral infection of the human joint causes a limited infection compared with mumps or varicella zoster.[76]

IMMUNODEFICIENCY

Human Immunodeficiency Virus Infection

All serotypes of adenovirus have been recovered from a variety of sites in patients with AIDS; no epidemiologic significance can be attributed to any one serotype.[77, 78] Viral isolates of subgenus A and C have been recovered from liver, lung, blood, urine, and stool. The isolates from subgenus B and D are mostly isolated from urine and stool, respectively. These viruses may contribute to long-term, debilitating illness in patients with AIDS.

Adenovirus has been recovered from the spinal fluid of a 4-year-old patient with encephalitis and in an adult with concurrent infection of the central nervous system caused by Ad2 and Epstein-Barr virus.[79, 80] The presence of the virus was confirmed by in situ hybridization.

Adenovirus has been isolated from the urine of patients with AIDS.[81] In this study, approximately 20% of patients with AIDS shed viruses in the urine. This finding differed markedly from that noted in the urine of other immunosuppressed patients, such as those with renal transplants, in whom only 4% of a series of 52 urine samples were adenovirus positive. The adenoviruses were similar to serotype 35 and ultimately were called type 34–35. Type 34–35 appears to be more common in immunocompromised hosts. Disseminated disease and concomitant hepatic necrosis have been described in patients with human immunodeficiency virus.[82] These adenoviruses belong primarily to serotypes 1, 2, 3, 5, and 7, and patients as young as 6 months have been described. Approximately one third of these patients had no interstitial pneumonia or pleural effusion with the accompanying extensive hepatic necrosis, underscoring the observation that adenovirus may cause disease without pulmonary involvement. Of those patients who suffered hepatic necrosis, two thirds had fever and coagulopathy and one third had gastrointestinal hemorrhage. Hence, adenoviruses were placed on the list of opportunistic agents capable of establishing infection in patients with AIDS.

Other Immunodeficiency States

Immunocompromised adenovirus-infected patients can have wide-ranging manifestations from asymptomatic viruria to fatal pneumonitis and hepatitis. Adenoviruses were recovered from 51 of 151 bone marrow transplants during a 6-year period.[83] Patients with types 11, 34, or 35 (subgenus B) had positive urine cultures. Approximately 20% of the 51 patients had invasive disease with pneumonia as a prominent manifestation. Moderate to severe graft-vs.-host disease was a risk factor for development of infection and severe adenovirus disease. Adenovirus type 21 was found in four of five bone marrow recipients with hemorrhagic cystitis out of a cohort of 502 patients.[71] Patients with autologous bone marrow transplantation showed progressive hemophagocytosis of normal hematopoietic progenitors resulting in aplasia. Adenovirus type II was isolated from bone marrow, urine, and stool cultures. Diagnosis of adenoviral infection should be considered in any bone marrow transplant recipient who exhibits evidence of secondary graft failure.[84] Adenoviruses also can cause infection in the setting of solid organ transplants. Hepatitis secondary to adenoviruses have been described in patients receiving liver transplants.[85]

Other manifestations of adenoviral infection in patients with immunodeficiency have included lesions resembling granuloma annulare, colitis, mycocarditis, and pneumonitis.[86-88]

OTHER IMPORTANT PROFILES

In a day-care center study, nasal washes were obtained from 1,416 children younger than 6 years; 8.2% of the specimens yielded adenovirus.[89] Eighty-one percent of those were adenovirus type 1 or 2. These infections were accompanied by significant antibody rises in more than 75% of the population. The risk of infection among nonindex cases was high (approximately 67%), suggesting a high secondary attack rate. Most infections occurred in children between ages 12 and 17 months (10 isolates per 100 children). Fever was prominent. Temperatures were greater than 39.4° C in 38% and between 38.7° C and 39° C in 32%; the remaining 30% had a history of fever. Abnormal respiratory tract findings were noted in 80%: cough in 50%, conjunctivitis in 12%, wheezes and rales in 8% and pharyngitis in 14.5%, and pneumonia in 6.8%.

Nosocomial spread of Ad3 has been described in pediatric patients in a respiratory care unit, crowded wards, and a transitional care facility.[39, 47, 90] These outbreaks were associated with restrictive or obstructive lung disease and fatalities among patients with bronchopulmonary dysplasia.

DIAGNOSIS

COLLECTION AND PREPARATION OF SPECIMENS

Swabs and washings from conjunctiva, nasopharyngeal aspirates, stool, urine, blood, and spinal fluid should be transported in a viral transport medium to the laboratory as soon as possible.[91]

ISOLATION OF VIRUS

Adenovirus are host specific and are best isolated in human cell lines such as primary HEK, an epithelial cell line (HEP-2), or a human carcinoma cell line (HeLa cells). Graham 293 cell lines are used for isolation of Ad40 and Ad41 in stool. A cytopathic effect, consistent with rounding up and clustering of infected cells, is seen by the tenth day. Serotyping of the isolated virus is not routinely done and requires standard pools of antibodies. Alternatively specimens can be sent to a reference laboratory.[91]

SEROLOGY

Neutralizing, hemagglutination inhibition (HAI), and CF antibodies appear 7 days after the infection. The level of CF antibodies decline 2 to 3 months after acute infection. The tests for CF antibodies are relatively insensitive, and negative results do not rule out infection. Neutralizing and HAI antibodies persists for years after infection. The tests for these antibodies, although sensitive, are cumbersome to perform.[91]

RAPID DIAGNOSIS OF ADENOVIRUS

Direct detection of antigen from specimens obtained from conjunctiva, respiratory tract, and stool can be done by ELISA using monoclonal antibodies. Other rapid methods include time-resolved fluoroimmunoassay (using europium and dot-dot hybridization) and polymerase chain reaction.[92–101] These methods can be useful in patients with severe keratoconjunctivitis or in suspected cases of nosocomial infection such as severe pneumonia, hepatitis, or gastroenteritis. Rapid tests such as adenovirus immune dot-blot have been used in planning and conducting control strategies for an outbreak of Ad8 keratoconjunctivitis.[102, 103]

PREVENTIVE STRATEGIES

Adenoviruses are of great importance in certain environments. In the armed forces Ad4 and Ad7 cause frequent incapacitating acute febrile respiratory tract infection. In this setting the bivalent, live, adenovirus vaccine with types 4 and 7 can be administered in lyophilized form in enteric-coated tablets. The vaccine has been shown to be safe, immunogenic, and 80% effective in reducing type-specific adenoviral disease in this population.[104] Although this vaccine has not been recommended for universal use due to the low incidence of type 4 or 7 adenoviral disease in the general population, it might be useful for immunization of high-risk populations, such as institutionalized children and adults. Transmissions of adenovirus can be successfully interrupted in chronic care facilities by prompt diagnosis, rapid antigen detection, strict infection control methods, suspension of new admissions, cohorting of residents, and use of disinfectants that inactivate adenovirus. Because water contamination with adenovirus has been responsible for outbreaks, methods for detection of these viruses in water and establishment of stringent quality standards of virus identification should be helpful in preventing infection.[105, 106]

REFERENCES

1. Rowe WP, Huebner RJ, Gillmore LK, et al: Isolation of a cytopathogenic agent from human adenoids undergoing spontaneous degeneration in tissue culture. *Proc Soc Exp Biol Med* 84:570–573, 1953.
2. Hilleman MR, Werner JH: Recovery of new agents from patients with acute respiratory illness. *Proc Soc Exp Biol Med* 85:183–188, 1954.
3. Schnurr D, Dondero MC: Two new candidates adenovirus serotypes. *Intervirology* 36:79–83, 1993.
4. Schmitz H, Wigand R, Heinrich W: Worldwide epidemiology of human adenovirus infections. *Am J Epidemiol* 117:455–466, 1983.
5. Huebner RJ, Rowe WP, Ward TG, et al: Adenoidal-pharyngeal-conjunctival agents, a newly recognized group of common viruses of the respiratory system.*N Engl J Med* 251:1077–1086, 1954.
6. Parrott RH, Rowe WP, Hubner RJ, et al: Outbreak of febrile pharyngitis and conjunctivitis associated with type 3 adenoviral-pharyngeal conjunctival virus infection. *N Engl J Med* 251:1087–1090, 1954.
7. Tyrrell DA, Balducci JD, Zaiman TE: Acute infections of the respiratory tract and the adenovirus. *Lancet* 2:1326–1330, 1956.
8. Green M, Mackey J, Wold WSM, et al: Thirty one human adenovirus serotypes (Ad1–Ad31) form five groups (A-E) based on upon DNA genome homologies. *Virology* 93:481–492, 1979.
9. Sussenbach JS: The structure of the genome. In Ginsberg HS (ed): *The Adenoviruses.* New York, Plenum Press, 1984, p 35.
10. Wadell G, Hammarskjold ML, Winberg, et al: Genetic variability of adenoviruses. *Ann N Y Acad Sci* 354:16–42, 1980.
11. Nermut MV: The architecture of adenovirus. In Ginsberg HS (ed): *The Adenoviruses.* New York, Plenum Press, 1984, p 5.
12. Nicholson F: Introduction to adenoviruses: An overview of morphology, classification and epidemiology. *Eye* 7(suppl):1–4, 1993.
13. Gooding LR, Wold WS: Molecular mechanisms by which adenoviruses counteract antiviral immune defense. *Crit Rev Immunol* 10:53–71, 1990.
14. Takiff HE, Straus SE, Garon CF: Propagation and in vitro studies of previously non-cultivable enteral adenoviruses in 293 cells. *Lancet* 832–834, 1981.
15. Takiff HW, Straus SE: Early replicative block prevents the efficient growth of fastidious diarrhea associated adenoviruses in cell culture. *J Med Virol* 9:93–100, 1982.
16. Graham FL: Transformation by and oncogenicity of human adenoviruses. In Ginsberg HS (ed): *The Adenoviruses.* New York, Plenum Press, 1984, p 339.

17. Cook JL, May DL, Lewis AM, et al: Adenovirus E1A gene induction of susceptibility to lysis by natural killers cells and activated macrophages in infected rodents cells. *J Virol* 61:3510, 1987.
18. Cook JL, Walker TA, Lewis AM, et al: Expression of the adenovirus E1A oncogene during cell transformation is sufficient to induce to susceptibility to lysis by host inflammatory cells. *Proc Natl Acad Sci U S A* 83:6965, 1986.
19. Pacini DL, Dubovi EJ, Clyde WA: A new animal model for human respiratory tract disease due to adenovirus. *J Infect Dis* 150:92–97, 1984.
20. Gurwith MJ, Horwith GS, Impellizzeri CA, et al: Current use and future directions of adenovirus vaccine. *Semin Respir Infect* 4:299–303, 1989.
21. Balley A, Levrero M, Buendia MA, et al: In vitro and in vivo synthesis of the hepatitis B virus surface antigen and of the receptor for polymerized human serum albumin from recombinant human adenoviruses. *EMBO J* 4:13B:3861–3865, 1985.
22. Haj-Ahmad Y, Graham FL: Development of a helper-independent human adenovirus vector and its use in the transfer of the herpes simplex virus thymidine kinanse gene. *J Virol* 57:267–274, 1986.
23. Hung PP, Chanda PK, Natuk RJ, et al: Adenovirus vaccine strains genetically engineered to express HIV-1 or HBV antigens for use as live recombinant vaccines. *Natl Immun Cell Growth Regul* 9:160–164, 1990.
24. Chandra PK, Natuk RJ, Dheer SK, et al: Helper independent recombinant adenovirus vectors: Expression of HIV env or HBV surface antigen. *Int Rev Immunol* 7:66–67, 1990.
25. Ginsberg HS: *Adenoviruses*. In Dulbecco R, Ginsberg HS (eds): *Virology*, ed 3. Philadelphia, JB Lippincott, 1988, pp 147–160.
26. Wright HT Jr, Beckwith JB, Gwinn JL, et al: A fatal case of inclusion body pneumonia in an infant infected with adenovirus type 3. *J Pediatr* 64:528–533, 1964.
27. Ginsberg HS, Prince GA: The molecular basis of adenovirus pathogenesis. *Infect Agents Dis* 3:1–8, 1994.
28. Ginsberg HS, Lundholm-Beauchamp U, Horswood RL, et al: Role of early region 3 (E3) in pathogenesis of adenovirus disease. *Proc Natl Sci U S A* 86:3823–3827, 1989.
29. Beutler B, Cerami A: Cachetin: More than a tumor necrosis factor. *N Engl J Med* 316:379–385, 1987.
30. Ginsberg HS, Moldanero II, Sehgal PB, et al: A unique animal model for studying the molecular pathogenesis of adenovirus pneumonia. *Proc Natl Acad Sci U S A* 88:1651–1655, 1991.
31. Duerksen-Hughes P, Wold WS, Gooding LR: Adenovirus E1A renders infected cells sensitive to cytolysis by tumor necrosis factor. *J Immunol* 143:4193–4200, 1989.
32. Gooding LR, Elmore LW, Tollefson AE, et al: A 14,700 mw protein from the E3 region of adenovirus inhibits cytolysis by tumor necrosis factor. *Cell* 53:341–346, 1988.

33. Gooding LR: Regulation of TNF-mediated cell death and inflammation by human adenoviruses. *Infect Agents Dis* 3:106–115, 1994.

34. Gooding LR, Aquino L, Duerksen-Hughes P, et al: The E1B 19,000-molecular-weight protein of group C adenovirus prevents tumor necrosis factor cytolysis of human cells but not of mouse cells. *J Virol* 65:3083–3094, 1991.

35. White E, Sabbatini P, Debbas M, et al: The 19-kilodalton adenovirus E1B transforming protein inhibits programmed cell death and prevents cytolysis by tumor necrosis factor. *Mol Cell Biol* 12:2570–2580, 1992.

36. Gooding LR, Ranheim TS, Tollefson AE, et al: The 10,400- and 14,500-dalton proteins encoded by region E3 of adenovirus function together to protect many but not all mouse cell lines against lysis by tumor necrosis factor. *J Virol* 65:4114–4123, 1991.

37. Forsyth BR, Bloom HH, Johnson KM, et al: Patterns of adenovirus infections in Marine corps personnel: II. Longitudinal study of successive advanced recruit training companies. *Am J Hyg* 80:343–355, 1964.

38. Brandt CD, Kim HW, Vargosko AJ, et al: Infections in 18,000 infants and children in a controlled study of respiratory tract disease: I. Adenovirus pathogenicity in relation to serologic type and illness syndrome. *Am J Epidemiol* 90:484–500, 1969.

39. D'Angelo LJ, Hierholzer JC, Keenlyside RA, et al: Pharyngoconjunctival fever caused by adenovirus type 4: report of a swimming pool–related outbreak with recovery of virus from pool water. *J Infect Dis* 140:42–47, 1979.

40. Jernigan JA, Lowry BS, Hayden FG, et al: Adenovirus type 8 epidemic keratoconjunctivitis in an eye clinic: risk factors and control. *J Infect Dis* 167:1307–1313, 1993.

41. Threlkeld AB, Froggatt JW III, Schein OD, et al: Efficacy of a disinfectant wipe method for the removal of adenovirus 8 from tonometer tips. *Ophthalmology* 100:1841–1845, 1993.

42. Kemp MC, Hierholzer JC, Cabradilla CP, et at: The changing etiology of epidemic keratoconjunctivitis: Antigenic and restriction enzyme analyses of adenovirus types 19 and 37 isolated over a 10 year period. *J Infect Dis* 148:24–33, 1983.

43. Janner D, Petru AM, Belchis D, et al: Fatal adenovirus infection in a child with acquired immunodeficiency syndrome. *Pediatr Infect Dis J* 9:434–436, 1990.

44. Ellaurie M, Schutzbank TE, Rakusan RA, et al: Spectrum of adenovirus infection in pediatric HIV infection. *Pediatr AIDS HIV Infect* 4:211–214, 1993.

45. Pacini D, Collier A, Henderson F: Adenovirus infections and respiratory illnesses in children in group day care. *J Infect Dis* 156:920–927, 1987.

46. Kotloff KL, Losonsky GA, Morris JG, et al: Enteric adenovirus infec-

tion and childhood diarrhea: An epidemiologic study in three clinical settings. *Pediatrics* 84:219–225, 1989.

47. Herbert F, Wilkinson D, Burchak E, et al: Adenovirus type 3 pneumonia causing lung damage in childhood. *Can Med Assoc J* 116:274–276, 1977.

48. Singh-Naz N, Brown M, Ganeshananthan M: Nosocomial adenovirus infection: Molecular epidemiology of an outbreak. *Pediatr Infect Dis J* 12:922–925, 1993.

49. Flewett TH, Bryden AS, Davies H, et al: Epidemic viral enteritis in a long-stay children's ward. *Lancet* 4–5, 1975.

50. Richmond SJ, Caul EO, Dunn SM, et al: An outbreak of gastroenteritis in young children caused by adenoviruses. *Lancet* 1178–1180, 1979.

51. Piedra P: Adenovirus infection: Epidemiology and clinical manifestations. *Contemp Pediatr* 11:15–27, 1994.

52. Andiman W, Jacobsen RI, Tucker G: Leukocyte-associated viremia with lower respiratory tract disease. *N Engl J Med* 297:100–101, 1977.

53. Ladisch S, Lovejoy FH, Hierholzer JC, et al: Extrapulmonary manifestations of adenovirus type 7 pneumonia simulating Reye syndrome and the possible role of an adenovirus toxin. *J Pediatr* 95:348–355, 1979.

54. Rodriguez WJR, Kim HW, Brandt CD, et al: Fecal adenovirus from a longitudinal study of families in Metropolitan Washington, D.C.: Laboratory, clinical and epidemiologic observations. *J Pediatr* 107:514–520, 1985.

55. Uhnoo I, Wadell G, Svensson L, et al: Importance of enteric adenoviruses 40 and 41 in acute gastroenteritis in infants and young children. *J Clin Microbiol* 20:365–372, 1984.

56. Bates PR, Bailey AS, Wood DJ, et al: Comparative epidemiology of rotavirus, subgenus F (types 40 and 41) adenovirus, and astrovirus gastroenteritis in children. *J Med Virol* 39:224–228, 1993.

57. Yolken RH, Lawrence F, Leister F, et al: Gastoenteritis associated with enteric type adenovirus in hospitalized infants. *Pediatr* 101:21–26, 1982.

58. Van Lierde S, Corbeel L, Eggermont E: Clinical and laboratory findings in children with adenovirus infections. *Eur J of Pediatr* 148:423–425, 1989.

59. Ruuskanen O, Meruman O, Sarkkinen H: Adenoviral disease in children: A study of 105 hospital cases. *Pediatrics* 76:79–83, 1985.

60. Bakaletz LO, Daniels RL, Lim DJ: Modeling adenovirus type 1–induced otitis media in the chinchilla: Effect of ciliary activity and fluid transport function of eustachian tube mucosal epithelium. *J Infect Dis* 168:865–872, 1993.

61. Zahradnik JM: Adenovirus pneumonia. *Semin Respir Infect* 2:104–111, 1987.

62. Abzug MJ, Beam AC, Gyorkos EA, et al: Viral pneumonia in the first month of life. *Pediatr Infect Dis J* 9:881–885, 1990.

63. Abzug MJ, Levin MJ: Neonatal adenovirus infection: Four patients and review of the literature. *Pediatrics* 87:890–895, 1991.

64. Matsuse T, Hayashi S, Kuwano K, et al: Latent adenoviral infection in the pathogenesis of chronic airways obstruction. *Am Rev Respir Dis* 146:177−184, 1992.

65. Becroft DM: Bronchiolitis obliterans, bronchiectasis, other sequelae of adenovirus type 21 infections in young children. *J Clin Pathol* 24:72−83, 1971.

66. Alice M: Ocular viral infections. *Pediatr Infect Dis J* 3:358−368, 1984.

67. Mitsui Y, Hanna L, Hanabusa J, et al: Association of adenovirus type 8 with epidemic keratoconjunctivitis. *Arch Ophthalmol* 61:891−898, 1959.

68. O'day D, Guyer B, Hierholzer JC, et al: Clinical and laboratory evaluation of epidemic keratoconjunctivitis due to adenovirus types 8 and 19. *Am J Ophthalmol* 81:207−215, 1993.

69. Adrian T, Brunnemann H, Wigand R: Adenovirus isolations from patients with conjunctivitis in Thuringia. *Int J Med Microbiol Parasitol Infect* 278:127−131, 1993.

70. Numazaki Y, Kumasaka T, Yano N, et al: Further study of acute hemorrhagic cystitis due to adenovirus type 11. *N Engl J Med* 289:344−347, 1973.

71. Ambinder RF, Burns W, Forman M, et al: Hemorrhagic cystitis associated with adenovirus infection in bone marrow transplantation. *Arch Intern Med* 146:1400−1401, 1986.

72. Brandt CD, Kim HW, Rodriguez WJ, et al: Adenoviruses and pediatric gastroenteritis. *J Infect Dis* 151:437−443, 1985.

73. Clarke EJ, Phillips IA, Alexander ER: Adenovirus infection in intussusception in children in Taiwan. *JAMA* 208:1671−1674, 1969.

74. Yunis EJ, Hashida Y: Electron microscopic demonstration of adenovirus in appendix vermiformis in a case of ileocecal intussusception. *Pediatrics* 51:566−570, 1973.

75. Yunis EJ, Atchison RW, Michaels RH, et al: Adenovirus and ileocecal intussusception. *Lab Invest* 33:347−351, 1975.

76. Huppertz HI, Niki NPH, Chantler JK: Susceptibility of normal human joint tissue to viruses. *J Rheum* 18:699−704, 1991.

77. Hierholzer JC, Wigand R, Anderson LJ, et al: Adenoviruses from patients with AIDS: a plethora of serotypes and a description of five new serotypes of subgenus D (types 43−47). *J Infect Dis* 158:804−813, 1988.

78. Horwitz MS, Valderrama G, Hatcher V, et al: Characterization of Adenovirus Isolates From AIDS Patients. *Ann N Y Acad Sci* 437:160−174, 1984.

79. West T, Papasian CJ, Park BH, et al: Adenovirus type 2 encephalitis and concurrent Epstein-Barr virus infection in an adult man. *Arch Neurol* 42:815−817, 1985.

80. Anders KH, Park CS, Cornford ME, et al: Adenovirus encephalitis and widespread ependymitis in a child with AIDS. *Pediatr Neurosurg* 16:316−320, 1990−1991.

81. De Jong PJ, Valderrama G, Spigland I, et al: Adenovirus isolates from urine of patients with acquired immunodeficiency syndrome. *Lancet* 11:1293–1296, 1983.

82. Krivlov LR, Rubin LG, Frogel M, et al: Disseminated adenovirus infection with hepatic necrosis in patients with human immunodeficiency virus infection and other immunodeficiency states. *Rev Infect Dis* 12:303–307, 1990.

83. Shields AF, Hackman RC, Fife KH, et al: Adenovirus infections in patients undergoing bone-marrow transplantation. *N Engl J Med* 213:529–533, 1985.

84. Levy J, Wodell RA, August CS, et al: Adenovirus-related hemophagocytic syndrome after bone marrow transplantation. *Bone Marrow Transplant* 6:349–352, 1990.

85. Koneru B, Jaffe R, Esquivels CO, et al: Adenoviral infection in pediatric liver transplant patients. *JAMA* 258:489–492, 1987.

86. Coldiron BM, Freeman RG, Beaudoing DL: Isolation of adenovirus from a granuloma annulare-like lesion in the acquired immunodeficiency syndrome related complex. *Arch Dermatol* 124:654–655, 1988.

87. Janoff EN, Orenstein JM, Manischewitz JF, et al: Adenovirus colitis in the Acquired Immunodeficiency Syndrome. *Gastroenterology* 100:976–979, 1991.

88. Lozinski GM, Davis GG, Krous HF, et al: Adenovirus myocarditis: Retrospective diagnosis by gene amplification from Formalin-fixed, paraffin-embedded tissues. *Hum Pathol* 25:831–834, 1994.

89. Edwards KM, Thompson J, Paolini J, et al: Adenovirus infections in young children. *Pediatrics* 76:420–424, 1985.

90. Porter JDH, Teter M, Traister V, et al: Outbreak of adenoviral infections in a long-term paediatric facility, New Jersey, 1986/87. *J Hosp Infect* 18:201–210, 1991.

91. Lennette EH, Schmidt NJ: *Diagnostic Procedures for Viral, Rickettsial and Chlamydial Infections*, ed 5. American Public Health Association, 1979, p 229.

92. Kidd AH, Harley EH, Erasmus MJ: Specific detection and typing of adenovirus types 40 and 41 in stool specimens by dot-blot hybridization. *J Clin Microbiol* 22:934–939, 1985.

93. Singh-Naz N, Naz RK: Development and application of monoclonal antibodies for specific detection of human enteric adenoviruses. *J Clin Microbiol* 23:840–842, 1986.

94. Singh-Naz N, Rodriguez WJ, Kidd AH, et al: Monoclonal antibody enzyme-linked immunosorbent assay for specific identificatoin of typing of subgroup f adenoviruses. *J Clin Microbiol* 26:297–300, 1988.

95. Herrmann JE, Perron-Henry DM, Blacklow NR: Antigen detection with monoclonal antibodies for the diagnosis of adenovirus gastroenteritis. *J Infect Dis* 155:1167–1170, 1987.

96. Scott-Taylor T, Ahluwalia G, Klisko B, et al: Prevalent enteric adenovirus variant not detected by commercial monoclonal antibody enzyme immunoassay. *J Clin Microbiol* 28:2797–2801, 1990.

97. Brown M: Laboratory identification of adenoviruses associated with gastroenteritis in Canada from 1983 to 1986. *J Clin Microbiol* 28:1525–1529, 1990.

98. Brown M, Shami Y, Zywulko M, et al: Time-resolved fluroimmunoassay for enteric adenoviruses using the europium chelator 4,7-bis(chlorosilfophenyl)-1,10-phenanthroline-2-9-dicarboxylic acid. *J Clin Microbiol* 28:1398–1402, 1990.

99. Allard A, Girones R, Juto P, et al: Polymerase chain reaction for detection of adenoviruses in stool samples. *J Clin Microbiol* 29:2659–2667, 1990.

100. Rousell J, Zajdel ME, Howdle PD, et al: Rapid detection of enteric adenoviruses by means of the polymerase chain reaction. *J Infect* 27:271–275, 1993.

101. Gleaves CA, Militoni J, Ashley RL: An enzyme immunoassay for the direct detection of adenovirus in clincial specimens. *Diagn Microbiol Infec Dis* 17:57–59, 1993.

102. Ankers HE, Klapper PE, Cleator GM, et al: The role of a rapid diagnostic test (adenovirus immune dot-blot) in the control of an outbreak of adenovirus type 8 keratoconjunctivitis. *Eye* 7(suppl):15–17, 1993.

103. Buffington J, Chapman LE, Stobierski MG, et al: Epidemic keratoconjunctivitis in a chronic care facilty: Risk factors and measures for control. *J Am Geriat Soc* 41:1177–1181, 1993.

104. Steinhoff MC: Viral vaccines for the prevention of childhood pneumonia in developing nations: Priorities and prospects. *Rev Infect Dis* 13(suppl 6):S562–S570, 1991.

105. Melnick JL, Gerba CP, Wallis C: Viruses in water. *Bull WHO* 56:499–508, 1978.

106. Ramia S: Transmission of viral infections by the water route: Implications for developing countries. *Rev Infect Dis* 7:180–188, 1985.

Helicobacter pylori in Infants and Children*

Steven J. Czinn, M.D.
Associate Professor, Department of Pediatrics, School of Medicine, Case Western Reserve University, Rainbow Babies and Children's Hospital, Cleveland, Ohio

Mark S. Glassman, M.D.
Professor, Department of Pediatrics, New York Medical College, Valhalla, New York

---

Twenty years ago it was thought that peptic ulcer disease rarely occurred in children. When a diagnosis of peptic ulcer disease was made, surgical intervention was often recommended. In 1982, Marshall and Warren[1,2] rediscovered *Helicobacter pylori* and confirmed the association of this organism with gastritis in adults. Three years later *H. pylori*–associated gastroduodenal disease was also being reported in children.[3–9] Although the relationship between *H. pylori* and primary chronic antral and fundic gastritis was suggested by many investigators, this relationship was ultimately confirmed in a pediatric study by Drumm et al.[10] Since that time, *H. pylori* has been identified in children with duodenal ulcers, gastric ulcers, and gastritis and may be a risk factor for the development of gastric cancer.[11–14] Although there is broad consensus that peptic ulcer disease is the result of multiple factors, *H. pylori* has been shown to be the primary cause of gastroduodenal disease (gastritis and duodenal ulcers) in both children and adults. Heredity and emotional stress are also thought to play a role in selected cases.

EPIDEMIOLOGY

Recent studies from all continents have documented the presence of *H. pylori* gastritis in infants and children.[15–27] *Helicobacter pylori* infection is less common in individuals born in the United States compared with similar populations in China or India. The

---

*This work was supported in part by Grant DK-46461-01 from the National Institutes of Health.

Advances in Pediatric Infectious Diseases®, vol. 11
© 1996, Mosby–Year Book, Inc.

higher prevalence in underdeveloped countries suggests that hygiene and nutritional status may be of significance in acquiring this infection. The method of acquisition and transmission of *H. pylori* is unclear; however, the most likely mode of transmission is fecal-oral. Evidence for this mechanism was demonstrated by Thomas et al.,[28] who isolated viable *H. pylori* microorganisms from the feces of infected individuals. In addition, *H. pylori* has been recovered from artificially contaminated milk or water.[29, 30] Finally, several pediatric studies have shown serologic evidence of infection in parents and siblings of *H. pylori*–infected children, corroborating reports of intrafamilial spread. Higher rates of *H. pylori* infection have also been noted for institutionalized children.[31] In adults, education and socioeconomic status influence the rate of bacterial colonization, whereas gender, smoking history, alcohol ingestion, and use of nonsteroidal anti-inflammatory drug use do not affect the rate of bacterial isolation from gastric tissue.[32] A recent report by Fiedorek et al.[14] indicates that many of these same epidemiologic factors affect the prevalence of *H. pylori* infection in children. There was an inverse relationship between both family income and socioeconomic status and the prevalence of serum antibodies against *H. pylori*. In addition, race-specific prevalence rates were also identified in their pediatric patients.

During the past 5 years, the association between gastric *H. pylori* infection and gastroduodenal inflammation in children has been confirmed by numerous investigators and include data on more than 1,000 children.[8–13, 22, 33–35] In the United States, *H. pylori* infection is rare in infants and children, increases during adolescence, and peaks at 65 years, when the infection rate approaches 45%. In asymptomatic children and adolescents, the prevalence of anti-*Helicobacter* antibodies, a marker of active infection, is 3.8%[22] and ranges from 80% in Algeria and the Ivory Coast to approximately 30% in Belgium, Spain, and Italy[17–19] and falls to 10% to 15% in France and Canada. Studies have also examined the prevalence of *H. pylori* infection in children with symptomatic abdominal pain. In asymptomatic children, the prevalence of *H. pylori* ranges from 60% in Finland to approximately 40% in Israel and falls to 5% to 10% in the United States, Netherlands, and Greece.[23–27] The most common presenting signs and symptoms include epigastric abdominal pain (50%), vomiting (40%), and hematemesis (16%). Although the clinical manifestation is not helpful in discriminating children with *H. pylori* gastritis from those with *H. pylori*–negative gastritis, pediatric patients with *H. pylori*

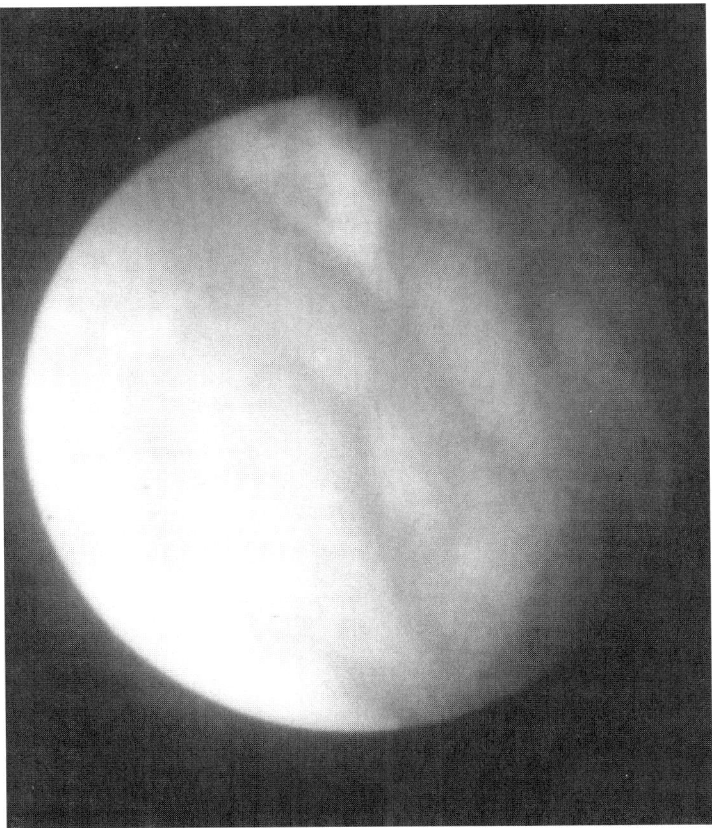

FIGURE 1.
Antral nodularity present in children with *Helicobacter pylori* gastritis.

gastroduodenal disease are usually more symptomatic than their adult counterparts.

ENDOSCOPIC FINDINGS

In children, the endoscopic appearance of *H. pylori* gastritis can vary from normal to the presence of gross ulcerations. In endoscopic studies, 50% of the children with gastritis or gastric ulcers had *H. pylori* infection, and 60% with duodenal ulcers had *H. pylori* infection. Interestingly, the majority of children with *H. pylori* infection had a nodular-appearing gastric antrum (Fig 1). This finding is pathognomonic for *H. pylori* infection in children and has only rarely been reported in any of the adult studies. Presently the cause of this finding is unclear, but it does not appear to correlate with the presence of submucosal lymphoid follicles.

RADIOLOGIC FINDINGS

Unlike adults with *H. pylori* gastroduodenal disease, children often have chronic vomiting or hematemesis. Although the digestive

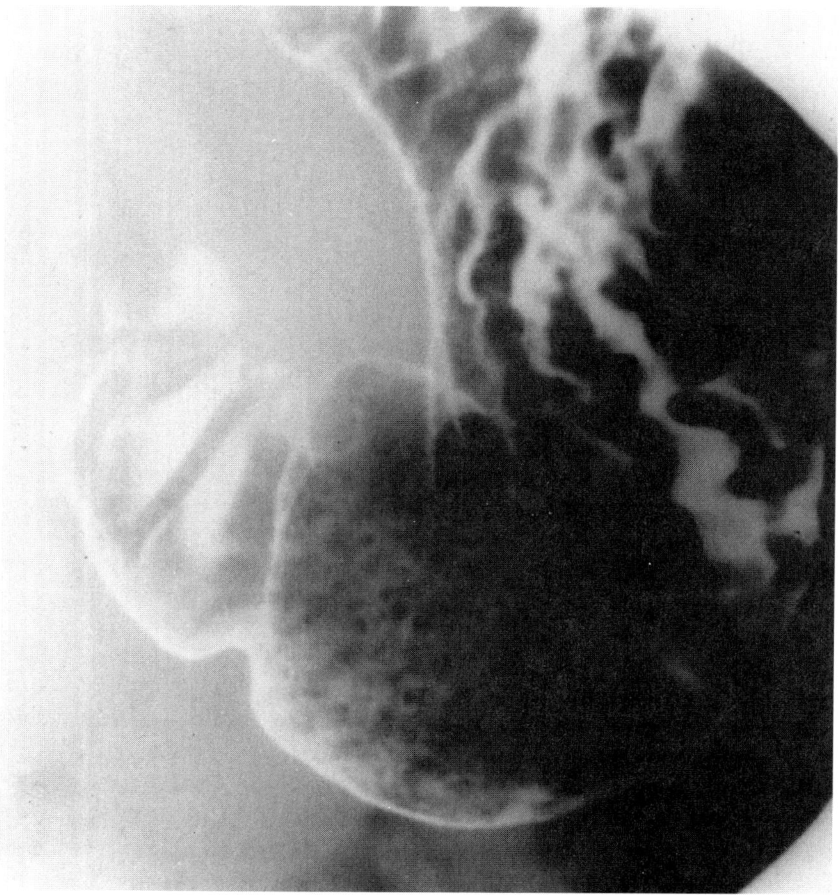

FIGURE 2.

Air-contrast examination of a child with *Helicobacter pylori* gastritis. Note the thickened folds in the body and antrum of the stomach. (From Morrison S, Dahms BB, Hoffenberg E, et al: *Radiology* 171: 819–821, 1989. Used by permission.)

tracts of these patients are usually endoscoped, initially they may undergo radiologic examination of the upper gastrointestinal tract at the time of manifestation. In one study, seven pediatric patients ultimately diagnosed with *H. pylori* infection were noted to have hypertrophic or enlarged gastric folds (Fig 2).[36] The mechanism by which *H. pylori* can cause hypertrophy of gastric folds was thought to be the result of the mucosal inflammation or edema associated with *H. pylori* infection. Transient protein-losing gastropathy, similar to that seen with Ménétrier's disease, has now also been reported in two pediatric patients with acute *H. pylori* infection.[37] Therefore, infection with *H. pylori* should be added to the list of causes for radiologic evidence of hypertrophic gastric folds in children, such as cytomegalovirus infection and Ménétrier's disease.

HISTOLOGIC FINDINGS

As noted in the adult population, the majority of children with *H. pylori* infection have moderate to severe antral gastritis. Children with *H. pylori* gastritis have a diffuse chronic gastritis with lymphocytes and plasma cells in the lamina propria, and, in the most severe cases, occasional foci of active inflammation in the glandular epithelium (Fig 3).[7] Most children with *H. pylori* have only a chronic inflammatory reaction within the lamina propria. The pediatric pattern of inflammation is also seen in the germ-free pig model of *H. pylori* infection.[38] This differs significantly from the descriptions of *H. pylori* gastritis in adults, where polymorphonuclear neutrophils are conspicuous within the lamina propria and gastric glandular epithelium. In our experience, lymphoid follicles are only occasionally present in the pediatric population and do not explain the gross antral nodularity seen at the time of endoscopy.

A definitive diagnosis of *H. pylori*–associated gastritis requires recovery of the microorganism from biopsy specimens or identification of the bacteria in tissue specimens. This can be accomplished through either direct or indirect means, as described later on.

Biopsy specimens obtained during endoscopy can be evaluated for the presence of *H. pylori* by culture, detection of urease activity, and through specific histologic staining techniques. The sensitivity of a culture diagnosis approximates 80% and is limited by the previous use of antibiotics and H_2 antagonists,[39] administration of local anesthetics during the endoscopy,[40] and biopsy sampling error. Histologic staining of the gastric mucosa with

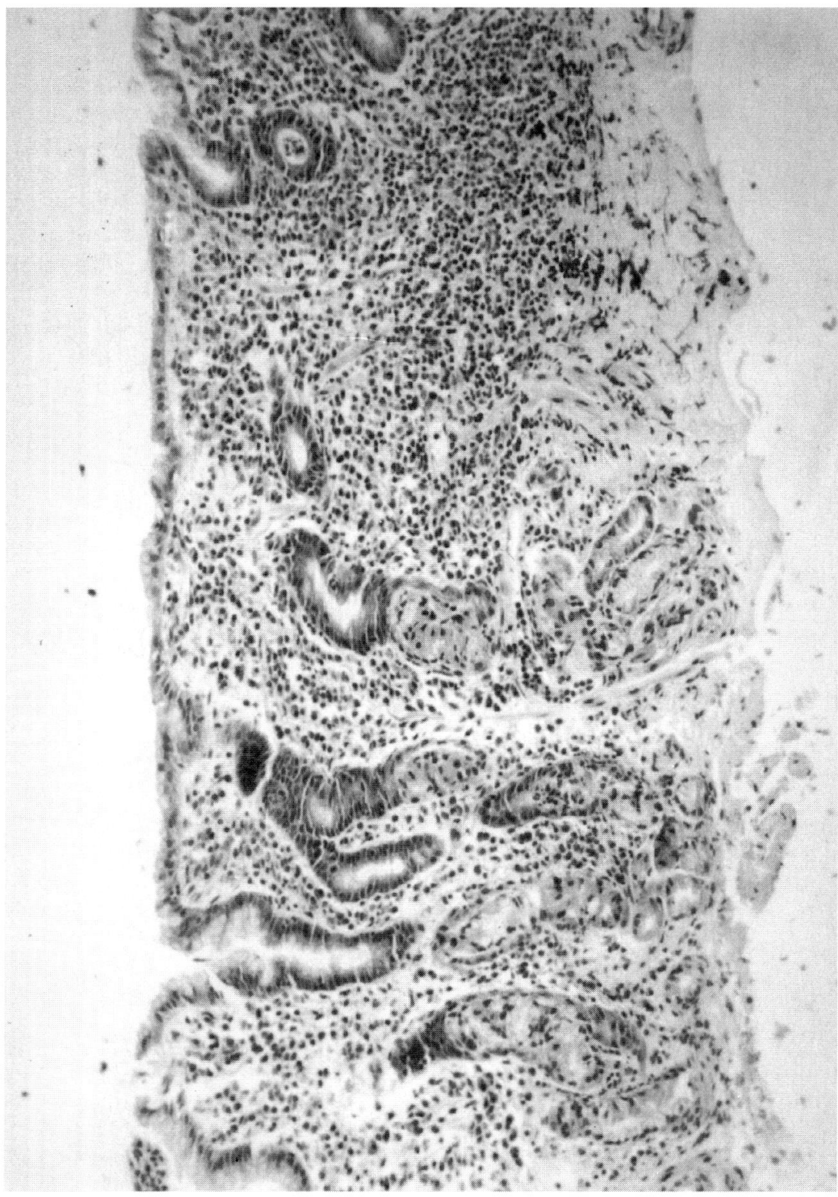

FIGURE 3.

Gastric biopsy specimen of a child with *Helicobacter pylori* gastritis. Note the diffuse chronic gastritis.

hematoxylin-eosin stain, Warthin-Starry silver stain, and Giemsa stain will detect *H. pylori* infection in virtually 100% of specimens. Reports by our laboratories indicate that the specificity and sensitivity of urease testing, histologic staining, and culture of gastric biopsies in the diagnosis of *H. pylori* in children is comparable with that noted in adult patients.[9, 34]

NONINVASIVE METHODS

Helicobacter pylori may be detected by the ingestion of urea labeled with stable isotopes of carbon 13 and carbon 14. The urease produced by *H. pylori* metabolizes these compounds and releases labeled carbon dioxide, which is then excreted in the breath. Analysis of the end-expiratory breath sample by gas chromatography/mass spectrophotometry has a sensitivity of 95% for the detection of gastric *H. pylori* in both adults and children.[41]

Pediatric patients infected with *H. pylori* produce both IgG and IgA antibodies against the five major proteins present in the outer membrane. We, and others, have demonstrated the utility of serologic techniques to identify infected individuals.[33, 42, 43] When sonicated whole-cell proteins are used as the detecting antigen in the enzyme-linked immunosorbent assay, the serum IgG and IgA antibody titer is a sensitive and specific method for identification of *H. pylori* infection. In addition, the serum IgG immune response in children appears to correlate directly with the degree of gastritis.

A latex agglutination test for antibodies to *H. pylori* combines the benefits of a noninvasive test with speed and low cost. Although this testing method has shown consistently high sensitivity and specificity in studies involving adult patients, it has produced mixed results in pediatric patients due to differences in the humeral immune response between children and adults.[44] Specifically, the mean optical density of *H. pylori*–positive pediatric samples is considerably lower than that seen in adults. Western blot analysis confirms the considerable variability in antibody response of pediatric patients to the highly antigenic outer membrane proteins of *H. pylori*.[45]

TREATMENT

Although most gastroenterologists acknowledge that the prevalence of *H. pylori* is high in patients with gastroduodenal inflammation, the treatment of *H. pylori*–positive patients remains controversial. In a majority of adult patients, eradication of *H. pylori* is associated with healing of the inflammatory lesion.[46-48] Reports have also documented continued gastrointestinal inflammation despite successful eradication of the organism.[49] Presently the National Institutes of Health Consensus Conference on *H. pylori* has recommended that anti–*H. pylori* therapy be reserved for adults with ulcer disease.

In adults with gastric *H. pylori* infection,[48] much attention has focused on bismuth compounds in combination with metronidazole and either amoxicillin or tetracycline to eradicate *H. pylori* infection. Although the only bismuth product available in the United States is bismuth subsalicylate, all bismuth salts have in vitro activity against *H. pylori*. The most commonly reported adverse effects of bismuth compounds are constipation and black stools. The black stools are a result of the bismuth salts reacting with hydrogen sulfide in the colon, producing bismuth sulfide. The most commonly reported adverse effects of metronidazole are nausea, headache, and an unpleasant metallic taste. In addition, carcinogenic and mutagenic activity have been noted in rodents or in in vitro assays. Finally, although amoxicillin and tetracycline are well tolerated, hypersensitivity to amoxicillin and permanent tooth discoloration from the use of tetracycline in children has been reported. The combination of bismuth, metronidazole, and amoxicillin or tetracycline has been used in numerous studies for periods varying from 2 weeks to 2 months. The side effects most often noted in patients treated with this triple therapy include nausea, vomiting, diarrhea, metallic taste, rash, and malaise. Although up to one third of individuals will suffer from minor side effects when treated with this protocol, most studies indicate less than 5% of individuals discontinued treatment because of them.

The role of omeprazole in combination with antimicrobial agents has recently received much attention as an alternate therapy for *H. pylori* infection. Omeprazole in combination with amoxicillin or clarithromycin has produced eradication rates as high as 90%. Recent data from studies in adults comparing omeprazole plus amoxicillin to omeprazole plus clarithromycin suggest the latter combination may be more effective in eradicating *H. pylori*. The short-term side effects of omeprazole are minimal. Long-term use of omeprazole leads to increased serum gastrin concentrations, which in research animals can lead to the development of carcinoid tumors of the stomach. The major side effects of this combined therapy include stomatitis, diarrhea, and rash.

Compliance appears to be a critical factor when eradication of *H. pylori* infection is attempted.[50] Both the triple therapy and omeprazole plus an antibiotic regimen pose a major problem when pediatric patients are treated, because it is difficult to administer two to three medications three to four times daily for 2 weeks to children.

Presently there is no consensus for the treatment of children with *H. pylori*–associated gastroduodenal disease. Kilbridge et al.[7] reported that treatment with H_2–antagonists, although effective in promoting initial clinical improvement in 80% of children with *H. pylori*, resulted in a high rate of symptom recurrence and reinfection (68%) after 2 years. The results of clinical trials using a single antibiotic for the treatment of pediatric gastric *H. pylori* infection have also been disappointing. De Giacomo et al.[51] found that children given 1 week of amoxicillin had no improvement of symptoms. Oderda et al.[6] reported a recurrence rate of 75% in 30 children who initially responded to 4 weeks of amoxicillin. Drumm et al.[52] used bismuth subsalicylate and amoxicillin to treat 16 children who had failed initial therapy with H_2 antagonists. They documented both clearance of gastric *H. pylori* and resolution of gastritis in 75% of their patients; however, long-term repeat gastric biopsy specimens were not obtained 1 month after completion of therapy to confirm eradication. In a later study, Oderda et al.[53] reported that therapy with amoxicillin and tinidazole resulted in resolution of symptoms in 94% and healing of gastritis in 84% of the children examined. The recurrence rate in this study was 16.6% after 6 months. Similar results were reported by De Giacomo et al.,[51] who found that after 4 weeks of amoxicillin and bismuth subcitrate administration, *H. pylori* was eradicated and gastritis had healed in 68%. Three of five patients who had remained symptomatic responded after tinidazole was added to the treatment protocol. Unfortunately, blinded placebo-controlled studies have not been done to confirm these findings.

The treatment of *H. pylori* gastrointestinal disease in children remains controversial. There may be compelling reasons to treat pediatric patients with *H. pylori* infection more aggressively than adults. First, pediatric patients infected with *H. pylori* usually have significant symptoms that include vomiting or hematemesis. Second, *H. pylori* infection may be a risk factor in the development of gastric carcinoma. The odds ratio for the risk of gastric cancer with *H. pylori* is as high as 6.0.[54] It appears that the acquisition of *H. pylori* infection and the concomitant gastritis at an early age are associated with an increased risk of gastric cancer. Third, in contrast to treatment outcomes in adult patients, data suggest that pediatric patients with symptomatic *H. pylori* infection treated with antimicrobial agents show significant and sustained symptomatic improvement.

Although antimicrobial therapy for children with *H. pylori*–associated gastroduodenal disease remains controversial, recent studies suggest that the majority of children suffering from *H. pylori* infection will remain asymptomatic after therapy. A survey of pediatric gastroenterologists in North America indicates the majority of respondents consider *H. pylori* to be a pathogen and are treating symptomatic children infected with *H. pylori*. Although prospective double-blind studies are needed to confirm the efficacy of antimicrobial therapy for these children, the present standard of care is to treat *H. pylori*–infected children who have symptoms. Treatment with Pepto-Bismol, metronidazole, and amoxicillin or omeprazole and amoxicillin or clarithromycin leads to resolution of symptoms and eradication of the organism in the majority of children and may ultimately prevent the development of gastric cancer. However, additional research is needed to identify the optimal duration, dose, and combination of agents to eradicate *H. pylori* with minimal side effects.

REFERENCES

1. Warren JR: Unidentified curved bacilli on gastric epithelium in chronic gastritis. *Lancet* 1:1273–1275, 1983.
2. Marshall B, Warren JR: Unidentified curved bacilli in the stomach of patients with gastritis and peptic ulceration. *Lancet* 1:1311–1314, 1984.
3. Czinn SJ, Dahms BB, Jacobs GH, et al: *Campylobacter*-like organisms in association with symptomatic gastritis in children. *J Pediatr* 109:80–83, 1986.
4. Mahony MJ, Wayatt JI, Littlewood JM: *Campylobacter pylori* gastritis. *Arch Dis Child* 63:654–655, 1988.
5. Drumm G, Sherman P, Chiasson D, et al: Treatment of *Campylobacter pylori*–associated antral gastritis in children with bismuth subsalicylate and ampicillin. *J Pediatr* 113:908–912, 1988.
6. Oderda G, Dell'Olio D, Morra I, et al: *Campylobacter pylori* gastritis: Long-term results of amoxicillin therapy. *Arch Dis Child* 64:326–329, 1988.
7. Kilbridge PM, Dahms BB, Czinn SJ: *Campylobacter pylori*–associated gastritis and peptic ulcer disease in children. *Am J Dis Child* 142:1149–1152, 1988.
8. Drumm B, O'Brien A, Cutz E, et al: *Campylobacter pylori*–associated primary gastritis in children. *Pediatrics* 80:192–195, 1987.
9. Glassman MS, Schwarz SM, Medow MS, et al: *Campylobacter pylori*–related gastrointestinal disease in children: Incidence and clinical findings. *Dig Dis Sci* 34:1501–1504, 1989.
10. Drumm B, Sherman P, Cutz E, et al: Association of *Campylobacter py*-

lori on the gastric mucosa with antral gastritis in children. *N Engl J Med* 316:1557–1561, 1987.

11. Tolia V, Chang CH, Brennan S, et al: Occurrence and diagnosis of *Campylobacter pylori* infection in children. *Int Pediatr* 5:37–41, 1990.

12. Queiroz DMM, Rocha GA, Mendes EN, et al: Differences in distribution and severity of *Helicobacter pylori* gastritis in children and adults with duodenal ulcer disease. *J Pediatr Gastroenterol Nutr* 12:178–181, 1991.

13. Hassall E, Dimmick JE: Unique features of *Helicobacter pylori* disease in children. *Dig Dis Sci* 36:417–423, 1991.

14. Fiedorek SC, Malaty HM, Evans DL, et al: Factors influencing the epidemiology of *Helicobacter pylori* in children. *Pediatrics* 88:578–582, 1991.

15. de Rafael L, Vascones F, Camarero C, et al: *Campylobacter pylori* and recurrent abdominal pain in children. Paper presented at the Workshop on Gastroduodenal Pathology and *Campylobacter pylori*, Bordeaux, France, October 1988.

16. De Giacomo C, Fiocca R, Bottino R, et al: A prospective study on the prevalence of *Campylobacter pylori*–positive and –negative gastritis in symptomatic and asymptomatic children. Paper presented at the Workshop on Gastroduodenal Pathology and *Campylobacter pylori*, Bordeaux, France, October 1988.

17. Cadranel S, Hennequin Y, Souayah H, et al: *Campylobacter pylori* (CP) in children: Is it frequent and what does it mean? Paper presented at the Workshop on Gastroduodenal Pathology and *Campylobacter pylori*, Bordeaux, France, October 1988.

18. Brassens-Rabbe MP, Kazmi M, Megraud F, et al: How common is *Campylobacter pylori* infection in children? A serological survey. Paper presented at the Fifth International Workshop on *Campylobacter* Infections, Puerto Vallarta, Mexico, Feb 25–March 1, 1989.

19. Chiesa C, Bonamico M, Pacifico L, et al: Identification of *Campylobacter pylori* in antrum and duodenum of children. Paper presented at the Fifth International Workshop on *Campylobacter* Infections, Puerto Vallarta, Mexico, Feb 25–March 1, 1989.

20. Maaroos H-I, Rago T, Sipponen P, et al: *Helicobacter pylori* and gastritis in children with abdominal complaints. *Scand J Gastroenterol* 26(suppl 186):95–99, 1991.

21. Jones DM, Lessells AM, Eldridge J: *Campylobacter*-like organisms on the gastric mucosa: Culture, histological and serological studies. *J Clin Pathol* 37:1002–1006, 1984.

22. Drumm B, Perez-Perez GI, Blaser MJ, et al: Intrafamilial clustering of *Helicobacter pylori* infection. *N Engl J Med* 322:359–363, 1990.

23. Maaroos I, Rago T, Sipponen P, et al: *Helicobacter pylori* in gastritis in children with abdominal complaints. *Scand J Gastroenterol* 26(suppl 186):95–99, 1991.

24. Bujanover Y: Nodular gastritis and *Helicobacter pylori*. *J Pediatr Gastroenterol Nutr* 11:41−44, 1990.

25. Fiedorek S, Casteel H, Pumphrey C: The role of *Helicobacter pylori* in recurrent functional abdominal pain in children. *Am J Gastroenterol* 87:347−349, 1992.

26. Van der Meer S, Forget P, Loffeld R: The prevalence of *Helicobacter pylori* serum antibodies in children with recurrent abdominal pain. *Eur J Pediatr* 151:799−901, 1992.

27. Mavromichalis I, Zaramboukas T, Richman P, et al: Recurrent abdominal pain of gastrointestinal origin. *Eur J Pediatr* 151:560−563, 1992.

28. Thomas JE, Gibson GR, Darboe MK, et al: Isolation of *Helicobacter pylori* from human faeces. *Lancet* 340:1194−1195, 1992.

29. Korin QN, Maxwell RH: Survival of *Campylobacter pylori* in artificially contaminated milk [letter]. *J Clin Pathol* 42:778, 1989.

30. West AP, Millar MR, Tompkins DS: Effect of physical environment on survival of *Helicobacter pylori*. *J Clin Pathol* 45:228−231, 1991.

31. Berkowicz J, Lee A: Person-to-person transmission of *Campylobacter pylori*. *Lancet* 2:680−681, 1987.

32. Graham DY, Malaty HM, Evans DG, et al: Epidemiology of *Helicobacter pylori* in an asymptomatic population in the United States: Effect of age, race, and socioeconomic status. *Gastroenterology* 100:1495−1501, 1991.

33. Glassman MS, Dallal S, Berzin SH, et al: Utility of enzyme-linked immunosorbent assay (ELISA) in the identification of *Helicobacter pylori* infection in children. *Dig Dis Sci* 35:993−997, 1990.

34. Czinn SJ, Carr H: Rapid diagnosis of *Campylobacter pyloridis*−associated gastritis. *J Pediatr* 110:569−570, 1987.

35. Oderda G, Vaira D, Helton J: *Helicobacter pylori* in children with peptic ulcer disease and their families. *Dig Dis Sci* 36:572−576, 1991.

36. Morrison S, Hoffenberg E, Dahms BB, et al: Enlarged gastric folds in association with *Campylobacter pylori* gastritis. *Radiology* 171:819−821, 1978.

37. Hill ID, Sinclair-Smith C, Lastovka AJ, et al: Transient protein losing enteropathy associated with acute gastritis and *Campylobacter pylori*. *Arch Dis Child* 62:212−219, 1987.

38. Krakowka S, Morgan DR, Kraft W, et al: Establishment of gastric *Campylobacter pylori* infection in the neonatal gnotobiotic piglet. *Infect Immunol* 55:2789−2796, 1987.

39. Price AB, Levi J, Dolby JM, et al: *Campylobacter pyloridis* in peptic ulcer disease: Microbiology, pathology and scanning electron microscopy. *Gut* 26:1183−1188, 1985.

40. Czinn SJ, Carr HS, Speck WS: Effects of topical anaesthetic agents on *Campylobacter pylori*. *J Pediatr Gastroenterol Nutr* 9:46−48, 1989.

41. Graham DY, Klein PD, Evans DG, et al: Rapid, non-invasive diagnosis of gastric *Campylobacter* by a 13 C-urea breath test. *Gastroenterology* 19:A1435, 1986.

42. Czinn SJ, Carr HS, Speck WT: Diagnosis of gastritis caused by *Helicobacter pylori* in children by means of an ELISA. *Rev Infect Dis* 13(suppl 8):S700–S703, 1991.

43. Evans DJ Jr, Evans DG, Graham DY, et al: A sensitive and specific serologic test for detection of *Campylobacter pylori* infection. *Gastroenterology* 96:1004–1008, 1989.

44. Westblom TU, Madan E, Gudipati S, et al: Diagnosis of *Helicobacter pylori* infection in adult and pediatric patients by using Pyloriset, a rapid latex agglutination test. *J Clin Microbiol* 30:96–98, 1992.

45. Czinn S, Carr H, Sheffler L, et al: Serum IgG antibody to the outer membrane proteins of *Campylobacter pylori* in children with gastroduodenal disease. *J Infect Dis* 159:586–589, 1989.

46. Glupczynski Y, Burette A: Drug therapy of *Helicobacter pylori* infection: Problems and pitfalls. *Am J Gastroenterol* 85:1545–1551, 1990.

47. Lambert T, Megraud F, Gerbaud G, et al: Susceptibility of *Campylobacter pyloridis* to 20 antimicrobial agents. *Antimicrob Agents Chemother* 30:510–511, 1986.

48. Marshall BJ, Goodwin CS, Warren JR, et al: Prospective double-blind trial of duodenal relapse after eradication of *Campylobacter pylori*. *Lancet* 2:1437–1441, 1988.

49. Ho J, Hui WM, Ng SC, et al: Natural history of *Campylobacter pylori* in duodenal ulceration treated with H_2 status antagonist. *Aliment Pharmacol Ther* 3:315–320, 1989.

50. Graham DY, Lew GM, Malata HM, et al: Factors influencing the eradication of *Helicobacter pylori* with triple therapy. *Gastroenterology* 102:493–496, 1992.

51. De Giacomo C, Fiocca R, Villani L, et al: *Helicobacter pylori* infection and chronic gastritis: Clinical, serological, and histologic correlations in children treated with amoxicillin and colloidal bismuth subcitrate. *J Pediatr Gastroenterol Nutr* 11:310–316, 1990.

52. Drumm G, Sherman P, Chiasson D, et al: Treatment of *Campylobacter pylori*–associated antral gastritis in children with bismuth subsalicylate and ampicillin. *J Pediatr* 113:908–912, 1988.

53. Oderda G, Holton J, Altare F, et al: Amoxicillin plus tinidazole for *Campylobacter pylori* gastritis in children. Assessment by serum IgG antibody, pepsinogen I and gastric level. *Lancet* 1:690–692, 1989.

54. Parsonnet J: *Helicobacter pylori* and gastric cancer. *Gastroenterol Clin North Am* 22:89–104, 1993.

Urinary Tract Infections in Infants and Children

Martin A. Nash, M.D.

Associate Professor of Clinical Pediatrics, Columbia University College of Physicians and Surgeons, Director of Pediatric Nephrology, Babies and Children's Hospital of New York, Columbia-Presbyterian Medical Center, New York, New York

Robert L. Seigle, M.D.

Assistant Professor of Clinical Pediatrics, Columbia University College of Physicians and Surgeons, Division of Pediatric Nephrology, Babies and Children's Hospital of New York, Columbia-Presbyterian Medical Center, New York, New York

---

Urinary tract infection (UTI) occurs relatively frequently in infants and children. By itself, it is, however, an infrequent cause of progressive renal failure and end-stage renal disease. In the North American Pediatric Renal Transplant Cooperative Study only 2% of more than 3,000 children receiving renal transplants had pyelonephritis or interstitial nephritis as the renal condition leading to end-stage renal disease, and a similar figure was found among children on dialysis.[1] Thus, the major significance of UTI in children is the accompanying morbidity and the possible association with anatomical abnormalities (obstruction, vesicoureteral reflux [VUR]) that may lead to progressive renal failure and may be amenable to medical therapy or surgical repair, if detected early. The underlying disease in 21% of children receiving renal transplants was obstructive uropathy or reflux nephropathy.[2] These anomalies may have been detected because of a UTI and, in concert with UTI, may have been important in the progression of disease. This is not to say that UTI may not cause renal morphologic changes (scarring) in the absence of anatomic abnormalities but that by itself UTI rarely leads to chronic renal insufficiency. Therefore, the focus of therapy and evaluation should be toward relieving symptoms associated with infection and toward detecting important underlying abnormalities of the urinary tract.

EPIDEMIOLOGY

In the newborn period, UTI is more frequent in boys than in girls. The infection may be blood borne and part of the general picture

Advances in Pediatric Infectious Diseases®, vol. 11
© 1996, Mosby–Year Book, Inc.

of sepsis. Anatomic abnormalities are not frequent. The prevalence of bacteriuria in the first year of life was found by Jodal et al.[3] to be 0.9% in girls and 2.5% in boys. In contrast, after infancy the prevalence of bacteriuria is 1.2% to 1.9% in girls and 0.03% in boys.[4-6] About 5% of girls will have bacteriuria by age 18 years. In later adulthood, UTI is again more frequent in men as partial obstruction from benign prostatic hypertrophy develops.

In more than 80% of urinary tract infections, *Escherichia coli* is the causative organism. This is particularly true of first infections and those not associated with an underlying anatomic abnormality. Other organisms are *Proteus* spp. (more common in boys), *Klebsiella pneumoniae, Staphylococcus saprophyticus* (especially in older girls), *Staphylococcus aureus,* and *Pseudomonas* spp. Adenovirus type 2 is associated with hemorrhagic cystitis.

ETIOLOGY AND PATHOGENESIS

Most UTIs occur by the ascending route with the possible exception of the newborn period. In this age group UTIs are often part of the larger clinical setting of sepsis. At times, UTI may be the source of sepsis. At other ages, the infecting organism is the same as that found in the rectum and in the periurethral area, implying movement into the urethra and upward. The short female urethra is thought to explain the predominant occurrence of UTI in girls and women. The high frequency of recurrent UTIs suggests a predisposition in some girls. After the first UTI, 65% to 80% of girls will experience a recurrence (almost always reinfection rather than relapse).[7]

Organisms move from the rectum to the vagina and periurethral area, perhaps aided by defecation and hygienic practices. They may then colonize the distal urethra, move up the urethra, and enter the bladder. Under the proper conditions, bacteria may multiply in the bladder and produce cystitis or migrate further to produce pyelonephritis. The factors that determine the occurrence of UTI relate to both bacterial virulence and host defense.

BACTERIAL VIRULENCE

For bacteria to colonize the urinary tract, they must avoid being swept away by the urinary stream during voiding. Some bacteria have properties that enable them to adhere to the genitourinary mucosa. Some *E. coli,* as well as some *Proteus, Klebsiella,* and *Pseudomonas* spp., exhibit pili, or fimbriae, on their surfaces containing adhesins that can bind to specific epithelial cell receptors, notably the disaccharide $\alpha(1 \rightarrow 4)$-galactose, β-galactose, or Gal-Gal (Fig 1).

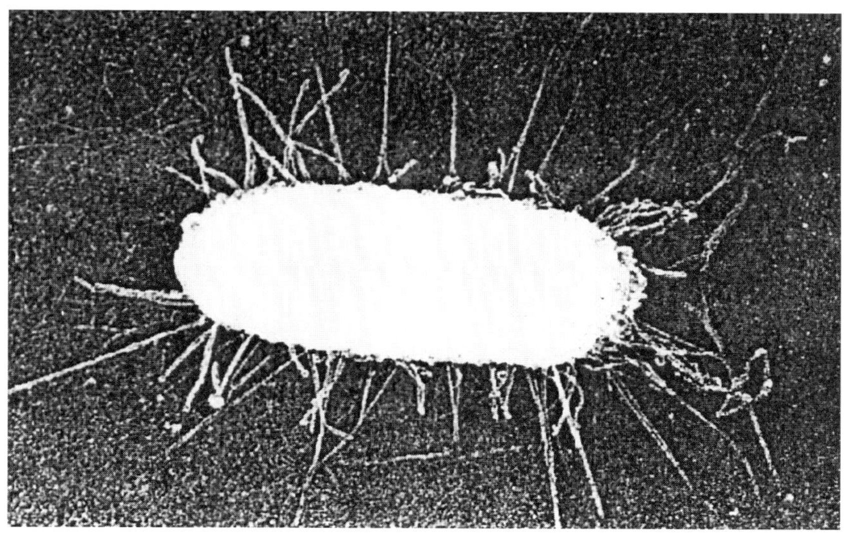

FIGURE 1.

Transmission electron micrograph of P-fimbriated *Escherichia coli* shadow cast with platinum-carbon. (Magnification ×56,000.) (From Roberts JA: *J Urol* 148:1721–1725, 1992. Used by permission.)

Fimbriated *E. coli* were found in 94% of children with pyelonephritis but in only 19% of those with cystitis.[8,9] These pili, or fimbriae, are also known as P fimbriae because of their specificity for the P1 blood group antigen on red blood cells (RBCs). In humans, 75% of the population have the P1 antigen and 25% have the P2 antigen. Lomberg et al.[10,11] showed that in girls without UTIs the expected 75% expressed the P1 antigen. However, in those with recurrent pyelonephritis, 97% had the P1 antigen. Infections in girls with VUR were not often associated with fimbriated *E. coli*, suggesting that factors other than adhesion are more important in this group. Thus, the P1 subgroup appears to be associated with susceptibility to UTIs, particularly pyelonephritis, and is related to a hemagglutinin on P fimbriae of *E. coli*. These fimbriae also contain an adhesin specific for the Gal-Gal receptor on urinary epithelium, which helps determine bacterial adhesion and localization. Adhesion is also associated with decreased ureteral peristalsis and ureteral dilatation.[12] Another feature associated with increased risk of UTI is the ABO secretory status. Women and girls who are unable to secrete into body fluids (urine and saliva) the water-soluble forms of the blood group antigens have a higher incidence of UTI and a greater inflammatory response.[13] The uroepithelium from nonsecretors has an increased affinity for the attachment of bacteria.[11] In secretors, the oligosaccharides of the blood groups may cover the bacterial receptors and render them unavailable for attachment.

Undoubtedly other factors influence bacterial virulence, but these have been less well studied than the P fimbriae. Bacteria must take up iron from their surroundings, and evidence suggests that the intensity of the inflammatory response in the urinary tract is directly related to this ability.[14] Some strains of *E. coli* contain a hemolysin, which, by causing destruction of RBCs, could increase the availability of free iron and thus the virulence of these bacteria.[15, 16] The presence of free iron could also favor the production of reactive oxygen metabolites with resulting tissue damage.[17] However, a recent study in infants and children with their first UTI[18] found no difference in the inflammatory response (fever, C-reactive protein, erythrocyte sedimentation rate [ESR], urinary white blood cell [WBC] count, and renal concentrating capacity) between children whose infecting organism was a hemolysin-producing *E. coli* and those in whom it was not. More important for inflammation in this study was the presence or absence of P fimbriae.

HOST FACTORS

The normal periurethral area in girls and women is colonized by an anaerobic microflora (mainly lactobacilli) that inhibits colonization by coliform organisms.[19] Winberg et al.,[20] using a monkey model, showed that alterations in this microflora by flushing with various antibiotics promoted vaginal colonization with *E. coli*. The protective effect of the microflora was not caused solely by lactobacilli because it could be only partially restored by instillation of lactobacilli. Vaginal antibodies also aid in the prevention of colonization by bacteria[21]; vaginal immunoglobulin levels are lower in girls with UTIs compared with controls.[22]

Complete emptying of the bladder removes most organisms that have gained access to it. Organisms remaining are killed by the bladder mucosa by a process that involves secretion of surface mucin.[23, 24] Factors that interfere with emptying (obstruction, neurogenic bladder, and dysfunctional voiding) predispose to UTI. Foreign bodies (catheters and stones) also favor the growth of bacteria.

Vesicoureteral reflux provides a means for organisms in the bladder to reach the renal parenchyma and also interferes with complete bladder emptying. Many, but not all, episodes of pyelo-nephritis are associated with reflux. Those that are not may reflect the intermittent nature of this process, the occurrence of blood-borne infection, or the ascent of P-fimbriated organisms by attachment to ureteral mucosa.

Uncircumcised male infants have a 10-fold greater risk of infantile UTI than circumcised infants.[25] Ginsburg and McCracken[26] and Wiswell et al.[27] found in 109 infants with UTI that most were boys and that 95% were uncircumcised. P-fimbriated *E. coli* predominantly, but also fimbriated *Proteus* and other uropathogenic organisms, can attach to the preputial mucosa and colonize in this area and in the terminal urethra.[28] From here pathogenic organisms can ascend to the bladder and renal parenchyma. It has been assumed that UTI in infants is usually blood borne rather than ascending. If this were so, the incidence of UTI should be the same in circumcised as in uncircumcised infants. The recent data on circumcision suggest that in this age group as well, many UTIs occur through the ascending route.[29] The advisability of neonatal circumcision remains controversial,[30, 31] because it is affected by social, ethnic, and economic issues, in addition to medical ones. However, consideration should be given on purely medical grounds for circumcision in male infants subject to UTIs or renal damage from infections. This would include those with obstructive uropathy, high grades of reflux, or both.[32]

Constipation has been associated with recurrent UTI in children.[33] Although this has not been carefully studied, personal experience supports the frequency of this association in girls referred for recurrent infections. Possible mechanisms include incomplete emptying of the bladder due to partial obstruction from the distended rectal segment, bladder distortion with stimulation of detrusor stretch receptors resulting in dysfunctional voiding (detrusor-sphincter dyssynergia), or vesicoureteral reflux from distortion of the bladder trigone.[34] Treatment of the constipation may improve bladder function and decrease the number of infections.[35]

Other associations, such as direction of wiping after defecation, swimming, wet swim suits, bubble bath, and tight clothing are either of dubious significance or have not been studied carefully.

ROLE OF REFLUX

Vesicoureteral reflux, UTI, and renal scars are closely associated.[36] However, the relationship is not as tight as was formerly believed. The conditions most favorable for the production of scars would be a preschool-age child with a UTI, especially if the UTI is caused by fimbriated *E. coli,* and high-grade reflux. The situation would be enhanced if the child were a nonsecretor of blood group antigens and had dysfunctional voiding leading to high intravesical pressure. The cause and effect relationship among these variables has been historically difficult to determine. Scars were often present at initial manifestation of UTI, at which time reflux was not always demonstrable but was presumed to have been present in the past. Reflux was thought to be the sine qua non for the development of renal scars in association with infected urine. The primacy of reflux was such that the term "atrophic pyelonephritis" to describe renal scars was discarded in favor of "reflux nephropathy." Scars, as determined from an intravenous (IV) urogram, were thought to originate almost exclusively in children younger than 5 years. They required the presence of both reflux and infection and could be prevented by either antibiotics to maintain sterile urine or correction of reflux. Renal parenchymal infection was produced by intrarenal reflux (pyelotubular backflow) that occurred in children who had compound renal calyces rather than simple calyces (Fig 2). The straight papillae of compound calyces allow free flow of infected urine into the renal parenchyma, as opposed to the angled papillae of simple calyces, which act as a shut-off valve.[37, 38]

Recent studies have challenged some of these tenets, or at least have rendered them less dogmatic. Several prospective studies of reflux and its therapy are now available.[39–41] In addition, the re-

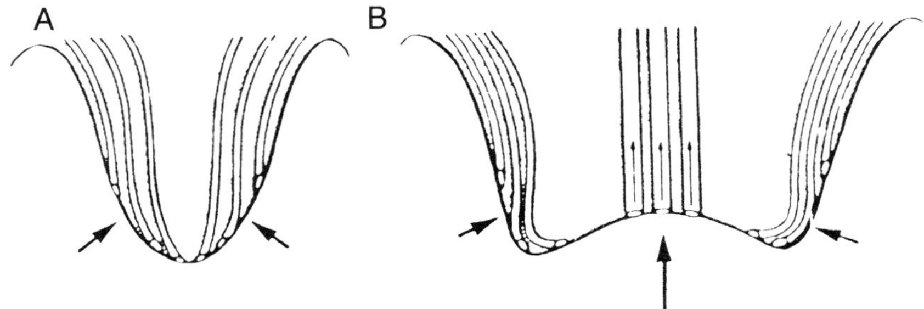

FIGURE 2.

Simple (nonrefluxing) papilla **(A)** and compound (refluxing) papilla **(B).** If pressure in the renal pelvis is sufficiently high, intrarenal reflux can occur through the circular orifices of the compound papilla. With the simple papilla, the oblique, slitlike orifices close when pelvic pressure increases and prevents intrarenal reflux. (From Ransley PG: *Urol Res* 5:61–69, 1977. Used by permission.)

cent use of dimercaptosuccinic acid (DMSA) renal scans has greatly enhanced the ability to detect and follow the development of renal scars.[42]

In general, reflux occurs in 20% to 35% of girls with bacteriuria.[7, 43] The prevalence of reflux decreases with age. In Kunin's[7] studies, reflux was found in 35% of infected girls age 5 to 9 years, only 15% of infected girls aged 10 to 14 years, and 3% of infected girls older than 15 years. With time, reflux disappears in 65% to 80%,[7, 44] more likely in milder degrees of reflux. It is rare in the black population, present in only 2% of black school children with bacteriuria.[7]

Smellie et al.[43] found renal scars in 10% of children with UTI (boys and girls). Scars were found in 31% of those with reflux but in only 1% of those without reflux. Studies of nephrectomy specimens confirm the association of intrarenal reflux with scars.[45] Recent studies using DMSA renal scans have also shown a high correlation between renal scars and gross reflux, but in children with pyelonephritis and in those with scarring, the majority of affected kidneys are drained by nonrefluxing ureters.[42, 46, 47] Thus, current studies suggest that although reflux is highly associated with the development of pyelonephritis and scarring, it is not a prerequisite.[48, 49] The organisms involved in those without reflux, however, remain the predominantly gram-negative bacteria found in the periurethral area. Therefore, the majority of episodes of pyelonephritis occur by the ascending rather than the hematogenous route, even in the absence of reflux.

In the absence of reflux, bacteria most likely ascend to the renal parenchyma through fimbriated attachment to the urothelium. This is facilitated by ureteral dilatation demonstrated in children with febrile UTI[50] and the absence of ureteral peristalsis seen in a monkey model of UTI.[51] Once bacteria reach the renal parenchyma, inflammation results with chemotaxis and release of leukocytic enzymes. Further tubulointerstitial damage can be produced by toxic oxygen radicals (superoxide, hydroxyl ion, hydrogen peroxide) released from the respiratory burst associated with phagocytosis and following reoxygenation (reperfusion) after ischemia from capillary obstruction.[52, 53] After pyelonephritis, segmental renal atrophy and fibrosis may produce scars in some children, perhaps related to virulence factors of the infecting organisms, recurrent pyelonephritis, and promptness and duration of antibacterial therapy.[48] Studies using DMSA scans have shown that these scars develop at the exact site in the kidney where infection was localized.[46] Although scars occur predominantly in children younger than 5 years, new scars can develop at all ages.[46, 39, 40] New scars appear to be more frequent in those with an abnormal bladder (obstructive or neuropathic) than in those with a normal bladder.[46] Studies in monkey models show that sterile intrarenal reflux causes scarring only if the intravesical pressure is high, as in posterior urethral valves or dysfunctional voiding. The mechanism is likely related to ischemia.[52, 54]

CLINICAL FEATURES

No single symptom complex is common to all patients with UTI. The signs and symptoms that bring the infected child to medical attention vary with the patient's age, the nature of associated abnormalities, if present, and the number of previous infections. The physician must maintain a high level of suspicion because the patient's complaints may be vague or may not immediately suggest the existence of disease of the urinary tract.

The diagnosis of UTI may easily be overlooked in affected infants. They may be apathetic, may be irritable, or may have anorexia or feeding difficulties. Fever is present in about two thirds of patients, and vomiting, with or without diarrhea, occurs in one third.[26] The vomiting may, in fact, be so impressive in its forcefulness and frequency as to focus the full attention on the gastrointestinal tract. Late-onset jaundice, due to elevation of both direct and indirect bilirubin concentrations, can be a manifestation of infantile UTI and is sometimes accompanied by hepatomegaly and hemolytic anemia. The cause of this curious complex is not entirely understood, but the syndrome occurs almost exclusively in association with UTI caused by *E. coli*. The physical examination of the infected infant may vary from an unremarkable examination to, at the other extreme, a moribund state. In many infants UTI is associated with congenital genitourinary anomalies, and some of these patients may have palpable flank or suprapubic masses. Laboratory evaluations will reveal that the urine culture is positive, but results of other studies, such as complete blood cell count, urinalysis, and ESR, may be normal or abnormal. A blood culture is frequently positive.

The older child with a UTI is more likely than the infant to have signs and symptoms that direct attention to the urinary tract. Voiding symptoms, such as frequency, dysuria, and urgency, are fairly common. However, some patients with UTI do not experience these symptoms, and many children with voiding complaints do not have a UTI. On physical examination, about half of the patients will have fever. Suprapubic tenderness is common, and costovertebral angle (CVA) tenderness can be elicited in some patients. As in the infant, laboratory results are inconstant from patient to patient, other than the obligatory positive urine culture.

In the majority of pediatric patients with UTI, clinical and routine laboratory data cannot distinguish between pyelonephritis and lower urinary tract disease. Although pyelonephritis is the likely diagnosis for a child who has a positive urine culture accompanied by voiding symptoms, high fever, flank pain, CVA tenderness, leukocytosis, pyuria, and prolonged ESR, renal involvement cannot be excluded even in the absence of many or most of these findings.[55] In addition, among patients with recurrent UTIs, the associated symptoms tend to be most intense during the first episode and become less pronounced with each subsequent infection.[56] Thus, a paucity of symptoms in a child with UTI should not be reassuring. The symptoms of *untreated* UTI persist for 1 to 2 weeks and then subside. Urine sediment usually normalizes within about 3 weeks, but the urine culture remains positive in virtually all patients. Thus, a history of even transient symptoms of UTI should be taken seriously.

Asymptomatic bacteriuria is the term that is used to describe the "positive" urine culture result that is obtained from urine culture screening of apparently well children. It occurs in 1% to 2% of young school-age girls but in only 0.03% of boys and, by definition, is not associated with symptoms that would prompt a visit to the physician.[57, 58] However, when girls who have positive cultures are questioned more closely, most report some history of subtle urinary tract symptoms, such as frequency or dysuria. About 50% of these girls will have abnormal imaging studies. In most, these findings are clinically unimportant because the majority of patients continue to do well over long periods of follow-up. Many have persistence of covert bacteriuria, which is sometimes punctuated by symptomatic UTIs.[59]

EVALUATION

The initial evaluation of a patient who manifests signs and symptoms of a possible UTI is aimed at confirming or refuting the diagnosis. If the presence of UTI is established on the basis of the results of such evaluations, further studies should be undertaken to uncover any anatomic urologic abnormalities that may exist.

URINE CULTURE

Historically the diagnosis of UTI has been made by evaluating the concentration of bacteria present in the urine. Normal bladder urine is a sterile product of the processes of glomerular filtration and tubular reabsorption and secretion. Thus, the presence of bacteria in urine implies either colonization or infection of the bladder urine or contamination of normal urine during the process of collection or evaluation. In the 1940s and 1950s, Kass[60] and others[61, 62] observed that the concentration of bacteria in urine collected by bladder catheterization of women was likely to be high in patients with symptoms suggestive of UTI and low among asymptomatic women. Several investigators have published data that have quantified the early observations in adults and expanded them to children so that we can now interpret the results of bacteriologic evaluation of urine obtained by a variety of methods from almost every pediatric patient population.

In his often-quoted paper from 1956, Kass[63] demonstrated a very good correlation between urinary tract symptoms in women and urine bacterial colony counts greater than 100,000 colonies/mL. On the other hand, the overwhelming majority of asymptomatic women had urine bacterial colony counts less than 10,000 colonies/mL. The group of patients with counts between 10^4 and 10^5 colonies/mL included both symptomatic and asymptomatic women, and so this range of colony counts was not predictive for the presence or absence of a UTI (Fig 3). As mentioned earlier, all of the urine specimens used in this study were obtained by bladder catheterization after a green soap cleansing of the perineum. It soon became clear that it was not necessary to subject women to bladder catheterization to diagnose a UTI and that an alternative method of urine collection, the clean-catch method, was equally effective.[64, 65] More recently, it has been demonstrated in women that an even simpler method of urine collection, the midstream specimen, gives culture results almost indistinguishable from those obtained from culture of the clean-catch urine.[66] This procedure eliminates the need for cleansing of the perineum and involves only the spreading of the labia by the patient, initiation of the urine stream into the toilet, and the subsequent collection of a portion of the middle of the voided urine. Thus, the results of quantitative bacteriologic evaluation of women's urine, whether obtained by catheter, clean-catch, or midstream collection, can be interpreted using the same paradigm: more than 100,000 colonies/mL diagnoses UTI; less than 10,000 colonies/mL rules out the diagnosis.

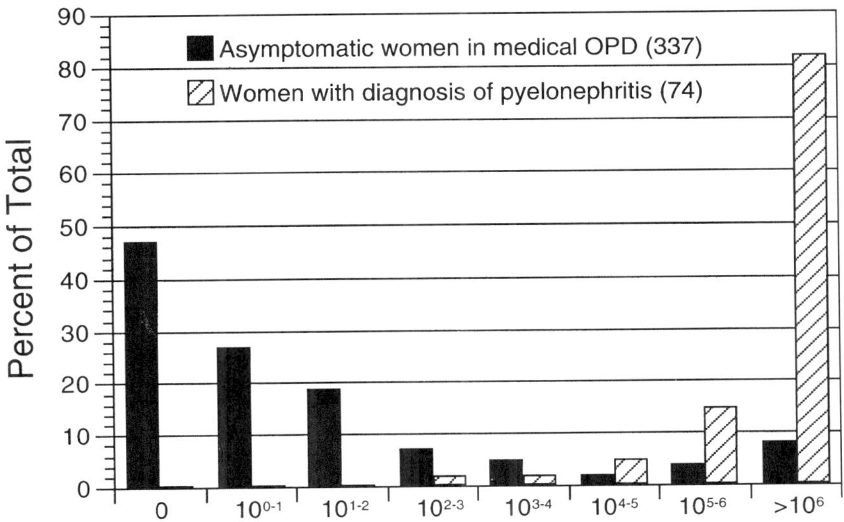

FIGURE 3.

Bacterial counts in catheterized urines from asymptomatic women and those with symptoms of pyelonephritis. (Redrawn from Kass EH: *Trans Assoc Am Phys* 69:59–64, 1956.)

Because of the anatomic differences of the periurethral area between the sexes, it seemed possible that voided urine specimens obtained from men would be less likely to be contaminated by skin flora than would voided urine obtained from women. Lipsky et al.[67] demonstrated that culture of clean-catch or midstream urine from asymptomatic men revealed no significant bacterial contamination. Therefore, in men, as in women, quantitative results from the culture of *voided* urine, whether collected by the clean-catch or the midstream method, can be interpreted using the same criteria as are used for evaluating culture results of urine obtained by bladder catheterization.

In the pediatric population, a study of more than 2,000 children younger than 2 years who were evaluated for fever demonstrated a urine colony count profile in urine obtained by bladder catheterization that was almost identical to the profile published by Kass.[63] The assumption about these young, febrile patients was that the fever was caused by a UTI in those whose catheterized urine colony counts were greater than 100,000 colonies/mL and that it resulted from some other source in those with bacterial concentrations less than 10,000 colonies/mL.

Hoberman et al.[68] suspected that the more appropriate lower limit for diagnosing UTI by bladder catheter in children may be 50,000 colonies/mL. Even this criterion for diagnosing UTI from catheterized urine is much higher than the values of 1,000 or 10,000 colonies/mL suggested by earlier authors.[69, 70] Thus, it may be prudent to suggest that UTI can be *suspected* in the symptomatic child younger than 2 years if a catheterized urine specimen yields a pure growth of a single species of the family Enterobacteriacae with a density greater than 10,000 colonies/mL. In such a situation, if a second culture also demonstrates pure growth of the same organism at a concentration in excess of 10,000 colonies/mL, UTI can be diagnosed. A single catheterized urine specimen can *confirm* the diagnosis of UTI if the microbiology laboratory reports a pure growth of any organism at a colony count greater than 100,000 colonies/mL.

As was the case among adult patients, data document that these same urine culture-based diagnostic criteria can be applied to colony count results obtained from culture of urine that is *voided* by children using the clean-catch midstream method (Fig 4).[71] Dodge et al.[72] obtained urine by the clean-catch method from approximately 4,000 healthy boys and 4,000 healthy girls, all between ages 6 and 9 years. "Positive" culture results (i.e., >100,000 colonies/mL) were reported in only 0.3% of boys and 2.4% of girls. Only about 50% of these positive results were duplicated in a second clean-catch urine specimen. Thus, even for children in these middle childhood years, the degree of contamination of bladder urine that may occur as a result of obtaining the specimen by the clean-catch technique is of such small magnitude as to be of negligible clinical significance. Indeed, some studies have demonstrated that urine collection techniques that are even less fastidious than the clean-catch method will provide urine specimens that are not significantly contaminated. Lohr et al.,[73] after evaluating the results of cultures of urine obtained from circumcised boys, reported that "cleansing of the urethral meatus prior to collecting a urine specimen for culture from circumcised boys has no demonstrable benefit." Others have substantiated the interpretability of cultures of casual urine specimens (i.e., neither clean-catch nor midstream collections) from children of both sexes.[4, 73, 74]

Thus, urine infection can be diagnosed in the symptomatic infant or child, as is the case in adults, by detection of a urinary bacterial colony count of more than 100,000 colonies/mL in specimens obtained by bladder catheterization. Urine infection is ruled out if the bacterial colony count is less than 10,000 colonies/mL in catheterized specimens; colony counts between 10,000 and 100,000 colonies/mL are suggestive of UTI if there is pure growth of a single organism. In girls and circumcised boys who can void on command, there is no significant difference in bacterial colony counts in urine obtained by clean-catch compared with urine obtained by catheter. Thus, for these children, bladder catheterization holds no advantage over the clean-catch voided technique in terms of the ability to interpret urine culture results and diagnose UTIs. The clean-catch technique provides a diagnostically and medically acceptable alternative to bladder catheterization, a procedure that is universally disliked by patients and their parents and one that can be associated with morbidities, such as urethral trauma and stric-

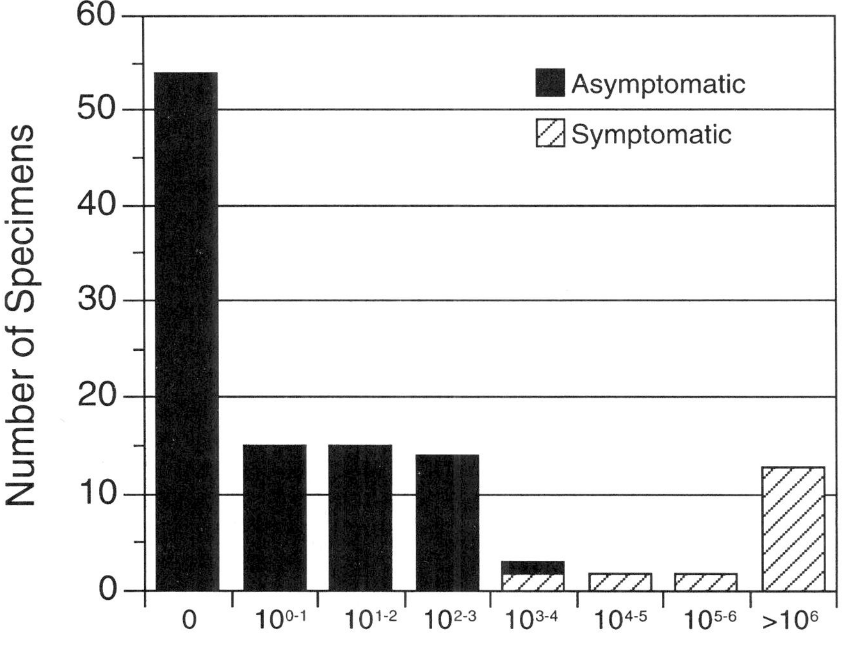

FIGURE 4.

Bacterial counts in clean voided urines from asymptomatic girls and those with clinical symptoms of UTI. (From Pryles CV, Steg NL: *Pediatrics* 23:441–452, 1959. Used by permission.)

ture, and iatrogenic infection of the bladder. The fact that it may not even be necessary to clean the periurethral area to obtain urine for culture and diagnosis may prove useful in the toddler or young child who may become frightened or agitated during the preparations involved in obtaining a clean-catch specimen. If this method of collection is employed, however, improved confidence in the results can be achieved by culturing two separate specimens voided at two different times.[72]

At times pediatric patients other than those described will need evaluation for possible UTI. These include uncircumcised boys, children who cannot void on command, and infants. The most problematic group is uncircumcised boys.

In males who have a foreskin that can be retracted to expose the urethral meatus, cleansing and drying of the periurethral area and the prompt collection of a midstream specimen will yield an uncontaminated aliquot of urine for culture. However, in a boy whose urethral orifice cannot be visualized, collection of a voided specimen may be associated with significant contamination with bacteria that normally colonize the glans underlying the prepuce.[28, 75] Bladder catheterization is not an acceptable alternative for such boys because it is unlikely to be successful if the urethral meatus cannot be visualized and because, if a blindly introduced catheter does happen to enter the urethra, it will likely carry with it preputial flora that can either contaminate the urine specimen or iatrogenically infect the bladder. The foreskin must not be forcibly retracted under any circumstance because this can cause paraphimosis acutely or can perpetuate phimosis into later life. In some circumstances, it may be appropriate to resort to suprapubic bladder puncture even in patients beyond infancy. However, this procedure is both technically more difficult and emotionally more traumatic when performed on a toddler than on a patient who is only several months old. If the specimen is to be collected by voiding, at least two, and if possible several, samples should be cultured. A negative result (i.e., <10,000 colonies/mL) on any voided specimen rules out the diagnosis of UTI. However, the risk of contamination of the voided urine is so high that it is best to assume that infection exists if all specimens grow more than 100,000 colonies/mL of one organism, even if there is growth of other species on the same culture plates.

For children who are not toilet trained and who therefore cannot provide a specimen on command, there is great temptation to use bladder catheterization to obtain urine for culture. This practice may be warranted in some circumstances, but it is not without morbidity, as discussed previously and, in most cases, it is not necessary. Infants are likely to void spontaneously when their diapers are removed. If a portion of this void can be collected in a sterile container, reliable culture results can be obtained.[76] An alternative method of obtaining voided urine specimens from infants and young toddlers is by applying a urine collection bag to the perineum. If the periurethral area is carefully washed and dried before the bag is affixed, the reservoir inspected every 10 to 15 minutes, and the urine removed in a sterile fashion as soon as it appears in the bag, uncontaminated urine cultures can be expected in approximately 75% of patients.[77] Thus, a negative culture result on a "bagged urine" specimen is useful. However, if treatment must be begun before the time when culture results are available, the initial specimen must be obtained by another method, one that is associated with a lower risk of contamination.

A special problem with regard to collection of urine for culture is presented by infants who are suspected of having UTI during the first few months of life. Urine infection at this early age may be hematogenous. Thus, a positive urine culture obtained from an infant during the first few months of life must be interpreted and acted on as if it were a positive blood culture. For this reason, even a small risk of bacterial contamination of the urine specimen is unacceptable; rapidly obtained specimens and accurate culture data are essential. Therefore, the only satisfactory method of obtaining urine for culture in early infancy is via suprapubic bladder puncture, as described by Nelson and Peters.[78] Because normal bladder urine should be sterile, the growth of *any* bacteria from urine obtained by this method is diagnostic of UTI.

In some special situations infection may exist, but colony counts may be unexpectedly low. Patients with underlying renal disease associated with a severe defect in renal concentrating ability (e.g., patients with congenital obstructive uropathy or adolescents or adults with sickle cell disease) may have such a high urine flow rate that there is both a decrease in duration of bacterial residence in the bladder and dilution of the density of organisms. Each of these factors may lower the colony count reported from urine culture. The presence in the urine of inhibitors of bacterial proliferation may also result in deceptively low urinary bacterial colony counts. Such inhibitors include low urinary pH, low urinary osmolarity, and antibiotics, administered by the parent without the physician's knowledge.

Furthermore, it may be that the urinary milieu is not the only factor that affects colony counts; the characteristics of the infecting organism are also important. Bollgren et al.[79] reported on six children, ages 6 months to 4½ years, who had fever and either UTI symptoms or leukocytosis and whose initial clean-catch urine cultures grew between 200 and 10,000 colonies/mL of P-fimbriated *E. coli*. Subsequent clean-catch cultures from all six patients demonstrated a bacterial concentration greater than 100,000 colonies/mL. These observations suggest that urine infection by P-fimbriated *E. coli* may cause symptoms and laboratory results that suggest UTI before the clean-catch urinary colony count has reached the diag-

TABLE 1.
Diagnosis of Urinary Tract Infection From Results of Urine Culture

1. Specimen obtained by suprapubic bladder tap.
   a. Method of choice for: symptomatic infants in the first several months of life.
   b. Useful for: confirming diagnosis in infants and young children when other methods of urine collection have yielded equivocal or uninterpretable culture results; initial evaluation of some symptomatic boys with nonretractable foreskins.
   c. Interpretation of urine culture results: the growth of any organism is significant.
2. Specimen obtained by bladder catheterization.
   a. Method of choice for: children with neurogenic or myogenic bladders. Such patients require special evaluation by a pediatric urologist or pediatric nephrologist.
   b. Useful for: some infants and toddlers from whom voided urine specimens cannot be obtained; some uncircumcised males.
   c. Interpretation of urine culture results:
      All patients: >100,000 colonies/mL of a single organism = UTI.
                      <10,000 colonies/mL = no UTI.
      Patients >2 yr: 10,000–100,000 colonies/mL = uninterpretable.
      Patients <2 yr: 10,000–100,000 colonies/mL, pure growth, single organism = suggestive of UTI; can be confirmed if a second culture gives similar results.
3. Specimen obtained by clean-catch method or midstream method:
   a. Method of choice for: most patients who can void on command.
   b. Useful for: many infants and toddlers who are not toilet trained.
   c. Interpretation of urine culture results:
      >100,000 colonies/mL of a single organism = UTI.
      <10,000 colonies/mL = no UTI.
      10,000–100,000 colonies/mL = uninterpretable.

4. Specimen obtained by casual collection:
   a. Method of choice for: not an optimal method of urine collection for any patient.
   b. Useful for: infants (spontaneous voiding), boys without retractable foreskin.
   c. Interpretation of urine culture results: most accurate if more than one void is cultured.
      <10,000 colonies/mL, pure growth, single organism = no UTI.
      >100,000 colonies/mL, pure growth, single organism = *probable* UTI.
      Other result = difficult to interpret.
5. Specimen obtained in adhesive urine bag:
   a. Method of choice for: no patient; this method of urine collection is associated with the highest risk of contamination.
   b. Useful for: the older infant who is not expected to require immediate antibiotic therapy.
   c. Interpretation of urine culture results:
      <10,000 colonies/mL = no UTI.
      >100,000 colonies/mL, pure growth, single organism = suggestive, but requires confirmation.
6. Special circumstances: polyuric states, infection with P-fimbriated *Escherichia coli*, infection with *Pseudomonas aeruginosa*, antibiotic pretreatment, acute urethral syndrome. For interpretation of urine culture results, see text.

---

nostic value of 100,000 colonies/mL. A similar problem may exist in the case of UTI due to *Pseudomonas aeruginosa*. In an experimental system, Mulvihill and Montgomerie[80] induced histologically proven *P. aeruginosa* pyelonephritis in mice. The urinary concentration of organisms, as determined by culture, was less than the urinary bacterial density usually associated with murine UTIs caused by other bacterial species. Other organisms, such as coagulase-negative staphylococci, do not multiply in urine as rapidly as do more common urinary pathogens and, as a result, may cause tissue infection even when urinary colony counts are low (10,000–100,000 colonies/mL).[81]

The acute urethral syndrome, which manifests with complaints of frequency and dysuria in women, is characteristically associated with low urinary colony counts, usually of *E. coli*.[82–84] This syndrome may occur in adolescent girls, and the diagnosis should be suspected in a symptomatic patient whose urine consistently grows more than 100 colonies/mL of a single enteric organism.

Table 1 summarizes the diagnosis of UTI in the pediatric patient from the results of urine culture.

Bacterial density in the urine can be artificially lowered if bactericidal agents such as povidone-iodine or hexachlorophene are washed into the collection container by the urine stream. Thus, during the cleansing of the periurethral area before bladder catheterization, care must be exercised so as not to allow the antiseptic agent to enter the lumen of the catheter. If the clean-catch technique is to be used to obtain the urine specimen, the perineum should be dried with a sterile pad before the patient is asked to void into the collection container.

Bacterial replication in urine does not cease after the specimen leaves the patient's bladder. Many enteric organisms, when stored at room temperature in a liquid medium such as urine, will increase in density by more than 100-fold over 6 hours.[85] Cooling the solution to a temperature of 4°C will completely inhibit bacterial replication.[86] Thus, factitious elevation of the urinary bacterial density can be avoided if the specimen is rapidly transported to the microbiology laboratory and expeditiously plated on culture media. If there must be a delay in delivering the specimen to the laboratory, the urine sample should be cooled to 4°C.

The diagnosis of UTI can be unequivocally made only by evaluation of the results of urine culture, as discussed earlier. Other studies may also be abnormal in patients with UTI, but the urine culture results hold primacy over all other evaluations. Unfortunately, 24 or 48 hours may elapse before the results of a urine culture are known, and there are frequent situations in which decisions about initiating therapy must be made earlier. A useful method that gives rapid results that correlate well with the urine culture is the microscopic examination of the urine for the presence of bacteria. Urine specimens that are to be evaluated for this purpose must be collected and transported using the same meticulous procedures that have been recommended for the handling of samples destined for the microbiology laboratory. Aliquots of *uncentrifuged* urine can be examined microscopically after they are air-dried on a glass slide and subsequently stained by the Gram method. The finding of one or more bacteria in each high-power field (HPF) suggests a urinary bacterial density of greater than 100,000 colonies/mL.[71, 87, 88] Comparable semiquantitative results can be obtained from urine samples of between 1 and 5 mL that have been *centrifuged* for 2 to 3 minutes at a speed of 2,000 to 3,000 rpm. The pellet that is produced by the centrifugation should be separated from the supernatant and resuspended in 0.25 to 0.5 mL of urine or isotonic saline solution. A drop applied to a glass slide and promptly examined through a cover slip will reveal less than 20 organisms per oil emersion field if there were fewer than 10,000 bacteria/mL in the original urine specimen.[86] A colony count greater than 10,000 colonies/mL can be suspected if large numbers of loosely packed bacteria are observed in every HPF, and more than 94% of urines demonstrating innumerable, closely packed bacteria in each HPF will have bacterial colony counts in a range that is consistent with UTI.[89] A urinalysis report of "many bacteria" from a casually collected urine that has been transported to the laboratory in an unsterile container and not examined promptly is of no value.

INDIRECT TESTS

Indirect tests for bacteriuria aimed at demonstrating the presence of bacterial *enzyme activity* in the urine have a poor correlation with results of urine cultures in children suspected of having UTI. The dip strip test for determining the presence of urinary nitrites is promoted as an assay that can detect bacteriuria. This indirect method is based on the observation that ingested dietary nitrates cannot be converted to nitrites by mammalian cells and are thus excreted intact in the urine. Because some bacteria, including many common urinary pathogens, possess enzyme systems that can convert urinary nitrates to nitrites, it is presumed that the presence of nitrites in the urine, as detected by a color change on the dip strip, implies that bacterial enzymes are present.[90] Although this assumption may be qualitatively correct, it is not always appropriate to assume that the detection of urinary nitrites means that urinary bacterial colony counts are of a magnitude sufficient to suggest the diagnosis of UTI. Although some reports suggest that in selected populations of adult patients there is an acceptable concordance between the presence of urinary nitrite, as determined from commercial rapid result dip strips, and "significant" bacteriuria,[87, 91] data from studies of pediatric patients strongly suggest that this screening test is of little predictive value in the symptomatic child. The dip strip test for urinary nitrite can give a negative result in as many as 50% of the specimens from symptomatic pediatric patients with UTI, as diagnosed by urine culture,[92] and positive results often do not predict that the urine culture colony count will be diagnostic of UTI.[93, 94] In addition, some microorganisms, such as *Pseudomonas,* lack the ability to convert nitrates to nitrites, and infection with one of these organisms will therefore give a negative nitrite test result.

Pyuria is commonly but mistakenly believed to be a marker for UTI in the symptomatic child. In a variety of studies, only between 50% and 60% of children with leukocyturia, defined as 5 or more WBCs/HPF in centrifuged urine, will also have a "positive" urine culture.[89, 94–96] The positive predictive value of pyuria for significant bacteriuria on culture is only 20% to 50%.[68, 97] In contrast, the presence of fewer than 5 WBCs/HPF (centrifuged urine) predicts, with between 95% and 98% confidence, that the urine culture will be negative. However, it would be imprudent to forgo urine culture in a symptomatic patient solely on the basis of absence of pyuria. In summary, many patients with pyuria do not have positive urine cultures. Conversely, the absence of pyuria strongly suggests that the patient does not have a UTI. Other methods of detecting pyuria offer sensitivities, specificities, and positive and negative predictive values similar to those described for the microscopic inspection of urine sediment. If *uncentrifuged* urine is examined in a counting chamber, the threshold for abnormal pyuria is 10 WBCs/mm^3. If the leukocyte density is below this threshold, UTI is unlikely, though a higher value is of no diagnostic assistance.[89] Indirect evidence of pyuria can be provided by the commercially available dip strip that detects the presence of leukocyte esterase in the urine. This enzyme is normally found in granulocytes and, when present in the urine, hydrolyzes a substrate on the dip strip to produce a pyrrole that, in turn, participates in a reaction that generates a purple-pink chromogen. A negative result predicts a negative urine culture with a probability of greater than 95%, but a positive result predicts that the patient has a UTI with only about a 25% probability. Urine cultures should be performed in symptomatic patients regardless of the results of any of these tests for pyuria.

Some investigators have proposed the use of various combinations of the aforementioned rapid urine evaluations to improve the sensitivity, specificity, and predictive values over those that can be provided by any one single test.[88] Though initial reports appear promising, it is premature to speculate whether similar results can be produced by busy clinical laboratories.

ANATOMIC EVALUATION

The diagnosis of UTI in a child identifies the patient as one who may have important underlying anatomic abnormalities of the urinary tract such as VUR or obstruction. In a study of 744 British children with symptomatic UTI who subsequently underwent IV pyelography (IVP) and fluoroscopic voiding cystourethrography

(VCUG), 47% were documented to have some detectable genitourinary abnormality.[43] Approximately 33% of the total group of infected patients were noted to have reflux, with or without other anomalies. Another 3% of the total population was found to have no reflux but had congenital abnormalities resulting in significant obstruction to urine flow. In the remaining 11%, other anomalies such as ectopia, agenesis, or horseshoe kidney were documented. Not all investigators have found such a high prevalence of genitourinary anomalies among pediatric patients with UTI, and values as low as 5% to 10% have been reported.[98] The disparities possibly may be accounted for by dissimilar referral patterns or by differences in the ages or ethnic backgrounds of the various patient populations studied (see later discussion). Even if the lower estimates are representative of patients with UTI, it is clear that genitourinary anomalies are sufficiently common among infected patients as to warrant an anatomic evaluation of the urologic system in all.

What evaluations should be done, and in which patients? The presence of high pressure in the upper urinary tract is inferred by finding dilatation of the calyces, renal pelvis, ureters, or combination thereof on IVP or renal ultrasound (RUSG). This elevation of hydrostatic pressure may be caused by either distal obstructing lesions or retrograde transmission via VUR of high pressure in the contracting bladder. Other anomalies, such as ectopia, renal duplication, or agenesis, may also be diagnosed or suspected from one of these studies. The conclusive diagnosis and grading of VUR and elucidation of the anatomy of the bladder and urethra can be accomplished only by performing the fluoroscopic VCUG. The *static cystogram*, that is, a radiograph taken after the bladder is filled with contrast but before voiding begins, may underdiagnose VUR, because in some children VUR occurs only with voiding.[99] In addition, the static cystogram provides no information about urethral anatomy, especially important in boys. Radionuclide cystography, an alternate method of diagnosing VUR that is often recommended because it is associated with significantly lower radiation exposure than the radiographic VCUG,[100] does not eliminate the need for bladder catheterization and cannot accurately define the anatomy of the refluxing ureter and pyelocalyceal system, nor can it demonstrate the contours of the bladder and urethra. It should be emphasized that VUR, even of moderate severity, cannot be conclusively ruled out on the basis of a normal RUSG or a normal IVP.[101]

The protocol that would be most likely to uncover the greatest number of structural lesions among children with UTI would include a VCUG and either RUSG or IVP in all children at the time of their first infection. This policy has been adopted by many pediatric nephrologists and, in fact, extended to include adolescents, with the possible exception of the sexually active, afebrile teenage girl whose symptoms are limited to voiding complaints (frequency, urgency, and dysuria). Such an approach would be acceptable were it not for the fact that the IVP and the VCUG both have a finite morbidity and, in the case of IVP, mortality.[102, 103] Discomfort, pain, and embarrassment are sentiments expressed by almost all "victims" of the VCUG who are old enough to voice their feelings.

Over the years, much effort has been expended in trying to minimize the risk and discomforts of the anatomic evaluation of the child with a UTI without compromising the ability to detect significant urologic abnormalities. Improvement in ultrasound technology has now made this technique as sensitive at demonstrating hydroureteronephrosis as the IVP. The utility of RUSG in this regard continues to be endorsed by most observers.[99, 104, 105]

Because of the invasive nature of the VCUG, it would be desirable to decrease the number of children subjected to this study. Every patient who is found to have hydronephrosis (either from IVP or RUSG) should undergo a VCUG because VUR will be detected in the majority.[99] However, a more difficult question is: who does not need a VCUG? Reflux occurring from a normal bladder at normal vesical pressure is of importance only because it serves as a potential route for ascent of bacteria to the kidney where tissue infection may develop. It is the pyelonephritis, not the VUR per se, that carries with it risks for long-term complications such as renal scarring, hypertension, and chronic renal failure. Thus, the argument has been advanced that the patient with UTI who does not have renal parenchymal involvement does not need to undergo investigation for VUR. Therefore, the infected child who may not need a VCUG is the child who does not have pyelonephritis. Unfortunately, there is no way to conclusively determine that a particular patient is free of renal parenchymal inflammation. Conclusive proof of a negative result is almost never obtainable. Consequently, the approach has been to search for findings that correlate with pyelonephritis and to assume that pyelonephritis does not exist in a patient who does not manifest these markers. For example, the UTI patient with high fever and costovertebral angle tenderness, particularly if accompanied by a leukocytosis and prolonged ESR, probably has pyelonephritis. However, the absence of these signs and symptoms does not preclude the possibility of kidney infection; symptoms and routine tests correlate poorly with the location of the disease.[106] More sophisticated evaluations have been equally disappointing in their ability to identify the level of infection. Evaluations such as the neomycin bladder washout test,[107] plasma concentrations of antibodies to *E. coli*,[108] antibody-coated bacteria in the urine,[109] renal concentrating capacity,[110] C-reactive protein,[111] or plasma[112] or urinary[113] lactic dehydrogenase, are rarely used. Some of these evaluations lack sensitivity and specificity, and others are invasive or difficult to perform. More direct evaluations, specifically imaging studies, might be expected to be more helpful in identifying areas of pyelonephritis. Histologic study of the lesion demonstrates an intense inflammatory response disproportionately involving the cortex and associated with interstitial edema and tubulitis.[114] Unfortunately, the changes in renal contour or echotexture of the parenchyma that result from this process are in most cases too subtle to be detected by IVP or RUSG.[104, 115]

In recent years, however, radioisotope renal scintigraphy has come to the fore as an imaging method that may hold greater potential for reliably locating areas of renal cortical inflammation. In addition, this is the most sensitive method for identifying areas of renal scarring, frequently evidence of prior episodes of pyelonephritis. The radionuclide that is used for this purpose is technetium 99m–DMSA, an agent that is not filtered and thus enters the postglomerular circulation. It is then transported into proximal tubule cells where it resides and emits radioactivity for several hours.[116] The isotope is relatively excluded from areas of acute inflammation and from renal scars, resulting in a "cold spot" on the scan.[117–119] The sensitivity for detecting areas of experimental pyelonephritis in piglets is about 90%, and false-positive results are exceedingly rare.[119] Among children with symptoms and signs suggesting acute pyelonephritis, the prevalence of scintigraphic evidence of acute renal inflammation is about 75%.[118–120] The DMSA scan is superior to other methods for diagnosing renal scars. Many studies have demonstrated that more than 50% of kidneys that demonstrate scars on scan would be mistakenly diagnosed as normal by RUSG or IVP.[101, 121–123] If the DMSA renal scan can demonstrate, with high sensitivity and specificity, evidence of renal parenchymal infection, either acute (pyelonephritis) or remote (renal scar), an argument could be made that VCUG need be performed only in those children with an abnormal scan; as mentioned earlier, VUR is probably important only when it results in pyelonephritis. This approach has, however, not gained universal endorsement because of concerns that the accuracy of the scan in detecting parenchymal disease, as reported in the literature, may not be achievable by all nuclear medicine departments, particularly when the study is performed on very small or uncooperative children.[124, 125] Because the kidneys of young patients seem to be more prone to developing pyelonephritic scars then do kidneys of older children,[126-128] technical difficulties of performing and interpreting a scan on an infant or toddler might result in serious underdiagnosis in a population at high risk for long-term complications. It may therefore be unwise to eliminate the VCUG from the evaluation of a young child with UTI solely on the basis of a normal DMSA scan.

It has been shown that black African children who are investigated as a result of the diagnosis of UTI have an exceedingly low prevalence of VUR.[7, 129, 130] We have made the same observation in a population of infected black American children in New York City. Accordingly, the risk/benefit ratio for VCUG in this population may be higher than for other patient groups.

There is no consensus about how to evaluate genitourinary anatomy in children with UTIs. At least three different approaches have been advocated, and a summary of these follows. Most investigators agree that in most situations the IVP can be replaced by the RUSG.

1. RUSG (or IVP) to uncover obstructing lesions and fluoroscopic VCUG for VUR and urethral anatomy in all infected patients except, perhaps, the sexually active adolescent girl with bladder symptoms only. This is the traditional approach.
2. RUSG (or IVP) and DMSA scan in all patients and subsequent fluoroscopic VCUG only if an abnormality is detected on scan.[131]
3. RUSG (or IVP) and DMSA scan on all patients; VCUG in all infants and young children, and VCUG in older patients if ultrasound or scan are abnormal.

Once the appropriate diagnostic studies have been planned for a particular pediatric patient with UTI, the next question is when to perform these studies. The RUSG (or, in some cases, the IVP) should be performed expeditiously. These evaluations are aimed at diagnosing obstructing lesions in the urinary tract; this assessment should be made as soon as possible because infection behind obstruction may require early surgical intervention.[87, 132] In contrast, there is disagreement as to when the VCUG should be performed. It has been suggested that the performance of the VCUG should be postponed for several weeks after the UTI has been successfully treated.[87, 133] This advice is based on the assumption that acute bacterial infection of the bladder wall can alter the anatomy of the vesicoureteral junction and thereby induce VUR in a system that would not normally reflux. The recommendation to delay performing the VCUG is made to allow the anatomy of the inflamed vesicoureteral junction to return to its basal configuration before the evaluation. It is hoped that by this means, detection of infection-induced VUR will be avoided. Opinions that argue against delaying the VCUG are based on the observation that there is no evidence in the literature to support the contention that cystitis can induce VUR in a nonrefluxing ureter subjected to physiologic bladder pressures. Furthermore, even if one assumes that bladder infection can actually induce VUR in some patients, the resulting combination of reflux and bacteriuria are the very components that can lead to renal parenchymal infection. Proponents of this view, therefore, advise that the VCUG be performed soon after the diagnosis of UTI is made in order to identify any patients who may have infection-induced reflux. However, because urethral catheterization in the presence of bacteriuria has potential for significant morbidity,[102] the VCUG should be postponed until antibiotic treatment has successfully sterilized the bladder urine; this is usually accomplished within the first several days after treatment is initiated.

Cystoscopy has no role in the initial evaluation of the pediatric patient with UTI and is only rarely indicated thereafter.[134] Even among patients with VUR, cystoscopic visualization of the ureteral orifice or assessment of the length of the ureteral submucosal tunnel[135] adds nothing to alter therapeutic decisions.[133] Older literature suggests that distal urethral stenosis diagnosed by cystoscopy is a common abnormality that is etiologically important in the development of UTI in girls.[136] Subsequent observations do not support this view.[137–140] Thus, diagnostic cystoscopy should be considered only in the unusual patient with complex urologic anomalies that cannot be adequately defined radiographically. It should never be performed on the patient whose imaging studies are normal.

VOIDING DYSFUNCTION

An important area that should be explored during the evaluation of a patient with UTI is dysfunctional voiding. Unfortunately, this is a subject that is unfamiliar to most pediatricians and, as noted by Koff,[141] one that is "sorely neglected in most recommended protocols for evaluation of urinary infection." This is unfortunate because there is ample evidence of an association between certain abnormal voiding patterns and UTI, with reports of prevalence ratios for UTI among dysfunctional voiders ranging from 50% to 94%.[142-148] Conversely, perhaps as many as 50% of children with a history of UTI, especially recurrent UTI, can be shown to manifest evidence of voiding dysfunction.[145] In some cases, the abnormal voiding will result in structural alterations observable on imaging studies as abnormal bladder configuration or VUR. That the coexistence of UTI and abnormal voiding patterns is not just a chance association is suggested by reports that successful therapy of the voiding dysfunction is associated with a significant decline in the incidence of UTI[149] and with accelerated rates of resolution of VUR.[150, 151] Thus, it is important to be familiar with the various clinical signs and symptoms that suggest that a patient with UTI may suffer from a functional disturbance of voiding.

Some abnormal voiding patterns are not associated with an increased incidence of UTI, whereas others place the patient at high risk for secondary changes in bladder and vesicoureteral functional anatomy, as well as for progressive renal scarring. The disorders under discussion are not caused by neurologic lesions. These behaviors are learned, either consciously or subconsciously, and subsequently may establish a vicious cycle of positive reinforcement for the maladaptive voiding pattern. This may result in perpetuation or even in progressive worsening of the behavior. With proper diagnosis and treatment, the cycle can be broken and normal bladder function regained. In contrast, true neurogenic abnormalities of bladder function will need vigilant long-term care and a different therapeutic approach.

Of the various forms of voiding dysfunction, two are not associated with an increased incidence of UTI, although many such patients undergo repeated urine cultures and may receive courses of antibiotics in the belief that their symptoms must be caused by bacteriuria. Pure nocturnal enuresis, the periodic, involuntary nighttime voiding of a large volume of urine without daytime incontinence, is not associated with a higher than expected incidence of UTI in some studies[152] or only a minimal increased risk in others.[153] A second disorder, the daytime urinary frequency syndrome,[154, 155] is also not associated with UTI, although the symptoms may strongly suggest bacteriuria. The abnormality is slightly more common in boys than in girls and has its onset usually in the winter months in previously toilet-trained children at about 5 years. The patients void several times an hour, but *are continent* and are usually able to sleep through the night without bed wetting or nocturia. Therapeutic interventions are usually unsuccessful, and the symptom often remits after a few months but may persist for up to 1½ years, much to the chagrin of patients and parents.

All of the dysfunctional voiding patterns associated with UTI are characterized by *daytime urinary incontinence.* On careful questioning, these patients or their parents can report that dampness or frank urinary saturation of the underwear and clothing occurs regularly. Patients with these functional symptom complexes can be divided into two groups: those who void infrequently and those who are frequent voiders, the latter group being distinguished from patients with the benign syndrome of daytime urinary frequency by the presence of daytime wetting. A voiding frequency of 3 to 5 micturitions each day is the norm for toilet-trained children.[155] Any significant variation more than or less than this range should be considered abnormal.

A history of *infrequent voiding* by the patient who is intermittently wet during the day should alert the practitioner to the diagnosis of "lazy bladder syndrome."[156] In these patients, usually girls, the syndrome manifests in later childhood or early adolescence. Voiding is infrequent and does not completely empty the bladder. Many of these patients are also constipated. Imaging studies demonstrate a large-capacity bladder, but there is usually no evidence of bladder wall trabeculation or of VUR. Despite radiographic evidence of a large bladder capacity, these patients experience daytime incontinence. The wetting usually occurs shortly after the abrupt onset of a sensation of bladder fullness; this phenomenon is termed "urge incontinence."

In contrast, there is another group of patients who also suffer from diurnal enuresis but whose pattern of urination is characterized by *frequency.* This symptom complex should suggest that there is a derangement in the relationship between detrusor contraction, which normally results in bladder emptying, and high levels of urethral resistance to urine flow, which normally prevents incontinence. If the irritable, or "unstable," bladder[157] contracts spontaneously at a time when the external urethral sphincter is not maximally constricted, urine will leak into the underwear. It will take only a few such episodes to prompt the child to develop a means of avoiding being wet. Maneuvers that can accomplish this include volitional contraction of the external sphincter, squatting so that the perineal urethra is compressed by the heel of a foot, or forcibly crossing the legs (Vincent's curtsy)[158] to increase urethral resistance. Though these efforts can often stem the flood tide of urine, a small volume of urine escapes before the gates can be closed; therefore, damp underwear may be the only hint of dysfunction. In other patients, involuntary and abnormal sphincter or pelvic floor contractions may occur during voiding resulting in hesitancy of the urine stream or staccato voiding (start-stop-start-stop).[159, 160] In these patients, wetting is caused by either ill-timed sphincter relaxation or overflow incontinence. In the potentially most severe form of functional voiding abnormality, so-called Hinman bladder,[161] or non-neurogenic neurogenic bladder, detrusor and sphincter contractions occur totally independently. Patients, usually boys, are wet, suffer from urge incontinence, must strain to void, are often constipated, and may give a history of fecal soiling. Radiographic evaluation reveals that a significant number of these patients have VUR, hydronephrosis, renal scars, or a combination thereof.[162]

All of the disorders of voiding characterized by frequent micturition, diurnal incontinence, and propensity for UTI are also associated with a high prevalence of constipation, sometimes even encopresis, a peak incidence during the later childhood years, a marked female preponderance (except for the Hinman bladder syndrome), and a psychosocial history characterized by a drive for overachievement and perfection, a compulsive fear of dirt and contamination, or a distant or alcoholic parent.

The desire of incontinent children to try to conceal their wetting may make it difficult to elicit the information that is needed to establish the diagnosis and characteristics of a particular dysfunctional voiding pattern in a child with UTI. It may be necessary to speak with the child and the parents separately and repeatedly. Attention should be directed toward ascertaining whether or not the patient experiences daytime wetting. Even occasional episodes of diurnal dampness may be significant. It is vital to determine the setting in which the wetting occurs. If involuntary voiding occurs only with hearty laughing, this is the benign disorder of older and adolescent girls termed "giggle incontinence." If, on the other hand, spontaneous micturition or dribbling occurs simultaneously with the abrupt onset of a strong urge to void, such urge incontinence suggests the presence of uninhibited detrusor contractions. Careful questioning should uncover any history of voiding postponement maneuvers such as squatting or curtsying. It is often surprisingly difficult to accurately assess the frequency of volitional voiding from a history. Suspicion that a patient may be an infrequent voider should be aroused if the patient or family reports that the child frequently fails to urinate soon after arising in the morning. One also should inquire about bowel habits, because many patients with pathologic voiding patterns will also suffer from constipation, and a few will manifest encopresis. Many of these questions can be more accurately answered by giving the family instructions for maintaining a 1-week diary of voiding, stooling, involuntary wetting, and the circumstances surrounding the "accident." It is also important to gain a clear picture of exactly what happens during a volitional urination. Is straining used to initiate the stream? Is Valsalva's maneuver required to maintain the flow of urine? Is the urine stream constant or interrupted (staccato)? Is bladder emptying complete, and if so, how large is the total volume voided? (Normal bladder capacity in fluid ounces is roughly equal to the child's age in years plus 2.)[163] If the patient is comfortable enough to void in the presence of the physician, these observations can be made directly. Frequently, however, the child is embarrassed or uncomfortable in such a setting, and, as a result, the void that is observed may not be representative of the child's usual micturitional behavior. With some instruction, the parents can often be taught how to evaluate the voiding effort of the child at home. Finally, because psychosocial factors seem to play an important role in the development and maintenance of voiding disturbances in many children, it is necessary to construct a picture of the family dynamics. What demands do the parents place on the child? Are the parents overly rigid or critical? Does the child throw himself or herself into a myriad of organized activities? Do family members abuse alcohol?

In most cases, careful observation and discussions with the patient and family will suffice to uncover evidence of voiding dysfunction in children with UTI. A treatment plan can often be formulated without resorting to more standardized and invasive evaluations. Occasionally, however, it is necessary to define more completely the abnormality in a given patient, and this can be accomplished in the urodynamics laboratory. This procedure involves placing catheters, electrical probes, and pressure transducers in the bladder, urethra, and rectum and monitoring changes during bladder filling and voiding. Certain patterns of abnormalities are characteristic of each of the types of voiding disturbances, and a great deal of information can be gained. The urodynamic evaluation may also be very important in monitoring the patient's response to therapy.

THERAPY

Antibiotic treatment must be employed in every symptomatic child who has a positive urine culture. As discussed earlier, the symptoms of a UTI will resolve even without treatment, but spontaneous resolution of bacteriuria is rare. It is often necessary to institute antimicrobial therapy before urine culture results are available. Particularly in infants and young children, it is important to begin antibiotics early rather than waiting for microbiologic confirmation of the diagnosis. Therapy can be discontinued if the urine culture result does not confirm the clinical impression of UTI. During the first several months of life UTI may be caused by bacteremia or sepsis. In this case, early and aggressive antimicrobial therapy is needed. Early institution of antibiotics may also benefit the older infant and young child. Experimental data suggest that in immature animals fewer scars develop if antibiotic therapy is initiated promptly after induction of pyelonephritis than if it is delayed for more than 48 hours.[164, 165] The decision about whether to use the oral or the IV route of antibiotic administration must be made based on the physician's opinion of the extent of the infection. Specifically, a judgment must be made as to whether the infection is confined to the kidney and lower urinary tract (genitourinary-limited infection) or whether there is a reasonable risk of concomitant bacteremia.

Many of the commonly used oral antibiotics, such as ampicillin, sulfonamides, and trimethoprim-sulfamethoxazole, reach very high concentrations in urine and the renal medulla despite relatively low concentrations in the blood. For example, urine obtained from a patient 2 hours after a single oral 50 mg/kg dose of sulfisoxazole contains the drug at a concentration more than 10 times that needed to kill sulfa-resistant *E. coli*. Urine and renal parenchymal antibiotic concentrations correlate more closely with therapeutic outcome of pyelonephritis than does the blood drug level.[166, 167] Therefore, infections limited to the kidney or lower urinary tract can, in most cases, be cured by a course of oral antibiotics. There are, however, situations in which oral therapy may not be appropriate for genitourinary-limited UTI. A parenteral route of administration is indicated for the patient who is vomiting. However, this situation does not necessarily mandate IV therapy; use of an initial, single intramuscular dose of antimicrobials can result in rapid cessation of vomiting and the ability to begin oral medication within 12 to 18 hours. Patients with decreased function of the infected kidney due to extensive renal involvement or the presence of ipsilateral obstruction or preexisting chronic scarring may require high *blood* antibiotic concentrations to achieve bacteriologic cure. Such children may benefit from IV therapy. The child who may have bacteremia must be treated in a manner that can result in therapeutic antibiotic *blood* levels. Therefore, patients whose infection is deemed to extend beyond the genitourinary system should receive IV antimicrobials. Urinary tract infection that occurs in patients during the first several months of life may be a consequence of bacteremic colonization of the kidney. Older patients with UTI who manifest clinical and laboratory evidence of systemic infection may have urosepsis. Intravenous antibiotic therapy should be instituted in both situations.

It is impossible to prove that a particular child with UTI does not have pyelonephritis. Therefore, the duration of antibiotic therapy used for all infected children should be long enough to effect a cure of renal parenchymal infection. A 10-day course of treatment with an appropriate antibiotic results in eradication of infection in almost 100% of patients.[168] As a result, this has become standard treatment. There has been recent interest in using shorter courses of antibiotics based on published experience in adults. A high percentage of women with UTIs and symptoms of pure lower tract infections can be cured by courses of antibiotics as short as 1 to 3 days.[169–171] If short-duration therapy fails to sterilize the urine, it is assumed that the patient has pyelonephritis. Some studies evaluating efficacy of short-term therapy in children (excluding infants) have demonstrated that truncating the duration of therapy does not decrease the likelihood of bacteriologic cure or increase the risk of recurrence.[172–176] In other studies, short-term treatment has been shown to be inferior to a 10-day course.[177, 178] In a composite review of 14 published studies of short-term therapy, Moffat et al.[179] concluded that there are insufficient data to allow endorsement of such an approach in children. It may be true that in children, as in adults, pure cystitis can be cured with a very brief course of antibiotics. However, because it is difficult to localize the level of infection in children, instituting single-dose or short-term therapy on the assumption that the UTI is limited to the lower urinary tract may result in inadequate or delayed treatment of what is actually pyelonephritis. This may, in turn, increase the risk that the area of renal inflammation will evolve into a pyelonephritic scar.

Asymptomatic bacteriuria should probably not be treated at all. About 80% of girls with covert bacteriuria will have a recurrence after a course of antibiotic therapy.[180, 181] This contrasts with a 30% recurrence rate during the first year after successful treatment of a symptomatic UTI. Furthermore, long-term follow-up of girls with screening bacteriuria showed that treatment provided no benefit with regard to renal size or function.[127] Treatment of asymptomatic bacteriuria using either short-duration therapy or long-term prophylaxis is associated with the subsequent development of symptomatic acute pyelonephritis in as many as 30% of girls.[182] Untreated patients, even those with preexisting renal scars, had a much lower incidence of symptomatic infection. The explanation for this perhaps paradoxical outcome is that the *E. coli* cultured from most patients with asymptomatic bacteriuria are untypable and without virulence factors. Treatment may eradicate these "benign" *E. coli* and promote intestinal overgrowth of more aggressive organisms that can infect the patient and cause symptomatic disease.

Selecting the appropriate antibiotic is easy if culture results are available before therapy is started. This is, however, usually not the case, and so the decision must often be made on the basis of indirect information. Because the normal kidney is capable of accumulating very high concentrations of a variety of antibiotics, it is possible that a drug to which an organism is relatively resistant may, in fact, succeed in curing the infection. Because UTI during the first several months of life may be a result of bacteremia or sepsis, the antibiotics used to treat a UTI should target the microbes that cause sepsis at this age. In 80% to 90% of girls and a slightly lower percent of boys who become infected after infancy, *E. coli* is the cause of UTI. These organisms are usually sensitive to a wide range of antibiotics unless the child has recently received a course of antimicrobial therapy, in which case resistant strains may be encountered. Resistant strains may also cause infection in patients who are receiving chronic antibiotic prophylaxis. In either situation, it would be unwise to begin treatment with a drug that is related to an antibiotic that the patient has recently received. Certain special circumstances can impact on drug selection. Infection with *Proteus* spp. is somewhat more common in older boys than in other groups. Sexually active females may become infected with coagulase-negative staphylococci. Patients being treated with clean intermittent bladder catheterization or those who have indwelling catheters may have *Klebsiella* spp., *Pseudomonas* spp., or enterococci in their urine. The choice of an appropriate antibiotic in each of these settings should be determined by the local patterns of drug sensitivities.

If antibiotic selection has been appropriate, symptoms should begin to subside within 24 to 48 hours, and a repeat urine culture, performed after 2 to 3 days of treatment, should be sterile. It is not always necessary to change the antibiotic regimen based on culture sensitivity results when they become available; if the culture at 48 to 72 hours is sterile, the drug may be continued to complete the course, even though another drug may appear, on paper, to be more effective. A third culture should be performed 1 to 2 weeks after completion of the 10-day course of antibiotics. Earlier "post-treatment" cultures may be misleading because many drugs continue to be excreted in the urine for days after the final dose has been taken.

REFLUX

If renal parenchymal infection is the primary factor leading to renal damage, as is now believed, and not VUR per se, the therapy of reflux becomes problematic. Theoretically the maintenance of sterile urine might suffice without surgical correction of reflux. This is all the more important because reflux, especially milder grades, tends to resolve with age. In one study,[41] 80% of grade I or II reflux and 46% of grade III reflux resolved after 5 years of follow-up. Several studies have prospectively evaluated prophylactic antibiotics alone as opposed to surgical correction.[39, 40, 183] Depending on whether one looks at the glass as being half empty or half full, both therapies were equally effective or neither therapy completely protected against renal damage. In the International Reflux Study, which included only children with grades III and IV reflux, there was no difference in the recurrence of UTI in the two groups during 5-year follow-up (38% in the medical group and 39% in the surgical group)[183] or in the development of new scars or progression of old scars.[40] The same was seen in the Birmingham Reflux Study.[183] However, pyelonephritis was more common in the medical (21%) than in the surgical (10%) group.

Thus, it appears that VUR in all but the most severe grade (grade V) can be adequately, if not ideally, managed by keeping the urine sterile with prophylactic antibiotics. This is especially important in younger children because scarring occurs more frequently in this age group. An indication for surgery would be breakthrough infections despite antibiotic prophylaxis. If the organism involved in the breakthrough infection is sensitive to the prophylactic antibiotic, the problem is likely to be one of noncompliance. If the organism is resistant, it is likely that either bladder residual volume is elevated because of dysfunctional voiding or bowel flora has been altered and replaced by resistant organisms due to an inappropriate prophylactic antibiotic or a dose of antibiotic that is too high.[44]

Suggested antibiotics for prophylaxis are trimethoprim-sulfamethoxazole (1−2 mg/kg trimethoprim daily) or nitrofurantoin (1–2 mg/kg daily) as a single bedtime dose. The Winberg et al.[20] study in adult monkeys has shown that amoxicillin disturbs the normal vaginal microflora and promotes vaginal colonization by *E. coli*. Some cephalosporins appear to have a similar effect. Therefore, these drugs should not be used for prophylaxis. Trimethoprim-sulfamethoxazole and nitrofurantoin did not have these effects and are therefore the agents of choice for prophylaxis.

A special problem has been the treatment of reflux persisting in girls into late childhood and adolescence. Some have suggested that reflux should be repaired to avoid pyelonephritis, fetal wastage, and maternal morbidity during pregnancy. However, studies have shown that reflux in pregnancy is not associated with increased fetal or maternal risk if renal function is not impaired,[184, 185] although there is an increased prevalence of bacteriuria. Women with reflux nephropathy and decreased renal function, however, are at risk for further decline in function during pregnancy, hypertension, preeclampsia, and fetal loss[186, 187] independent of the presence or absence of reflux.

VOIDING DYSFUNCTION

The treatment of voiding dysfunction is an important component of the management of children with UTIs. Many patients with recurrent UTIs will have pathologic voiding abnormalities. Treatment of the dysfunctional voiding pattern can result in a decrease in the frequency of UTIs for many of these patients. Several therapeutic interventions are useful for most patients. In some, additional maneuvers are required.

Because non-neurogenic voiding abnormalities are, in part, learned behaviors, initial attempts at treatment should be aimed at retraining the bladder. Establishing a timed voiding schedule, usually at 2-hour intervals, begins to recreate a more normal and regulated pattern of micturition. "Voiding by the clock" also helps to prevent complete filling of the bladder and thereby minimizes the frequency of spontaneous contractions due to overdistention. Antibiotic prophylaxis against recurrence of UTI aids in the program of bladder retraining because cystitis can cause frequency of urination and spontaneous bladder spasms, both of which work against the redevelopment of normal voiding patterns.

Stool retention is common among patients with abnormal voiding patterns. It has been implicated as an important factor that perpetuates the voiding dysfunction and predisposes to UTI. Aggressive bowel catharsis with enemas and maintenance of a pattern of daily defecation is vital to the therapy of most patients. Short-term laxative therapy and dietary advice are often useful.

In some patients, drug therapy is required. Oxybutynin chloride, a smooth muscle relaxant with anticholinergic effects, can reduce or eliminate spontaneous bladder contractions. It is particularly effective in patients with unstable bladder contractions during filling. Patients who maintain an inappropriately high external sphincter tone during voiding may benefit from treatment with a skeletal muscle relaxant such as diazepam or baclofen. These drugs are, however, not universally effective and can cause unacceptable side effects. Frequently the psychosocial situation contributes significantly to the problem and should be dealt with through psychotherapy or family counseling. Such interventions can accelerate the rate of resolution.

In the patients with the most severe anatomic abnormalities, such as the Hinman bladder, it is sometimes necessary to resort to surgical treatment of VUR or obstruction to prevent progressive renal damage. Unfortunately, the failure rate for surgery is high when the voiding dysfunction is not corrected.

REFERENCES

1. Avner ED, Chavers B, Sullivan EK, et al: Renal transplantation and chronic dialysis in children and adolescents: The 1993 annual report of the North American Pediatric Renal Transplant Cooperative Study. *Pediatr Nephrol* 9:61–73, 1995.
2. North American Pediatric Renal Transplant Cooperative Study: *1994 Annual Report*. Unpublished.
3. Jodal U, Hellström M, Mårild S, et al: Bacteriuria during the first year of life. In Kass EH, Svanborg-Edén C (eds): *Host-Parasite Interactions in Urinary Tract Infections*. Chicago, University of Chicago Press, 1989, pp 23–25.
4. Kunin CM, Southall I, Paquin AJ: Epidemiology of urinary tract infections. A pilot study of 3057 school children. *N Engl J Med* 263:817–823, 1960.
5. Kunin CM, Zacha E, Paquin AJ: Urinary tract infections in school children. Prevalence of bacteriuria and associated urologic findings. *N Engl J Med* 266:1287–1296, 1962.
6. Verrier-Jones K, Sacks S, Roberts R, et al: Covert bacteriuria: Long-term outcome and effect on subsequent pregnancy. In Kass EH, Svanborg-Edén C (eds): *Host-Parasite Interactions in Urinary Tract Infections*. Chicago, University of Chicago Press, 1989, pp 26–33.
7. Kunin CM: Epidemiology and natural history of urinary tract infection in school age children. In Edelmann CM Jr (ed): *The Pediatric Clinics of North America*. Philadelphia, WB Saunders, 1971, pp 509–528.
8. Kallenius G, Svenson SB, Mollby R, et al: Structure of carbohydrate part of receptor on human uroepithelial cells for pyelonephritogenic *Escherichia coli*. *Lancet* 2:604–606, 1981.

9. Harber MJ, Asscher AW: Virulence of urinary pathogens. *Kidney Int* 28:717–721, 1985.
10. Lomberg H, Hanson LA, Jakobsson B, et al: Correlation of P blood group, vesicoureteral reflux, and bacterial attachment in patients with recurrent pyelonephritis. *N Engl J Med* 308:1189–1192, 1983.
11. Lomberg H, Hellström M, Jodal U, et al: Virulence-associated traits in *Escherichia coli* causing first and recurrent urinary tract infection in children with or without vesicoureteral reflux. *J Infect Dis* 150:561–569, 1984.
12. Mårild S, Hellström M, Jacobsson B, et al: Influence of bacterial adhesion on ureteral width in children with acute pyelonephritis. *J Pediatr* 115:265, 1989.
13. Lomberg H, Jodal U, Leffler H, et al: Blood group non-secretors have an increased inflammatory response to urinary tract infection. *Scand J Infect Dis* 24:77–83, 1992.
14. Finkelstein RA, Scirotino CV, McIntosh MA: Role of iron in microbic-host interactions. *Rev Infect Dis* 5:S759–S777, 1983.
15. Hughes C, Hacker J, Roberts A, et al: Hemolysin production as a virulence marker in symptomatic and asymptomatic urinary tract infections caused by *Escherichia coli*. *Infect Immun* 39:546–551, 1983.
16. Fried FA, Vermeulen CW, Ginsburg MJ, et al: Etiology of pyelonephritis: Further evidence associating the production of experimental pyelonephritis with hemolysin in *Escherichia coli*. *J Urol* 106:351–354, 1971.
17. Keane WF, Welch R, Gekker G, et al: Mechanism of *Escherichia coli* α-hemolysin-induced injury to isolated renal tubular cells. *Am J Pathol* 126:350–357, 1987.
18. Connell H, de Man P, Jodal U, et al: Lack of association between hemolysin production and acute inflammation in human urinary tract infection. *Microb Pathog* 14:463–472, 1993.
19. Chan RCY, Reid G, Randall TI, et al: Competitive exclusion of uropathogens from human uroepithelial cells by lactobacillus whole cells and cell wall fragments. *Infect Immun* 47:84–89, 1985.
20. Winberg J, Herthelius-Elman M, Möllby R, et al: Pathogenesis of urinary tract infection—experimental studies of vaginal resistance to colonization. *Pediatr Nephrol* 7:509–514, 1993.
21. Stamey TA, Wehner A, Mihara G, et al: The immunologic basis of recurrent bacteriuria: Role of cervico-vaginal antibody in enterobacterial colonization of the introital mucosa. *Medicine (Baltimore)* 57:47–56, 1978.
22. Tuttle JP Jr, Sarvas H, Koistinen J: The role of vaginal immunoglobulin A in girls with recurrent urinary tract infections. *J Urol* 120:742–744, 1978.
23. Parsons CL, Greenspan C, Mulholland SG: The primary antibacterial defense mechanism of the bladder. *Invest Urol* 13:72–76, 1975.
24. Parsons CL, Shrom SH, Hanno PM, et al: Bladder surface mucin. Ex-

amination of possible mechanisms for its antibacterial effect. *Invest Urol* 16:196–200, 1978.

25. Wiswell TE, Smith FR, Bass JW: Decreased incidence of urinary tract infections in circumcised male infants. *Pediatrics* 75:901–903, 1985.
26. Ginsburg CM, McCracken GH: Urinary tract infections in young infants. *Pediatrics* 69:409–412, 1982.
27. Wiswell TE, Enzenauer RW, Holton ME, et al: Declining frequency of circumcision: Implications for changes in the absolute incidence and male to female sex ratio of urinary tract infections in early infancy. *Pediatrics* 79:338–342, 1987.
28. Wiswell TE, Miller GM, Gelston HM Jr, et al: Effect of circumcision status on periurethral bacterial flora during the first year of life. *J Pediatr* 113:442–446, 1988.
29. Wiswell TE: John K Lattimer Lecture. Prepuce presence portends prevalence of potentially perilous periurethral pathogens. *J Urol* 148:739–742, 1992.
30. Poland RL: The question of routine neonatal circumcision [editorial]. *N Engl J Med* 332:1312–1315, 1990.
31. Schoen EJ: Sounding board: The status of circumcision of newborns. *N Engl J Med* 322:1308–1311, 1990.
32. Winberg J: Is routine circumcision advised in boys with obstructive uropathy in order to prevent urinary tract infection? *Pediatr Nephrol* 5:178, 1991.
33. Dohil R, Roberts E, Jones KV, et al: Constipation and reversible urinary tract abnormalities. *Arch Dis Child* 70:56–57, 1994.
34. Yazbeck S, Schick E, O'Regan S: Relevance of constipation to enuresis, urinary tract infection and reflux. A review. *Eur Urol* 13:318–321, 1987.
35. O'Regan S, Yazbeck S, Schick E: Constipation, bladder instability, urinary tract infection syndrome. *Clin Nephrol* 23:152–154, 1985.
36. Smellie JM, Normand ICS: Bacteriuria, reflux, and scarring. *Arch Dis Child* 50:581–585, 1975.
37. Ransley PG, Risdon RA: Reflux and renal scarring. *Br J Radiol* (suppl 14):1–35, 1978.
38. Tamminen TE, Kaprio EA: The relation of the shape of renal papillae and of collecting duct openings to intrarenal reflux. *Br J Urol* 49:345–354, 1977.
39. Birmingham Reflux Study Group: Prospective trial of operative versus non-operative treatment of severe vesicoureteric reflux in children: Five years' observation. *Br Med J (Clin Res)* 295:237–241, 1987.
40. Weiss R, Duckett J, Spitzer A: Results of a randomized clinical trial of medical versus surgical management of infants and children with grades III and IV primary vesicoureteral reflux (United States). *J Urol* 148:1667–1673, 1992.
41. Arant BS Jr: Medical management of mild and moderate vesicoureteral reflux: Follow-up studies of infants and young children. A prelimi-

nary report of the Southwest Pediatric Nephrology Study Group. *J Urol* 148:1683–1687, 1992.

42. Rushton HG, Majd M: Dimercaptosuccinic acid renal scintigraphy for the evaluation of pyelonephritis and scarring: A review of experimental and clinical studies. *J Urol* 148:1726–1732, 1992.

43. Smellie JM, Normand ICS, Katz G: Children with urinary infection: A comparison of those with and those without vesicoureteric reflux. *Kidney Int* 20:717–722, 1981.

44. Smellie JM: Reflections on 30 years of treating children with urinary tract infections. *J Urol* 146:665–668, 1991.

45. Bernstein J, Arant BS Jr: Morphological characteristics of segmental renal scarring in vesicoureteral reflux. *J Urol* 1712–1714, 1992.

46. Rushton HG, Majd M, Jantausch B, et al: Renal scarring following reflux and non-reflux pyelonephritis in children: Evaluation with 99m technetium-dimercaptosuccinic acid scintigraphy. *J Urol* 147:1327–1332, 1992.

47. Jakobsson B, Berg U, Svenson L: Renal scarring after acute pyelonephritis. *Arch Dis Child* 70:111–115, 1994.

48. Winter AL, Hardy BE, Alton DJ, et al: Acquired renal scars in children. *J Urol* 129:1190–1194, 1983.

49. Roberts JA, Suarez GM, Kaack B, et al: Experimental pyelonephritis in the monkey: VII. Ascending pyelonephritis in the absence of vesicoureteral reflux. *J Urol* 133:1068–1075, 1985.

50. Hellström M, Jodal U, Mårild S, et al: Ureteral dilatation in children with febrile urinary tract infection or bacteriuria. *AJR* 148:483–486, 1987.

51. Roberts JA: Experimental pyelonephritis in the monkey: III. Pathophysiology of ureteral malfunction induced by bacteria. *Invest Urol* 13:117–120, 1975.

52. Roberts JA: Vesicoureteral reflux and pyelonephritis in the monkey: A review. *J Urol* 148:1721–1725, 1992.

53. Roberts JA: Etiology and pathophysiology of pyelonephritis. *Am J Kidney Dis* 17:1–9, 1991.

54. Mendoza JM, Roberts JA: Effect of sterile high pressure vesicoureteral reflux on the monkey. *J Urol* 130:602–606, 1983.

55. Busch R, Huland H: Correlation of symptoms and results of direct bacterial localization in patients with urinary tract infections. *J Urol* 132:282–285, 1984.

56. Cohen M: Urinary tract infections in children: I. Females aged 2 through 14, first two infections. *Pediatrics* 50:271–278, 1972.

57. Lindberg U, Claesson I, Hanson LA, et al: Asymptomatic bacteriuria in schoolgirls: I. Clinical and laboratory findings. *Acta Pediatr Scand* 64:425–431, 1975.

58. Newcastle Asymptomatic Bacteriuria Research Group: Asymptomatic bacteriuria in school children in Newcastle-upon-Tyne. *Arch Dis Child* 50:90–102, 1975.

59. Verrier-Jones K, Asscher AW, Verrier-Jones ER: Long-term aspects of covert bacteriuria: A 10 year follow-up of Cardiff schoolgirls. In Brodehl J, Ehrlich HH (eds): *Pediatric Nephrology.* New York, Springer Verlag, 1984, pp 302–305.

60. Kass EH: Bacteriuria and the diagnosis of infections of the urinary tract. *Arch Intern Med* 100:709–714, 1957.

61. Marple CD: The frequency and character of urinary tract infections in an unselected group of women. *Ann Intern Med* 14:2220–2239, 1941.

62. Sanford JP, Favour CB, Mao FG, et al: Evaluation of the positive urine culture. *Am J Med* 20:88–93, 1956.

63. Kass EH: Asymptomatic infections of the urinary tract. *Trans Assoc Am Phys* 69:59–64, 1956.

64. Hart EL, Magee MJ: Collecting urine specimens. *Am J Nurs* 57:1323–1326, 1957.

65. Boshell BR, Sanford JP: A screening method for the evaluation of urinary tract infections in female patients without catheterization. *Ann Intern Med* 48:1040–1045, 1958.

66. Immergut MA, Gilbert EC, Frensilli FJ, et al: The myth of the clean-catch urine specimen. *Urology* 17:339–340, 1981.

67. Lipsky BA, Inui TS, Plorde JJ, et al: Is the clean-catch midstream void procedure necessary for obtaining urine culture specimens for men? *Am J Med* 76:257–262, 1984.

68. Hoberman A, Wald ER, Reynolds EH, et al: Pyuria and bacteriuria in urine specimens obtained by bladder catheter from young children with fever. *J Pediatr* 124:513–519, 1994.

69. Durbin WA Jr, Peter G: Management of urinary tract infections in infants and children. *Pediatr Infect Dis* 3:564–574, 1984.

70. McCracken GH Jr: Diagnosis and management of acute urinary tract infections in infants and children. *Pediatr Infect Dis J* 6:107–112, 1987.

71. Pryles CV, Steg NL: Specimens of urine obtained from young girls by catheter versus voiding. *Pediatrics* 23:441–452, 1959.

72. Dodge WF, West EF, Fras PA, et al: Detection of bacteriuria in children. *J Pediatr* 74:107–110, 1969.

73. Lohr JA, Donowitz LG, Dudley SM: Bacterial contamination rates for non-clean-catch and clean-catch midstream urine collections in boys. *J Pediatr* 109:659–660, 1986.

74. Lohr JA, Donowitz LG, Dudley SM: Bacterial contamination in voided urine collections in girls. *J Pediatr* 114:91–93, 1989.

75. Bollgren I, Winberg J: The periurethral aerobic bacterial flora in healthy boys and girls. *Acta Paediatr Scand* 65:74–80, 1976.

76. Cruickshank G, Edmond E: "Clean-catch" urines in the newborn: Bacteriology and cell excretion patterns in first week of life. *Br Med J (Clin Res)* 4:705–707, 1967.

77. McCarthy JM, Pryles CV: Clean voided and catheter neonatal urine specimens. *Am J Dis Child* 106:85–90, 1963.

78. Nelson JD, Peters PC: Suprapubic aspiration of urine in premature and term infants. *Pediatrics* 36:132−134, 1965.
79. Bollgren I, Engstrom CF, Hammarlind M, et al: Low urinary counts of P-fimbriated Escherichia coli in presumed acute pyelonephritis. *Arch Dis Child* 59:102−106, 1984.
80. Mulvihill S, Montgomerie JZ: Correlation of tissue infection with bacteriuria. *J Infect Dis* 145:917, 1982.
81. Kunin CM: *Detection, Prevention and Management of Urinary Tract Infections*, ed 4. Philadelphia, Lea & Febiger, 1987, p 59.
82. Stamm WE, Wagner KF, Amset R, et al: Causes of the acute urethral syndrome in women. *N Engl J Med* 303:409−415, 1980.
83. Stamm WE, Counts GW, Running KR, et al: Diagnosis of coliform infection in acutely dysuric women. *N Engl J Med* 307:463−468, 1982.
84. Tapsall JW, Bell SM, Taylor PC, et al: Relevance of "significant" bacteriuria to aetiology and diagnosis of urinary-tract infection. *Lancet* 2:637−638, 1975.
85. Asscher AW: *The Challenge of Urinary Tract Infections*, New York, Academic Press, 1980.
86. Sen S, Moudgil A: Urinary tract infections in children: Epidemiology, etiology, and diagnosis. *Indian Pediatr* 28:1353−1358, 1991.
87. Sherbotie JR, Cornfeld D: Management of urinary tract infections in children. *Med Clin North Am* 75:327−338, 1991.
88. Hoberman A, Wald ER, Penchansky L, et al: Enhanced urinalysis as a screening test for urinary tract infection. *Pediatrics* 91:1196−1199, 1993.
89. Pryles CV, Eliot CR: Pyuria and bacteriuria in infants and children. *Am J Dis Child* 110:628−635, 1965.
90. Cruickshank J, Moynes JM: The presence and significance of nitrites in the urine. *Br Med J (Clin Res)* 2:712−713, 1914.
91. Mills SJ, Ford M, Gould FK, et al: Screening for bacteriuria in urological patients using reagent strips. *Br J Urol* 70:314−317, 1992.
92. Powell HR, McCredie DA, Ritchie MA: Urinary nitrite in symptomatic and asymptomatic urinary infection. *Arch Dis Child* 62:138−140, 1987.
93. Kunin CM, DeGroot JE: Sensitivity of a nitrite indicator strip method in detecting bacteriuria in preschool girls. *Pediatrics* 60:244−245, 1977.
94. Goldsmith BM, Campos JM: Comparison of urine dipstick, microscopy, and culture for the detection of bacteriuria in children. *Clin Pediatr* 29:214−218, 1990.
95. Cannon HJ Jr, Goetz ES, Hamoudi SC, et al: Rapid screening and microbiologic processing of pediatric urine specimens. *Diagn Microbiol Infect Dis* 4:11−17, 1986.
96. Weinberg AG, Gan VN: Urine screen for bacteriuria in symptomatic pediatric outpatients. *Pediatr Infect Dis J* 10:651−654, 1991.
97. Lohr JA: Use of routine urinalysis in making a presumptive diagnosis

of urinary tract infection in children. *Pediatr Infect Dis J* 10:646–650, 1991.

98. Winberg J, Andersen HJ, Bergstrom T, et al: Epidemiology of symptomatic urinary tract infection in childhood. *Acta Pediatr Scand* 252(suppl):1–20, 1974.

99. Conway JJ, King LR, Belman AB, et al: Detection of vesicoureteral reflux with radionuclide cystography. A comparison study with roentgenographic cystography. *Am J Roentgenol* 115:720–727, 1972.

100. Willi U, Treves S: Radionuclide voiding cystography. *Urol Radiol* 5:161–173, 1983.

101. Rickwood AM, Carty HM, McKendrick T, et al: Current imaging of childhood urinary infections: Prospective survey. *Br Med J (Clin Res)* 304:663–665, 1992.

102. Jones KV, Asscher AW: Urinary tract infection and vesicoureteral reflux. In Edelmann CM Jr (ed): *Pediatric Kidney Disease.* Boston, Little, Brown, 1992, pp 1943–1991.

103. Dunbar JS, Nogrady B: Excretory urography in the first year of life. *Radiol Clin North Am* 10:367–391, 1972.

104. MacKenzie JR, Fowler K, Hollman AS, et al: The value of ultrasound in the child with an acute urinary tract infection. *Br J Urol* 74:240–244, 1994.

105. Huang FY, Huang YC, Tsai TC, et al: Is IVP necessary in children with urinary tract infection? *Acta Pediatr Sin* 33:257–263, 1992.

106. Spenser JR, Schaeffer SJ: Pediatric urinary tract infections. *Urol Clin North Am* 13:661–672, 1986.

107. Fairley KF, Bond AG, Brown RB, et al: Simple test to determine the site of urinary tract infection. *Lancet* 2:427–428, 1967.

108. Winberg J, Andersen HJ, Hanson LA, et al: Studies of urinary tract infections in infancy and childhood: I. Antibody response in different types of urinary tract infections caused by coliform bacteria. *Br Med J (Clin Res)* 8:524–527, 1963.

109. Thomas V, Skelokov A, Forland M: Antibody-coated bacteria in the urine and the site of urinary tract infection. *N Engl J Med* 290:588–590, 1974.

110. Winberg J: Renal functional studies in infants and children with acute non-obstructive urinary tract infections. *Acta Pediatr Scand* 48:577–589, 1959.

111. Jodal U, Lindberg U, Lincoln K: Level diagnosis of symptomatic urinary tract infections in childhood. *Acta Pediatr Scand* 64:201–208, 1975.

112. Carvajal HF, Passey RB, Berger M, et al: Urinary lactic dehydrogenase isoenzyme 5 in the differential diagnosis of kidney and bladder infections. *Kidney Int* 8:176–184, 1975.

113. Hellerstein S: Urinary LDH enzyme activity and site of urinary tract infections. *Pediatr Infect Dis J* 7:180–185, 1988.

114. Heptinstall RH: *Pathology of the Kidney,* ed 2. Boston, Little, Brown, vol 2, 1974, pp 880–881.

115. Jakobsson B, Soderlundh S, Berg U: Diagnostic significance of 99m Tc-dimercaptosuccinic acid (DMSA) scintigraphy in urinary tract infection. Arch Dis Child 67:1338–1342, 1992.
116. Handmaker H: Clinical experience with 99m Tc-DMSA (dimercaptosuccinic acid): A new renal imaging agent. *J Nucl Med* 16:28–32, 1975.
117. Majd M, Rushton HG: Renal cortical scintigraphy in the diagnosis of acute pyelonephritis. *Semin Nucl Med* 22:98–111, 1992.
118. Björgvinsson E, Majd M, Eggli KD: Diagnosis of acute pyelonephritis in children: Comparison of sonography and 99m Tc-DMSA scintigraphy. *AJR* 157:539–543, 1991.
119. Jakobsson B, Nolstedt L, Svensson L, et al: 99m Technetium-dimercaptosuccinic acid scan in the diagnosis of acute pyelonephritis in children: Relation to clinical and radiological findings. *Pediatr Nephrol* 6:328–334, 1992.
120. Benador D, Benador N, Slosman DO, et al: Cortical scintigraphy in the evaluation of renal parenchymal changes in children with pyelonephritis. *J Pediatr* 124:17–20, 1994.
121. Conway JJ: The role of scintigraphy in urinary tract infection. *Semin Nucl Med* 18:308–319, 1988.
122. Shanon A, Feldman W, McDonald P, et al: Evaluation of renal scars by technetium-labeled dimercaptosuccinic acid scan, intravenous urography, and ultrasonography: A comparative study. *J Pediatr* 120:399–403, 1992.
123. Tasker AD, Lindsell DR, Moncrieff M: Can ultrasound reliably detect renal scarring in children with urinary tract infection? *Clin Radiol* 47:177–179, 1993.
124. Smellie JM: The DMSA scan and intravenous urography in the detection of renal scarring. *Pediatr Nephrol* 3:6–8, 1989.
125. Brem AS: Cortical scintigraphy in the evaluation of urinary tract infections. *J Pediatr* 125:334–336, 1994.
126. Savage DCL, Wilson MI, McHardy M, et al: Covert bacteriuria of childhood. *Arch Dis Child* 48:8–20, 1973.
127. Newcastle Covert Bacteriuria Research Group: Covert bacteriuria in schoolgirls in Newcastle upon Tyne: A 5-year follow-up. *Arch Dis Child* 56:585–592, 1981.
128. Smellie JM, Ransly PG, Normand ICS, et al: Development of new renal scars: A collaborative study. *Br Med J (Clin Res)* 290:1957–1960, 1983.
129. Kala UK, Jacobs DW: Evaluation of urinary tract infection in malnourished black children. *Ann Trop Pediatr* 12:75–81, 1992.
130. Askari A, Belman AB: Vesicoureteral reflux in black girls. *J Urol* 127:747–748, 1982.
131. Rosenberg AR, Rossleigh MA, Brydon MP, et al: Evaluation of acute urinary infection in children by dimercaptosuccinic acid scintigraphy: A prospective study. *J Urol* 148:1746–1749, 1992.

132. Rubin MI: Infection of the urinary tract. In Rubin MI, Barratt TM (eds): *Pediatric Nephrology*. Baltimore, Williams & Wilkins, 1975, pp 607–645.
133. Levitt SB, Weiss RA: Vesicoureteral reflux. In Kelalis PP, King LR, Belman BA (eds): *Clinical Pediatric Urology*, ed 2. Philadelphia, WB Saunders, 1985, pp 355–380.
134. Johnson DK, Kroovand RL, Perlmutter AD: The changing role of cystoscopy in the pediatric patient. *J Urol* 123:232–233, 1980.
135. Ireland GW, Cass AS: The clinical measurement of the ureteral submucosal tunnel. *J Urol* 107:564–566, 1972.
136. Lyon RP, Tanagho EA: Distal urethral stenosis in little girls. *J Urol* 93:379–387, 1965.
137. Forbes PA, Drummond KN, Nogrady MB: Meatotomy in girls with meatal stenosis and urinary tract infections. *J Pediatr* 75:937–942, 1969.
138. Robson AM, Manley CB: Pediatric renal disease. *Curr Probl Pediatr* 1:1–48, 1970.
139. Immergut M, Culp D, Flocks RH: The urethral caliber in normal female children. *J Urol* 97:693–695, 1966.
140. Kaplan GW, Sammons TA, King LR: A blind comparison of dilatation, urethrotomy and medication alone in the treatment of urinary tract infection in girls. *J Urol* 109:917–919, 1973.
141. Koff SA: A practical approach to evaluating urinary tract infection in children. *Pediatr Nephrol* 5:398–400, 1991.
142. Herman F: Urinary tract damage in children who wet. *Pediatrics* 54:143–150, 1974.
143. Van Gool JD, Kuijten RH, Donckerwolcke RA, et al: Bladder-sphincter dysfunction, urinary infection and vesicoureteral reflux—with special reference to cognitive bladder training. *Contrib Nephrol* 39:190–210, 1984.
144. Snodgrass W: Relationship of voiding dysfunction to urinary tract infection and vesicoureteral reflux in children. *Urology* 38:341–344, 1991.
145. Hansson S: Urinary incontinence in children and associated problems. *Scand J Urol Nephrol* 141(suppl):47–55, 1992.
146. Hjalmas K: Functional daytime incontinence: definitions and epidemiology. *Scand J Urol Nephrol* 141(suppl):39–44, 1992.
147. Van Gool JD, Vijverberg MA, de Jong TP: Functional daytime incontinence: Clinical and urodynamic assessment. *Scand J Urol Nephrol* 141:58–69, 1992.
148. Williams MA, Noe HN, Smith RA: The importance of urinary tract infection in the evaluation of the incontinent child. *J Urol* 151:188–190, 1994.
149. Koff SA, Murtagh DS: The uninhibited bladder in children: Effect of treatment on recurrence of urinary infection and on vesicoureteral reflux resolution. *J Urol* 130:1138–1141, 1983.

150. Homsy YL, Nsouli J, Hamberger B, et al: Effects of oxybutynin on vesicoureteral reflux in children. *J Urol* 134:1168–1171, 1985.
151. Seruca H: Vesicoureteral reflux and voiding dysfunction: Prospective study. *J Urol* 142:494–498, 1989.
152. Jones B, Gerrard JW, Skokeir MK, et al: Recurrent urinary infections in girls: Relation to enuresis. *Can Med Assoc J* 106:127–130, 1972.
153. Dodge WF, West EF, Bridgeforth EB, et al: Noctural enuresis in 6 to 10 year old children: Correlation of bacteriuria, proteinuria and dysuria. *Am J Dis Child* 120:32–35, 1970.
154. Koff SA: Evaluation and management of voiding disorders in children. *Urol Clin North Am* 15:769–775, 1988.
155. Koff SA, Byard MA: The daytime urinary frequency syndrome of childhood. *J Urol* 140:1280–1281, 1988.
156. Casale AJ: Functional voiding disorders of childhood. *J Ky Med Assoc* 91:185–191, 1993.
157. Bauer SB, Retik AB, Colodny AH, et al: The unstable bladder of childhood. *Urol Clin North Am* 7:321–336, 1980.
158. Vincent SA: Postural control of urinary incontinence: The curtsy sign. *Lancet* 2:631–632, 1966.
159. Griffiths DJ, Scholtmeijer RJ: Detrusor-sphincter dyssynergia in neurologically normal children. *Neurourol Urodyn* 2:27–37, 1983.
160. Van Gool J, Tanagho E: External sphincter activity and recurrent urinary tract infections in girls. *Urology* 10:348–353, 1977.
161. Hinman F, Baumann FW: Vesical and ureteral damage from voiding dysfunction in boys without neurologic or obstructive disease. *Trans Am Assoc Genitourin Surg* 64:116–121, 1972.
162. Bauer SB: Neuropathology of the lower urinary tract. In Kelalis PP, King LR, Belman AB (eds): *Clinical Pediatric Urology*, ed 3. Philadelphia, WB Saunders, 1992, p 399.
163. Koff SA: Estimating bladder capacity in children. *Urology* 21:248, 1983.
164. Miller T, Phillips S: Pyelonephritis: The relationship between infection, renal scarring, and antimicrobial therapy. *Kidney Int* 19:654–662, 1981.
165. Ransley PG, Risdon RA: Reflux nephropathy: Effects of antimicrobial therapy on the evolution of the early pyelonephritic scar. *Kidney Int* 20:733–742, 1981.
166. Stamey TA, Pfau A: Some functional, pathologic, bacteriologic and chemotherapeutic characteristics of unilateral pyelonephritis in man: II. Bacteriologic and chemotherapeutic characteristics. *Invest Urol* 1:162–172, 1963.
167. Stamey TA, Govan DE, Palmer JM: The localization and treatment of urinary tract infections. *Medicine (Baltimore)* 44:1–36, 1965.
168. Winberg J, Bergstrom T, Jakobsson B: Morbidity, age and sex distribution, recurrences and renal scarring in symptomatic urinary tract infection in childhood. *Kidney Int* 213(suppl):101–106, 1975.

169. Sigurdsson JA, Ahlmen J, Berglund L, et al: Three-day treatment of acute lower urinary tract infection in women. *Acta Med Scand* 213:55–60, 1983.
170. Bailey RR, Keenan TD, Eliott JC, et al: Treatment of bacterial cystitis with a single dose of trimethoprim, co-trimazole, or amoxycillin compared with a course of trimethoprim. *N Z Med J* 98:387–389, 1985.
171. Kallenius G, Winberg J: Urinary tract infections treated with a single dose of short-acting sulphonamide. *Br Med J (Clin Res)* 1:1175–1176, 1979.
172. Khan AJ, Kumar K, Evans HE: Three-day antimicrobial therapy of urinary tract infection. *J Pediatr* 99:992–994, 1981.
173. Lohr JA, Hayden GF, Gleason CH, et al: Three-day therapy of lower urinary tract infections with nitrofurantoin macrocrystals: A randomized clinical trial. *J Pediatr* 99:980–983, 1981.
174. Pitt WR, Dyer SA, McNee JL, et al: Single-dose trimethoprim-sulphamethoxazole treatment of symptomatic urinary infection. *Arch Dis Child* 57:229–239, 1982.
175. Kornberg AE, Sherin K, Veiga P, et al: Two-day therapy with cefuroxime axetil is effective for urinary tract infections in children. *Am J Nephrol* 14:169–172, 1994.
176. Khan AJ: Efficacy of single-dose therapy of urinary tract infection in infants and children: A review. *J Natl Med Assoc* 86:690–696, 1994.
177. McCracken GH, Ginsburg CM, Namasonthi V, et al: Evaluation of short-term antibiotic therapy in children with uncomplicated urinary tract infections. *Pediatrics* 67:796–801, 1981.
178. Avner ED, Ingelfinger JR, Herrin JT, et al: Single-dose amoxicillin therapy of uncomplicated pediatric urinary tract infections. *J Pediatr* 102:623–627, 1983.
179. Moffat M, Embree J, Grimm P, et al: Short-course antibiotic therapy for urinary tract infection in children: A methodological review of the literature. *Am J Dis Child* 142:57–61, 1988.
180. Kunin CM, Deutscher R, Paquin A: Urinary tract infection in school children: An epidemiologic, clinical and laboratory study. *Medicine (Baltimore)* 43:91–130, 1964.
181. Lindberg U: Asymptomatic bacteriuria in schoolgirls: V. The clinical course and response to treatment. *Acta Pediatr Scand* 64:718–724, 1975.
182. Hansson S, Jodal U, Noren L: Treatment versus non-treatment of asymptomatic bacteriuria in girls with renal scarring. In Kass EH, Eden CS (eds): *Host-Parasite Interactions in Urinary Tract Infections*. Chicago, University of Chicago Press, 1986, pp 289–291.
183. Jodal U, Koskimies O, Hanson E, et al: Infection pattern in children with veiscoureteral reflux randomly allocated to operation or long-term antibacterial prophylaxis. *J Urol* 148:1650–1652, 1992.
184. el-Khatib M, Packham DK, Becker GJ, et al: Pregnancy-related complications in women with reflux nephropathy. *Clin Nephrol* 41:50–55, 1994.

185. McGladdery SL, Aparicia S, Verrier-Jones K, et al: Outcome of pregnancy in an Oxford-Cardiff cohort of women with previous bacteriuria. *Q J Med* 83:533–539, 1992.
186. Jungers P, Forget D, Houillier P, et al: Pregnancy in IgA nephropathy, reflux nephropathy, and focal glomerular sclerosis. *Am J Kid Dis* 9:334–338, 1987.
187. Kincaid-Smith P, Fairley KF: Renal disease in pregnancy. Three controversial areas: Mesangial IgA nephropathy, focal glomerular sclerosis (focal and segmental hyalinosis and sclerosis) and reflux nephropathy. *Am J Kid Dis* 9:328–333, 1987.

Diagnosis and Treatment of Congenital Toxoplasmosis*

Kenneth M. Boyer, M.D.
Director, Section of Pediatric Infectious Diseases, Rush-Presbyterian-St. Luke's Medical Center, Professor and Associate Chairman, Department of Pediatrics, Rush Medical College of Rush University, Chicago, Illinois

C ongenital toxoplasmosis results from transplacental infection by the coccidian parasite *Toxoplasma gondii* during gestation. An estimated 400 to 4,000 cases occur in the United States each year. Most often the consequence of asymptomatic infection in pregnant women, congenital infection ranges in its manifestations from subclinical to devastating. Involvement may be apparent at birth or become evident only months to years later. The disease eventually will manifest in virtually all congenitally infected infants.[1, 2]

Treatment of a mother can prevent congenital infection. Treatment of an infected fetus or newborn infant can prevent involvement of vital organs or can arrest disease progression. Treatment of recrudescent disease can preserve vision and neurologic function. Although current therapies are not ideal, several recent studies indicate a substantial improvement in long-term outcomes for treated infants. Despite these advances, congenital toxoplasmosis exacts a considerable emotional and financial toll on affected children, their families, and society.[3]

ETIOLOGY AND PATHOGENESIS

Toxoplasma gondii is a protozoan whose full life cycle has been understood since the early 1970s. Three developmental stages of the organism are known. Tachyzoites are metabolically active and can proliferate rapidly in all mammalian cell types. They are the pathogenic stage of the parasite and are susceptible to both immune surveillance and killing by physical and pharmacologic means.

By contrast, bradyzoites are metabolically inactive. They pro-

*Supported in part by Grant RO-1-AI-27530 from the National Institute of Allergy and Infectious Diseases.

Advances in Pediatric Infectious Diseases®, vol. 11
© 1996, Mosby–Year Book, Inc.

liferate only slowly within cysts that evolve from intracellular tachyzoites (schizogony), particularly in the retina, brain, myocardium, and skeletal muscle. Bradyzoites within cysts account for the lifelong parasite latency that occurs after primary infection. They are relatively remote from immune surveillance and resist killing by physical and pharmacologic means.

Sporozoites develop as a consequence of the sexual portion of the parasite's life cycle (gametogony), which can occur only in the gastrointestinal tract of domestic cats and other feline species.[4,5] They are excreted in cat feces within oocysts, another physically hardy form capable of prolonged survival in soil.

Bradyzoites in raw or undercooked meat and sporozoites in soil or cat litter are the most common forms of *T. gondii* whose ingestion leads to primary infection during pregnancy. Other less obvious pathways of primary infection occasionally are documented, such as playing with a child in a sandbox, frequenting a riding stable, butchering a deer, or indulging in unusual foods at an expensive restaurant. Reactivation of toxoplasmosis is an important mechanism of infection in the immunocompromised host and also in the congenitally infected infant but is rarely the mechanism of infection in a pregnant woman.

Congenital toxoplasmosis in general is a consequence of primary infection during pregnancy. There are exceptions to this rule, as in women whose primary infections occur periconceptionally or even up to 6 months before conception, but such instances are rare. Mandated serologic surveillance during pregnancy in France has permitted analysis of the risks of fetal infection by trimester of maternal infections.[6] First-trimester seroconversion carries the lowest probability of congenital infection (14%) but the highest risk of severe disease. Conversely, third-trimester seroconversion carries a high probability of congenital infection (59%), but most infants will have mild or subclinical involvement at birth. Second-trimester seroconversion yields intermediate risks of both congenital infection (29%) and clinically overt neonatal disease.

When a pregnant woman acquires *T. gondii*, tachyzoites are spread hematogeneously to the placenta. The organism can then be spread transplacentally directly to the fetus during gestation or at birth. It is possible that differences in rates of transmission during gestation depend on placental size, virulence of the *T. gondii* strain, the number of organisms spread to the placenta, and genetic differences in susceptibility. As in other congenital infections, the greater severity of toxoplasma infection acquired early in gestation relates to the sensitivity of early fetal tissues to damage by intracellular parasites, the placental barrier separating the fetus from the mother's hormonal and cell-mediated immune responses, and the fetus's intrinsic immunologic immaturity. The most profoundly affected infants frequently show specific immunologic tolerance in the perinatal period.[7]

EPIDEMIOLOGY AND INCIDENCE

The epidemiology of congenital toxoplasmosis is determined by the risk of a woman experiencing primary infection with *T. gondii* while pregnant. This risk depends, in turn, on three factors: the age-specific incidence of primary infection in the population during childbearing years, the age distribution of pregnant women in the population, and the fetal transmission rate in primary infection. A theoretical analysis based on these three factors by Frenkel,[8] assuming a childbearing age group of 20 to 29 years and an overall fetal transmission rate of 40%, showed that maximum risk occurs when the age-specific incidence rate in a population is 3% to 5% per year, which corresponds to prevalences of seropositivity of 50% to 80% in women of childbearing age. In such a population, the predicted prevalence of congenital toxoplasmosis would be 44 to 46 per 10,000 pregnancies. At higher age-specific incidences, rates of congenital toxoplasmosis would be lower because nearly all pregnant women would already be chronically infected. At lower incidences, rates would also be lower but because of less frequent exposure.

The incidence of congenital toxoplasmosis in the United States is probably declining at the present time, although accurate data collected over time do not exist. This may relate in part to widespread public awareness of the "dangers of kitty litter" to women who are pregnant. People are less informed about the potential for disease transmission from raw or undercooked meat. However, the common practice of freezing commercial meats before releasing them for sale, combined with the use of home freezers, may also be having a beneficial effect. Recent estimates are that about 8% of commercial beef, 20% of commercial pork, and 25% of commercial lamb contain toxoplasma bradyzoites.[9]

In the United States, the prevalence of seropositivity in women of childbearing age is inferred from studies of military recruits and from seroprevalence studies in major cities. In the early 1960s, the overall prevalence in military recruits was 14%, with lowest rates in the mountain (3%) and Pacific (8%) states, highest in the northeastern (20%) and southeastern states (19%).[10] Urban studies of

U.S. women of childbearing age have yielded variable rates: Denver, 3%; Palo Alto, 10%; Chicago, 12%; Boston, 14%; and Birmingham, 30%.[1, 2] Internationally rates are also quite variable: Thailand, 3%; Australia, 4%; Japan, 6%; Scotland, 13%; London, 20%; Poland, 36%; Belgium, 53%; and Paris, 73%.[2]

The strongest prospective data regarding current incidence in the United States are derived from screening of 635,000 newborns in Massachusetts and New Hampshire using the IgM enzyme-linked immunosorbent assay (ELISA) as applied to filter paper blood samples.[11, 12] The incidence of confirmed positive results in this study was approximately 1:12,000. Note that this incidence figure is comparable to other congenital defects for which neonatal screening is mandated by law: phenylketonuria (1:12,000), congenital hypothyroidism (1:5,000), and congenital adrenal hyperplasia (1:15,000).

CLINICAL MANIFESTATIONS
MATERNAL INFECTION
Primary infections with *T. gondii* in otherwise healthy pregnant women are asymptomatic in 80% to 90% of cases.[13] When disease is clinically apparent, the most common manifestation is lymphadenopathy, occasionally with heterophile-negative mononucleosis.[14] Cervical nodes are most frequently involved. They may be tender or nontender. They are often firm, discrete, smooth, and mobile, they do not suppurate or ulcerate. Lymphoma or other malignancy is generally a differential diagnostic consideration. Although exclusion of malignancy by biopsy is a priority for the pathologist, the implications of a diagnosis of lymphadenopathic toxoplasmosis in a woman who is pregnant or could become so should not be minimized.

Pregnant women with human immunodeficiency virus (HIV) infection and acquired immunodeficiency syndrome (AIDS) are an emerging risk group for progressive *Toxoplasma* infection, most often in the form of encephalitis. Infants born to these women may have both pediatric AIDS and congenital toxoplasmosis. In reported dual infections, fulminant and rapidly fatal courses have been observed.[15] Maternal HIV infection is the only situation in which reactivation of latent *Toxoplasma* infection is likely to lead to congenital infection.

CONGENITAL INFECTION
In infants the classic features of congenital toxoplasmosis are the triad of chorioretinitis, intracranial calcifications, and hydrocepha-

lus. However, unless hydrocephalus is already advanced at birth, none of these findings is likely to be detected on a routine newborn physical examination. Thus, it is not surprising that most cases of congenital toxoplasmosis are unrecognized or considered to be subclinical in the neonatal period.[12] Even a careful examination, including dilated indirect ophthalmoscopy and imaging of the brain by ultrasound or computed tomography (CT), may fail to show abnormalities. However, 80% to 90% of seemingly unaffected newborns with toxoplasmosis will develop eye or neurologic disease by adulthood.[16–18]

In a large early series, Eichenwald[19] somewhat arbitrarily divided his 152 patients into two groups: those with neurologic disease and those with generalized disease. As a rule, the 44 patients with generalized disease developed symptoms within the first months of life; the 108 patients with neurologic disease developed symptoms later. When the two groups were combined, 86% of the children had chorioretinitis, 37% had intracranial calcifications (on routine skull radiograph), and 20% had hydrocephalus. Other noteworthy features included abnormalities of cerebrospinal fluid (CSF; most often elevated protein levels), splenomegaly, convulsions, and microcephaly. In a similar retrospective series from France, Couvreur and Desmonts[20] made the diagnosis of congenital toxoplasmosis in only 105 of 300 patients (35%) during the first year of life. Among the 300, 76% had eye disease, 33% had intracranial calcifications, and 26% had hydrocephalus or microcephaly.

Regardless of age at diagnosis, most chorioretinitis due to toxoplasmosis is a consequence of congenital infection. In infants, the most common manifestation is strabismus, first noted by the parents. In children or adolescents, "floaters" or defects in acuity are the most common complaints. Funduscopic examination shows chorioretinal lesions that may be active (with indistinct borders and associated vitritis) or quiescent (with gray-white central areas and sharply demarcated hyperpigmented borders). Unfortunately, the macula is the most common focus of retinal involvement; accordingly, vision is often threatened.[21] Chorioretinal lesions may be single or multiple, unilateral or bilateral. Microphthalmia, glaucoma, and retinal detachment may be seen in eyes with extensive involvement. In some patients, eye lesions are stable. In others, repetitive episodes of reactivation disease with progressive loss of vision may occur over decades.

Neurologic abnormalities range from subtle findings to severe encephalitis. Intracranial calcifications are best seen by brain CT. Hydrocephalus may be the only manifestation of congenital toxoplasmosis and may be compensated or require shunt placement. Like eye disease, it may be seen in the perinatal period, later in infancy, or rarely up to adulthood. A variety of different seizure patterns may occur in the perinatal period and later in life. Central focal motor deficits have been noted, as have signs of spinal or bulbar involvement. Microcephaly in untreated infants is generally associated with diminished cognitive functioning. In Eichenwald's[19] follow-up studies of 101 mostly untreated patients, 87% were mentally retarded, 82% had seizures, 71% had spasticity and palsies, 62% had severely impaired vision, and 15% were deaf. Only 11% of these children were "normal." Like eye disease, reactivation of central nervous system (CNS) disease can occur but is less likely to be considered as a reason for clinical deterioration.

The prognosis for children with congenital toxoplasmosis at present is undoubtedly better than in earlier studies for two reasons. First, infants with infection but without overt disease can now be identified by prospective study of pregnant women or newborns. Second, treatment can substantially improve their outcome and may actually prevent the development of clinically overt disease.[21] Two recent studies show changes in the clinical spectrum of congenital infection by *T. gondii* with prospective identification of cases. Couvreur et al.[22] described the spectrum of signs and symptoms in infected newborn infants whose mothers were identified in a systematic screening program for seroconversion. Only 10% of these infants had substantial ocular, CNS, or systemic involvement; 34% had normal clinical examinations with the exception of retinal scars or isolated calcification; and 55% had no abnormalities detected. Similarly, Guerina et al.[12] identified and studied 52 infected newborn infants by filter paper blood testing for IgM antibodies. Two had obvious abnormalities, and 50 had "normal" newborn examinations. On careful reexamination after recognition of their serologic status, 19 (40%) of 48 apparently normal infants had retinal lesions or CNS abnormalities. Improved outcomes in such asymptomatic or mildly affected infants and in others with overt disease will be discussed later in the chapter.

DIAGNOSIS

SPECIFIC TESTS

Toxoplasmic lymphadenitis has a distinctive histopathology characterized by reactive follicular hyperplasia, irregular clusters of epithelioid histiocytes, and monocytoid cells that distend the subcapsular and trabecular lymph node sinuses.[23] Tachyzoites are only rarely seen in affected nodes.

Intraperitoneal inoculation of tissue (amniotic fluid, fetal blood, and, most reliably, placenta) into laboratory mice is the most definitive diagnostic technique for fetal or congenital infections.[24] Maternal treatment reduces the sensitivity of this test, but a negative result also can be a useful indicator of an effective regimen.

Serologic testing is the usual approach to maternal, fetal, and infant diagnosis. A formidable array of tests is available (Table 1).[1, 2, 24] None is without problems of technique or interpretation. A combination of tests is generally best, with confirmation of results in a reference laboratory. The major problems of serologic diagnosis are determining acuity (in maternal infection) and differentiating endogenous from transplacentally acquired antibodies (in fetal or neonatal infection).

The gold standard for serologic tests is the dye test developed in the 1940s by Sabin and Feldman.[25] In the presence of complement and specific antibodies, *T. gondii* tachyzoites lose their ability to be stained with the vital dye alkaline methylene blue. The range of positive results is great. In general, acute infection is associated with high titers, chronic infection with lower titers. Immunofluorescence and ELISA tests for IgG antibodies are used in most hospital and commercial laboratories because of their simplicity and, in the case of ELISA, ease of automation. Results with these tests, particularly with strongly positive sera, correlate well with the result of the dye test. Lower titers or absorbencies are not as reliable.

Endogenous antibodies in a fetus or newborn or recently acquired infection in a mother can be detected with tests for IgM-, IgA-, and IgE-specific antibodies. The double-sandwich IgM ELISA developed by Naot et al.[26] has had considerable use in the United States. If results are positive in a baby, it indicates fetal or congenital infection. However, 25% of congenitally infected infants will have negative results in this assay. Strong positives are also reliable indicators of recent maternal infection. The IgM immunosorbent agglutination assay (IgM ISAGA), used extensively in France, is somewhat more sensitive than the IgM ELISA but is less available in the United States.[27] Detection of IgM antibodies by indirect immunofluorescence (IgM IFA) is widely available in this country. It is a significantly less sensitive test than the ELISA and ISAGA and is subject to false-positive results caused by rheumatoid factor and antinuclear antibodies. Guidelines for interpreting results are summarized in Table 1.

Other serologic tests that may be used to identify fetal or recent maternal infection include the IgA and IgE ELISAs and immunofiltration assays.[28, 29] Differences in immunoblot antibody

TABLE 1.

Guidelines for Interpretation of Serologic Tests for Toxoplasmosis*

Test†	Positive Titer‡	Titer in Acute Infection	Titer in Chronic Infection	Duration of Elevation of Titer
IgG				
Sabin-Feldman dye test	Undiluted	1:4 to ≥1:1,000 (usual)	1:4 to 1:2,000	Years
Direct agglutination test	≥1:20	Rises slowly from negative to low titer to high titer (1:512)	Stable (≥1:1,000) or slowly decreasing titer	≥1 yr
IgG IFA	≥1:10	≥1:1,000	1:8 to 1:2,000	Years
IHA test	≥1:16	≥1,000	1:16 to 1:256	Years
Complement fixation	≥1:4	Varies among laboratories	Negative to 1:8	Years
IgM				
IgM IFA	≥1:2, infants ≥1:10 adults	≥1:80	Negative to 1:20	Weeks to months, occasionally years

Double-sandwich IgM ELISA	≥0.2, newborn infant, fetus ≥1.7, older children, adults	≥6	Negative to 1.7 (older children, adults)	Can be >1 yr
IgM ISAGA	≥8, adult 1–7, indeterminate	≥8	Negative to 1	Unknown, can be ≥1 yr
IgA				
IgA ELISA	≥1.0 infants ≥1.3 adults	>1.0, infants >1.3, adults	Negative to <1.0 Negative to <1.3	Weeks to months, occasionally longer
IgE				
IgE ELISA	≥1.9	≥1.9	Negative	Weeks to months
IgE ISAGA	≥4	≥4	Negative	Weeks to months
AC/HS	See Dannemann et al.[31]	See Dannemann et al.[31]	See Dannemann et al.[31]	Usually <9 mo
PCR	Positive	Positive	Negative	Only when *Toxoplasma* DNA present

*Adapted from McLeod R, Wisner J, Boyer KM: Toxoplasmosis. In Krugman S, Katz SL, Gershon AA, et al (eds): *Infectious Diseases of Children*, ed 9. St Louis, Mosby, 1992, pp 518–550.

†IFA = immunofluorescence assay; IHA = indirect hemagglutination; ELISA = enzyme-linked immunosorbent assay; ISAGA = immunosorbent agglutination assay; AC/HS = acetone/formalin differential agglutination test; PCR = polymerase chain reaction.

‡Values are those of one reference laboratory; each laboratory must provide its own standards and interpretation of results in each clinical setting.

patterns between maternal serum and infant serum are suggestive of congenital infections.[30] The acetone/formalin (AC/HS) differential agglutination test is a helpful adjunct to assay of IgM, IgA, and IgE antibodies in determining the acuity of maternal infection.[31]

Transformation of lymphocytes exposed to lysates of *Toxoplasma* organisms indicates acquisition of cell-mediated immunity.[7, 32] Amplification of parasite DNA in amniotic fluid by the polymerase chain reaction (PCR), followed by probing with specific complementary DNA sequences, is a promising approach to diagnosis of intrauterine infections.[33, 34]

EVALUATION OF THE PREGNANT WOMAN WITH SUSPECTED ACUTE TOXOPLASMOSIS

The diagnosis of acute toxoplasmosis in a pregnant woman is most often suspected based on a set of TORCH (toxoplasmosis, rubella, cytomegalovirus, and herpes simplex) titers performed in a hospital or commercial laboratory or occasionally based on histologic results of an involved cervical lymph node. In the former case, the result is most likely to represent old or chronic infection. However, acuity must be established by reexamining serum in a reference laboratory using the dye test together with one or more reliable indicators of recent infection, such as IgM-, IgA-, IgE-specific antibodies, or the AC/HS differential agglutination test. At present, the most experienced U.S. laboratory for confirmation is the Research Institute, Palo Alto Medical Foundation (860 Bryant St, Palo Alto, CA 94301, telephone 415-326-8120).

If results indicate acute maternal infection, establishment of fetal involvement becomes the critical issue. Ultrasound evaluation of the fetus for gestational age and to screen for abnormalities is the usual starting point. Although fetal blood sampling can be a definitive test for fetal infection, it is risky.[35] This complex and invasive approach is now being replaced by PCR examination of amniotic fluid obtained by routine amniocentesis. Based on the results of PCR, the mother (and fetus) should be treated as described later on or pregnancy termination can be considered.

EVALUATION OF THE NEWBORN INFANT WITH SUSPECTED CONGENITAL TOXOPLASMOSIS

In addition to a careful examination, the suspect newborn should have serologic studies (in a pair with maternal serum) by the dye test and by assays for specific IgM, IgA, and IgE antibodies. Cerebrospinal fluid should be examined for routine cells, glucose levels, and protein levels. In addition, CSF serologic studies should be performed by dye test and IgM ELISA. Other common causes of congenital infection, particularly cytomegalovirus, should be excluded by viral culture and serologic evaluation. If the diagnosis of congenital toxoplasmosis was anticipated before delivery, inoculation of placental tissue and cord blood into mice is desirable.

If serologic results suggest congenital toxoplasmosis, a full evaluation of the infant should include dilated indirect funduscopic examination, a careful neurologic examination, and a brain CT scan. Baseline blood counts and liver function tests should be performed before initiation of therapy.

THERAPY

Pregnant women with acute toxoplasmosis and infants with congenital toxoplasmosis should be treated.[1, 2] In the former instance, the goal is prevention of fetal infection or initiation of treatment for an infected fetus before delivery. In the latter, the goal is termination of tissue destruction by proliferating tachyzoites and prevention of long-term morbidity. Current therapies are not effective against encysted bradyzoites and therefore may not prevent establishment of latency or late reactivation of disease. Longitudinal treatment trials are currently under way to evaluate optimal regimens and long-term outcome.

Two drug regimens are used in maternal and congenital toxoplasmosis (Table 2). Spiramycin is a macrolide antibiotic available to physicians through the Food and Drug Administration (telephone 301-443-9553). Side effects are usually minimal but have included gastrointestinal distress, local vasospasm, dysesthesias, dizziness, and allergy. There are no known deleterious effects on the fetus. Given to a mother, spiramycin appears to effectively control placental infection. Early studies, in which the fetus was not evaluated in utero, showed a reduction in transmission rates by 60% with treatment.[37] Detailed pharmacologic studies of transplacental passage and fetal blood levels of spiramycin do not exist. By analogy to other macrolides, fetal levels are probably not high. Spiramycin is currently indicated for treatment of a pregnant woman with acute infection whose fetus either does not have infection or whose evaluation for fetal infection is pending.

The drug regimen of choice for proven fetal or congenital toxoplasmosis is the combination of pyrimethamine (Daraprim) and sulfadiazine, with folinic acid (Leucovorin). Pyrimethamine and sulfadiazine antagonize folic acid synthesis by synergistic inhibi-

TABLE 2.

Treatment of Congenital Toxoplasmosis*

Manifestation of Disease	Therapy	Dosage (Oral Unless Specified)	Duration
Congenital toxoplasmosis†	Pyrimethamine†	Loading dose: 2 mg/kg/day for 2 days, then 1 mg/kg/day for 2 or 6 mo, then this dose on each Mon, Wed, and Fri	1 yr
	and sulfadiazine†	100 mg/kg/day in 2 daily divided doses	1 yr
	and leucovorin (folinic acid)†	5–10 mg 3 times weekly	1 yr
	Spiramycin‡	100 mg/kg/day in divided doses used in alternate months in place of pyrimethamine/ sulfadiazine/leucovorin in France	1 yr
	Corticosteroids (prednisone)§	1 mg/kg/day in 2 daily divided doses	Until resolution of elevated (≥1 g/dL) CSF protein level or active chorioretinitis that threatens vision

In pregnant women with acute toxoplasmosis first 21 wk of gestation or until term if fetus not infected	Spiramycin‡	1.5 g q12h without food	Until fetal infection documented or excluded at 21 wk; if documented, replace with pyrimethamine, leucovorin, and sulfadiazine
If fetal infection confirmed after 17th wk of gestation or if infection acquired in last few weeks of gestation	Pyrimethamine	Loading dose: 100 mg/day in divided doses for 2 days, followed by 50 mg/day	Until delivery
	and sulfadiazine	Loading dose: 75 mg/kg/day in 2 divided doses (maximum, 4 g/day) for 2 days, then 100 mg/kg/day in 2 divided doses (maximum, 4 g/day)	Until delivery
	and Leucovorin¶	5–20 mg qd	Until delivery

*Adapted from McLeod R, Wisner J, Boyer KM: Toxoplasmosis. In Krugman S, Katz SL, Gershon AA et al (eds): *Infectious Diseases of Children*, ed 9. St Louis, Mosby, 1992, pp 518–550.

†Optimal dosage and feasibility currently being evaluated in ongoing National Collaborative Treatment Trial (312-791-4152).

‡Available only on request from the Food and Drug Administration (301-443-9553).

§Corticosteroids should be continued until signs of inflammation (high CSF protein level ≥1 g/dL) or active chorioretinitis that threatens vision have subsided, dosage then can be tapered and discontinued; use only in conjunction with pyrimethamine, sulfadiazine, and leucovorin.

‖CSF = cerebrospinal fluid.

¶Monitor blood counts and platelets weekly, adjust for megaloblastic anemia, granulocytopenia, or thrombocytopenia.

tion of dihydrofolate reductase and dihydrofolate synthetase, respectively. The combination of the two drugs does not have a high therapeutic ratio. Marrow suppression, manifested by granulocytopenia, thrombocytopenia, and megaloblastic anemia, is frequent. However, folinic acid selectively overcomes the marrow suppressive effects of pyrimethamine and sulfadiazine, without compromising therapeutic efficacy against toxoplasma tachyzoites.[38] Use of the combination of three drugs is well tolerated by most patients. Close (i.e., weekly) hematologic monitoring is desirable, but marrow suppression generally is easily reversed with increased dosage of folinic acid or short-term interruption of pyrimethamine and sulfadiazine.

French physicians have had considerable experience treating fetal infection in utero with pyrimethamine, sulfadiazine, and folinic acid.[39] It appears from this experience, based on comparison with historical controls, that outcome is substantially improved by maternal and fetal treatment. Of the 52 infants with first- or second-trimester fetal infection whose mothers received treatment from 1982 to 1988, only 1 (2%) had evidence of severe organ system damage at birth, whereas 15 (21%) of 72 comparable infants whose mothers were not treated during 1972 to 1981 had severe involvement.

Antibiotic treatment of infected newborn infants after birth also appears to be beneficial. French experience with a 1-year regimen in which spiramycin was alternated monthly with pyrimethamine and sulfadiazine showed a reduction in recurrent eye lesions.[40] The U.S. National Collaborative Treatment Trial now underway in Chicago, although still incomplete, has so far shown substantial improvement in outcomes. Long-term (1-year) treatment with varying doses of pyrimethamine/sulfadiazine and folinic acid has been used.[21] Compared with Eichenwald's[19] historical series, improvements in outcome with long-term treatment have included reduction in sensorineural hearing loss[41] and in neurodevelopmental[42–44] and visual handicaps.[45] Infants with congenital toxoplasmosis or mothers with acute infection can be referred to this study by telephoning 312-791-4152.

Supportive therapy for affected infants is also a key aspect of management. Prednisone should supplement antiparasitic therapy for infants with elevated CSF protein levels (≥ 1 g/dL) or with active, vision-threatening chorioretinitis. Careful surveillance for ventricular enlargement and ventriculoperitoneal shunting for hydrocephalus should be pursued aggressively for infants with expanding head circumferences, increasing ventricular dimensions, or neurologic deterioration. Patching and prismatic or corrective spectacles may help to achieve maximum visual potential. In addition, any child with significant eye involvement (unilateral or bilateral) should always wear protective glasses.

Future considerations in treating toxoplasmosis will undoubtedly involve development of agents capable of eliminating parasite latency by their activity against encysted bradyzoites.[46] Such agents would have the potential to eliminate the reactivations of toxoplasmic eye and neurologic disease, which contribute to long-term morbidity. Several new agents that appear promising in this regard are atovaquone (Mepron), azithromycin (Zithromax), clarithromycin (Biaxin), and aprinocid.

PREVENTION

Toxoplasmosis can be avoided primarily through an awareness of its transmission mechanisms. Physicians responsible for the care of pregnant women should inform them of simple measures for prevention.[47] Educational brochures can be obtained from the March of Dimes (312-435-4007). In recent years, educational efforts of this sort have resulted in a 50% reduction in the incidence of congenital toxoplasmosis in France. The goals are the avoidance of the ingestion or inhalation of oocysts in cat feces and ingestion of encysted bradyzoites in raw meat.

Surveillance for seroconversion in pregnant women is mandated in France and Austria.[48] In these countries where congenital toxoplasmosis occurs at high incidence and where the majority of pregnant women are already chronically infected, this approach is cost effective. The lower incidence of toxoplasmosis in the United States makes routine maternal screening more controversial.[49-51] Some obstetricians screen women with a history of cat contact or if there is a suggestion of a high-risk pregnancy. However, there is no agreed-upon standard of care in this regard. Symptomatic pregnant women with lymphadenitis, mononucleosis, or unexplained fever, however, should always be tested for toxoplasmosis. Identification of seroconversion or acute toxoplasmosis enables a rational approach to managing pregnancy with the highest likelihood of therapeutic benefit. A simple approach that needs to be evaluated could involve screening during pregnancy with IgM-, IgA-, or IgE-specific serologic tests.

Identification of congenital toxoplasmosis by neonatal screening after birth probably misses about 25% of cases.[11, 12] However, the growing awareness that treatment of affected infants can be carried out safely and that it improves their condition, as well as the simplicity and low cost of this approach, is creating medical and economic justification for such screening.

REFERENCES

1. McLeod R, Wisner J, Boyer KM: Toxoplasmosis. In Krugman S, Katz SL, Gershon AA, et al (eds): *Infectious Diseases of Children*, ed 9. St Louis, Mosby, 1992, pp 518–550.
2. Remington JS, McLeod R, Desmonts G: Toxoplasmosis. In Remington JS, Klein JO (eds): *Infectious Diseases of the Fetus and Newborn*, ed 4. Philadelphia, WB Saunders, 1994, pp 140–263.
3. Featherstone H: *A Difference in the Family*. New York, Penguin, 1981.
4. Frenkel J, Dubey JP, Miller NL: *Toxoplasma gondii* in cats. Fecal stages identified as coccidian oocysts. *Science* 167:893–896, 1970.
5. Ruiz A, Frenkel JK: *Toxoplasma gondii* in Costa Rican cats. *Am J Trop Med Hyg* 29:1150, 1980.
6. Desmonts G, Couvreur J: Congenital toxoplasmosis: A prospective study of the offspring of 542 women who acquired toxoplasmosis during pregnancy. Pathophysiology of congenital disease. In Thalhammer O, Baumgarten K, Pollak A (eds): *Perinatal Medicine. Sixth European Congress*. Stuttgart, Germany, Thieme, 1979, p 51.
7. McLeod R, Mack DG, Boyer KM, et al: Phenotypes and functions of lymphocytes in congenital toxoplasmosis. *J Lab Clin Med* 116:623–635, 1990.
8. Frenkel JK: Breaking the transmission chain of *Toxoplasma*: A program for the prevention of human toxoplasmosis. *Bull N Y Acad Sci* 50:228–235, 1974.
9. Dubey JP, Beattie CP: *Toxoplasmosis of Animals and Man*. Boca Raton, Fla, CRC, 1988, pp 1–220.
10. Feldman HA: A nationwide serum survey of United States military recruits: VI. Toxoplasma antibodies. *Am J Epidemiol* 81:385–391, 1965.
11. Hoff R, Weiblen BJ, Reardon LA: Screening for congenital toxoplasma infection. In Bellisario R, Mizejewski GJ (eds): *Transplacental Disorders: Perinatal Detection, Treatment and Management (Including Pediatric AIDS)*. New York, Liss, 1990, pp 169–182.
12. Guerina N, Hsu H-W, Meissner HC, et al: Neonatal serologic screening and early treatment for congenital *Toxoplasma gondii* infection. *N Engl J Med* 330:1858–1863, 1994.
13. Koppe JG, Kloosterman GJ, deRoever-Bonnet H, et al: Toxoplasmosis and pregnancy, with a long-term follow-up of the children. *Eur J Obstet Gynecol Reprod Biol* 413:101–110, 1974.
14. McCabe RE, Brooks RG, Dorfman RF, et al: Clinical spectrum in 107 cases of toxoplasmic lymphadenopathy. *Rev Infect Dis* 9:754–774, 1987.
15. Mitchell CD, Erlich SS, Mastrucci MT, et al: Congenital toxoplasmo-

sis occurring in infants perinatally infected with human immunodeficiency virus 1. *Pediatr Infect Dis J* 9:512–518, 1990.

16. Saxon SA, Knight N, Reynolds DW, et al: Intellectual deficits in children born with subclinical congenital toxoplasmosis: A preliminary report. *J Pediatr* 82:792–797, 1973.

17. Koppe JG, Loewer-Sieger DH, DeRoever-Bonnet H: Results of 20-year follow-up of congenital toxoplasmosis. *Lancet* 1:254–256, 1986.

18. Wilson CB, Remington JS, Stagno S, et al: Development of adverse sequelae in children born with subclinical congenital *Toxoplasma* infection. *Pediatrics* 66:767–774, 1980.

19. Eichenwald HG: A study of congenital toxoplasmosis, with particular emphasis on clinical manifestations, sequelae, and therapy. In Siim JC (ed): *Human Toxoplasmosis.* Copenhagen, Munksgaard, 1960, pp 41–49.

20. Couvreur J, Desmonts G: Congenital and maternal toxoplasmosis. A review of 300 congenital cases. *Dev Med Child Neurol* 4:519–530, 1962.

21. McAuley JB, Boyer KM, Patel D, et al: Early and longitudinal evaluations of treated infants and children and untreated historical patients with congenital toxoplasmosis: The Chicago Collaborative Treatment Trial. *Clin Infect Dis* 18:38–72, 1994.

22. Couvreur J, Desmonts G, Tournier G, et al: Study of a homogeneous series of 210 cases of congenital toxoplasmosis in infants aged 0 to 11 months detected prospectively. *Ann Pediatr* 31:815–819, 1984.

23. Dorfman RF, Remington JS: Value of lymphnode biopsy in the diagnosis of acute acquired toxoplasmosis. *N Engl J Med* 289:878–881, 1973.

24. Wilson M, McAuley JB: Laboratory diagnosis of congenital toxoplasmosis. *Clin Lab Med* 11:923–939, 1991.

25. Sabin AE, Feldman HA: Dyes as microchemical indicators of a new immunity phenomenon affecting a protozoan parasite *(Toxoplasma).* *Science* 108:660–663, 1948.

26. Naot Y, Desmonts G, Remington JS: IgM enzyme-linked immunosorbent assay test for the diagnosis of congenital *Toxoplasma* infection. *J Pediatr* 98:32, 1981.

27. Desmonts G, Naot Y, Remington JS: Immunoglobulin M–immunosorbent agglutination assay for diagnosis of infectious diseases: Diagnosis of acute congenital and acquired *Toxoplasma* infections. *J Clin Microbiol* 14:486–491, 1981.

28. Stepick-Bick P, Thullicz P, Araujo FG, et al: IgA antibodies for diagnosis of acute congenital and acquired toxoplasmosis. *J Infect Dis* 162:270–273, 1990.

29. Wong SY, Hajdu MP, Ramirez R, et al: The role of specific immunoglobulin E in the diagnosis of acute *Toxoplasma* infection and toxoplasmosis. *J Clin Microbiol* 31:2952–2959, 1993.

30. Remington J, Araujo FG, Desmonts G: Recognition of different *Toxo-*

plasma antigens by IgM and IgG antibodies in mothers and their congenitally infected newborns. *J Infect Dis* 152:1020–1024, 1985.

31. Dannemann BR, Vaughan WC, Thulliez P, et al: The differential agglutination test for diagnosis of recently acquired infection with *Toxoplasma gondii*. *J Clin Microbiol* 28:1928–1933, 1990.

32. Wilson CB, Desmonts G, Couvreur J, et al: Lymphocyte transformation in the diagnosis of congenital *Toxoplasma* infection. *N Engl J Med* 302:785–788, 1980.

33. Grover CM, Thulliez P, Remington JS, et al: Rapid prenatal diagnosis of congenital *Toxoplasma* infection by using polymerase chain reaction and amniotic fluid. *J Clin Microbiol* 28:2297–2301, 1990.

34. Hohlfeld P, Daffos F, Costa J-M, et al: Prenatal diagnosis of congenital toxoplasmosis with a polymerase-chain-reaction test on amniotic fluid. *N Engl J Med* 331:695–699, 1994.

35. Daffos F, Forestier F, Capella-Pavlovsky M, et al: Prenatal management of 746 pregnancies at risk for congenital toxoplasmosis. *N Engl J Med* 318:271–275, 1988.

36. McLeod R, Boyer KM, Roizen N, et al: Treatment of congenital toxoplasmosis. 17th International Congress on Chemotherapy, Berlin, abstract 1933, 1991.

37. Couvreur J, Desmonts G, Thulliez P: Prophylaxis of congenital toxoplasmosis. Effect of spiramycin on placental infections. *Antimicrob Chemother* 22:193–200, 1988.

38. McLeod R, Mack D, Foss R, et al: The Toxoplasmosis Study Group. Levels of pyrimethamine in sera and cerebrospinal and ventricular fluid from infants treated for congenital toxoplasmosis. *Antimicrob Agents Chemother* 36:1040–1048, 1992.

39. Hohlfeld P, Daffos F, Thulliez P, et al: Fetal toxoplasmosis: Outcome of pregnancy and infant follow-up after in utero treatment. *J Pediatr* 115:765–769, 1989.

40. Couvreur J, Desmonts G, Aron-Rosa D: Le pronostic oculaire de la toxoplasmose congenitale: Role du traitement. *Ann Pediatr* 31:855–858, 1984.

41. McGee T, Wolters C, Stein L, et al: Absence of sensorineural hearing abnormalities in treated infants with congenital toxoplasmosis. *Otolaryngol Head Neck Surg* 106:75–80, 1992.

42. Roizen N, Swisher CN, Stein MA, et al: Neurologic and developmental outcome in treated congenital toxoplasmosis. *Pediatrics* 95:11–20, 1995.

43. Swisher CN, Boyer KM, McLeod R, et al: Congenital toxoplasmosis. *Semin Pediatr Neurol* 1:4–25, 1994.

44. Guerina NG, Ware J, Burbridge J, et al: Neurodevelopmental outcomes for infants with congenital *Toxoplasma* infection from a newborn serologic screening and treatment program. *Pediatr Res* 37:292A, 1995.

45. Mets MB, Toxoplasmosis Collaborative Study Group: Ophthalmologic findings in congenital toxoplasmosis. *Assoc Res Vision Ophthalmol* abstract 2876, 1992.

46. Huskinson-Mark J, Araujo FG, Remington JS: Evaluation of the effect of drugs on the cyst form of *Toxoplasma gondii. J Infect Dis* 164:170–177, 1991.
47. Wilson CB, Remington JS: What can be done to prevent congenital toxoplasmosis? *Am J Obstet Gynecol* 138:357–363, 1980.
48. Aspock P: Prevention of congenital toxoplasmosis by serological surveillance during pregnancy: Current strategies and future perspectives. In Marget W, Lang W, Gabler-Sandberger E (eds): *Parasitic Infections, Immunology, Mycotic Infections, General Topics*, vol 3. Munich, MMV Medizin Verlag, 1986, pp 69–72.
49. McCabe RE, Remington JS: Toxoplasmosis: The time has come. *N Engl J Med* 318:313–315, 1988.
50. Frenkel JK: Prevention of toxoplasma infection in pregnant women and their fetuses. *Clin Infect Dis* 20:727–728, 1995.
51. Schoen EJ, Cohen D, Black S: Should we screen for congenital toxoplasmosis? *Pediatr Res* 37:188A, 1995.

Index

A

Acetone/formalin differential agglutination test, for toxoplasmosis, 457, 458
Acinetobacter, 32
Acquired immune deficiency syndrome (*see also* Human immunodeficiency virus infection)
  adenovirus infection in, 379
  aspergillosis and, 213
  Pneumocystis carinii pneumonia prophylaxis, 165–166
    adverse reactions to trimethoprim-sulfamethoxazole, 173–174
  Toxoplasma infection in, 452
Acute urethral syndrome, 419
Adenoviral infections, 365–388
  clinical significance, 374–376
    acute otitis media, 376
    conjunctivitis and keratoconjunctivitis, 377–378
    gastroenteritis, 378
    joints, 378
    pneumonia, 376–377
    urinary tract, 378
  diagnosis, 380–381
  epidemiology, 374
  immunodeficiency, 379–380
  molecular biology, 365–371
  pathogenesis, 371–373
  prevention, 381–382
  serotypes and diseases, 366–367
Adolescents, cytomegalovirus infection in, 137
Aeromonas, food and water contamination by, 118–119
Aerosol pentamidine, for *Pneumocystis carinii* pneumonia prophylaxis, 165–166, 170, 171–172, 179–180

Agar dilution, in antibiotic susceptibility, 81
AIDS (*see* Acquired immune deficiency syndrome)
Albendazole, 306, 321, 322, 323–324
Alkaline water, water contamination by, 108
Allergic bronchopulmonary aspergillosis, 208, 210–211
Allylamines, 258–259
AmBisome, 204, 245, 246
Amidase, pneumococci and, 66–67, 75, 76
Amikacin, for CSF shunt infections, 44, 47
Aminoglycosides
  amphotericin B and, 243
  for CSF shunt infections, 42, 44
Amoxicillin
  for *Helicobacter pylori* infection, 396, 397, 398
  for otitis media, 87
  pneumococcal resistance, 74
  urinary tract infection and, 436
Amphocil, 245
Amphotericin B
  flucytosine with, 246, 248
  for fungal infections of respiratory tract, 208, 209, 210
  lipid formulations, 244–246
  properties, 240–244
  for specific invasive infections
    aspergilloma, 212
    aspergillosis, 220–222, 223
    Candida, 194, 195, 197, 200, 201, 203, 204, 205
    coccidioidomycosis, 232
    cryptococcosis, 236–237
    disseminated histoplasmosis of infancy, 229–231
    disseminated *Trichosporon* infections, 237–238

B

X

Xylohypha bantiana, 226

Y

Yersinia enterocolitica, food and
water contamination by, 104,
109, 117–118

Z

Zoonotic filariases, 314–315
Zygomycetes, angioinvasion, 215
Zygomycosis, 208, 224–225